Cardiovascular Manual for the Advanced Practice Provider

Richard Musialowski • Krista Allshouse
Editors

Cardiovascular Manual for the Advanced Practice Provider

Mastering the Basics

Springer

Editors
Richard Musialowski
Sanger Heart and Vascular Institute
Atrium Health
Charlotte, NC, USA

Krista Allshouse
Atrium Health
Levine Childrens' Congenital Heart Center
Charlotte, NC, USA

ISBN 978-3-031-35818-0 ISBN 978-3-031-35819-7 (eBook)
https://doi.org/10.1007/978-3-031-35819-7

This Springer imprint is published by the registered company Springer Nature Switzerland AG
The registered company address is: Gewerbestrasse 11, 6330 Cham, Switzerland

Foreword

It is with honor that I write this foreword to the first *Cardiovascular Manual for the Advanced Practice Provider*. In my over thirty-year cardiovascular career, I have witnessed the inception, acceptance, growth, indispensability, and leadership of advanced practice providers (APPs) to the cardiovascular care (CV) team. This is corroborated now by nearly 7000 CV team members in the American College of Cardiology (ACC) worldwide. Recent innovative new pathways to both associate (AACC) and fellow (FACC) status ensure this continued growth and leadership. These designations are awarded each year at ACC's annual scientific sessions convocation and emphasize the importance of APPs to the College's mission to "transform cardiovascular care and improve heart health for all." Furthermore, the APP numbers continuing global growth will promote the College's vision of "a world where science, knowledge, and innovation optimize cardiovascular care." In short, APPs are now essential to the CV team, and this manual will aid in the best care of complex cardiovascular patients as well as filling a previously unmet clinical need.

Much appreciation goes to Richard Musialowski, MD, FACC, Director of CV Education at Sanger Heart and Vascular Institute/Atrium Health, and Krista Allshouse, PA-C, who conceived and kick-started this manual. Much credit goes to Amy Winiger, DNP, FACC, who has shown the far-reaching possibilities that APPs can achieve in cardiology today, as well as Kathy Venable, PA-C, who trailblazed and has led our own APP program at Sanger Heart and Vascular Institute/Atrium Health for over 30 years. This program now employs over 120 APPs. Nationally, George Rodgers, MD, MACC, Eileen Handberg, Ph.D., FACC, and Janet Wyman, DNP, FACC, have led the ACC CV Team section to become one of the strongest forces for advocacy and advancement of the ACC in the past decade.

I close with admiration and awe for all those who have contributed not only to the writing of this manual but to the acceleration of APP leadership within the CV team. This manual will become an invaluable resource in the optimal care of all our cardiovascular patients.

Sanger Heart & Vascular Institute/Atrium Health B. Hadley Wilson
Charlotte, NC, USA
Clinical Professor of Medicine, Wake Forest University-Atrium Health,
Charlotte, NC, USA
President, American College of Cardiology, Washington, DC, USA
May 1, 2022

Letter from Editor

Dear Readers,

Why was this manual created? It was the brainchild of the editors after many long discussions about how advanced practice providers (APPs) are currently used in the healthcare setting, the future of our work, and APP education. How can we best prepare a new graduate from PA/NP school, a resident, or an APP changing specialties to practice in cardiology? In today's environment of ultra-specialized APPs, how can we best give them a broad knowledge base in cardiology? Then it hit us! Write a Cardiovascular Manual **BY** APPs working in cardiology **FOR** these new APPs. What would these seasoned providers want their new colleagues to know in each of their areas of expertise? And the book was born: *Cardiovascular Manual for the Advanced Practice Provider*.

There were many discussions regarding other learning, outside of books. It is critical for new providers to learn from the entire healthcare team. Each aspect of patient care is important and a provider can learn from each of these specialties, especially nursing. Nurses provide patient care for hours on end, whether that is an 8, 10, or 12 h shift and gain an exorbitant amount of information about the patient during this time. Listen to them! They will always know the patient better than you. Respect everyone in the care team; they all have different jobs to do, but are equally important. The more you talk to and ask questions to the care team, the more likely they will come to you with concerns or questions, which will improve patient care and communication. You do not want to be unapproachable.

You also should become a leader in your field and to the entire care team. Everyone is busy but as a provider, you should be the guide for care and take responsibility of the patient. Lead by doing. Be a leader in the way you direct care, create a team-based care team, and educate. Accept education gladly from other care providers. It is all a learning experience. Don't be afraid to be vulnerable and admit you don't know something. It is the only way to learn. Put the effort in to educate yourself outside of the job—go to conferences, read and LISTEN!

We hope this publication serves you well in your journey to becoming a well-rounded and spectacular Cardiovascular APP!

Thank you to Dr. Ronald Sing for jump starting our idea by allowing us to help with his book *Interventional Critical Care*. We appreciate the opportunity to be involved.

We also want to thank the following people for their help obtaining images for this work:

Tom Johnson, M.D. F.A.C.C., F.A.S.E.
Markus Scherer, M.D. F.A.C.C., F.A.S.E.
Kristi Johnson, RDCS, F.A.S.E.
Cody Frye, RDCS, F.A.S.E.
Amar Parikh, M.D.
Joshua Lisenby
Shannon Culver
Nainesh Patel, M.D., F.A.C.C., F.S.C.A.I.

Sincerely,
Richard Musialowski and Krista Allshouse

Contents

Part I

Introduction

1 Cardiac Anatomy, Physiology, and Exam

Richard Musialowski and Krista Allshouse

Embryologic Development

The fetal heart begins as a simple tube in the third week of gestation and develops to a four chambered beating structure by approximately week 7 to 8 [1]. Valves develop according to their location in the embryonic tube and differentiate from the ventricle they arise within. The right ventricle (RV) will always produce a three to four leaflet tricuspid valve (TV). The left ventricle (LV) will always produce a two-leaflet mitral valve (MV). Septation occurs dividing both the atria and ventricles into two separate and genetically different pairs.

Septation of the embryonic atria creates two independent chambers with a small residual communication called the foramen ovale. Placental blood (oxygenated) is preferentially shunted across this structure into the left atrium, LV, and into the fetal aorta. At delivery, the LA pressure exceeds the RA pressure and closes this connection. Fifteen percent of the population will have a persistent patent foramen ovale (PFO) into adulthood.

The great vessels (aorta and pulmonary artery) arise from the aortic arch. Through septation, the pulmonary artery and aorta divide into two separate vessels. These tubes are in continuation with the developing and rotating ventricles. These vessels create the semilunar valves seen in the aortic and pulmonic positions. The coronary arteries arise above the semilunar valves in the developing aorta. A connection persists between the aorta and pulmonary artery during fetal development, called the ductus arteriosus. This structure empties blood from the uninflated fetal lungs and pulmonary artery into the aorta in utero. The spontaneous breathing of the infant after birth causes a subsequent fall in the pulmonary vascular resistance (PVR) and the removal of the placenta causes an increase in systemic vascular resistance (SVR), resulting in abrupt closure of the ductus, creating two separate circuits: pulmonary (unoxygenated) and systemic (oxygenated).

Abnormalities during development can occur at any point, resulting in a variety of congenital cardiac defects. The advancement of surgical techniques and medical therapies have improved the survival of patients with congenital heart disease, and many are now living well into adulthood (see Chap. 29).

R. Musialowski
Sanger Heart and Vascular Institute, Atrium Health, Charlotte, NC, USA
e-mail: Richard.musialowski@atriumhealth.org

K. Allshouse (✉)
Atrium Health, Levine Childrens' Congenital Heart Center, Charlotte, NC, USA
e-mail: Krista.allshouse@atriumhealth.org

R. Musialowski, K. Allshouse (eds.), *Cardiovascular Manual for the Advanced Practice Provider*,
https://doi.org/10.1007/978-3-031-35819-7_1

Excitation Contraction Coupling (ECC)

Each cardiac cycle is a rapid process of electrical depolarization and muscle contraction with active electrical repolarization and muscle relaxation. The timing is well organized, and deviations of this process may result in distinct cardiac dysfunction (Diagram 1).

ECC begins with the spontaneous phase 4 depolarization of pacemaker cells due to the influx of sodium and calcium ions, i.e. the funny current [2]. This is known as automaticity and cells with this characteristic are present within the sinoatrial node (SAN), atrial tissue, atrioventricular (AV) node, and ventricular myocytes. The speed of spontaneous depolarization determines the heart rate, and thus the P-to-P interval. Once the depolarization meets a threshold, phase 0 of the action potential begins (Fig. 1.1). Propagation of the electrical impulse on the cell membrane alters the chemical structure of transmembrane proteins called voltage-gated channels. These channels are ion-specific and allow additional sodium and calcium ions into the cell, specifically at the T-tubule. The impulse then spreads to surrounding cells via gap junctions, microtubule structures that allow sodium and calcium ions to rapidly flow to the next cell. This ion flow spreads rapidly throughout the whole heart so that when one cell is depolarized, all cells become depolarized at a speed of 0.5 m/s!

At this point, the electrical excitation is completed, and repolarization begins with shifts of other ions (mainly potassium) out of the cell. This reset of the transmembrane potential or refractory period is essential for the next impulse to occur. This is seen as phase 3 on the action potential and is associated with the QT interval on EKG. Energy expenditure in the form of ATP within the membrane exchange pumps is essential in this process. When the calcium enters the cell in phase 2 of the action potential, it binds to

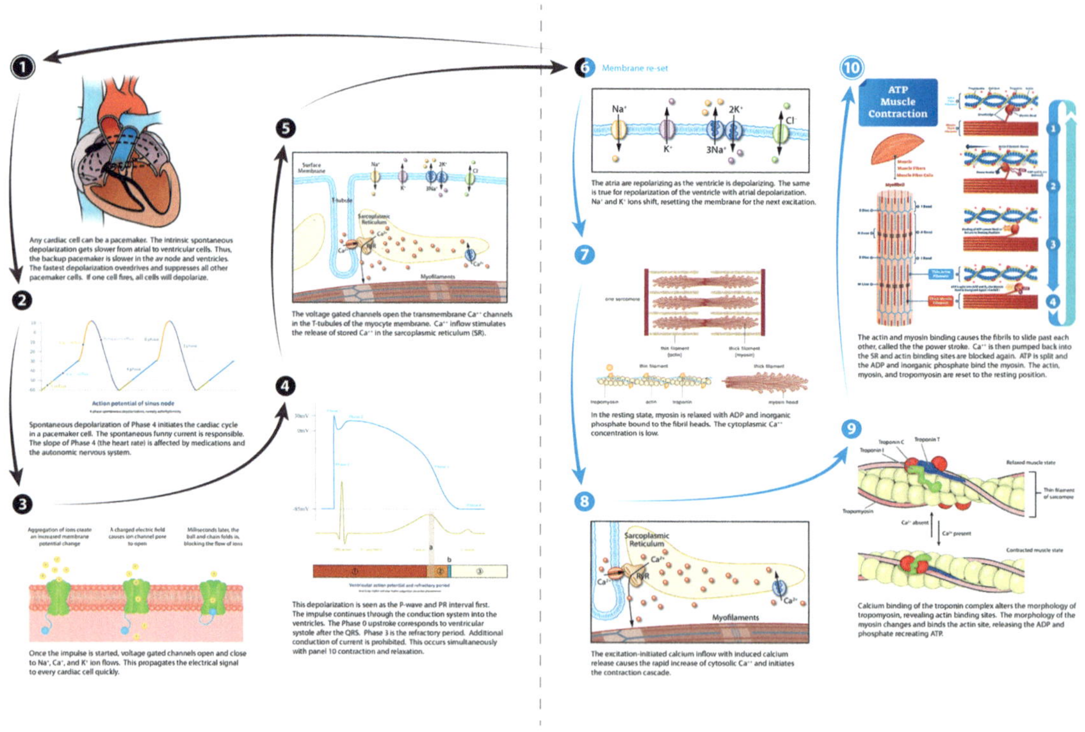

Diagram 1

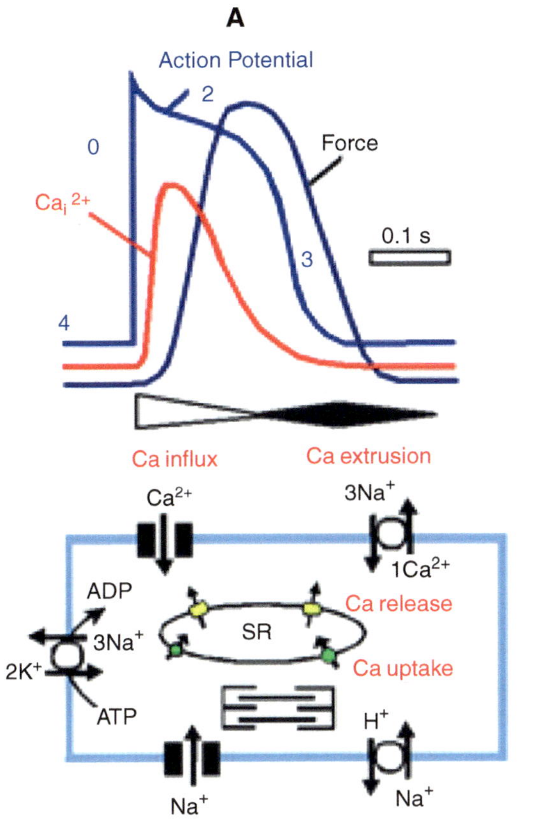

Fig. 1.1 Phase 4 depolarization is spontaneous due to the funny current that determines the heart rate [2]. Phase 0 depolarization is due to rapid sodium influx that occurs after opening of voltage-gated channels due to the funny current depolarization. During phase 2, calcium ions influx as well. These calcium ions are essential to cause the muscle contraction necessary for cardiac function. The force line is the representation of muscle contraction. Electrical repolarization (phase 3) is occurring during mechanical contraction. Calcium homeostasis is regulated by the sarcoplasmic reticulum that releases and resets the gradients for the next contraction [3]. Adapted from Figure 1Cell calcium 2020 Jan; 85:102129

the ryanodine receptors on sarcoplasmic reticulum which releases a flood of calcium throughout the muscle cells (Diagram 1).

Cardiac muscle fibrils are made up of thick myosin and thin actin filaments. Intertwined between these two structures is a protein complex called tropomyosin. This structure is composed of multiple proteins with specific responsibilities. Troponin T is bound to the tropomyosin, troponin C, and troponin I. Troponin I can restrict the actin and myosin interaction while in the resting state. Troponin C binds the excitation released calcium ions causing a loosening of the troponin I/actin complex revealing the myosin-binding sites.

In the resting state, the myosin heads have ADP and inorganic phosphate bound to them. The calcium-troponin directed transformation of tropomyosin causes the presentation of the actin binding sites. Interaction of the actin and myosin heads releases the bound ADP and inorganic phosphate creating cytosolic ATP. This release causes a conformational change in the myosin head resulting in the sliding of the actin and myosin by each other called the "power stroke" and contraction results. Contraction is coordinated in every cell at the same time! The reformed cytosolic ATP now binds to the contracted myosin heads and the molecule is split back to ADP and phosphate. This energy expenditure results in myosin conformation changes and the fibrils slide back, thus establishing the resting state. Calcium is pumped back into the SR against a gradient by sarcoplasmic reticulum calcium ATPase (SERCA2A), occurring during phase 3 and repolarization of the action potential (Diagram 1).

This whole process from the initiation within the sinus node to propagation to the AV node takes less than 180 ms, or the PR interval. This is the moment the atria contract. This same impulse proceeds into the ventricle in the same ECC process with resultant QRS of 80 ms and ventricular contraction. The repolarization of the ventricle (refractory period) takes about 300 ms and corresponds to the QT interval. Phase 4 of the action potential is reached and the cycle begins again.

Alterations in the SERCA2 calcium homeostasis are pathologic in HfrEF and the diastolic dysfunction of HFpEF [4]. Since diastole requires molecular energy, disease states that reduce cellular energy (i.e., ischemia) alter calcium homeostasis and impair diastolic function (see Sect. 5). Sympathetic nervous system innervation alters calcium flows thus increasing heart rate and contractility. Antiarrhythmic medications alter the action potential resulting in changes in conduction, repolarization, and ekg morphology (see Chap. 7).

Conduction System

The specialized cells of the sinoatrial node (SAN) are located in the upper portion of the right atrium near the entrance to the superior vena cava. The impulse arises due to automaticity of these cells and propagates through the atria. In the crux or center of the heart, there is fibrous tissue surrounding the atrioventricular node (AVN). This fibrous tissue acts as a brake to slow down and organize the impulse. The organized impulse proceeds through the bundle of His and continues down the right and left bundles. The left bundle then splits into the left anterior fascicle which is a relatively organized structure and a diffuse left posterior fascicle. These bundles are cardiac cells that have differentiated for electrical conduction [5]. Blood supply is important to the function of this system and coronary ischemia can cause electrical abnormalities resulting in both tachycardia and bradycardia. Metabolic abnormalities can also alter function of this system (see the EP Section).

Electrocardiogram (EKG or ECG)

The normal QRS complex on an EKG is seen in Fig. 1.2. This is a graphic representation of the electrical impulse and conduction of a cardiac cycle. The P wave originates in the SA node and is the first waveform of the cardiac cycle. It is associated with atrial contraction. The beginning of the P wave to the deflection of the QRS is called the P-R interval. This is the time the impulse starts in the sinus node, propagates across the atria, and is slowed down in the AV node. This interval approximates AV node function. Normal is less than 200 ms. (Longer than this time suggests AV node dysfunction.)

The QRS is the impulse proceeding through to the right and left bundles to depolarize the ventricles, normally taking 80–100 ms. Pathology of the conduction system and ventricles causes this interval to widen. Medication and abnormal metabolic states also affect the QRS duration.

The QT segment corresponds to phase 3 of the action potential and is associated with repolarization of the ventricle. Atrial repolarization is hidden in the QRS complex. This interval is heart rate dependent. It is also influenced by many medications, pathology, and autonomic influences. This interval is important in the assessment and management of ventricular arrhythmias.

The P to P and R to R intervals are used to discuss rhythm interpretation. These intervals link different cardiac cycles together.

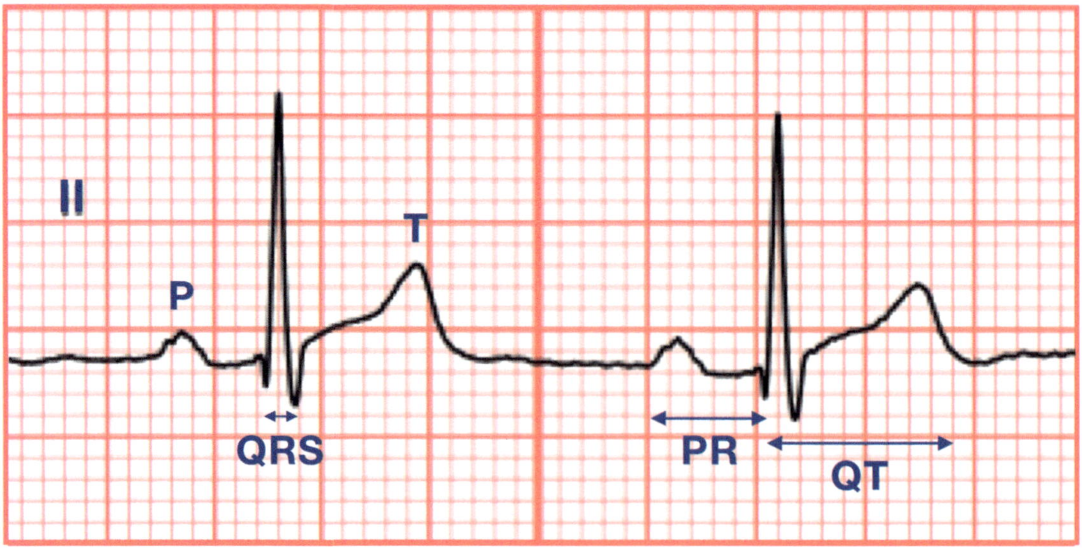

Fig. 1.2 Normal EKG with intervals

Cardiac Anatomy

As stated in the embryology section, two separate circuits are created during development. The right atrium (RA) and ventricle (RV) are separated by a three to four leaflet structure called the tricuspid valve (TV). The RV is continuous with the pulmonary artery and its pulmonary valve. Deoxygenated blood enters the RA and is pumped to the lungs for oxygenation. After pulmonary capillary oxygenation, the blood collects into the left atrium (LA) from the pulmonary veins. The left ventricle (LV) receives the oxygen-rich blood after it crosses a two leaflet valve called the mitral valve (MV). Ventricular systole moves blood through the left ventricular out flow tract (LVOT) into the aorta opening the aortic valve. Tissue perfusion throughout the body occurs and the deoxygenated blood returns to the RA through the superior (SVC) or inferior vena cava (IVC) (Fig. 1.4). A detailed discussion of the important hemodynamic features is contained in Chap. 2.

The atrioventricular valves (AV) and its apparatus have specific functions necessary to generate stroke volume and thus cardiac output. Papillary muscles are structures that are part of the myocardial wall whose role is to contract during ventricular systole and pull the valve leaflets close to avoid regurgitation of blood backward into the atria. The mitral valve has two muscles, one medially and one laterally. The anterior and posterior leaflets are attached to the papillary muscles by chordae tendineae. The leaflets of the MV are further described by their individual cusps (Fig. 1.3). Abnormalities in any part of this apparatus will result in pathology of the valve opening and closure. This is discussed in detail in the Sect. 4 on structural heart disease.

The tricuspid valve is similar with papillary muscles, chordae tendineae, and leaflets. There is a septal, anterior, and posterior leaflet.

The center or crux of the heart is an important crossroad of electrical and mechanical cardiac function (Fig. 1.4). The AVN is located within the membranous septum. It is located near the septal leaflet of the TV and below the right and non-coronary cusps of the AV annulus. Also, the septal attachments of the MV anchor here as well. In Fig. 1.3, the approximation of the atrioventricular and semilunar valves is seen. These valves are all anchored in the fibrous crux.

This anatomy is important when infection occurs as multiple valves may be involved, increasing mortality. Also, aortic valve endocarditis is associated with acute conduction interruption (see Chap. 19). Intervention of the aortic valve annulus can be complicated by disruption of the AVN and bundle branches (see Sect. IV).

Coronary Arteries

Normal coronary artery anatomy is seen in Fig. 1.5 with three epicardial arteries. The left main artery gives rise to the left anterior descending (LAD) and left circumflex (LCX).

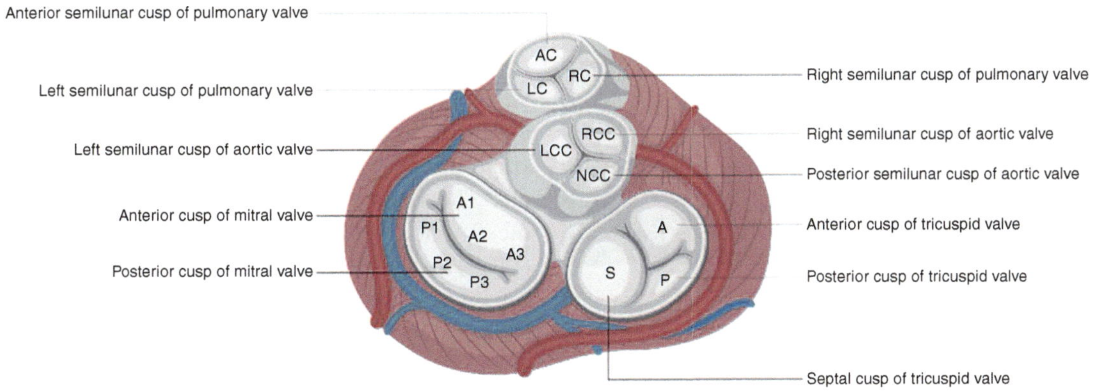

Fig. 1.3 Nomenclature of the cardiac valves

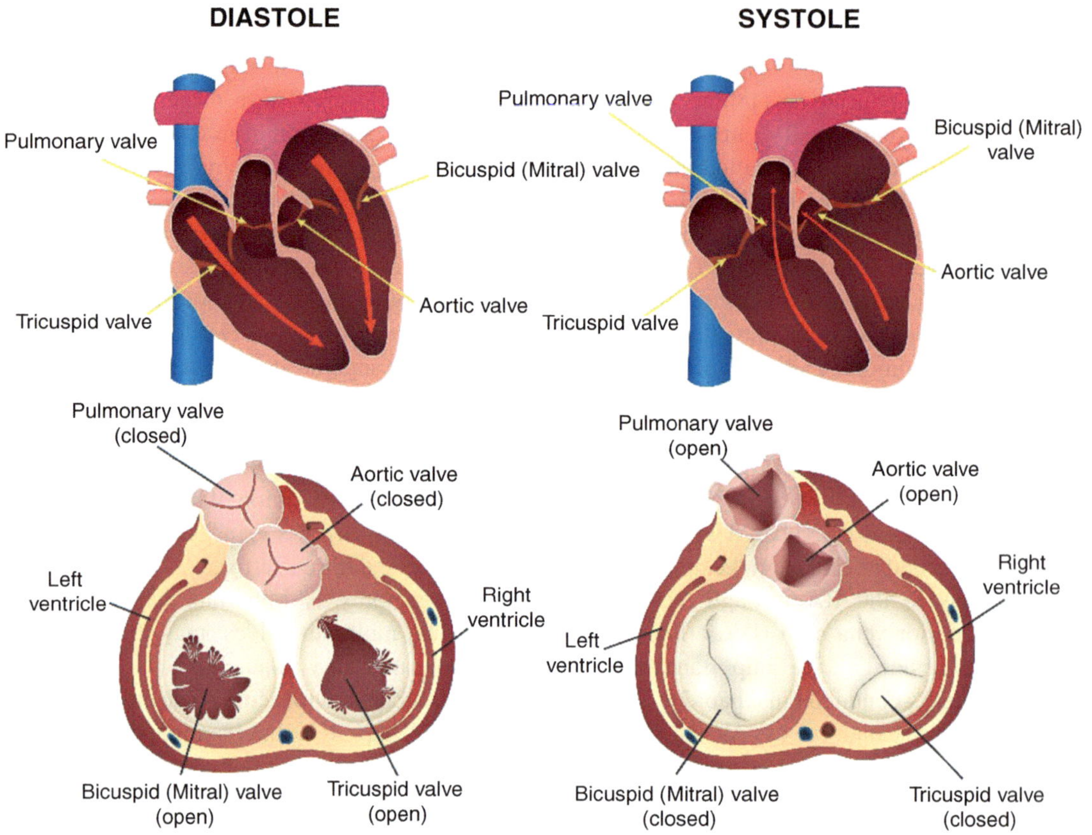

Fig. 1.4 Work of the heart valves

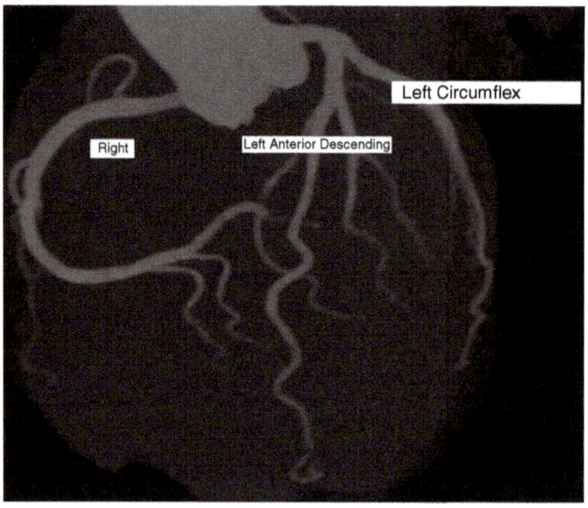

Fig. 1.5 Normal coronary anatomy

The LAD branches into diagonal vessels. This vascular distribution is the most important as it supplies the ventricular septum, which is very important during ventricular systole to generate stroke volume and cardiac output. The LCX branches into marginal vessels. This distribution is important in blood supply to the posterior medial papillary muscle supporting the mitral valve. Ischemia of the RCA and LCX is associated with ischemic mitral regurgitation due to a single blood supply from the PDA to this muscle. The right coronary artery (RCA) supplies the SA node. The posterior descending artery (PDA) arises from the right coronary 80% of the time and supplies the AV node. Ischemia in the RCA often results in bradycardia due to ischemia in these nodes.

Physical Examination of the Cardiovascular System: Pearls and Techniques

The stethoscope has two options to listen to the patient. The flat surface is called the diaphragm. It is best utilized for higher pitched sounds, including lung and bowel sounds. The other side, the bell, does not have a diaphragm over the contact area and is open to air. This is best utilized for lower pitched sounds including S3 and bruits. It is good practice to listen over an area of interest with both the bell and the diaphragm to assess for all frequency of sounds [7]. There are specific locations on the chest wall to best hear specific valves. Figures 1.6 and 1.7 demonstrate the best anatomic location and correlation with specific valves. Every heart sound has different characteristics that need to be assessed during auscultation (Tables 1.1 and 1.2).

The first heart sound (S1) is at the beginning of ventricular systole. The movement of blood within the heart results in a closure of the mitral and tricuspid valves. If these atrioventricular valves are incompetent, blood flows back into the atria and a murmur will result. The specific pathology causing the incompetence will decide the characteristics of the murmur. Mitral and tricuspid regurgitation are traditionally described as holosystolic as they begin immediately after S1. The quality is flat since the pressure generated in the ventricles is constant. Mitral valve regurgitation traditionally radiates toward the axilla from the apex. Tricuspid regurgitation often does not radiate but increases in intensity with inspiration. Antegrade systolic flow across a stenotic aortic and pulmonic valve creates a murmur that increases in intensity as flow across the valve increases (crescendo). As the ventricle completes its contraction, the pressure decreases and the intensity of the murmur decreases (decrescendo). Radiation of the systolic murmur is essential to determine if the pathology is atrioventricular or semilunar valve.

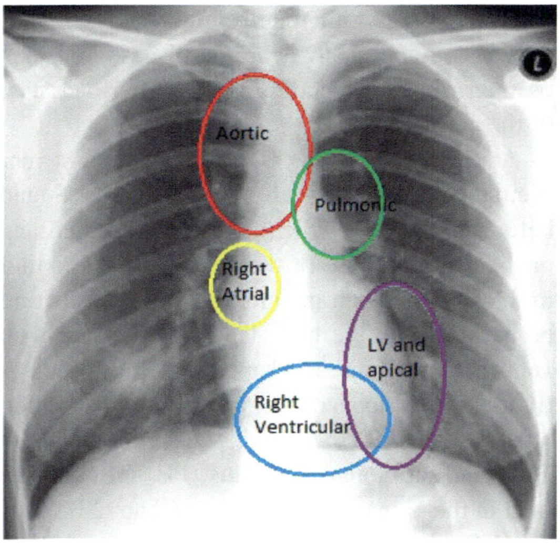

Fig. 1.6 Areas of auscultation

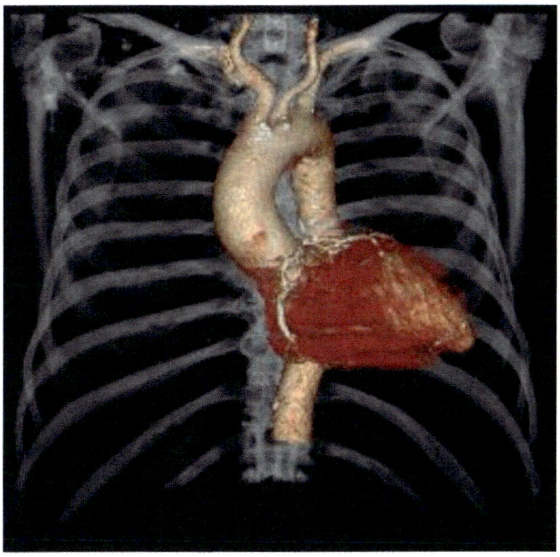

Fig. 1.7 Heart location within thorax

Table 1.1 Murmur descriptions

Location	Area Best Heard (see Fig. 1.6)
Timing	Systole or diastole: use radial pulse to assist
Pitch	High or low
Radiation	Where is it directed: neck, back, axilla, anterior, posterior
Duration	Early diastole Holosystolic Mid or late systolic
Intensity	1–4 for diastolic (1–3 most common) 1–6 for systolic (2–3/6 most common)
Quality	Harsh, soft, blowing, crescendo, decrescendo

Table 1.2 Heart Sounds, Respiration, and the Cardiac Cycle

Systolic Murmur	AS, PS, MR, TR
Diastolic murmur	AI, PI
Both systolic and diastolic	AS/AI, PS/PI, patent ductus arteriosus (PDA) "machine like"
Diastolic sound	Softer S3 after S2, louder S4 before S1
Second heart sound and respiration A2-P2 interaction	Normal splits with inspiration due to temporary delay P2 closure Paradoxical splits in expiration due to LBBB and delayed A2 closure Fixed split and independent of respiration due to fixed delay of P2 closure from pulmonary hypertension
Pericardial friction rub	Rarely heard and commonly has a systolic component sounding like velcro™
Right-sided murmurs PS, PI, TR	All increase in intensity with inspiration

After the ventricle begins to relax, it causes negative pressure, opening the AV valves, closing the pulmonic and aortic (semilunar) valves, and making the second heart sound (S2). This relaxation is ventricular diastole and all sounds after S2 are diastolic. Incompetence of the semilunar valves will cause flow backward into the ventricles immediately following S2 causing a short diastolic murmur. Diastolic atrioventricular murmurs are rare and out of the scope of this discussion.

Murmurs should be described by the terms included in Table 1.1 and should be recorded in the medical record as such. These include timing, pitch, radiation, location, duration, quality, and intensity. Diastolic murmurs are graded on a scale of 1–4 and systolic murmurs on a scale 1–6. Grade 1 is barely audible, grade 2 is louder, grade 3 is loud but no thrill is present. Grade 4 is loud with an associated thrill and grade 5 has a thrill and can be heard with the stethoscope partially off the chest. Grade 6 is the loudest, with a thrill and heard with the stethoscope completely off the chest.

Remember, normal inspiration causes an increase in the venous return to the right side of the heart. This increase in volume and flow increases the intensity of all right-sided murmurs. Increased venous return prolongs the right ventricular ejection time, prolonging pulmonic valve closure (P2) and thus normally splits the second heart sound. During exhalation, the RV flow decreases and P2 can disappear with only A2 heard. A LBBB causes the RV to contract and closes the PV first. At expiration, the sounds will be split. With inspiration, the P2 is delayed and merges with the A2 component and thus no longer split with inspiration. This is paradoxical splitting. If the pulmonary blood flow or pressure is chronically elevated, the P2 component is permanently delayed, or fixed, in the cardiac cycle. This is a common finding in ASD or pulmonary hypertension.

Since the QRS on the EKG is ventricular systole, the first heart sound occurs shortly after the QRS, while the diastolic second sound occurs during ventricular repolarization and after the T wave (see Fig. 1.8).

A fourth heart sound (S_4) is usually located near the heart's apex over the mitral area. S_4 is relatively short in duration and may occur only intermittently. It commonly sounds like a split S_1 but is located at the apex, away from the atrioventricular valves. It has a lower pitch than S_1 and is best appreciated with the bell. S_4 associated with left atrial systole and is caused by blood entering a left ventricle already having elevated end diastolic and volume. Therefore, it is appreciated prior to S_1 and within the PR interval. It is associated with hypertensive cardiac disease and may be intermittent depending on the afterload state of the patient.

A sequence of S_1, S_2, S_3 is referred to as a ventricular gallop. The S_3 is heard shortly after S_2 and before the P wave which is during the rapid and passive filling phase of the ventricles. It is softer in intensity and can be intermittently present and best heard with the bell. This is associated with ventricular volume and pressure overload. A right-sided S_3 appears and varies with inspiration due to isolated RV overload as seen in pulmonary HTN and pulmonary embolus (PE). This is best herd in the epigastric region (see Chap. 22). Left-sided S_3 does not vary with respiration and is associated with HFrEF (see Chap. 20).

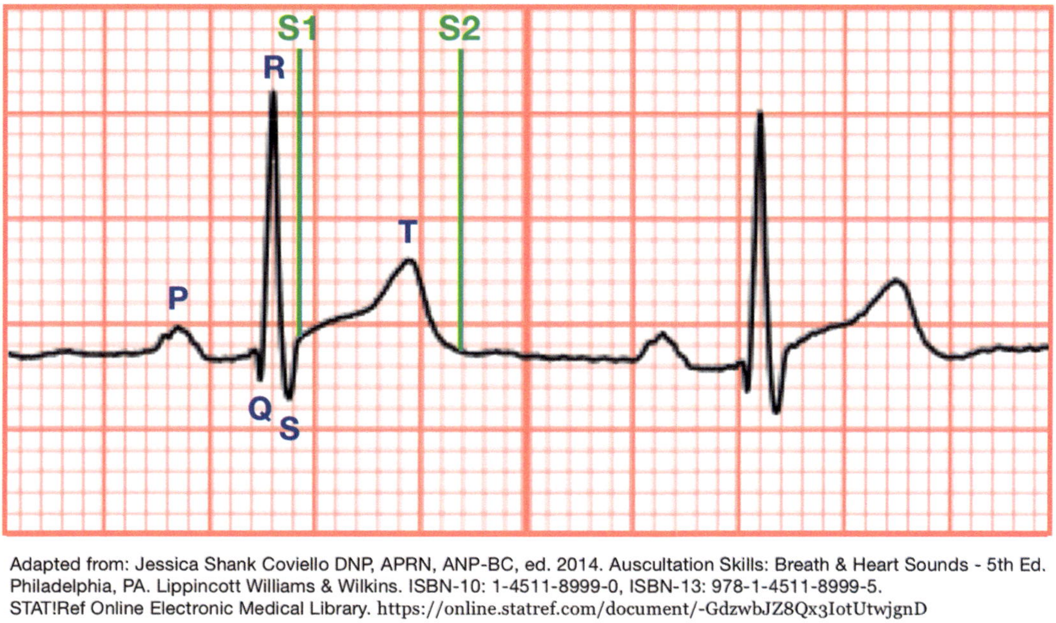

Fig. 1.8 Heart sounds in relation to EKG. Adapted from: Jessica Shank Coviello DNP, APRN, ANP-BC, ed. 2014. Auscultation Skills: Breath & Heart Sounds - 5th Ed. Philadelphia, PA. Lippincott Williams & Wilkins. ISBN-10: 1–4511–8999-0, ISBN-13: 978–1–4511-8999-5. STAT!Ref Online Electronic Medical Library. https://online.statref.com/document/-GdzwbJZ8Qx3IotUtwjgnD

Bruit:

Blood flow within a vessel that is obstructed creates a sound due to the higher velocity and turbulence created by the obstruction. It is like obstructing the flow at the end of a garden hose. The sound is higher pitched and radiated toward the direction of flow. It is not a murmur since this examination is occurring in the neck, legs, or abdominal location. It is systolic in nature. Rarely, diastolic or continuous sounds can be heard. When listening to the neck vessels, the bruit must be distinguished from aortic stenosis (AS) since this murmur will often radiate to the carotid arteries (see Chaps. 16 and 26).

Pulse Assessment

A scale from 0 to 4 is utilized. No palpable pulse is 0/4 with normal being 4/4. Commonly, the extremities are evaluated in assessment for peripheral arterial disease (PAD). Signs of chronic arterial insufficiency and specific arterial examination are discussed in Chap. 27. The pulses can be described as bounding in hyperdynamic states or in clinical presentation with prolonged runoff due to low afterload (see Chap. 16).

Peripheral Edema:

This is displacement of serous fluids outside the vascular space into the interstitial tissues. It is characterized based on the severity when depressed on a scale from 1 to 4. Commonly seen in the legs but can progress in some disease states like Cor pulmonale (see Chap. 22). If it is present diffusely throughout the body of the patient, it is called anasarca.

References

1. Sadler TW. Langman's medical embryology. 14th ed. Philadelphia: Wolters Kluwer; 2019.
2. DiFrancesco D. The role of the funny current in pacemaker activity. Circ Res. 2010;106:434–46.

3. Hilgemann DW. Control of cardiac contraction by sodium: Promises, reckonings, and new beginnings. Cell Calcium. 2020;85:102129.
4. Chien KR, Ross J Jr, Hoshijima M. Calcium and hert failure: the cycle game. Nat Med. 2003;9:508–9.
5. Josephson's Clinical Cardiac Electrophysiology: Techniques and Interpretations 6th Edition by Dr. David Callans. Publisher, LWW.
6. Zipes DP, Libby P, Bonow RO, Mann DL, Tomaselli GF, Braunwald E, editors. Braunwald's heart disease: a textbook of cardiovascular medicine, Single Volume. 11th ed. Philadelphia, PA: Elsevier; 2019.
7. Coviello JS, editor. Auscultation skills: breath & heart sounds. 5th ed. Philadelphia, PA: Lippincott Williams & Wilkins; 2014.

Basic Hemodynamics

2

Courtney Bennett and Amanda Solberg

Cardiac Cycle

The cardiac cycle is divided into two phases: systole and diastole (Fig. 2.1). The Wiggers diagram demonstrates the pressure and volume changes throughout the cardiac cycle and how these changes correlate with the ECG and cardiac auscultation (S1-S4).

Systole occurs when the AV valves close (S1) and the ventricles begin to contract (see Chap. 1). During systole, ventricular pressure increases through isovolumetric contraction and rapid ejection, and then begins to fall during isovolumetric relaxation. The onset of systole correlates with the R-wave on the ECG. Blood volume is ejected through the pulmonic and aortic valves (sometimes referred to as semilunar valves) into the systemic and pulmonary vasculature. Stroke volume (SV) is the amount of blood pumped out of the ventricle during each systolic contraction. A normal stroke volume is 70–80 mL. The volume of blood remaining in the ventricular chamber after ejection is called the end systolic volume.

The cardiac output (CO) is the SV times the heart rate (HR). CO is the volume of blood pumped by both ventricles per unit of time. In a normal resting heart, this would be approximately 5–6 L per minute. Cardiac index (CI) is the cardiac output divided by body surface area (L/min/M sq). This is a standardization tool used especially in the management of cardiogenic shock and transplantation.

The ejection fraction (EF) is the proportion of end-diastolic volume that is ejected during each systolic contraction and is commonly used as a noninvasive assessment of stroke volume. Afterload, or the pressure the ventricle pumps against, can affect stroke volume. Systemic vascular resistance (SVR) impacts the left ventricle while pulmonary vascular resistance (PVR) impacts the right. These pressures are calculated using the mean arterial pressure minus the CVP or mean pulmonary artery pressure minus the PCWP divided by the CO. These measurements and calculations are obtained from a right heart catheterization or pulmonary artery catheter (Swan-Ganz) catheter placement. Normal hemodynamic values are listed in Table 2.1.

$$\mathrm{CO}\left(\mathrm{L/min}\right) = \mathrm{SV} \times \mathrm{HR}$$

$$\mathrm{SVR}\left(\mathrm{Wood\,U}\right) = \frac{\mathrm{MAP} - \mathrm{CVP}}{\mathrm{CO}}$$

$$\mathrm{PVR}\left(\mathrm{Wood\,U}\right) = \frac{\mathrm{mPAP} - \mathrm{PCWP}}{\mathrm{CO}}$$

$$\mathrm{EF}\left(\%\right) = \frac{\mathrm{SV}}{\mathrm{EDV}} \times 100$$

Diastole occurs when the ventricles relax and pressure within the ventricles decreases. The ini-

C. Bennett · A. Solberg (✉)
Mayo Clinic, Rochester, MN, USA
e-mail: Bennett.Courtney@mayo.edu;
Solberg.Amanda@mayo.edu

R. Musialowski, K. Allshouse (eds.), *Cardiovascular Manual for the Advanced Practice Provider*,
https://doi.org/10.1007/978-3-031-35819-7_2

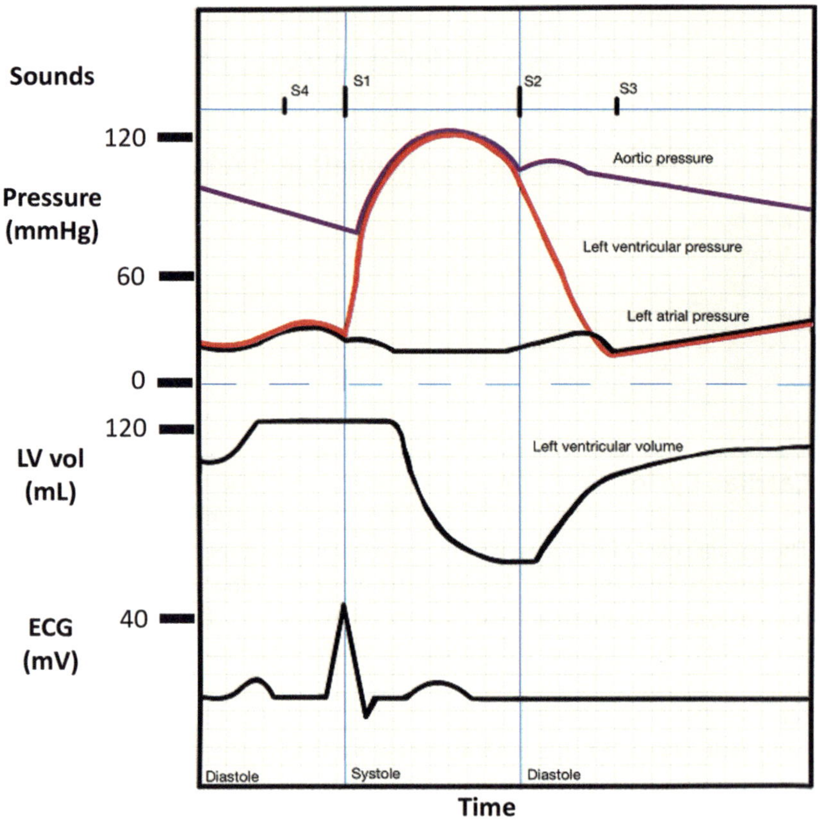

Fig. 2.1 Wiggers diagram showing a visual representation of the cardiac cycle showing heart sounds, pressure, left ventricular (LV) volume, and ECG comparison during. Permission from http://creativecommons.org/licenses/by/4.0/

Table 2.1 Normal hemodynamic values

RA pressure	0–8 mmHg
PA diastolic	15–30 mmHg
PA systolic	4–12 mmHg
PA mean	10–20 mmHg
PCWP	6–15 mmHg
CO	4–7 L/min
CI	2.5–3.6 L/min/m^2
SVR	800–1200 dynes/cm^5
SVRI	1970–2390 dynes/cm^2/m^5
PVR	0.5–2 Woods units (W.U.)
SvO2	65–75%

tial phase of diastole is passive filling of the ventricles from the atria after opening of the atrioventricular (AV) valves due to ventricular relaxation. In a normal heart, most ventricular filling occurs during this passive phase of diastole. Atrial contraction occurs following passive ventricular filling and correlates with the P-wave on the ECG. This contributes up to 20–30% of the end diastolic volume of the ventricles. End diastolic volume is the amount of blood the ventricles can hold at the end of diastole as the AV valves close (S2). The end diastolic volume of an average adult heart is approximately 130 mL of blood.

This end-diastolic volume is also known as preload and is defined as the degree of stretching that occurs in the ventricles at the end of diastole. A pulmonary capillary wedge pressure (PCWP) obtained from a pulmonary artery catheter is used to measure left ventricular end-diastolic pressure as a marker of left ventricular preload. End-diastolic volume can also be measured by 2-D echocardiogram and Doppler echocardiography can be used to estimate left ventricular filling pressures. Central venous pressure (CVP) from a central venous catheter or right atrial pressure (RAP) from a pulmonary artery catheter are used to estimate right ventricular preload in the absence of significant tricuspid valve pathology. Both PCWP and RAP pressure tracings consist of positive and negative deflections (Fig. 2.2).

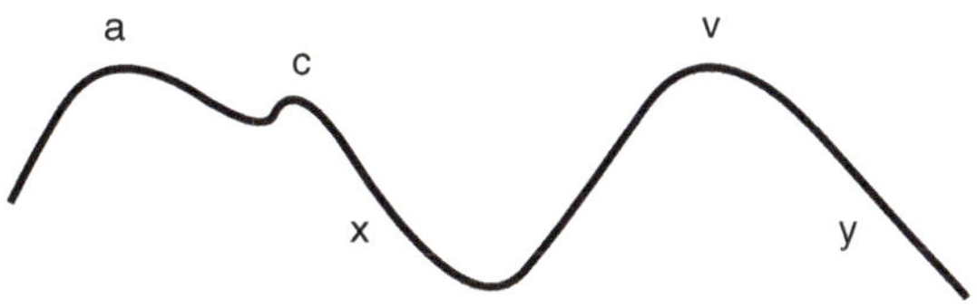

Fig. 2.2 Atrial pressure tracing; a-, c-, and v-waves and x- and y-descent

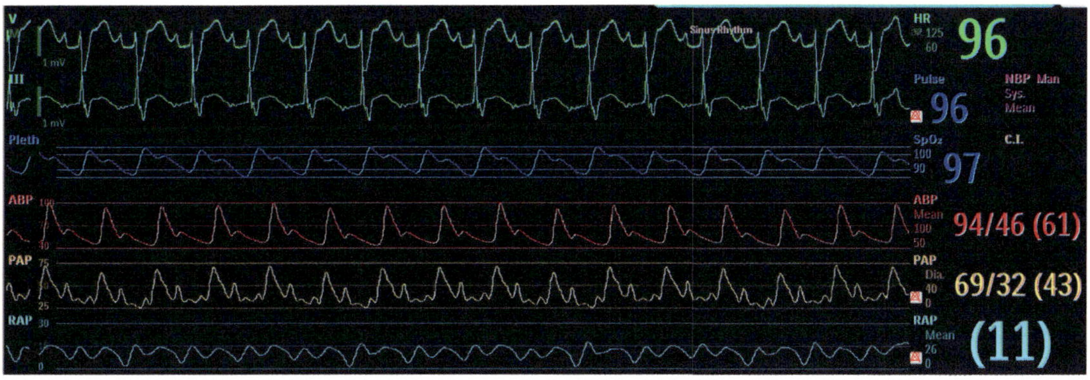

Fig. 2.3 RA tracing (light blue) and PA tracing (yellow) compared to the ECG and radial arterial tracing (red)

The a-wave follows the P-wave on the ECG and correlates with atrial contraction. At the bedside, the a-wave of the PCWP tracing is slightly delayed when compared to the a-wave seen on the RA tracing. This is due to the longer fluid filled tubing used while obtaining the PCWP tracing. Pressure falls within the atria as they empty into the ventricles and correlates with the x-descent. A c-wave or "bump" can sometimes be appreciated in the right atrium as the tricuspid valve begins to close. This finding is not seen on a PCWP tracing because the signal is diminished as the pressure is transmitted a further distance within the pulmonary artery catheter. The v-wave correlates with atrial filling during ventricular systole. The y-descent occurs during early ventricular diastole after the AV valves open and atrial pressure begins to decrease.

Using these measurements to evaluate patients in real-time can be valuable in the management of advanced heart failure and cardiogenic shock as an adjunct to standard care. Figure 2.3 shows the pulmonary artery pressure (PAP) and RAP with ECG and arterial line data.

The Frank-Starling Law represents the relationship between stroke volume and ventricular end-diastolic volume. As the volume of the blood in the ventricles increases, stroke volume increases until the volume or myocardial stretch exceeds the ability to contract effectively. When cardiac dysfunction occurs, ventricular end-diastolic volume increases, and stroke volume decreases due to decreased contractility. Figure 2.4 shows graphically representation of the relationship of pressure and volume during the cardiac cycle.

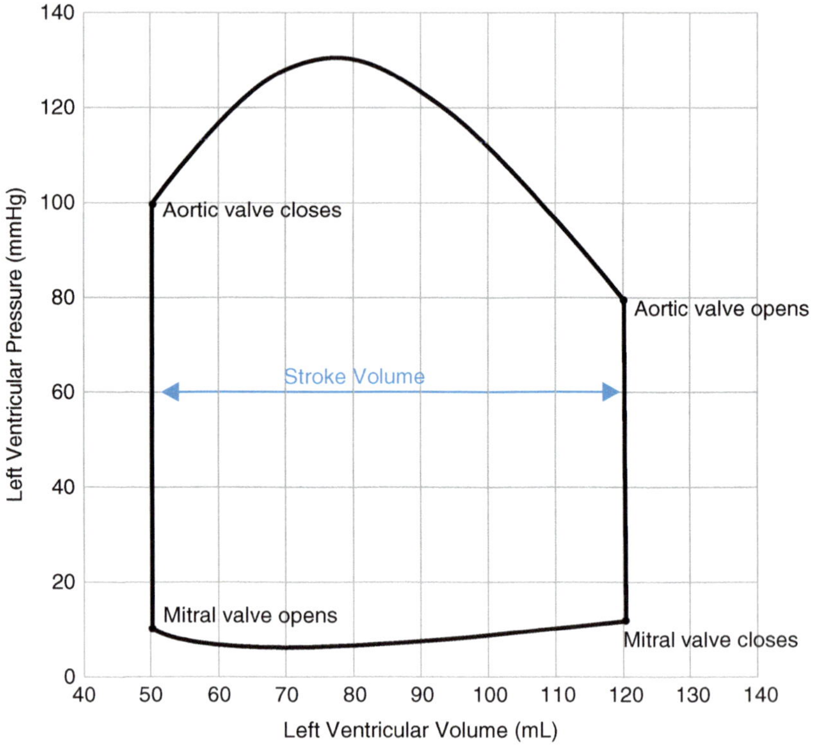

Fig. 2.4 Pressure-volume loop of the cardiac cycle

Part II

Coronary Artery Disease

Amy Winiger George P. Rodgers

Introduction

Atherosclerosis is the development of plaques made up of fatty and pro-inflammatory material in and on the walls of arteries. This may affect any arterial bed, but it is especially problematic when it affects the coronary arteries. Coronary atherosclerosis is the number one cause of death in the USA. There are several risk factors for coronary atherosclerosis. The non-modifiable risk factors are age, male gender, and family history of premature coronary artery disease. Premature onset is defined as the onset in a first-degree relative male before the age of 55, or first-degree relative female before the age of 65.

There are, however, several modifiable risk factors, which include hyperlipidemia, hypertension, diabetes mellitus, metabolic syndrome, cigarette smoking, obesity, a sedentary lifestyle, and heavy alcohol intake. There are many laboratory and imaging markers of coronary atherosclerosis, and these include elevated lipoprotein (a), hyper-homocystinuria, elevated high-sensitive C-reactive protein, and coronary artery calcification seen on multi-detector CT.

The current paradigm of atherosclerosis is an injury/inflammation paradigm. First consider the structure of the artery. The intima (tunica intima) is one layer of endothelium over the media (tunica media). The media layer consists of smooth muscle cells. Finally, the adventitia (tunica externa) is the outermost layer separated from the medial layer by fibrous elastic lamina (Fig. 1).

A. Winiger
Atrium Health/Sanger Heart and Vascular Institute, Charlotte, NC, USA
e-mail: Amy.Winger@atriumhealth.org

G. P. Rodgers
Ascension Texas Cardiovascular, Austin, TX, USA
e-mail: grodgers@austin.utexas.edu

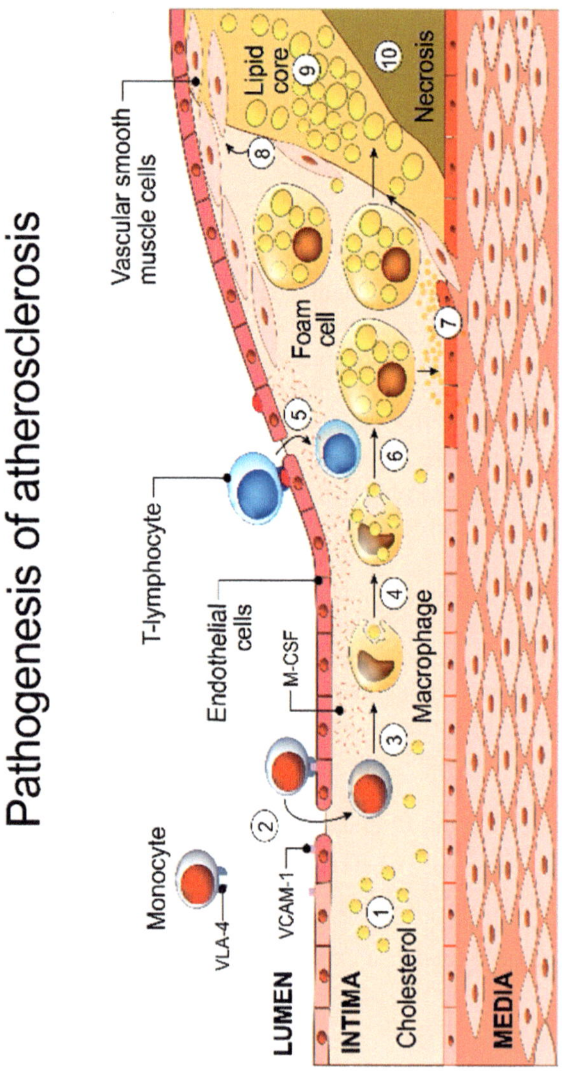

Fig. 1 Development of atherosclerotic plaque

The development of coronary atherosclerosis begins early in life. Fatty streaks, which are mainly intracellular lipid accumulation, are the first pathologic evidence of atherosclerosis. These occur within the intimal lining of the aorta and are sometimes evident within the first decade of life. By the third decade of life, these intracellular lipid accumulations have developed into small extracellular pools of lipids that are the first evidence of atheromas.

In the fourth decade of life, these emerging atheromas may become hardened and sclerotic with fibrosis, thus referred to as fibroatheroma. These lesions further transform through increased smooth muscle and collagen deposition and develop into mature atherosclerotic plaque (Fig. 1). Thus far, the development of coronary atherosclerosis has been silent; the individual has no symptoms. However, if the mature plaque becomes very large, it may obstruct the coronary artery to a degree (>70%) so that flow to the myocardium is reduced during exercise. This would produce myocardial ischemia and the individual may experience symptoms referred to as stable exertional angina (Fig. 2).

If an atherosclerotic plaque becomes significantly inflamed, it may exhibit a thinning of the fibrous cap that covers the extracellular pool of lipids. This is referred to as a "vulnerable plaque" because if the thinned fibrous cap becomes unroofed or ruptures, it will expose the lipid pool to the circulating blood elements. This results in immediate thrombus formation. Thrombus begets more thrombus such that the lumen of the coronary artery at this site may become seriously obstructed. This is the underlying pathophysiology of acute coronary syndrome (Type I MI).

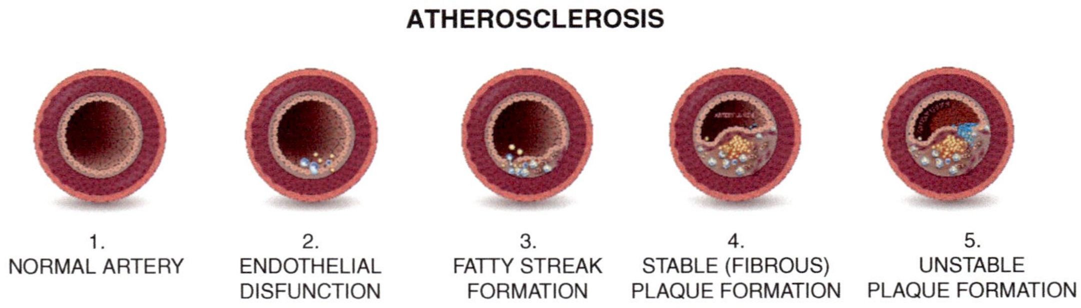

Fig. 2 Progression of atherosclerosis over time

Acute Coronary Syndrome (ACS) ST Segment Elevation Myocardial Infarction

3

Amy Winiger and George P. Rodgers

Anatomy and Physiology

Coronary arteries supply oxygenated blood to the myocardium of the heart. They are located on the outer surface of the heart (epicardial), originating from the aorta (see Chap. 1). The left main (LM) coronary artery originates at the left coronary cusp and bifurcates into the left anterior descending, or LAD, and the left circumflex artery (LCX). The LAD supplies the left ventricle anterior wall, anterior portion of the intraventricular septum and a portion of the right ventricular wall. The diagonal branches arise from the left anterior descending. The circumflex artery supplies the lateral and posterior regions of the left ventricle (LV). The obtuse marginal (OM) branches arise from the circumflex artery. The right coronary artery supplies the right ventricle and the posterior lateral branch. The right coronary artery (RCA) also supplies the sinoatrial node (SA node) and the atrial ventricular node (AV node) (see Fig. 3.1).

Coronary blood flow occurs during ventricular diastole. The myocardial oxygen requirement is influenced by the oxygen demand of the tissues: the faster the heart rate, the higher the oxygen demand. In addition, an increase in left ventricular contractility and left ventricular wall stress caused by an elevation in blood pressure increases the myocardial demand for more oxygen. This balance between the oxygen demand of the myocardium and the ability to supply the oxygen, through coronary blood flow, will determine whether the downstream myocardium becomes under-perfused, or ischemic. Different clinical coronary syndromes can be described based on the condition of the coronary arteries and hemodynamic requirements.

Definition of STEMI

> "in the absence of left ventricular (LV) hypertrophy or left bundle branch block (LBBB) is defined by the European Society of Cardiology/ACC/AHA/World Heart Federation Task Force for the universal definition of Myocardial Infarction as new ST elevation of the J point in at least 2 contiguous leads of ≥(0.2 mV in men or ≥1.5 mm (0.15) mV in women in leads V2–V3, and/or of ≥1 mm (0.1 mV) in other contiguous chest leads, or limb leads" [8, p. e83].

The definition of acute coronary syndrome (ACS) is suspicion or confirmation of acute myocardial ischemia or infarction [1]. There are three types of ACS: ST elevation MI (STEMI), non-ST elevation MI (NSTEMI), and unstable angina pectoris (UAP) [1]. The definition of a STEMI is

A. Winiger (✉)
Atrium Health/Sanger Heart and Vascular Institute, Charlotte, NC, USA
e-mail: Amy.Winger@atriumhealth.org

G. P. Rodgers
Ascension Texas Cardiovascular, Austin, TX, USA
e-mail: grodgers@austin.utexas.edu

R. Musialowski, K. Allshouse (eds.), *Cardiovascular Manual for the Advanced Practice Provider*,
https://doi.org/10.1007/978-3-031-35819-7_3

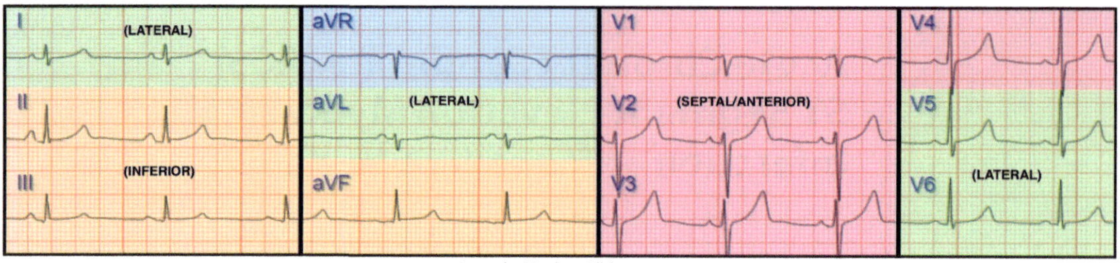

Image by Matthew Allshouse

EKG Location	Coronary Distribution
Anterior-V1-4	LAD
Septal-V1-V2	Prox. LAD
Lateral-I, aVL, V5-V6	LCx
Inferior-II, III, aVF	RCA (85%) or LCx (15%)
Posteriolateral-V7, V8, V9	RCA or LCx
Right Ventricle-V1, V4R	RCA

adapted from *Localization of the occluded vessel in acute myocardial infarction.* R. Samir, K. Amr. Published 18 February 2020. Medicine.

Fig. 3.1 EKG localization and related coronary distribution. (Image by Matthew Allshouse)

symptoms of myocardial ischemia with an EKG revealing ST elevation with the release of biomarkers, the result of myocardial injury.

As discussed in the introduction, a STEMI describes the rupture of the atherosclerotic plaque in a coronary artery due to disruption of the fibrous cap and the lipid core becoming exposed to the blood stream [2]. This instantly incites thrombosis, which may completely occlude the lumen of the artery and stop the blood flow and oxygen delivery downstream. This cessation of distal blood flow causes muscle cell death, referred to as myocardial infarction. This is a medical emergency. "Time is muscle" because with every minute that passes, there is more necrosis and progressive permanent injury to the heart muscle.

Evaluation

Any encounter with a patient begins with a history and physical exam. The initial bedside evaluation should occur very quickly in a patient with suspected ACS. The goal should be to complete the interview and evaluation within 5 min. A rapid, focused history should be obtained using the OLD CARTS format [3]. Ask about the patient's symptoms. These include pain Onset, Location, Duration (does it wax and wane?), Character (description of what they feel, "elephant on their chest?", sharp, dull, heavy), Aggravating/Alleviating Factors (activity, position, medication), Radiation, Timing (when did it start and what were you doing? How long did it last?) and Severity (1–10 with 10 being worst pain ever felt). OPQRST is an alternative way to perform rapid questioning regarding symptoms which includes: Onset, Provoking, Quality, Radiation, Severity, Timing of the pain (see Chap. 31).

Also, the patient's chart should be reviewed, paying special attention to prior coronary artery bypass surgery or percutaneous revascularization (PCI). The provider should attempt to obtain past procedure notes to determine grafts and/or stenting previously performed. It is important to note if the patient was fully revascularized. Prior testing should be reviewed including echocardiograms, stress tests, MRI/CTs, etc. Old EKGs and medications should be reviewed.

Symptoms

The patient presenting with STEMI will often display classic signs and symptoms including extreme pressure-like chest discomfort that is substernal, associated shortness of breath, diaphoresis, and potential nausea/vomiting on presentation to the emergency department. Differential diagnosis of severe anterior chest pain may include pericarditis, aortic dissection, costochondritis, gastroesophageal reflux, peptic ulcer disease, esophageal spasm, pulmonary embolism, biliary colic, pneumonia, or coronary vasospasm (Chap. 31).

Physical Exam

Prior to entering the patient's room, assess: how does the patient look? Does the patient appear to be in pain (clutching his/her chest with Levine's sign) [3]? Is the patient diaphoretic, anxious, or nauseous/vomiting [4]? Rapid physical exam should be performed including special focus on heart sounds (are there extra heart sounds indicating valve dysfunction or heart failure), jugular venous distention, or rales [5]. While completing the rapid physical exam, specific questions should tailored to the catheterization lab. These may include whether the patient is followed by a physician for any chronic medical problems such as undergoing treatment for cancer. Do they have any upcoming surgeries which may influence anticoagulation and antiplatelet decisions? The patient should be asked if they have had any history of bleeding including stroke or GI bleeding, and if so, was this due to dual antiplatelet therapy (DAPT)? If there is any question of whether the patient should be taken to the catheterization lab, communicate with the interventional cardiologist. It is always better to over communicate rather than under communicate. It may also be necessary to take the lead in the ED to coordinate and get the patient to the catheterization lab in an urgent manner. Do not be afraid to direct the healthcare team!

Diagnostics

A STAT EKG, and labs, including high sensitivity troponin, electrolytes, kidney and liver function, CBC, and INR should be performed. Troponin elevation is very specific for cardiac cellular death. The levels vary based on which type of troponin your facility uses. Any elevation above normal is due to cell death. The more elevated, the more muscle necrosed. The troponin levels may not be elevated initially but will elevate over hours to days, and thus should be trended.

A skillset that is critical to any cardiovascular practitioner is interpretation of acute coronary syndrome locations on the electrocardiogram. Figure 3.1 will assist you with remembering what each lead of the 12-lead EKG represents. A STEMI is characterized by one or more millimeters of ST elevation in two or more contiguous leads [6]. Contiguous refers to leads that are assessing a certain territory of the heart. Typically, the contiguous leads are fed by a single coronary artery.

The EKG correlates with the coronary anatomy. The anterior precordial leads V2-V4 correspond to the anteroseptal walls of the heart supplied by the LAD (Fig. 3.1). In this example, EKG (Fig. 3.2), urgent cardiac catheterization confirmed type I MI in the LAD distribution (Fig. 3.3) and primary stenting was completed (Fig. 3.4).

Limb leads 1 and aVL view the lateral aspect of the heart. This distribution is often perfused by the LCX. The distal anterior precordial leads V5 and V6 correspond with the apex and can be supplied by the LAD, LCX, or PDA. Notice the ST depression of V1-V2 in Fig. 3.5. If these depressions are seen with STEMI in the inferior leads, this is a posterior extension of the STEMI and not reciprocal changes. This is large and high-risk MI and is at risk for decompensation to cardiogenic shock. Figures 3.6 and 3.7 show the cardiac catheterization films of the left circumflex occlusion and percutaneous coronary intervention (PCI).

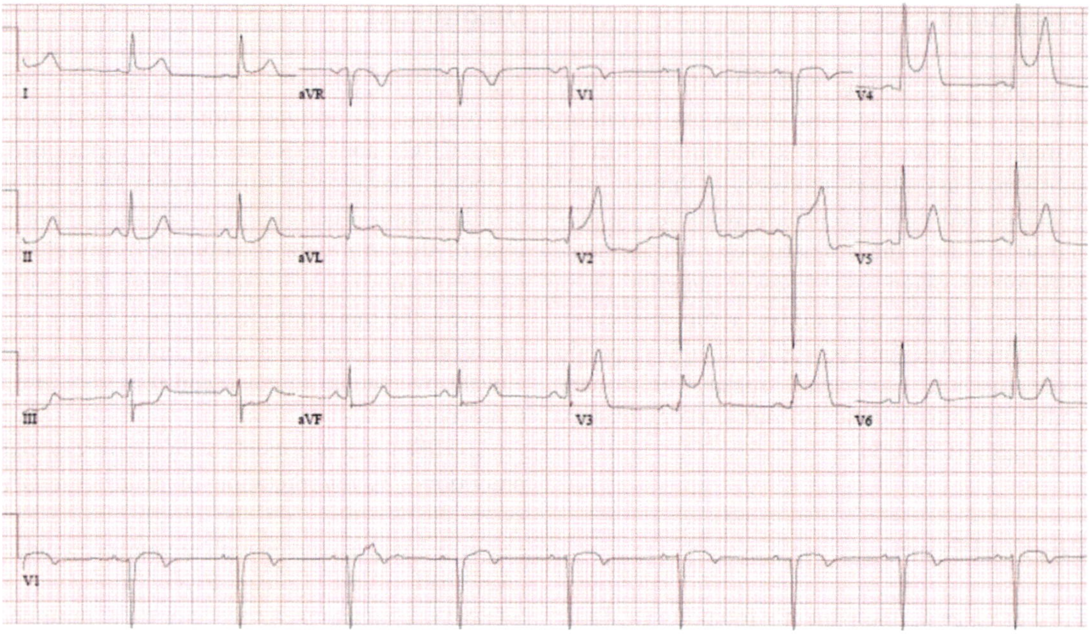

Fig. 3.2 STEMI in anterior leads V1-V5 with reciprocal changes

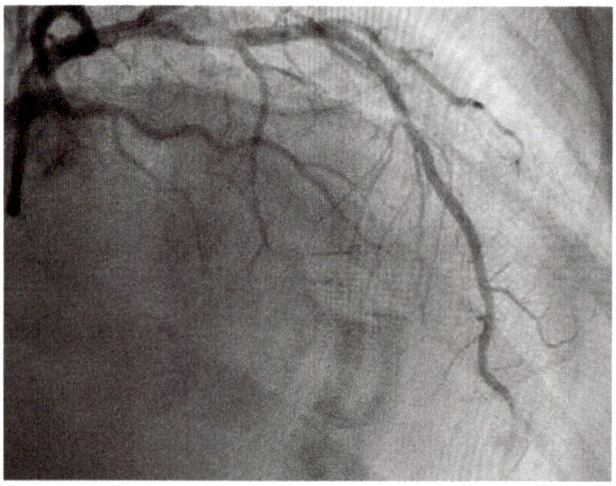

Fig. 3.3 Type I MI in LAD

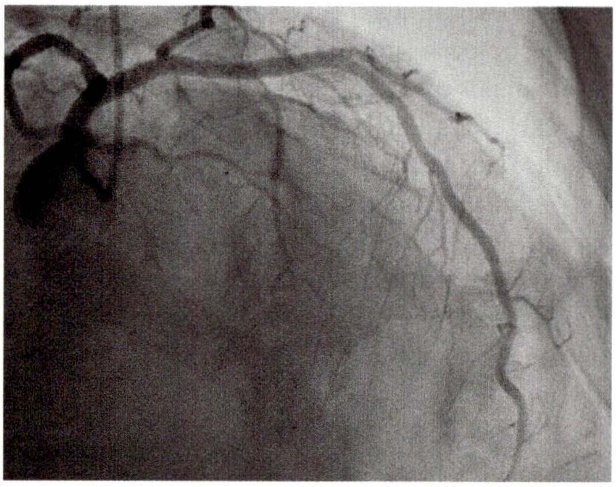

Fig. 3.4 LAD after PCI

Limb leads II, III, and aVF are evaluating the inferior portion of the heart corresponding to the posterior descending artery (PDA). Vessel dominance is described as the vessel that gives rise to the PDA. In 80% of patients, this vessel arises from the RCA (right dominant) with 20% arising from the LCX (left dominant). Type I STEMI of the RCA causes ST segment elevation of these inferior leads (Fig. 3.8).

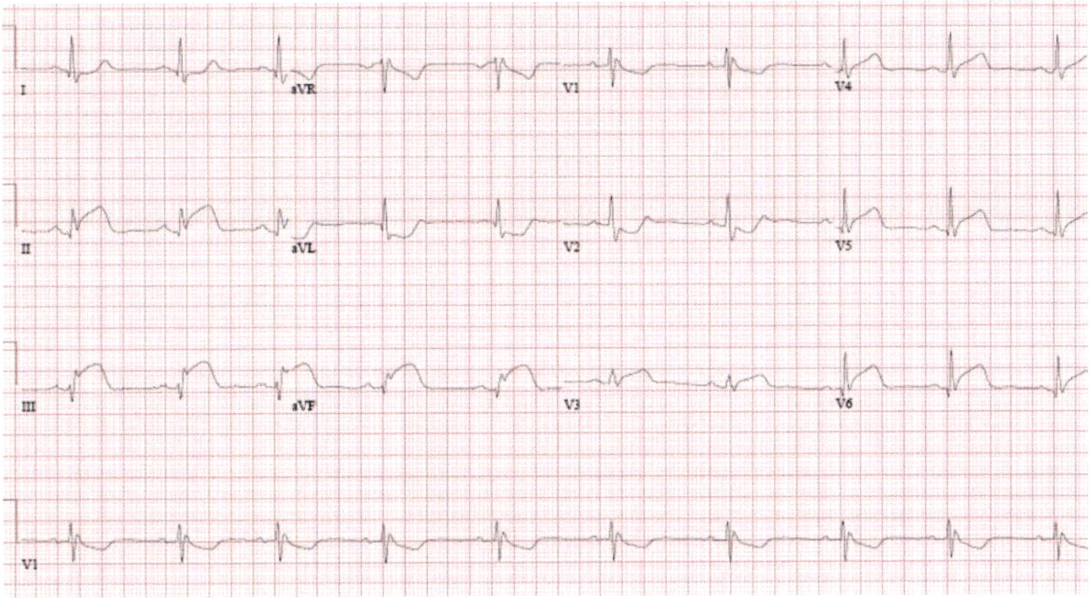

Fig. 3.5 Inferior and posterolateral STEMI

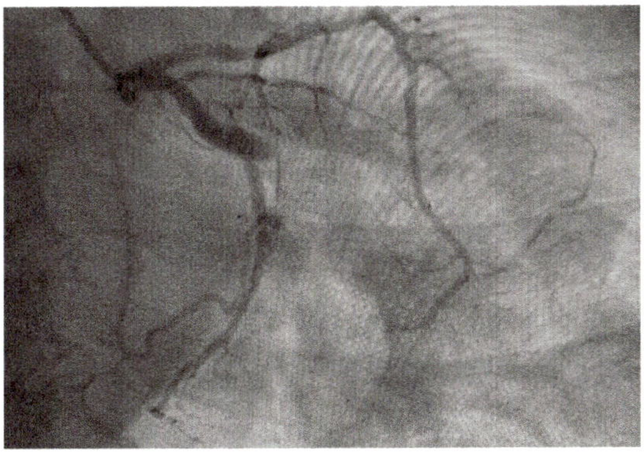

Fig. 3.6 Left circumflex occlusion

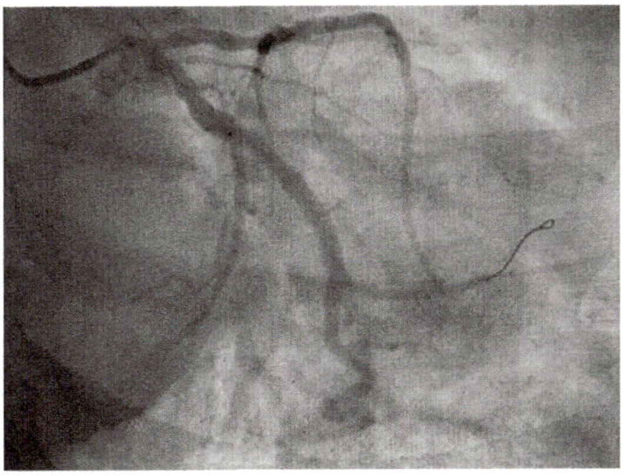

Fig. 3.7 Primary PCI of left circumflex

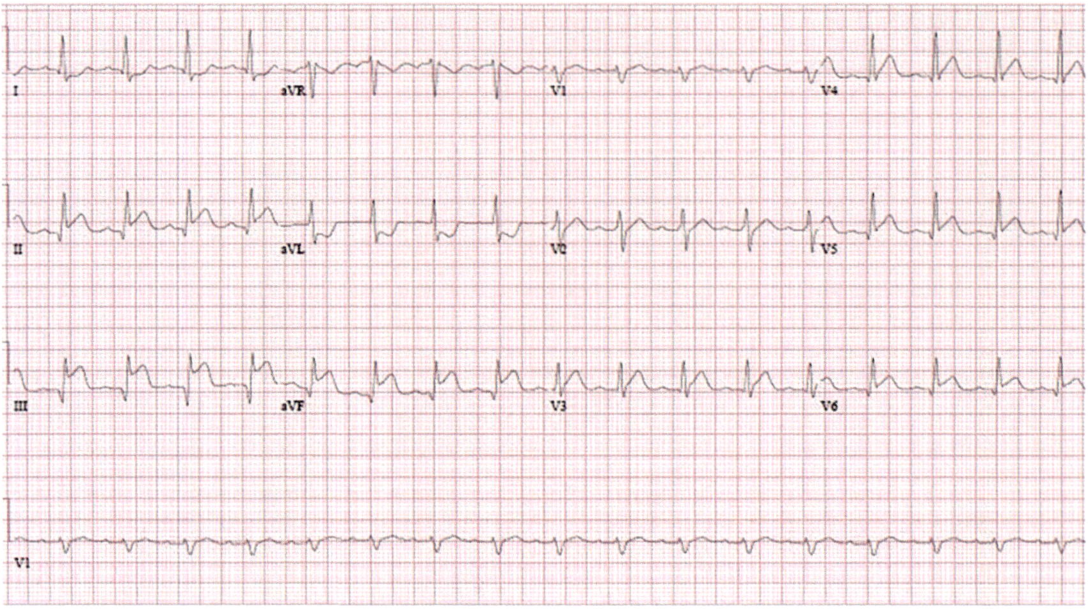

Fig. 3.8 STEMI inferior leads

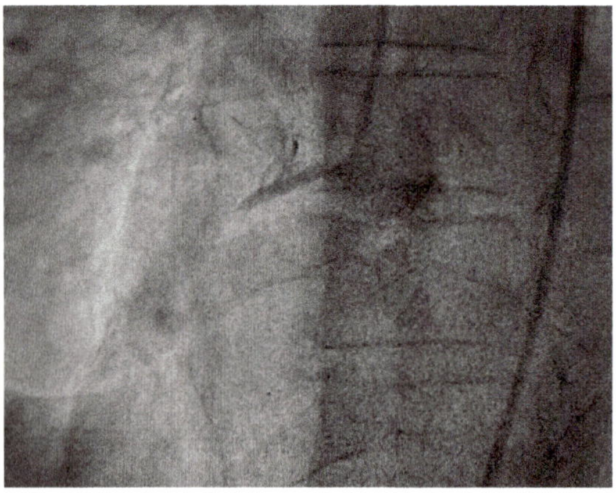

Fig. 3.9 RCA occlusion

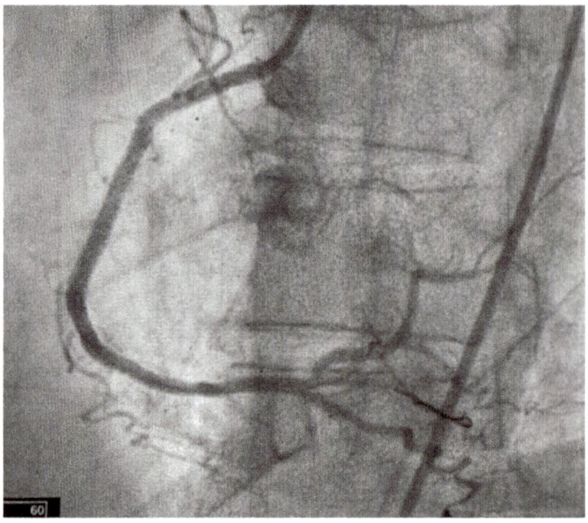

Fig. 3.10 RCA post intervention

Figures 3.9 and 3.10 show the catheterization films of inferior STEMI.

Imaging/Management

Once the diagnosis of STEMI has been confirmed, the interventional cardiologist should be alerted, and the catheterization laboratory notified. The lab and physician are sometimes activated prior to the patient's arrival in the ED by EMS if symptoms and EKG are consistent with a STEMI. It has been found that it is critical to open the affected artery and restore blood flow as quickly as possible. Percutaneous coronary intervention (PCI) or coronary balloon angioplasty and stenting is the most effective way to open an occluded artery. Timeliness is critically important with "door to balloon time" used as the metric throughout the world. This is the time from when the patient arrives at the hospital (door time) to when the first inflation of the angioplasty balloon occurs (balloon time). The goal of the "door to balloon time" is to open the artery within 90 min. This is derived from an important observational study showing that the best results with the lowest mortality rates for STEMIs occur in patients with a door to balloon time of less than 90 min [7]. Nationally, this is the target for any STEMI. After 12 h of total occlusion time of a coronary artery, the myocardial infarction is complete and there is little tissue left to salvage, and late revascularization may be dangerous leading to complications of the STEMI (Table 3.2).

A cardiac catheterization involves bringing the patient to the catheterization laboratory. Conscious sedation may be administered as per physician preference. Arterial access sites are prepped (radial vs. femoral artery). The interventional cardiologist accesses the artery with a needle, and a sheath is placed in the artery. Since the complication rate of femoral access is higher, radial artery access is preferred. A catheter over a guidewire is advanced to where the coronary arteries originate off the aorta. Contrast dye is injected into the coronary arteries while fluoroscopy (x-ray) is used to take pictures of the arteries (angiogram). In a STEMI, the angiogram will show an abrupt cut-off of the coronary artery or complete occlusion. The occlusion can be crossed with a coronary wire and using this wire as a monorail, a balloon is placed at the site of the occlusion and is inflated to open the artery. Next, another balloon with a stent crimped on it is brought into the coronary artery over the coronary wire and expanded into the walls of the artery, stenting open the artery. Unfractionated heparin is given during the procedure. This is called primary angioplasty and has been shown to reduce mortality in STEMI (see images of PCI). PCI requires a skilled interventional cardiologist and team of catheterization lab staff to perform the procedure safely. This is usually performed at tertiary hospitals.

In some settings, PCI is not available, and thrombolytic therapy must be used to medically open the coronary artery. The choice between PCI or thrombolytic therapy using tissue plasminogen activator (TPA), or TNK, has been carefully studied. In several head-to-head trials, PCI was shown to be superior to thrombolytics. However, thrombolysis may be more practical in rural settings where PCI is not universally available (greater than 2 h away for primary PCI).

After PCI, medical therapy is essential. Dual anti-platelet therapy is essential for reducing thrombosis within the stented artery. Typically, the patient is loaded with antiplatelet medication, which includes a P2Y12 inhibitor (clopidogrel, prasugrel, or ticagrelor) as well as low dose aspirin. This dual antiplatelet therapy (DAPT) will be continued for 12 months. High-potency statins (Atorvastatin 40–80 mg daily or Rosuvastatin 20–40 mg daily) and beta blockers are prescribed in the post STEMI setting according to the guidelines. If a patient has a reduced ejection fraction (EF), LVEF less than 50 percent, typically an angiotensin converting enzyme inhibitor (ACE inhibitor) or angiotensin receptor blocker (ARB) is added to the regimen. If the LVEF is less than 40 percent, Entresto (angiotensin receptor blocker and neprilysin inhibitor (ARNI), ACE inhibitor or an ARB is used. In addition, Spironolactone, a mineral corticoid receptor antagonist (MRA) might be added to the regi-

Table 3.1 Complication of cardiac catheterization and PCI

Hematoma at arteriotomy site	Bleeding: GI bleeding, intracranial hemorrhage
Pseudoaneurysm	CVA/TIA
Retroperitoneal hematoma	Local nerve injury at arteriotomy site
Vascular compromise distal to arteriotomy	Embolization atheromatous material
Complications of closure device-infection	

Table 3.2 Complications of STEMI

Cardiogenic Shock	Arrhythmia (VT, Torsade's)
Ventricular septal defect	Papillary muscle rupture and acute mitral regurgitation
Ventricular free wall rupture	Apical ventricular thrombus and embolization
Ischemic cardiomyopathy	Ventricular aneurysm
Pericarditis (Dressler's syndrome)	AV node injury and heart block

men. All have been shown to reduce mortality and reduce hospital readmissions in STEMI patients with severe depression of LV systolic function (LVEF <40%) [8].

It is essential that the patient is closely monitored for potential complications post PCI. Complications of cardiac catheterization can include peri-procedural bleeding which is the most frequent complication of PCI and associated with poor clinical outcomes (Table 3.1) [9].

Age, kidney function, and cardiogenic shock increase risk for bleeding complications [10, 11]. Use of multiple antithrombotic and anticoagulants increase the incidence of periprocedural bleeding. Women have an increased risk of bleeding complications due to the smaller size of the femoral artery [12, 13, 14]. Obesity is also a higher risk due to decreased ability to recognize bleeding. Hematomas at the arteriotomy site may form. The patient may develop a pseudoaneurysm if the site heals inappropriately. The pseudoaneurysm is diagnosed with ultrasound (US) and may require thrombin injection to manage this complication. Retroperitoneal hematoma is a potentially life-threatening complication where bleeding occurs in the retroperitoneal space. Acute lower abdominal pain after femoral access requires consideration for retroperitoneal bleeding, and this is diagnosed with CT scan of the abdomen [15]. Vascular compromise distal to the arterial access may occur, especially in patients who already have a large amount of peripheral vascular disease. This complication would be seen as loss of distal pulses, pain, and pallor and may occur after deployment of a vascular access occlusion device at the end of the PCI. Urgent Vascular Surgery consultation is needed. Finally, nerve injury may occur following PCI. Less common complications may include GI bleeding evidenced by a drop in Hgb with hematemesis or melena, or intracranial hemorrhage diagnosed with head CT after change in neurologic status is observed due to anticoagulation therapy during the PCI. The APP should evaluate for hematoma or pain at the access site, decreased distal pulses to the access site, abdominal or back pain, if femoral access is used [16]. Vitals must be monitored looking for tachypnea, tachycardia which results from increased oxygen demand in the setting of acute blood loss. The patient may also appear pale, cold, and clammy if they are losing blood and hemorrhagic shock is developing. Rapid and direct communication with the interventionalist and vascular surgeon is essential if bleeding is suspected.

STEMI complications may be significant (Table 3.2). The first is impairment of LV function which may be transient or permanent. This occurs due to ischemia or infarction of the muscle tissue of the ventricle. Transmural tissue necrosis complications may present 3–5 days after the myocardial infarction, especially in situations where the patient did not have the benefit of early PCI or thrombotic therapy. This necrosis can result in papillary muscle infarction, resulting in severe mitral regurgitation due to a flail mitral valve leaflet. This event may lead to flash pulmonary edema due to acute severe mitral regurgitation. If the necrosis occurs within the

LV septum, there can be ventricular septal wall rupture resulting in a VSD and heart failure symptoms with a new loud murmur. Ischemic VSD is a surgical emergency. A free wall rupture may result which is usually fatal. Occasionally, blood will fill the pericardium resulting in tamponade without death and is a surgical emergency. A rupture may cause a pseudoaneurysm, and the patient is fortunate to have survived. Severe damage to the heart muscle may result in a permanent reduction in LV function, called ischemic cardiomyopathy. If the infarct is localized to the apex, the patient may develop an LV aneurysm which may cause ventricular arrhythmias. Many of these complications require surgical intervention.

Another significant complication from acute MI is tachyarrhythmia and bradyarrhythmia. See Part III for arrhythmia details. Ventricular tachycardia, and ventricular fibrillation may result from acute ischemia and may cause sudden cardiac death (SCD) early in STEMI.

Follow-Up

Post MI, the patient is often admitted to the cardiac ICU for monitoring to include the above stated complications. An echocardiogram will likely be completed to evaluate the heart function and valves. The patient will be on continuous telemetry monitoring for arrhythmias. Assessment for post procedural complications is very important in the first 24 h after STEMI presentation.

All patients that have suffered acute coronary syndrome, and especially STEMI have a class 1 indication for cardiac rehab. This is a supervised program that is three 1-hour sessions per week for 12 weeks. The intradisciplinary healthcare team of RNs, exercise physiologists, and dieticians educate the patient on their medications, exercise regimen, and Mediterranean diet. The patients also meet others who have coronary artery disease; they form a support system for each other.

Clinical Pearls

- Family history of premature CAD is male <55 or first-degree relative women female <65.
- Time is muscle: the longer an area is ischemic, the more muscle dies.
- It is critical to know if an AMI patient had prior CABG or stents and the location of these.
- Goal door to balloon time is <90 min!!
- Review any old EKGs if possible. Pay particular attention to previous LVH with strain, left bundle branch blocks, or Q-waves.
- Quickly assess patients' history of bleeding (GIB or head bleed) and history of prior TIA or CVA to guide management with antiplatelets.
- Remember to consider alternative causes for ST elevations, particularly if the clinic picture is not consistent with ST-elevation MI, and if indicated rule out dissection or obtain head CT prior to cath lab (aortic dissection, cocaine induced vasospasm, pulmonary embolism, subarachnoid hemorrhage, etc.).
- Patients treated with 324 mg aspirin, 80 mg atorvastatin, 4000 U IV heparin prior to transfer to PCI facility. Loading with Plavix per PCI center protocol. Caution with nitroglycerin in RCA infarct.
- When discussing patient's pertinent medical history with referring provider, inquire about any significant comorbidities that patient is currently being treated for. If the patient is being treated for cancer, review their notes for treatment plan and prognosis. If possible, talk to the provider directly. Overall prognosis can help guide clinical decision making.
- Obtain patient's EMR and date of birth. If time allows, review previous medical records, including if patient has previous cardiac history, and any previous cardiac imaging. Review of patient's labs—particularly creatinine prior to taking to cath lab.
- Standard guideline directed medical therapy post intervention includes DAPT (unless patient on systemic OAC), high dose statin

therapy, beta-blocker, and when indicated ACE/ARB/ARNI when LVEF <40% or anterior MI.

- If patient is on novel oral anticoagulation (NOAC), ask rationale for treatment plan. If patient is on NOAC, provide detailed documentation and plan of care for anticoagulation going forward. For example, DAPT therapy for 1 month, in addition to NOAC, then discontinue aspirin.
- Arrange follow-up appointments prior to discharge. Include patient in discussion, they are more likely to follow up if office is closer to their home. Prescribe enough refills for antiplatelet medication for 1 year.

References

1. Kumar V, et al. Robbins and Cotran pathologic basis of disease. 9th ed. Philadelphia, PA: Elsevier.
2. DeLemos J, Omland T. Chronic coronary artery disease. A companion to Braunwald's heart disease. Philadelphia, PA: Elsevier; 2018.
3. Lilly LS. Pathophysiology of heart disease. 5th ed. Wolters Kluwer; 2021.
4. Benjamin IJ, et al. Andreoli and Carpenter's Cecil essentials of medicine. 9th ed. Philadelphia, PA: Elsevier.
5. Schiffman FJ, Wing EJ. Cecil essentials of medicine. 10th ed. Elsevier; 2022.
6. Bielinsky J. 2022. Contiguous leads and the EKG. https://cme4life.com/acute-care-cme/contiguous-leads-ekg/.
7. McNamara RL, et al. Effect of door-to-balloon time on mortality in patients with ST segment elevation myocardial infarction. J Am Coll Cardiol. 2006;47(6):2180–6.
8. O'Gara PT, et al. 2013 AACF/AHA guideline for the management of ST-elevation myocardial infarction. J Am Coll Cardiol. 2013;61(4):e78–e140.
9. Ferrante et al. (2016). Radial versus femoral access for coronary interventions across the entire spectrum of patients with coronary artery disease: a meta-analysis of randomized trials. JACC Cardiovasc Interv, 9(14), 1419–1434.
10. Chhatriwalla AK, et al. Association between bleeding events and in-hospital mortality after percutaneous coronary intervention. J Am Med Assoc. 2013;3903(10):1022–9.
11. Kubler P, et al. In patients undergoing percutaneous coronary intervention with rotational atherectomy radial access is safer and as efficient as femoral access. J Interv Cardiol. 2018;31:471–7.
12. Daughtery SL, et al. Patterns of use and comparative effectiveness of bleeding avoidance strategies in men and women following percutaneous coronary interventions. J Am Coll Cardiol. 2013;61(20):2070–8.
13. Kwok CS, et al. Effect of access site, gender, and indication on clinical outcomes after percutaneous coronary intervention: insights from the British Cardiovascular Intervention Society. Am Heart J. 2015;170(1):164–172.e5.
14. Ndrepepa G, et al. Bleeding after percutaneous intervention in women and men matched for age, body mass index, and type of antithrombic therapy. Am Heart J. 2013;166(3):534–40.
15. Sorajja P, Holmes DR. 2021. Periprocedural bleeding in patients undergoing percutaneous coronary intervention. Up to Date.
16. Rodgers GP, et al. 2020 ACC clinical competencies for nurse practitioners and physician assistants in adult cardiovascular medicine: a report of the ACC Competency Management Committee. J Am Coll Cardiol. 2020;2020(75):2483–517.

ACS Non-ST Elevation Myocardial Infarction (NSTEMI)

4

Michelle Ross and John Cedarholm

Introduction

The term acute coronary syndrome (ACS) refers to ST elevation MI (STEMI), NSTEMI, and unstable angina (UA.) STEMI and NSTEMI are caused by acute disruption of a coronary plaque resulting in partial or complete obstruction of flow through a coronary artery by a superimposed thrombus. The diminished blood flow and reduction in oxygen supply results in ischemia and ultimate infarct of myocardium. This usually causes symptoms of angina at rest (unstable angina), may cause ECG changes, and results in elevated troponins. Unstable angina without infarction may have a similar presentation to NSTEMI, but without a troponin release.

Type I and Type II Myocardial Infarction

As stated in the Chap. 3, Myocardial infarction can be classified as type I and type II. This is important distinction for patient care and prognosis. An elevated troponin occurring secondary to plaque rupture or erosion is considered a Type I MI (this includes STEMI and NSTEMI). Myocardial injury occurring due to acute oxygen supply and demand mismatch, without plaque rupture, is defined as a Type II MI. In this case, myocardial cell death occurs because of the inability to meet the oxygen demand of the tissue or in the presence of profound metabolic derangement. The patient may have chest pain, ECG changes with or without the presence of CAD. Examples can be seen in patients presenting with a COPD exacerbation, rapid atrial fibrillation, severe anemia, along with many other presentations (*see* Table 4.1). It is very important to make this distinction as the mortality rate of type II MI is higher than type I and type II may not require invasive evaluation [1] Treatment of the underlying cause of the Type II MI is the best treatment option, not an invasive evaluation or anticoagulation.

Table 4.1 Etiologies of myocardial cell death in Type II MI

CKD/ESRD
Heart failure (acute and/or chronic)
Sepsis/critical illness
Pulmonary embolism
Myocarditis
Stress cardiomyopathy (Takotsubo)
Cardiotoxic drugs
CPR/defibrillator shocks
Chest trauma (cardiac contusion)
Stroke
Anemia

M. Ross (✉)
Atrium Health/Sanger Heart & Vascular Institute, Charlotte, NC, USA
e-mail: michelle.ross@atriumhealth.org

J. Cedarholm
Lake Norman Regional Medical Center, Mooresville, NC, USA
e-mail: John_cedarholm@lnrmc.com

R. Musialowski, K. Allshouse (eds.), *Cardiovascular Manual for the Advanced Practice Provider*,
https://doi.org/10.1007/978-3-031-35819-7_4

Assessment and Diagnosis

History

A good history and physical exam will often help to expedite therapy and avoid unnecessary testing. Below are the standard questions rapid assessment questions (see Chaps. 3 and 31).

- Duration—Onset of symptoms.
- Location—radiation.
- Have these symptoms occurred before?
- Have the symptoms changed in frequency, duration, associated symptoms, or ease of onset?
- Aggravating or alleviating factors.
- Recent changes in medications.

Patients that present with possible ACS should all undergo rapid assessment (as mentioned in the STEMI chapter) to determine hemodynamic stability, evaluate for shock, critical arrhythmia, or other etiology that would require emergent stabilization or additional emergent treatment.

Patients can have a myriad of symptoms which may or may not include actual chest pain. Many patients struggle to describe their symptoms (*see* Table 4.2). In many cases, the patient has been having episodes of angina or an anginal equivalent for days or even weeks. It is important to ask the patient about a broad range of symptoms that typically present with activity and resolve upon rest. It is common for a patient to say that they have no "pain." Asking the patient if they have chest pain, pressure, fullness, or tightness will often help the patient describe their angina. Offering different locations such as the chest, either shoulder, under shoulder blades, upper back, neck, or jaw is also important to elucidate how they feel their pain. Patients often think that if they do not have an elephant sitting on their left chest, a cardiac etiology is unlikely. Additionally, increased dyspnea with exertion and/or easy fatigability may be present. In some patients, such as women or those who have diabetes, dyspnea may be the only presenting symptom.

Table 4.2 Key historical questions summarized

1. Symptoms
(a) What made you decide to come to be evaluated today? What changed?
(b) What were you doing when these symptoms started?
(c) Is it the first time you have had them? Have they changed?
(d) What makes them better or worse? Deep inspiration, being recumbent, getting anxious/upset, stretching, or palpation?
(e) Are there associated symptoms? Nausea, vomiting, dizziness, palpitations, dyspnea?
2. Do you have any history of CAD, MI, previous stent, or CABG?
(a) If so, when was this? Obtain reports of catheterization and/or specifics of how many bypass grafts are present and where they are located
3. Does this feel like what you experienced prior to any previous coronary event?
4. Have you had to adjust your daily activities to accommodate your symptoms?
5. Any recent medication changes? (Did an antianginal therapy get stopped? Did the patient stop any medications on their own?)
6. HTN, dyslipidemia, diabetes, tobacco abuse (when and how long), family history of early onset CAD?
(a) Often patients will say they have no medical issues. Remember that this may simply be because they haven't seen a physician in years
7. Any recent illnesses?
8. Hx of CVA, GIB, contraindications for DAPT/heparin?
9. Recent changes in daily activities (eating out, exercise, travel, illness, missing medications)

Patients who have a history of coronary disease or myocardial infarction may have a clear description of their prior symptoms. Always ask if their current discomfort is like what they experienced with their previous coronary event or intervention. Patients presenting with UA or NSTEMI may have had atypical anginal symptoms, such as believing they were having reflux. A timeline of change in symptoms is important. Is the discomfort different from a month ago? Is it happening more frequently over the last few days or weeks? Has it started occurring at rest or woken the patient from sleep? Did it begin coming and going over the last couple days?

Physical Exam

The physical exam on a patient with an NSTEMI may be normal if they have already received therapy for their anginal symptoms. Often, the patient has received aspirin and nitroglycerin in tablet or paste form. Findings may be much more subtle than in patients presenting with a STEMI. However, in the patient stating that they no longer have chest pain or dyspnea, physical exam is still important for your differential diagnosis. Physical exam findings may be correlated with the elevated troponin, adding to likelihood of the diagnosis. This includes findings such as significant tachycardia, new arrythmia, significant elevation above their baseline blood pressure or significant anemia.

Diagnostics

EKG—An EKG should be obtained for patients with angina or possible anginal equivalent. ACS/NSTEMI may present with new T wave inversion (Fig. 4.1), ST-segment depression >1 mm which may be horizontal or down sloping (Fig. 4.2). These changes are present within adjacent leads and correspond to a coronary artery vascular distribution. Arrhythmias including Torsades may suggest ischemia, especially if there are other ischemic changes noted (Fig. 4.2). Arrhythmias and ischemic ST and T-wave changes demonstrate a high-risk EKG, and urgent management is indicated. The EKG changes may change when anginal symptoms are treated or resolve. The ST and T waves may not completely normalize but have persistent abnormalities. Wellen's sign or syndrome is biphasic T wave segments that persist after the resolution of anginal symptoms (see Fig. 4.3). It is suggestive that the artery was occluded with spontaneous resolution within the past 24 h. This is a high-risk EKG finding and suggestive of unstable plaque and repeat occlusion is probable. It is important to compare the current EKG with any prior ECGs available to assess for an acute change. Patients may have very abnormal EKG findings; however, they may be unchanged from historical EKGs. If the EKG is normal, serial EKGs should be obtained to evaluate for developing ischemic changes [1]. Occasionally, an EKG that is abnormal at baseline may appear

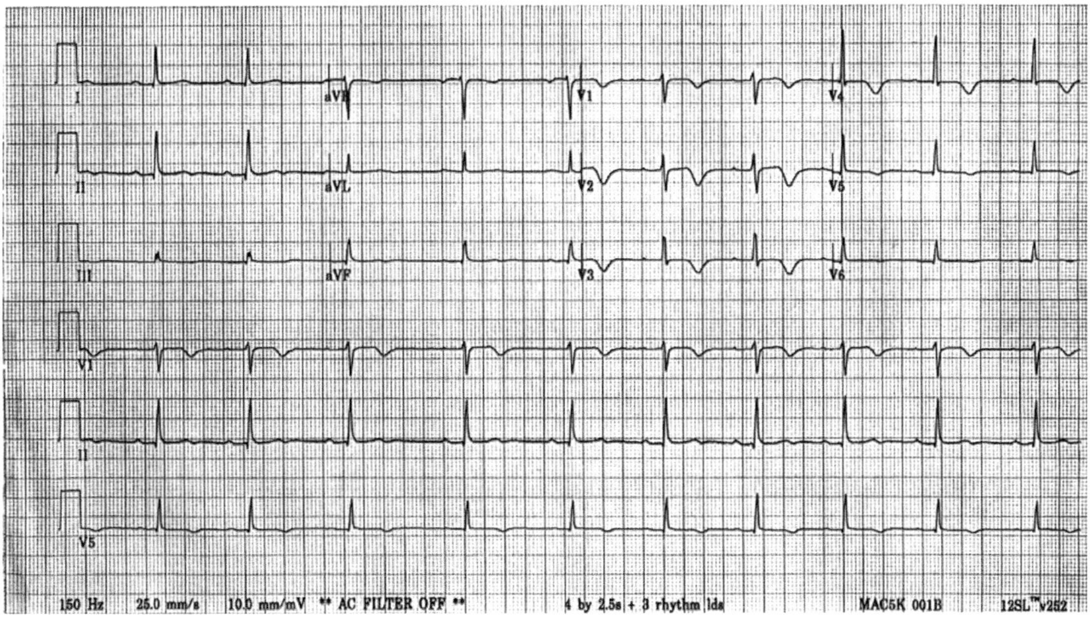

Fig. 4.1 Isolated T wave inversion in a vascular distribution

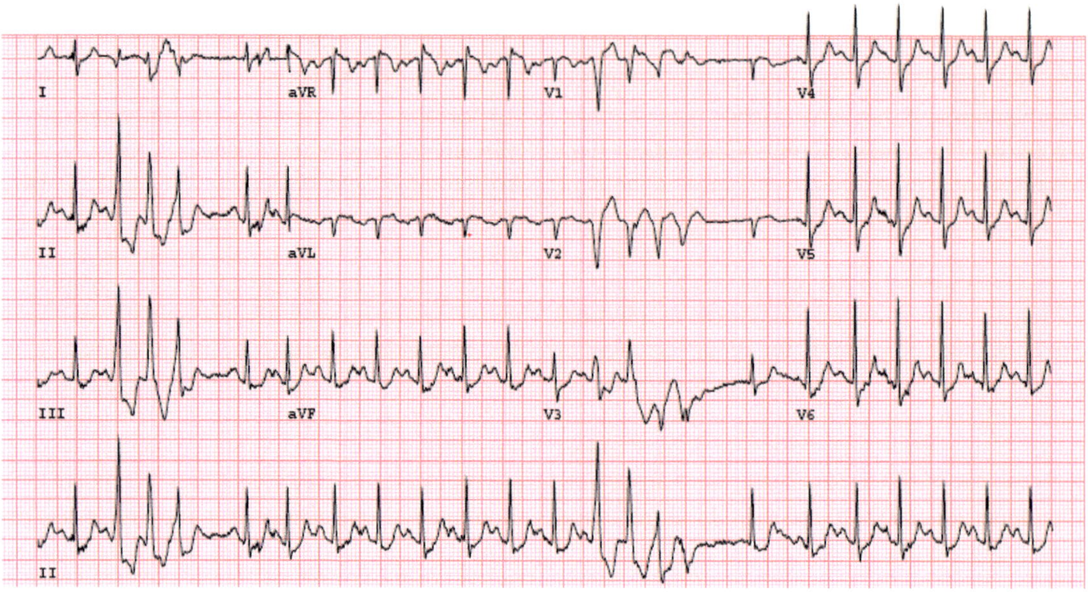

Fig. 4.2 High risk ischemic EKG with Torsades and ST depression

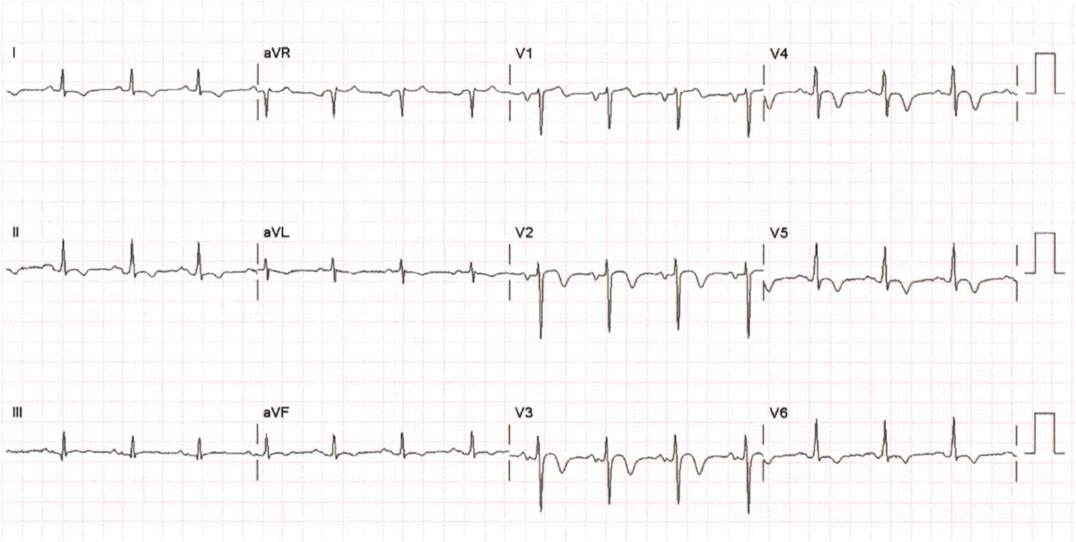

Fig. 4.3 Wellens Sign with biphasic T wave seen in leads V2-V5

"more normal" with an ACS. This is called pseudo normalization. *A normal ECG does NOT rule out an ACS/NSTEMI.*

NSTEMI patients may also be found to have arrythmias. Atrial fibrillation or flutter with rapid ventricular response (RVR) can result from NSTEMI and cause further chest discomfort and elevate troponin levels. These arrhythmias with RVR may also cause a type II MI in a patient with CAD due to supply-demand mismatch. Both arrythmias and critical laboratory results should be addressed (severe anemia) before directing the patient for further cardiac testing or invasive management.

Troponin Trending

The trending of troponin value is a key part of the initial assessment. Early detection of an elevated level allows for a rapid diagnosis of a possible ACS. Troponin should be measured on presentation and again between 3–6 h later. If using a high sensitivity troponin, visible upward trends may be seen in as early as 2 h. It is not uncommon for the initial troponin in the ACS patient to be negative, so trending troponin is important for determining NSTEMI (Type I MI).

The timing of symptom onset and the initial troponin result can be helpful with your differential. If the patient is unable to say what time the symptoms began, the time of ER presentation should be used. High sensitivity troponin (hsT) elevation is not diagnostic for an ACS. High sensitivity troponins may stay relatively low and may remain level over multiple samples which can be indicative of a diagnosis other than NSTEMI, like type II MI. However, a troponin level trending upward or significantly elevated on presentation is suspicious of a NSTEMI. The clinical presentation is very important to guide decision making. It is essential to determine if the presentation is type I or type II MI since the management and prognosis are very different.

Management

Initial Medical Therapy and Stabilization

STEMI and the need for immediate primary PCI must be excluded first (see Chap. 3). Once STEMI is excluded, stabilization of the patient and reduction of ongoing ischemia is essential.

If ACS (type I MI) is suspected, four 81 mg aspirin should be chewed upon arrival, provided there are no strong contraindications. These are generally given by medics or the ER prior to cardiology evaluation. Aspirin decreases platelet activation. The 4 × 81 mg aspirin should be given even if the patient takes 81 mg aspirin daily. The patient should also receive Atorvastatin 80 mg. Statin therapy is not only beneficial for lipid lowering but has a pleiotropic effect of decreasing the inflammatory response within the endothelium. This also aids in protecting the cardiac endothelium during coronary intervention. Statin is given regardless of the patient being on daily statin therapy. Patients who have not tolerated statin therapy in the past (not a true allergy) can generally tolerate the one-time dose of pre-procedural statin. This should be evaluated on a case-by-case basis. If the patient has a true allergy to aspirin, the case should be discussed with your attending physician prior to administration (Table 4.3) [2].

Once a Type I MI NSTEMI is diagnosed, a heparin bolus should be administered and ACS-dose heparin drip initiated, unless there is a contraindication. There is no indication for anticoagulation for a type II MI. It is reasonable to initiate full anticoagulation on presentation if the type of MI is unclear. Once type I has been excluded, early discontinuance is recommended to avoid bleeding complications. A risk assessment must be completed before administering heparin. Has the patient had any recent surgery, head injury, CVA, or another comorbidity that may increase the risk of bleeding? Is the patient on an anticoagulant, if so, what for, when was the last dose? Chronic anticoagulation will likely not contraindicate the use of heparin in the setting of ACS but may affect the timing of cardiac catheterization and short-term anticoagulation therapy.

Enoxaparin verses unfractionated heparin: Though full dose subcutaneous enoxaparin at 1 mg/kg bid has been shown to improve outcomes in ACS, IV unfractionated heparin is the preferred anticoagulant during acute presentation. In the catheterization laboratory, activated

Table 4.3 ACS/NSTEMI initial treatment guidelines

Four 81 mg Aspirin—chewed
Heparin bolus
Initiation of ACS dose heparin drip
Atorvastatin 80 mg PO
Documenting all the above, including what was given by medic or ER
If any of the initial treatments cannot be administered, you must document why you could not give them [1]

clotting times (ACTs) are used to measure the appropriate dose of IV heparin to prevent coronary and stent thrombosis during the procedure and to guide sheath removal. There is no reliable method to determine the dose of supplemental enoxaparin needed in the catheterization lab. Converting from weight-based enoxaparin to IV heparin in the catheterization laboratory has been shown to significantly increase bleeding risks associated with the procedure and should be avoided.

Glycoprotein 2B3A Inhibitors (eptifibatide or tirofiban): Historically, these agents were used prior to intervention to stabilize patients with ACS. However, due to increased bleeding risks, these agents are usually reserved for severe refractory ischemia prior to catheterization or for patients who cannot undergo an emergent procedure due to logistics. 2B3AIs are occasionally started in the catheterization laboratory due to significant thrombus burden and may be continued post-catheterization for up to 12 h.

Antiplatelet agent prior to catheterization (clopidogrel or ticagrelor): This is an area of controversy. ACC guidelines have encouraged preprocedural loading with either ticagrelor or clopidogrel in patients with clear-cut ACS/NSTEMI. However, if a patient requires CABG, this process may result in very high bleeding rates at CABG or a delay in surgery for up to 5 days due to a required drug to wash out period.

Ticagrelor has been shown to have early mortality benefit and is clearly the preferred agent over clopidogrel. There are no FDA indications for preprocedural loading of prasugrel in ACS as it has not been evaluated in this setting. Prasugrel should be loaded in the catheterization laboratory once PCI is planned. [3]

Once the history, physical exam, and initial testing are completed, the results should be discussed with the patient. Treatment options based on evidence-based guidelines should be discussed in shared decision making with the patient and family or healthcare POA as appropriate. Keep in mind that while providers may make these diagnoses and decisions daily, often our patients have never been in this situation. Educating the patient in the setting of new or old diagnoses, so that they can participate in their care is critical.

Invasive Verses Noninvasive Evaluation

If after a history, examination, ECG and Troponin evaluation, there is a strong suspicion for NSTEMI or UA, then an invasive workup (cardiac catheterization) should be pursued urgently rather than a noninvasive workup. If the patient is stabilized without ongoing chest pain or ECG changes, this can often wait up to 24 h. Noninvasive testing when ACS/NSTEMI has clearly been diagnosed may be contraindicated.

Timing of invasive strategy becomes a factor for those patients who present with significant comorbidities. Patients with heart failure exacerbation, abnormal renal studies, abnormal CBC findings, or chronic anticoagulation are some comorbidities that may delay invasive testing. In certain cases, the catheterization lab may not be readily available, due to location or timing of presentation. Patients may present with ACS/NSTEMI in the middle of the night, over a weekend or to a hospital that has no catheterization lab, etc. A thoughtful approach looks at the entire case on order to determine what plan of care is the safest and most appropriate. Criteria for early invasive strategy are demonstrated in Table 4.4.

Delayed invasive strategy, defined as >24 but <72 h is recommended for patients with diabetes mellitus, renal insufficiency, LVEF <40% or congestive heart failure, recent PCI, prior CABG, post-infarction angina, or GRACE risk score of >109 and <140 [1].

Table 4.4 Early invasive strategy <24 h from presentation

Rise in troponin consistent with type I MI
Dynamic ST segment and T wave changes
Hemodynamic instability-shock
Electrical instability
Persistent unstable symptoms on optimal medical therapy
GRACE score > 140

Cardiac Catheterization (Fig. 4.4)

Conscious sedation may be administered as per physician preference in the catheterization laboratory. Arterial access sites are prepped (radial or femoral artery). The interventional cardiologist accesses the artery with a needle, and a sheath is placed in the artery. Since the complication rate of femoral access is higher, radial artery access is preferred. Radial artery access has been shown to decrease mortality by reducing the risk of bleeding and vascular complications. A catheter over a guidewire is advanced to where the coronary arteries originate off the aorta. Contrast dye is injected into the coronary arteries while fluoroscopy (x-ray) is used to take pictures of the arteries (angiogram). The individual cardiac arteries are injected with contrast dye and visualized by the interventional cardiologist in real time. Once the coronary anatomy has been visualized, revascularization may be considered. Commonly, percutaneous coronary revascularization is performed in the same setting as diagnostic catheterization. However, depending on anatomy, medical therapy or CABG may be recommended. There are risks to this invasive procedure. Severe risks include death, stroke of type I MI (Table 4.5).

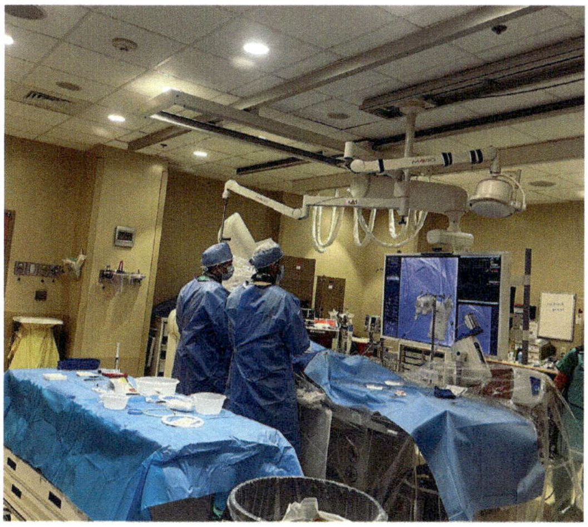

Fig. 4.4 Interventional cardiologist performing a cardiac catheterization in the lab

Table 4.5 Risks of cardiac catheterization

- Allergy to contrast
  - Premedication with 40 mg of prednisone the evening prior and the morning of the procedure, diphenhydramine 50 mg PO or IV 1 h prior to procedure
  - Emergent management is administration of methylprednisolone 40 mg or hydrocortisone sodium succinate 200 mg IV Q4 hours prior to procedure and diphenhydramine 50 mg PO or IV 1 h prior to procedure. (ref)
- Contrast-induced nephropathy
  - Risk is 2.5% with Cr < 2 mg/dL, but rises to 30.6% with Cr > 3.0 mg/dL
  - Minimizing contrast given and volume expansion with pre-procedure NS helps to mitigate this risk
- Vascular complication
  - Pseudoaneurysm
  - Detected as a pulsatile mass with bruit
  - Best diagnosed by arterial US
- Bleeding
  - Localized large hematoma
  - Retroperitoneal hemorrhage
- Thromboembolism
  - Distal to access site is cool to the touch, pale in color, pulses absent, changes in sensation
  - Emergent vascular surgery consultation
- Periprocedural myocardial infarction
  - Incidence is greatly influenced by comorbidities and extent of coronary disease
- CVA
  - <1% risk
  - Secondary to micro embolism post PCI
- Coronary artery perforation
  - <1% risk
  - A large proportion of these require a surgical intervention
- Death
  - <1% risk in elective PCI [4]

Percutaneous Coronary Intervention (PCI) Figs. 4.5 and 4.6

There are multiple forms of percutaneous coronary intervention (PCI): placement of coronary stents (bare metal stent—BMS or drug eluting stent—DES), plain old balloon angioplasty (POBA), and atherectomy by laser or rotational device. Not all areas of stenosis are treated by PCI. The primary goal of the procedure is to treat the lesion that is causing the ischemia and associated symptoms. If coronary intervention is pursued in the setting of ACS, complete

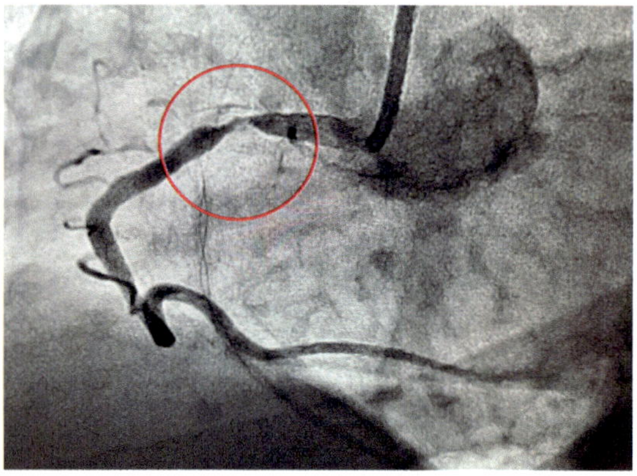

Fig. 4.5 Right coronary artery with proximal region of stenosis

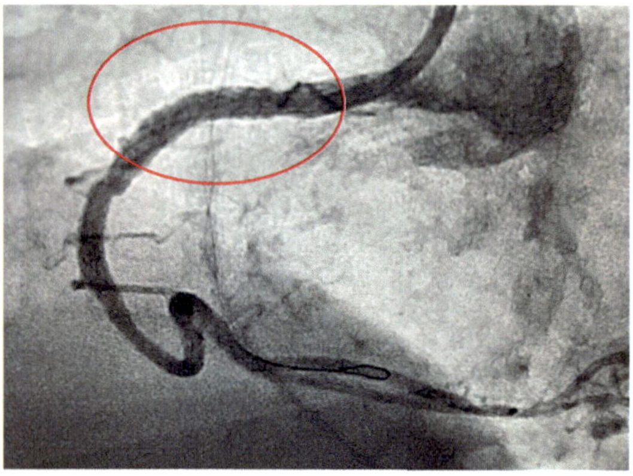

Fig. 4.6 Right coronary artery post percutaneous coronary intervention and stent placement

revascularizing of other significant lesions will be considered, either in the same procedure or in a later "staged" setting. PCI for ACS has been shown to improve mortality in addition to improving symptoms.

Surgical revascularization or Coronary Artery Bypass Grafting (CABG) will be considered if patient has complex coronary blockages such as 3 vessel CAD in a diabetic, left main disease, or complex and diffuse lesions not easily amenable to PCI (see Chap. 6). Sometimes lesions are not amenable to either PCI or CABG. Maximal medical therapy may be required with the administration of two anti-anginal therapies (see Chap. 5).

At the end of the PCI, femoral arteriotomy closure may be achieved by various strategies. The method of closure does not decrease the risk-bleeding complication. Suture-based devices such as Perclose® may be used to approximate edges of the arteriotomy. There are metallic clips such as StarClose® which are also a method to physically approximate the edges of the arteriotomy. Dissolving collagen plugs can be used, such as Angioseal®. Collagen plugs can often be felt by the patient and may be a source of concern; however, the ability to palpate the collagen device is normal and not an indication for alarm. It will dissolve over time. The method of closure is determined in the lab and not usually a primary focus for the advanced care practitioner, however, the method of closure used can aid in the determination of future access if the patient requires a repeat catheterization.

Post-catheterization procedure protocols are based on the site accessed, the procedure completed, and the physician preference. Primarily this involves rest, stabilization of the access site with compression. Radial access sites use a band that goes around the wrist and is inflated with air, to hold pressure. Increments of air are released from the band at specified intervals to avoid bleeding until it can be totally removed. One of the most immediate and potentially life-threatening complications is bleeding. The patient may begin developing a swollen area under the access site. This may be very firm to the touch and expands suddenly or there may be bleeding from the site. The most important action at this point is to put heavy pressure on the catheterization incision site manually until an alternative option is available. Additionally, examination to assess the limb distal to the arteriotomy is critical. Should a distal extremity become pale and pulseless, the circulation has been compromised and limb ischemia occurs. This requires emergent evaluation by Vascular Surgery to re-establish circulation. [4–7] Pseudoaneurysms can also form and may be found prior to discharge or at follow-up. A pseudoaneurysm is formed when blood leaks out into the surrounding tissue of the arteriotomy after closure. These can be felt as a swollen and often pulsatile enlarged area around the catheterization access site (radial or femoral artery). This requires urgent ultrasound of the area to assess if there is a pseudoaneurysm present. If present and depending on size, some may resolve on their own. Others require injection of thrombin under ultrasound guidance by interventional radiology. Some may require consultation from the vascular surgery team.

Medical Therapy at Discharge of Patients with ACS

Betablockers—should be used in all patients with ACS at discharge depending on HR and BP. Most commonly, this will be metoprolol tartrate 12.5–50 mg bid. Alternatively, metoprolol succinate can be used once per day at 25–100 mg. Beta blocker should be continued for at least 1 year. During a myocardial infarction, the sympathetic nervous system is stimulated, increasing the workload on the heart. This can lead to expansion of the infarcted area and increase risks for arrythmias. Betablockers serve to decrease the effect of the sympathetic nervous systems response to the infarct. They continue to do this while the heart is healing, post infarct. If a patient has a reduced EF of less than 40%, metoprolol succinate or carvedilol are the preferred betablockers to be used at discharge, to help prevent ventricular remodeling and improve mortality (see Chap. 20).

ACEI/ARBs/ARNI—all patients with EF ≤40% should also be placed on one of these agents at discharge and titrated up to maximal dose as an outpatient (see Chap. 20). These drugs help improve cardiac remodeling and decrease afterload.

Aldosterone Antagonists—should be considered in all patients with EF of ≤40% but can be considered also at first post hospital follow-up (see Chap. 20).

Aspirin (non-coated) 81 mg per day. 325 mg only increases bleeding risk, so 81 mg is the preferred dose. This is also important for patients on ticagrelor as high dose aspirin can decrease ticagrelor's efficacy. If the patient has a true aspirin allergy, there are aspirin desensitization protocols that can be completed. This may require ICU monitoring. This protocol may be completed prior to intervention or after but should be evaluated on a case-by-case basis with your attending physician. [5, 8, 9]

High dose/high potency statin—atorvastatin 40 or 80 mg, rosuvastatin 20 or 40 mg are the recommended statins post ACS. Please see previous discussion in this chapter.

Antiplatelet agents: All patients should be on DAPT for 1 year post ACS whether they received a PCI, CABG, or will be treated medically. These agents reduce the risk of thrombotic events in coronary arteries in Type I MI, with and without a stent placement. This includes aspirin and one other agent listed below. Ticagrelor or prasugrel are the preferred agents in patients with ACS. Notably clopidogrel is the least expensive agent but is also not as effective in ACS patients. Prasugrel is generic and generally less expensive but has multiple contraindications as noted below. Ticagrelor is indicated but a high percentage of patients complain a sense of breathlessness due its chemical similarity to adenosine (see Table 4.6). [3]

Table 4.6 Commonly used antiplatelet agents

P2Y12 receptor inhibitors	
Clopidogrel (Plavix)	• 300 mg or 600 mg loading dose • 75 mg daily • 5 days wash out period before a surgical procedure • *Rash is likely presentation if patient has an allergy*
Prasugrel (Effient)	• 60 mg loading dose • 10 mg daily • 7 days wash out before surgical procedure • *Contraindicated in patient with CVA or TIA history* • *Contraindicated if weight less than 60 kg or age over 75 years* • *NOT indicated for patients being treated medically for ACS*
Ticagrelor (Brilinta)	• 180 mg loading dose • 90 mg BID • 5 days wash out period before surgical procedure • *Dyspneic sensation in some people deter its use* • Aspirin dose must be only 81 mg QD if also on Ticagrelor (aspirin doses above 100 mg decrease efficacy of Ticagrelor) • Some patients, generally older, have additional GI upset or generalized sensations of feeling unwell • May cause bradyarrhythmia or pauses in some patients

Cardiac Rehabilitation

These programs are strongly encouraged in all patients who have been diagnosed with ACS. Patients receive initial education while inpatient. This is followed by an organized exercise program that lasts approximately 12 weeks. Patients are monitored with telemetry and vital signs as they resume physical activity in cardiac rehab. It also includes education consisting of dietary management, stress management, and assistance with overall risk factor modification. Those that participate have been shown to have reductions in mortality and reinfarction.

Patient Education Prior to Discharge

For many patients, ACS/CAD is a new diagnosis and can be very traumatic, especially to younger patients. It is important to clarify test results and answer any questions. Anxiety and depression are often present at discharge. Affirmation of their fears and reassurance of improvement with cardiac rehab is important. Having the patient write down questions to bring to their first outpatient appointment can be very helpful. Discussing tobacco cessation plans with patients who smoke should happen prior to discharge as well. The patient is a captive audience and has likely not smoked in about 48 h since admission. Use this opportunity to guide them to cessation. Ideally these patients are discharged with follow-up within 7–10 days. Early follow-up helps to address fears, questions, and new concerns. It allows early titration of goal directed medical therapy or changes in medical therapy due to intolerance. This helps avoid medical non-compliance and return ED visits. [4]

Clinical Pearls

- EKG with new T wave inversion, ST segment horizontal or down sloping depression in two contiguous leads can be indicative of ischemia. Deep T waves (or biphasic) in V1 and V2 can indicate proximal LAD disease.
- ASA 324 mg chewed, atorvastatin 80 mg, heparin bolus are the initial medications on presentation.
- Post-catheterization: bleeding at catheterization site.
  - hold pressure constant → obtain assistance from catheterization lab and nursing,
  - distal pulses, pallor, numbness → emergent vascular surgery eval,
  - pulsatile, enlarged catheterization site → US for pseudoaneurysm,
  - increased pain on right flank or lower back after femoral access may indicate possible retroperitoneal bleed,
- Antiplatelet dosing:
  - Clopidogrel 75 mg Daily.
  - Prasugrel 10 mg daily—NOT for previous CVA patient, <60 kg, or medical management without PCI.
  - Ticagrelor 90 mg BID—patients may have feelings of dyspnea or overall general weakness (more in elderly).
- High dose statin—Atorvastatin 40 mg–80 mg, Rosuvastatin 20 mg–40 mg.
- GDMT for Ejection fraction 40% or less in addition to ACS management.
- DAPT × 1 year with statin and ASA therapies lifelong.
- If on anticoagulation for other comorbidity, recommendations to stop aspirin and only use clopidogrel with the full anticoagulation agent. After 1 year discontinue clopidogrel and initiate aspirin 81 mg in its place.

References

1. Amsterdam E, Wenger N, Brindis R, et al. 2014 AHA/ACC guideline for the management of patients with non–ST-elevation acute coronary syndromes: a report of the American College Of Cardiology/American

Heart Association task force on practice guidelines. Circulation. 2014;130(25):e344–426. http://ovidsp.ovid.com/ovidweb.cgi?T=JS&NEWS=n&CSC=Y&PAGE=fulltext&D=ovft&AN=00003017-201412230-00017. https://doi.org/10.1161/CIR.0000000000000134.

2. Patti G, Pasceri V, Colonna G, et al. Atorvastatin pretreatment improves outcomes in patients with acute coronary syndromes undergoing early percutaneous coronary intervention. J Am Coll Cardiol. 2007;49(12):1272–8. https://www.clinicalkey.es/playcontent/1-s2.0-S0735109707006614. https://doi.org/10.1016/j.jacc.2007.02.025.
3. Schüpke S, Neumann F, Menichelli M, et al. Ticagrelor or prasugrel in patients with acute coronary syndromes. N Engl J Med. 2019;381(16):1524–34. https://doi.org/10.1056/NEJMoa1908973.
4. Mancini GBJ, Hartigan PM, Shaw LJ, et al. Predicting outcome in the COURAGE trial (clinical outcomes utilizing revascularization and aggressive drug evaluation): coronary anatomy versus ischemia. JACC Cardiovasc Interv. 2014;7(2):195–201. https://www.ncbi.nlm.nih.gov/pubmed/24440015. https://doi.org/10.1016/j.jcin.2013.10.017.
5. Tavakol M, Ashraf S, Brener SJ. Risks and complications of coronary angiography: a comprehensive review. Global. J Health Sci. 2012;4(1):65–93. https://www.ncbi.nlm.nih.gov/pubmed/22980117. https://doi.org/10.5539/gjhs.v4n1p65.
6. Chiarito M, Cao D, Nicolas J, et al. Radial versus femoral access for coronary interventions: an updated systematic review and meta-analysis of randomized trials. Catheter Cardiovasc Interv. 2021;97(7):1387–96. https://onlinelibrary.wiley.com/doi/abs/10.1002/ccd.29486. https://doi.org/10.1002/ccd.29486.
7. Levine GN, Bates ER, Blankenship JC, et al. 2011 ACCF/AHA/SCAI guideline for percutaneous coronary intervention. J Am Coll Cardiol. 2011;58(24):e44–e122. https://www.clinicalkey.es/playcontent/1-s2.0-S0735109711028762. https://doi.org/10.1016/j.jacc.2011.08.007.
8. Schwartz GG, Olsson AG, et al. Effects of atorvastatin on early recurrent ischemic events in acute coronary syndromes the MIRACL study: a randomized controlled trial. JAMA. 2001;285(13):1711–8. https://doi.org/10.1001/jama.285.13.1711.
9. Pasceri V, Patti G, Nusca A, et al. Randomized trial of atorvastatin for reduction of myocardial damage during coronary intervention: results from the ARMYDA (atorvastatin for reduction of MYocardial damage during angioplasty) study. Circulation. 2004;110(6):674–8. http://circ.ahajournals.org/cgi/content/abstract/110/6/674. https://doi.org/10.1161/01.CIR.0000137828.06205.87.

5 Outpatient Management of Coronary Artery Disease

Michelle Ross and John Cedarholm

Introduction

Patients who have been diagnosed with coronary disease and ischemic symptoms will follow-up with a cardiologist. It is important to know the following to guide further management: (a) Has the patient ever had a coronary intervention or surgery? (b) When and what interventions were done? (c) What are the indications of the cardiac medications? It is important to keep in mind that medications can serve multiple purposes, such as an antihypertensive medication also serving as an antianginal agent. Medication therapies should be used as appropriate to manage angina, heart rates, and hypertension.

The patient's baseline level of functioning helps us understand the level of stress they put on the heart. Are they always sedentary? Were they active and walking miles daily, but now walking minimally only a few days a week? The patient needs to be seen as a full picture, not only diagnostic images, and comorbidities.

M. Ross (✉)
Atrium Health/Sanger Heart & Vascular Institute, Charlotte, NC, USA
e-mail: Michelle.ross@atriumhealth.org

J. Cedarholm
Lake Norman Regional Medical Center, Mooresville, NC, USA
e-mail: John_cedarholm@lnrmc.com

Assessment and Diagnosis

History obtained for the visit should include asking about any recent hospitalizations and a review of the inpatient chart. Medications should be reviewed carefully. They are often changed at discharge from the hospital and patients are often unclear of the doses. Always encourage a review of the medication bottles specifically. Specific attention should be paid to antiplatelet therapies, anticoagulants, and lipid medications. Is the patient on guideline-directed therapies? Should they be on dual antiplatelet therapy? Any of their other cardiac medications changed?

Patients may present for an evaluation of new symptoms because a medication was altered by another provider. For example, a medication being stopped due to hypotension, resulting in a change in anti-anginal coverage. Are they using SL NTG? How often? More than usual? Asking if the patient has had chest pain, pressure, fullness, or any symptoms like their anginal equivalent is important. Inquire about their activities and any changes in their activity tolerance. Are their symptoms consistent with what they experienced prior to a previous coronary event/intervention? Keep in mind that some patients have only fatigue or dyspnea as a symptom. Table 5.1 explains the classification of angina. This standardization is important for long-term surveillance to determine a change in characteristic of symptoms.

R. Musialowski, K. Allshouse (eds.), *Cardiovascular Manual for the Advanced Practice Provider*,
https://doi.org/10.1007/978-3-031-35819-7_5

Table 5.1 Classes of angina

CLASS 1—angina only present with prolonged or very strenuous activity
CLASS 2—angina only with moderate activity, slightly limiting daily activities
CLASS 3—angina with minimal activity, activities of daily living, moderately limiting
CLASS 4—angina with any activity or at rest, severely limiting [1]

Regular visits should include a full physical examination, including weight and height (BMI), blood pressure, heart rate, and oxygen saturation. Patients should be encouraged to monitor their blood pressure at home, as it may be falsely elevated at a medical office. Frequency of measurement can be recommended based on the individual patient. If medications are being titrated to a maximum tolerated dose, such as a beta blocker after a myocardial infarction, more frequent measurements can be obtained. Patients benefit from directions on obtaining appropriate blood pressure measurement (see Chap. 30). Patients should have both feet on the floor, arm resting in an elevated position, such as on a table. The cuff should not be placed over clothing and the patient should be encouraged to rest for a few minutes prior to measuring and to remain still and silent while it is being measured.

Diagnostics

Cardiovascular testing may need to be considered. If the patient is having symptoms of concern, an ECG should be obtained to evaluate for signs of ischemia, arrythmia, or new infarct. Evaluate for new t-wave inversion, new q-waves, ST-segment depression, heart block, or arrhythmia. If a patient was recently discharged from the hospital after a coronary event, an ECG should be obtained. After a myocardial infarction, the ECG can change considerably from the hospital discharge to the follow-up visit.

If further testing is being considered, consider what you will do with the results, knowing that the patient must live with those results. A person may develop significant anxiety if they have an area of ischemia or stenosis, even if there is no indication for invasive evaluation. They often describe feeling as if they are "just waiting to have a heart attack." This can cause anxiety levels that interfere with daily functioning, so discussion of why you are doing a test and what you may find should be had before testing. This allows the patient to be part of shared decision making.

Stress Testing in Intermediate-Risk Chest Pain

Bayes rule postulates that the posttest probability of CAD is a function of the pretest probability of disease. If there is a low probability of CAD, then anything abnormal could be a false positive and testing is not recommended. Conversely, if there is a high likelihood of CAD, a negative test would not rule out disease [1]. Testing done with intermediate pretest probability has the greatest benefit. Pretest probability can be estimated based on age of the patient, gender, and type of chest pain. The discussion below is the assessment of intermediate-risk patients in which a true positive or true negative will alter patient care.

As stated earlier in this section, coronary artery narrowing of >70% is the degree of narrowing that causes symptoms. The assessment tools discussed here are designed to assess for lesions of 70% or greater. These assessment tools will guide further workup and management.

There are many tools to assess for symptomatic CAD. The first decision that needs to be made is whether structural or physiologic testing is needed. Physiologic testing will show ischemic significance, but not severity. Sometimes, both modalities are needed in clinical decision making. Examples of structural and physiologic testing are given in Table 5.2.

Table 5.2 Noninvasive mechanism to evaluate for symptomatic CAD

Structural	Physiologic
Cardiac CT	cMRI Nuclear Echocardiography Stress EKG

Structural Imaging

The test of choice in this category is coronary artery CT imaging. Cardiac CT will determine if there is a structural lesion of 70% or greater but the physiology of true ischemia is not easily obtained from the images. The resolution of this modality has markedly improved for the assessment of CAD. The images appear similar to those obtained from invasive evaluation in the cardiac catheterization laboratory. The true benefit of this test is the negative predictive value. A normal scan without CAD rules out ischemia as the cause of chest pain. There is predictive value as well. The cardiovascular event rate is low over the next 10 years in patients with negative scans. The limitations of this modality are listed in Table 5.3. The most important limitation is previous stenting or significant coronary calcifications, which would cause this test to be read as non-diagnostic. In this situation, a physiologic imaging modality should be considered. The coronary CT scan protocol may require beta blocker therapy to slow the heart rate into the 50-bpm range to optimize image quality. This test should be used with caution in patients with newly diagnosed cardiomyopathies as the administered beta blocker may cause cardiovascular collapse and cardiogenic shock in decompensated patients. Cardiac catheterization is often the best and safer test for ischemic evaluation in these patients.

Physiologic Testing

The cornerstone of physiologic testing is evaluating for myocardial ischemia by increasing myocardial oxygen consumption. The modalities differ in the assessment of the ischemia, and the interpretation of abnormalities is test specific. Additional imaging is required to assess the severity of ischemia. Sometimes, more than one modality may be used in evaluation of the same patient. The different ischemia-inducing modalities are listed in Table 5.4.

Table 5.3 Limitations to coronary CT interpretation

Previous stenting	Blooming artifact limits accuracy of stenosis severity
Coronary artery calcification	Blooming artifact
Renal failure	Dye-induced nephropathy
Morbid obesity	Impaired image resolution
Patient compliance	Impaired image resolution
Severe decompensated HFrEF	Beta blocker administration may cause cardiovascular collapse

Table 5.4 Options to assess for symptomatic CAD

Stress modality	Imaging
Treadmill	EKG tracing Nuclear Echocardiography
Vasodilator Adenosine/regadenoson	cMRI Nuclear
Chronotropic enhancement Dobutamine	Echo

Treadmill stress testing is the hallmark of physiologic testing. Exercise is preferred if possible as this provides prognostic information along with ischemia evaluation. Using this modality, myocardial oxygen consumption is increased by increasing both heart rate and blood pressure.

$$\text{Rate pressure product}(\text{RPP}) = \text{Peak heart rate} \times \text{Peak systolic blood pressure}$$

A value of >20,000 is suggestive of adequate myocardial stress and is used to assure the predictive value of the test. A second proxy of adequate myocardial stress is the target heart rate. A heart rate of 85% maximal predicted heart rate (MPHR) is the standard. As a reminder, the formula is:

$$\text{MPHR} = 220 - \text{age}$$

Treadmill stress testing can be used alone to assess for ischemia, but the sensitivity and specificity are low. Often, additional imaging is needed to improve the positive and negative predictive values. The most predictive result from the treadmill is duration of exercise as it is an assessment of functional capacity. The standard exercise protocol is called the Bruce Protocol with each stage being 3 min at an increasing treadmill speed and incline. Completion of a stage determines the degree of oxygen consumption, measured in metabolic equivalents or METS. This value is important for standardization of activities and utilized for many clinical decisions like preoperative cardiac risk assessment and candidacy for cardiac transplantation. The longer exercise time and higher METS achieved on the treadmill confer improved cardiovascular mortality risk, even if CAD is present. This is the main reason anyone who can navigate the treadmill should be stressed in this fashion. Some studies suggest that even in patients with an abnormal stress test, if 10 METS is achieved, medical management has the same outcome as revascularization and medical therapy should be considered.

If the baseline EKG is acceptable, the EKG tracing can be interpreted for ischemia. Resting LBBB, ST segment depression, or paced rhythm precludes EKG interpretation, and additional imaging should be added to the treadmill evaluation. Table 5.5 lists the criteria to determine a positive treadmill stress test.

ST segment elevation is a strongly positive finding, and the test should be terminated immediately to avoid risk of death. The location of the elevation correlates with the location of the ischemic distribution. In Fig. 5.1, the elevation is in the LAD distribution. ST segment depression does not correlate with the location of CAD but is a marker of ischemia. In Fig. 5.2, the ST segment depression is across multiple vascular distributions and nonspecific. The multifocal VT seen on the exercise tracing is also high risk for sudden death. 1:10,000 stress patients have cardiac arrest during treadmill stress testing. Severe aortic stenosis is a contraindication to treadmill testing due to the risk of sudden death.

Pharmacologic stress testing is used when treadmill utilization is not an option. Table 5.6 includes the main indications for pharmacologic testing. The pharmacologic agents utilized are adenosine and, less commonly, dobutamine. Dobutamine is a positive ionotropic and chronotropic agent. This combination increases myocardial oxygen demand but has significant side effects and an increased risk of inducing tachyarrhythmias.

Adenosine and its analogues do not increase myocardial oxygen demand but alters oxygen delivery. Adenosine is a coronary artery vasodilator. Atherosclerotic disease prevents the dilation of the diseased segment. The vasodilator will create a drop in pressure across the stenosis by dilating the normal arterial segments. Flow across a coronary artery lesion is also reduced. These vasodilators must be used with imaging modalities to assess the reduction in flow and determine ischemia. The images that are obtained will suggest ischemia in different ways.

Single Photon Emission Computed Tomography (SPECT) has been the main imaging modality for many years. A radioisotope of the element technetium is attached to a red blood cell with an agent called sestamibi. The red blood cell is tagged and can be evaluated to assess blood flow. Images are obtained at rest and after reinjected stress images. Comparing the images will determine if there is limited uptake at rest which is suggestive of scar. Reduction of radioactive counts after stress suggests ischemia. Examples of these findings are seen in Fig. 5.3.

The gamma rays emitted from the technetium are captured by a gamma camera and computerized. This program will assess the counts within specific coronary artery vascular distributions. By convention, the distribution with the highest counts is deemed "normal" by the program. The other vascular distributions are then compared to the "normal" distribution. The flaw of this process is when all arteries are equally diseased, and the scan can be falsely **normal** when multivessel disease is present. This can occur in up to 15% of all scans. Patient selection will reduce the risk of these false-negative results. This is one of the main reasons to assure the appropriate selection of patients based on pretest probability and assure true positive and negative results.

Attenuation artifact is due to the physics of gamma rays. Soft tissue will prevent counts in a

Table 5.5 Criteria for positive EKG stress test

Flat or down sloping ST segments lasting into recovery
ST segment elevation in a vascular distribution
Reproduction of exertional angina
Exercise-induced hypotension
Exercise-induced Torsades/VT

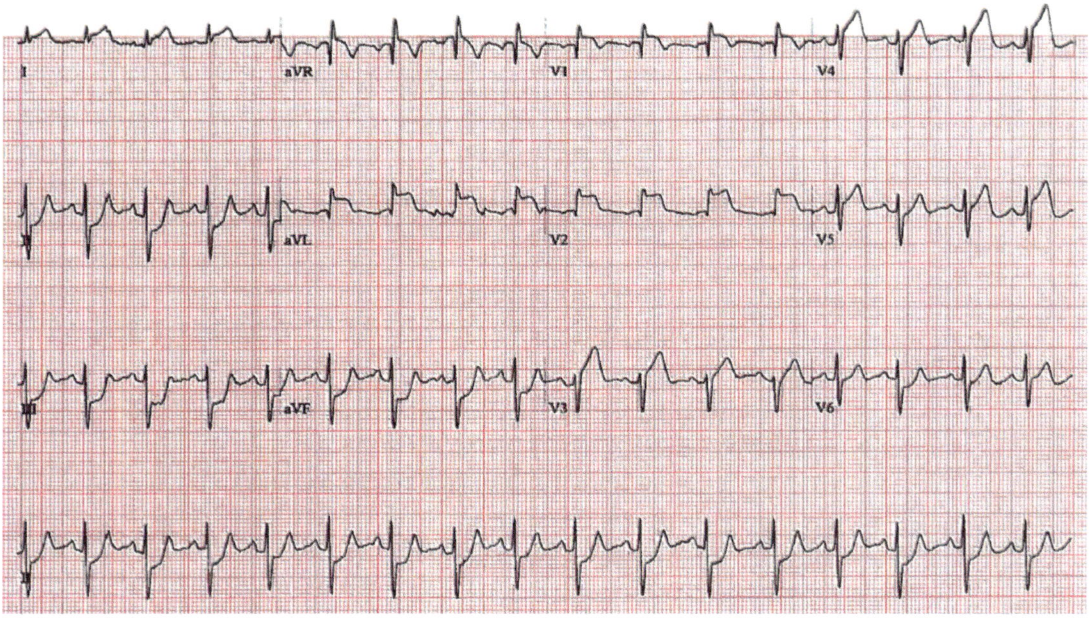

Fig. 5.1 EKG showing ST segment elevation in early treadmill stress testing

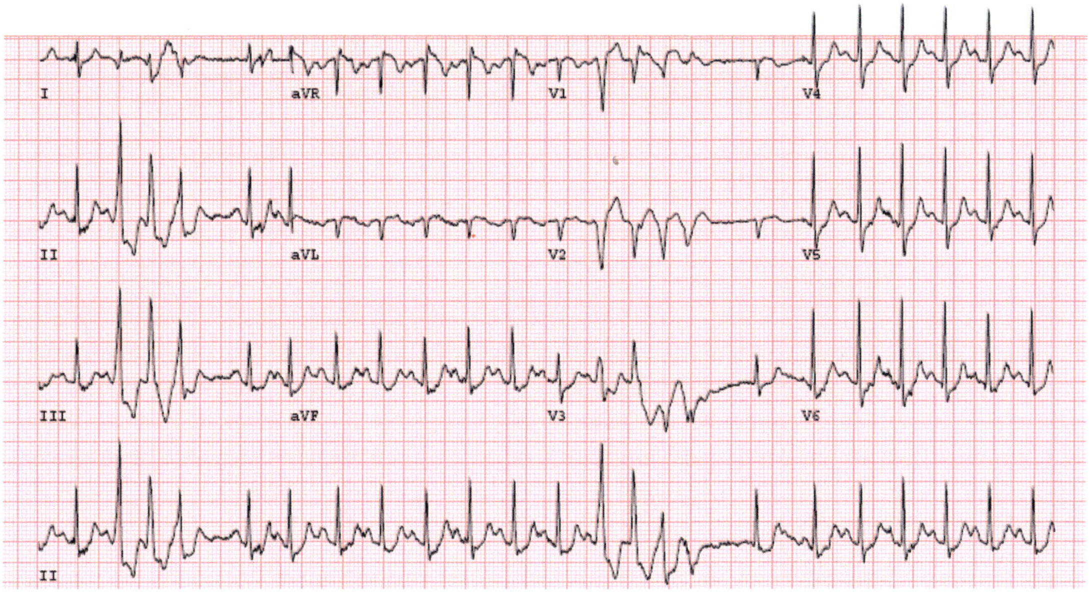

Fig. 5.2 EKG showing salvos of torsades during treadmill stress testing

Table 5.6 Pharmacologic stress testing

Indications	Contraindications
Left bundle branch block (LBBB)	Bronchospasm
Ventricular pacemaker	Bradycardia/heart block
Inability to navigate treadmill	Tachyarrhythmias—AFIB with RVR, VT
Chronotropic incompetence	

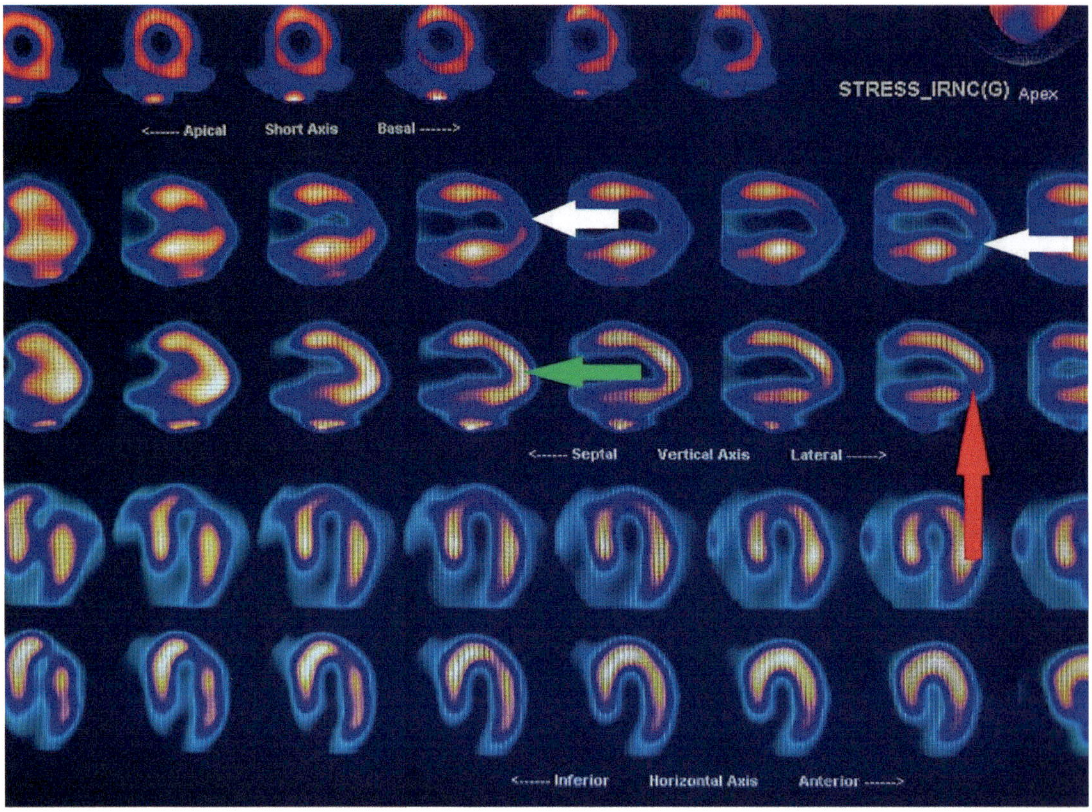

Fig. 5.3 Abnormal SPECT nuclear images. Green arrow shows normal LAD distribution perfusion at rest. Red arrow shows a reduction of counts in the apical segment at rest suggestive of remote infarction. White arrows show a LAD distribution of counts after exercise suggestive of ischemia. The white arrow on the left shows complete reversibility when compared to the green arrow and suggests CAD >70%. The right arrow appears worse when compared to the red arrow suggesting ischemia superimposed on previous infarct

vascular distribution from reaching the gamma camera. These areas can be misinterpreted as ischemia or infarction. Commonly, the reader will be able to determine if these areas are, in fact, artifact or a true defect. This attenuation artifact contributes to the false-positive tests associated with this modality. Anterior attenuation artifact is more common in women due to breast tissue interference. Inferior artifact is more common in males due to a thicker diaphragm adjacent to the inferior walls of the myocardium.

Stress MRI is emerging as an excellent alternative to SPECT testing. Adenosine is still used to vasodilate, but MRI imaging and parameters can assess tissue flow with gadolinium administration. In addition to stress data, a large amount of structural data can be seen with high resolution in an MRI scan. Specific coronary artery lesions are not seen with MRI. This stress modality is a physiologic test with respect to the coronary arteries. The MRI does give structural information about the rest of the heart. Due to the requirements of an MRI scanner, availability is often limited.

In a patient with an ischemic defect, the size of the imaging defect can be prognostic. However, unless the defect involves a significant section of myocardium, the risk of invasive coronary intervention may outweigh the benefit. This group can include patients being evaluated prior to a noncardiac surgery, elderly patients who are at higher risk for cardiac catheterization, and persistent anginal symptoms with known areas of unrevascularized disease including chronic total occlusion (CTO). Stress testing is generally not done for asymptomatic surveillance. However, if patient had an absence of symptoms with a previous MI or significant coronary lesion and is >2 years since invasive evaluation, testing should be considered. In patients with history of surgical bypass, the test free period is approximately 5 years, but should be evaluated on a case-by-case basis [2].

One other form of stress testing should be mentioned. Stress echoes can be done for very specific reasons such as evaluation of hypertrophic cardiomyopathy gradients across the LVOT obstruction. Stress echo is not used commonly due to its limitations and feasibility. It is completed by doing a baseline echo, having the patient exercise, and then laying them down for another echo while HR is still elevated. There is difficulty with obtaining images while the heart is still "stressed," and a correct interpretation is dependent on appropriate image acquisition.

Echocardiogram—Ischemic symptoms can be nonspecific and mimic valvular or CHF symptoms. Complaints may include increased fatigue, lack of endurance, or dizziness. An echocardiogram can evaluate for a change in wall motion abnormalities, ejection fraction, and valvular dysfunction to further guide therapy.

Cardiac catheterization may be considered in patients having anginal symptoms despite medical therapy. The initial plan involves titration and addition of anti-anginal therapies. If the patient is on two antianginal therapies that have been appropriately up titrated and are still experiencing anginal symptoms or their previously stable symptoms have increased in severity, frequency, or duration, then catheterization is appropriate [2].

Management

Antiplatelet Therapy

Lifelong aspirin 81 mg daily is recommended. Aspirin at 325 mg does not additionally reduce mortality but increases bleeding risk. Aspirin is an irreversible antiplatelet agent, helping prevent thrombosis within arteries [3]. See Chap. 4 for full discussion on antiplatelet agents.

Cholesterol Lowering Agents

HMGCoA reductase inhibitors are commonly referred to as Statins (see Table 5.1). Statins bind to receptors on a reductase enzyme, inhibiting the production of LDL by the liver. This production occurs primarily overnight, and therefore statins are most effective if administered in the evening. All coronary patients should remain on statin therapy life-long to aid in lowering lipid levels. Additionally, statins have a pleiotropic benefit of decreasing the inflammatory response within endothelium and stabilizing plaque that has already been formed. Side effects of statins include muscle pain, usually in the proximal large muscle groups, bilaterally. The symptoms generally resolve once the statin has been stopped. A lower dose or a weaker statin can be tried and may not have the same side effects. If the patient develops significant muscle pain, they should discontinue the statin and have laboratory evaluation for rhabdomyolysis. This is a rare side effect.

Immediately after a coronary event or intervention, high dose statin therapy consisting of atorvastatin 40–80 or rosuvastatin 20–40 mg should be initiated (Table 5.7). For patients who have had multiple cardiac events or one major event and multiple comorbidities, a goal LDL of <70 mg/dL is recommended. If the patient is also a diabetic, an LDL goal of <50 mg/dL should be considered. Ezetimibe 10 mg can be added if LDL goal is not achieved on the highest tolerated statin dose. Ezetimibe inhibits cholesterol absorption in the small intestine, lowering available

Table 5.7 Statin intensity and dosing

% of LDL lowering	≥50% - high intensity	30–49% moderate intensity	<30% low intensity
Statin	Atorvastatin 40–80 mg Rosuvastatin 20–40 mg	Atorvastatin 10–20 mg Rosuvastatin 5–10 mg Simvastatin 20–40 mg Pravastatin 40–80 mg Lovastatin 40–80 mg	Simvastatin 10 mg Pravastatin 10–20 mg Lovastatin 20 mg

cholesterol for the liver. This agent has minimal side effects and is very well tolerated. There is no mortality benefit of this agent alone without the high dose/high potency stain therapy.

Should the goal LDL not been met with these two therapies, then a PCSK-9 inhibitor should be considered. PCSK-9 inhibitors block the molecule that helps break down LDL receptors. This agent results in more LDL receptors being available to clear LDL from the bloodstream. The medication comes prepared in single use injections that are self-administered every 2 weeks. The cost of these medications must be considered before prescribing as the cost can be prohibitory. In patients with coronary artery disease who are unable to tolerate high dose statin therapy, moderate dose therapy can be initiated. The goal LDL reduction is 30–49%. If a PCSK-9 inhibitor is used, the patient should stay on the highest tolerated dose of statin and ezetimibe. It is used as an adjunct therapy, not a replacement [4].

Antianginal Therapy

Antianginal therapies are important for the management of ongoing coronary symptoms. Patients with CAD not amenable to revascularization and/or microvascular dysfunction (MVD) are the main indications for antianginal therapy. The different classes of medications lower myocardial oxygen consumption and improve oxygen delivery to the working myocardium. The patients' observations of their symptoms can help guide the need for antianginal adjustment. Patients are encouraged to regularly engage in cardiac exercise. This activity helps patients to monitor their symptoms by assessing their overall functional status. If they are regularly exercising, they can watch for changes in their capacity. These symptoms may include increased dyspnea, early fatigue, dizziness or palpitations, discomfort in their chest or upper back that may resolve with rest. Patients can monitor their blood pressure and heart rate at home looking for any changes that occur over time. Annual ischemic testing is no longer recommended. Patients should be educated that exercise is their method of "stress testing" themselves.

Beta-blockers—decrease heart rate and lower blood pressure, thereby reducing cardiac oxygen demand. Optimally, metoprolol or carvedilol is used as a first-line antianginal therapy. These should be titrated to maximal tolerated levels. They are often limited by bradycardia or patient developing a side effect, such as fatigue and erectile dysfunction (ED).

Calcium channel blockers—control the influx of calcium into smooth muscle cells of the vascular system, limiting contraction, and promoting vasodilation. These agents improve oxygen delivery and reduce oxygen consumption by lowering blood pressure (afterload). Amlodipine is often initiated as a second-line agent. This improved BP control but does not affect heart rate. The primary side effect reported is lower extremity edema. It is generally most pronounced at higher doses and does resolve upon cessation of the medication.

Nitrates—Nitroglycerine (NTG) relaxes smooth muscle cells resulting in vasodilation. Nitrates work in the venous system reducing ventricular preload and by decreasing afterload in the arteriole system. This leads to decreased workload on the heart and increased blood flow to coronary arteries. This group of medications is the class of choice for patients with MVD and symptoms rapidly improve with these agents. Isosorbide is a long-acting nitrate that will lower blood pressure but will not affect heart rate; however, often patients develop headaches. The headache improves with continued administration and should be discussed with the patient during the initiation of the medication. Nitroglycerine preparations are also contraindicated in patients who take medications for erectile dysfunction as concomitant use can result in extreme refractory hypotension. Patients may still use sublingual (SL NTG) in addition to long-acting NTG if they have discomfort that is consistent with exertional angina. They may use it prior to activity to prevent angina. One tablet should be placed under the tongue every 5 min, for a maximum of three doses, until the anginal symptoms have resolved. If symptoms do not resolve, then medical attention may be required. The effects of SLNTG are short acting. Tablets should burn under the tongue and if not are likely expired. Often patients need reassurance as to when it is safe to administer NTG. It is beneficial to remind the patient that they will likely need to lay down due to blood pressure drop. Also, nitroglycerine is not a traditional pain medication and is not addictive. It may also resolve symptoms aside from cardiac discomfort such as gastrointestinal discomfort, and the relief is not diagnostic for a cardiac etiology of symptoms.

Ranolazine—works primarily for smaller vessel disease. One benefit of this medication is that it does not decrease blood pressure or heart rate. This makes it beneficial when trying to treat ischemic chest pain in patients limited by hemodynamics. It also does not increase risk of arrythmia. Often patient's will have an awareness that their symptoms have improved or become less severe within a few days of starting the medication. The administration of ranolazine is entirely for anti-anginal symptoms, so it is reasonable to discontinue it, if there is no improvement. It is exceptionally well tolerated. It does prolong the QT interval and is contraindicated in liver disease [5].

Behavior Modification

Exercise and dietary recommendations can be made. Address modifiable risk factors (HTN, lipids, DM, tobacco, obesity) at each visit, educating the patient on the goals and what needs to be done to maintain or achieve them.

Pearls

- Complete versus incomplete revascularization is important information to know in an outpatient with chest pain.
- Medical management for stable chest pain may reduce the need for invasive procedures.
- Attention to hospitalization discharge medications is important to avoid complications in the outpatient setting.
- There are minimal indications for asymptomatic stress testing in patients with CAD and should be avoided.
- Pretest probability of each patient should be assessed to order the correct test and minimize false-positive and false-negative results.
- If you won't believe the result, or it won't change management, DON'T order the test!
- If symptoms are clearly cardiac or non-cardiac, no testing is required because the test may result in false-positive or negative results.
- Always walk the patient on a treadmill, if possible, to obtain functional capacity and prognostic data.
- The addition of imaging improves the positive predictive value of testing.
- If there is known CAD or stented segments, coronary CT is usually not the correct test for chest pain evaluation.
- MVD may have the same exertional symptoms, abnormal stress testing, and response to medical therapy without epicardial CAD.
- Lifelong antiplatelet and statin therapies are important GDMT for long-term management of CAD.

References

1. Gibbons RJ, Chatterjee K, Daley J, et al. ACC/AHA/ACP-ASIM guidelines for the management of patients with chronic stable angina: executive summary and recommendations: a report of the American college of cardiology/American heart association task force on practice guidelines (committee on management of patients with chronic stable angina). Circulation. 1999;99(21):2829–48. http://circ.ahajournals.org/cgi/content/extract/99/21/2829. https://doi.org/10.1161/01.CIR.99.21.2829.
2. Conti CR. Grading chronic angina pectoris (myocardial ischemia). Clin Cardiol. 2010;33(3):124–5. https://onlinelibrary.wiley.com/doi/abs/10.1002/clc.20766. https://doi.org/10.1002/clc.20766.
3. Grundy SM, Stone NJ, Bailey AL, et al. 2018 AHA/ACC/AACVPR/AAPA/ABC/ACPM/ADA/AGS/APhA/ASPC/NLA/PCNA guideline on the management of blood cholesterol: executive summary: a report of the American college of cardiology/American heart association task force on clinical practice guidelines. J Am Coll Cardiol. 2019;73(24):3168–209. https://www.ncbi.nlm.nih.gov/pubmed/30423391. https://doi.org/10.1016/j.jacc.2018.11.002.

4. Gulati M, Levy PD, Mukherjee D, et al. 2021 AHA/ACC/ASE/CHEST/SAEM/SCCT/SCMR guideline for the evaluation and diagnosis of chest pain: executive summary: a report of the American college of cardiology/American heart association joint committee on clinical practice guidelines. J Am Coll Cardiol. 2021;78(22):2218–61. https://www.ncbi.nlm.nih.gov/pubmed/34756652. https://doi.org/10.1016/j.jacc.2021.07.052.
5. Amsterdam E, Wenger N, Brindis R, et al. 2014 AHA/ACC guideline for the management of patients with non–ST-elevation acute coronary syndromes: a report of the American college of cardiology/American heart association task force on practice guidelines. Circulation. 2014;130(25):e344–426. http://ovidsp.ovid.com/ovidweb.cgi?T=JS&NEWS=n&CSC=Y&PAGE=fulltext&D=ovft&AN=00003017-201412230-00017. https://doi.org/10.1161/CIR.0000000000000134.

6 Surgical Management of Coronary Artery Disease

Elisabeth A. Powell and Larry Watts

Coronary artery bypass grafting is a surgical procedure performed to reestablish blood flow to the diseased coronary arteries. Atherosclerosis develops within the artery walls creating narrowing of the artery. Blood flow and myocardial perfusion are decreased distal to the areas of stenosis, resulting in ischemia and potentially, myocardial infarction. In coronary artery bypass grafting (CABG), an artery or vein is used as a conduit to deliver blood distal to the stenosis, bypassing the disease (Fig. 6.1).

A multitude of factors are considered when determining the best modality for coronary revascularization. Numerous studies have compared percutaneous coronary intervention (PCI) to coronary artery bypass grafting (CABG) for revascularization. These studies assessed risk to benefit ratios, long term patency, and overall survival rates. Although PCI is an appropriate option when stenting is feasible, CABG is the gold standard for revascularization in patients with left main disease, significant multivessel coronary artery disease (CAD) with decreased LV function, or when stenting is unsuccessful.

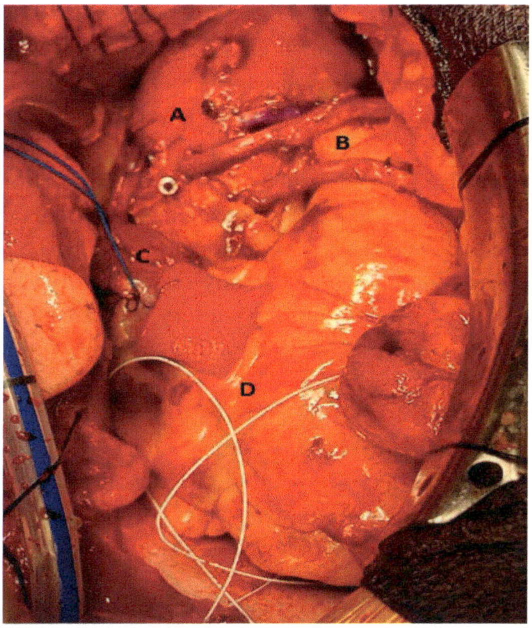

Fig. 6.1 CABG. (**a**) Ascending aorta (**b**) Bypass grafts coming off aorta (**c**) Right atrium (**d**) Right ventricle

E. A. Powell (✉)
Banner University Medical Center, Tucson, AZ, USA
e-mail: elisabeth.powell@bannerhealth.com

L. Watts
Atrium Health/Sanger Heart and Vascular Institute, Charlotte, NC, USA
e-mail: Larry.Watts@atriumhealth.org

R. Musialowski, K. Allshouse (eds.), *Cardiovascular Manual for the Advanced Practice Provider*,
https://doi.org/10.1007/978-3-031-35819-7_6

Indications for CABG

In general, patients are considered for CABG if they have one of the following:

- Left main disease >50%.
- Diffuse 3 vessel CAD (disease >50% in the LAD, circumflex, and right territories).
- 2 vessel CAD with significant stenosis in the proximal LAD (categorized as ≥70%)
- Significant stenosis, but coronary is not amenable to PCI.
- Patient is undergoing another cardiac operation and coronary artery disease is present.

Consideration for surgical revascularization is multifactorial and a diseased artery's eligibility for bypass depends on both the severity and location of the stenosis. The severity of the stenosis in the native vessel must be >50% to be eligible for bypass, and >70% to be considered a significant stenosis. Moderate to high grade stenosis ensures blood will flow preferentially down the bypass graft and into the coronary artery without competing with the natural flow from the proximal native artery.

The location of the stenosis is also important. The area of myocardium that is supplied by the coronary artery is directly proportional to the benefit gained from bypassing the artery. For comparison, the left anterior descending artery provides blood flow to a large portion of the left ventricle extending all the way to the apex. The diagonal artery, in contrast, only supplies a small area of the anterior and lateral left ventricle. A bypass placed to the proximal left anterior descending artery (LAD) revascularizes a larger area of myocardium than bypassing a stenosis at the distal end of a diagonal artery. Proximal or mid-vessel stenoses will yield more benefit from bypass than a distal stenosis given the territory the vessel feeds beyond the blockage.

Guidelines published by The American College of Cardiology (ACC) and American Heart Association (AHA) are available to assist in medical decision making and are demonstrated in Fig. 6.2. These guidelines are based on a comprehensive literary review on studies, trials, and evidence-based medicine which evaluate both indications to improve symptoms and anatomic indications to improve survival [1]. In patients with significant left main stenosis and complex disease unable to be safely stented, studies have shown that CABG is the gold standard for revascularization and portends an improved survival over PCI and medical therapy [1]. CABG has also shown to be superior to PCI in multivessel CAD with ischemic cardiomyopathy and EF ≤50% [1]. If multivessel CAD is present with an EF ≥50%, surgical revascularization is still reasonable for improved survival, especially with the presence of Diabetes [1].

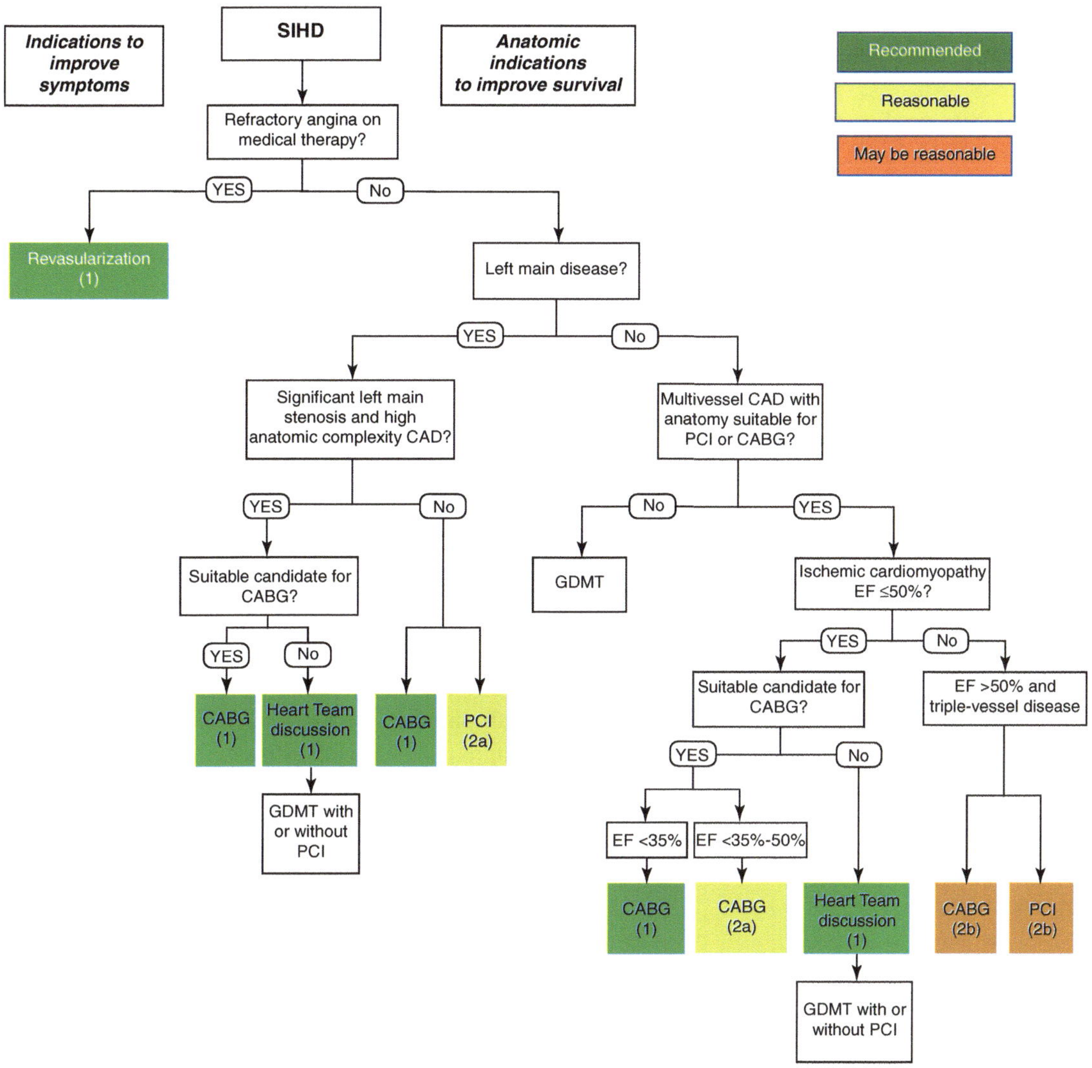

Fig. 6.2 Revascularization in patients with Stable Ischemic Heart Disease (SIHD) CABG indicates coronary artery bypass graft; CAD, coronary artery disease; EF, ejection fraction; GDMT, guideline-directed medical therapy; PCI, percutaneous coronary intervention; and SIHD, stable ischemic heart disease. This algorithm summarizes the recommendations in this guideline for the care of patients with stable CAD. It is not meant to encompass every patient scenario or situation, and clinicians are encouraged to us a Heart Team approach when care decisions are unclear and to see the accompanying supportive text for each recommendation. Additionally, in situations that lack sufficient data to make formal recommendations for care. (Adapted from [1])

The current guidelines by the ACC and AHA recommend a multidisciplinary approach to surgical decision making. The heart team consists of the cardiologist, interventionalist and cardiothoracic surgeon. Prior to intervention, a discussion with the entire team ensures a well-rounded and balanced analysis towards high-risk patients with supportive decision making. This is beneficial if the decision between high-risk surgical revascularization versus PCI vs medical management is unclear [1].

Preoperative Assessment and Calculating Risk

In addition to cardiac catheterization, preoperative work up includes a comprehensive history and physical, laboratory tests, and various imaging modalities. Every preoperative patient should begin with the same basic work up to assess baseline function and any abnormalities. Refer to Table 6.1.

A carotid artery duplex is recommended to assess for carotid stenosis in patients with neurological symptoms or a history of a CVA to ensure appropriate blood flow during cardiopulmonary bypass (see Table 6.2). Pulmonary disease or significant smoking history should be assessed with an arterial blood gas (ABG) and pulmonary function tests in consideration of intubation. Prior to undergoing cardiac surgery, a transthoracic echocardiogram should also be completed to assess heart and valve function. Consultation for surgical clearance should be made to respective specialist groups for underlying comorbidities at risk with surgery. Preoperative assessment is both patient and surgeon specific and additional testing should be considered to investigate various disease processes.

Table 6.1 Baseline preoperative testing

Comprehensive metabolic panel
Complete blood count
Prothrombin time (PT-INR)
Partial thromboplastin time (PTT)
Hemoglobin A1C
Type and screen
Pregnancy test (if female, childbearing age)
MRSA nasal swab
Urinalysis-potential
Electrocardiography
Chest xray

Table 6.2 Other potential preoperative testing

TSH
Platelet mapping
Vein mapping
Pulmonary function testing
Arterial blood gas
Carotid duplex
Upper extremity arterial duplex
Consults to medical specialists

Determining surgical risk is vital in determining if a patient is an appropriate candidate for cardiac surgery. The Society of Thoracic Surgeons (STS) has developed a risk calculator which allows providers to determine the mortality risk along with various morbidities for certain cardiac surgeries [2]. These surgeries include CABG, isolated aortic valve replacement (AVR), isolated mitral valve repair (MVr), isolated mitral valve replacement (MVR), CABG + AVR, CABG +MVr, and CABG+MVR. This calculator provides percentages of predicted risk in nine different categories based on STS data and research [3]. Refer to Table 6.3.

The risk calculator is available on the STS website: https://riskcalc.sts.org/stswebriskcalc/calculate

This calculator is meant to aid in, not define, decision making. This tool should be combined with physical assessment, frailty testing, clinical judgment, and discussions with both members of the care team and patient to determine if patient is an appropriate surgical candidate. The calculator is based on a database of greater than 30 years of patient information. It is utilized to help predict risks of cardiac surgery. Common categories utilized are 30-day mortality, risk of prolonged ventilation, risk of requiring post operative dialysis, stroke, among many other categories. A surgical mortality risk of >8% is considered high. These high-risk patients often require Heart Team discussions to determine optimal medical care and delivery. This may include a hybrid of surgical revascularization and PCI.

Table 6.3 STS risk calculator categories

Mortality
Stroke
Renal failure
Prolonged ventilation or reintubation (>24 h)
Mediastinitis/deep sternal wound infection
Need for reoperation during hospital stay
Major morbidity or mortality
Long length of stay (longer than 14 days)
Short length of stay (shorter than 6 days)

Conduit Selection

The primary objective of coronary bypass is to revascularize the myocardium. This reduces symptoms, increase survival rates, and decreased mortality. To obtain these goals, a vital part of the planning process prior to surgery is conduit and target vessel selection. The conduits used in CABG to provide blood supply to the coronary arteries are the internal mammary arteries, radial artery, greater and lesser saphenous vein, and less commonly, the gastroepiploic artery.

Extensive literary reviews and meta-analysis have demonstrated the superiority of arterial conduits versus venous conduits in CABG. Arterial conduits have demonstrated greater patency rates, quality, and durability over time leading to greater survival rates and decreased morbidities. This increased patency is due to many physical and biological factors. When compared to venous conduits, arterial conduits have similar functional and structural properties to the coronary artery, the ability to sustain arterial pressure on a cellular level, decreased rates of thrombosis, and significantly decreased evidence of atherosclerosis at the time of follow-up [4].

Although arterial conduits have shown improved patency and durability, venous conduits are still accepted and utilized in given circumstances. Conduit selection for CABG is multifactorial and depends on both clinical factors of the patient and anatomical characteristics of the physical stenosis. Best practices for conduit selection and surgical decision making are outlined in Table 6.4.

Table 6.4 Bypass conduit recommendations. Adapted from [1]

Best practices for the use of bypass conduits in CABG
• Objectively assess palmar arch completeness and ulnar compensation before harvesting the radial artery. Use the arm with the best ulnar compensation for radial artery harvesting
• Use radial artery grafts to target vessels with subocclusive stenoses
• Avoid the use of the radial artery after transradial catheterization
• Avoid the use of the radial artery in patients with chronic kidney disease and a high likelihood of rapid progression to hemodialysis
• Use oral calcium channel blockers for the first postoperative year after radial artery grafting
• Avoid bilateral percutaneous or surgical radial artery procedures in patients with coronary artery disease to preserve the artery for future use
• Harvest the internal mammary artery using the skeletonization technique to reduce the risk of sternal wound complications
• Use an endoscopic saphenous vein harvest technique in patients at risk of wound complications
• Use a no-touch saphenous vein harvest technique in patients at low risk of wound complications
• Use the skeletonized right gastroepiploic artery to graft right coronary artery target vessels with subocclusive stenosis if the operator is experienced with the use of the artery

Internal Mammary Artery

The internal mammary artery is the number one most utilized conduit in cardiac surgery. This artery has a low rate of atherosclerosis making it very durable with greater long-term patency rates when compared to other conduits. The location of the mammary artery along the sternum provides for easy accessibility and harvest is obtained without the need of an additional incision. The left internal mammary artery (LIMA) is the gold standard for grafting of the left anterior descending artery (LAD). The LIMA lies in proximity to the LAD and is grafted onto the LAD while remaining attached to the left subclavian artery (in situ). Given the importance of the LAD and the superiority of the IMA, this graft has shown to greatly increase survival, decrease mortality and morbidities, and increase graft patency rates after CABG [5].

The Society of Thoracic Surgeons recommends the use of bilateral IMAs for CABG if the degree and location of the stenosis is agreeable and there is no excessive risk of sternal complications [5]. Sternal complications of infection, nonunion, or poor healing with the harvest of bilateral IMAs are a potential risk given the decrease of arterial blood supply to the sternum after removal of the arteries. This risk is greatest in patients with diabetes due to a higher risk for infection and slower wound healing. This risk can be reduced if the IMA is harvested skeletonized, leaving the

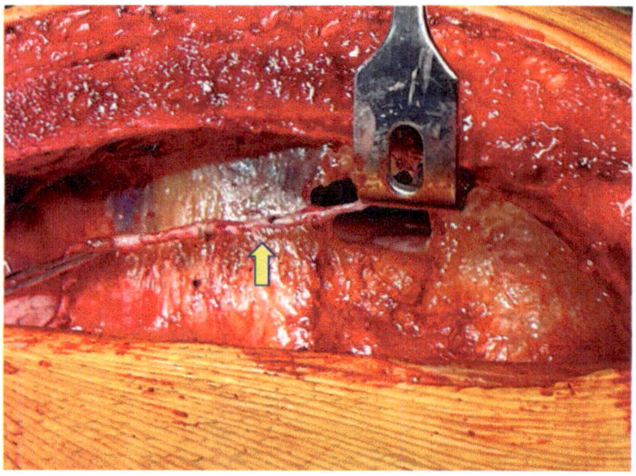

Fig. 6.3 Skeletonized left internal mammary artery in-situ

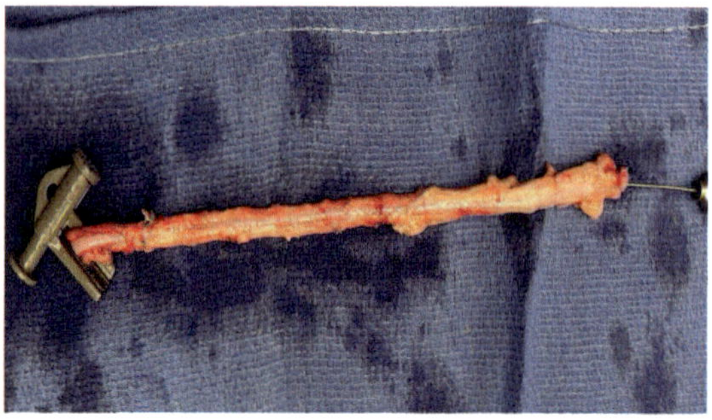

Fig. 6.4 Endoscopically harvested radial artery. Photo Credit: Roy Keller, CSFA

surrounding vasculature behind and intact on the chest wall. Demonstration of a skeletonized IMA harvest is shown in Fig. 6.3. Counseling on smoking cessation to decrease vasoconstriction, strict glycemic control to reduce risk of infection, and consideration of enhanced sternal stabilization with sternal closure all aid in sternal healing and decrease risk of complications [5].

Radial Artery

The radial artery is the second preferred conduit over the IMAs in CABG for longevity and quality. Advancements in postoperative medical therapy to prevent radial spasm with calcium channel blockers and improvement in target selection have greatly improved patency rates of radial conduits [5]. The selected target for the radial artery must be a coronary artery with significant stenosis (>70% stenosis for left sided grafts, >90% stenosis for right sided grafts) to prevent radial spasm, competitive flow, and early graft failure. With these improvements, recent studies have demonstrated greater patency rates and survival benefits for the radial artery when compared to the saphenous vein conduit [1]. The radial artery is now recommended as conduit choice for the most important vessel requiring bypass, second to the LAD [1]. It should be considered in patients <75 years old, women, and patients with preserved renal function [1]. If patients have chronic renal failure or known need for hemodialysis in the future, radial artery utilization is not recommended. A radial artery that has been harvest endoscopically is demonstrated in Fig. 6.4.

Before harvesting the radial artery, it is important to ensure the patient's hand will continue to have an arterial blood supply via the ulnar artery and an intact palmer arch. This can be assessed physically by performing a modified Allen's Test. To complete this test, the patient elevates their hand and clenches their fist while the provider occludes both the ulnar and radial artery to exsanguinate the hand. While still occluding the arteries, the patient opens their hand which should appear blanched. The ulnar artery pressure is then released while still compressing the radial artery. If the hand regains color, blood flow has re-entered the hand, demonstrating a patent ulnar artery and complete arch. This same test may be completed using a pulse oximeter or doppler. Completion of the palmer arch may be assessed more specifically with an arterial duplex study.

Greater and Lesser Saphenous Vein

Guidelines from the ACC, AHA, and STS recommend utilization of arterial conduits over venous, yet the greater saphenous vein (GSV) remains the second highest used conduit for CABG next to the LIMA. This is due to its accessibility, length, versatility, and relative ease of use. Although the long-term patency rate for saphenous vein grafts

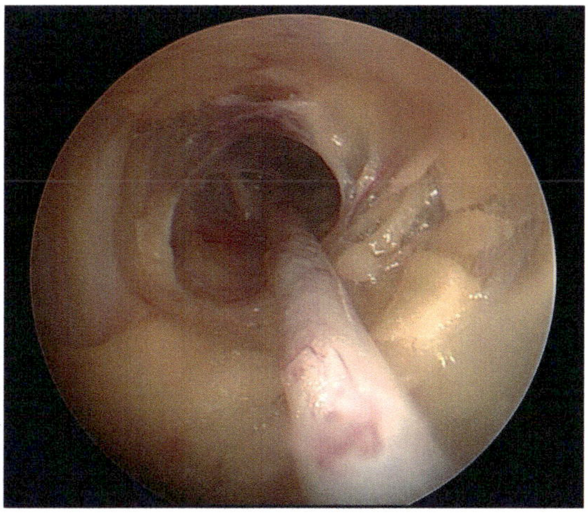

Fig. 6.5 Greater saphenous vein during endoscopic harvest

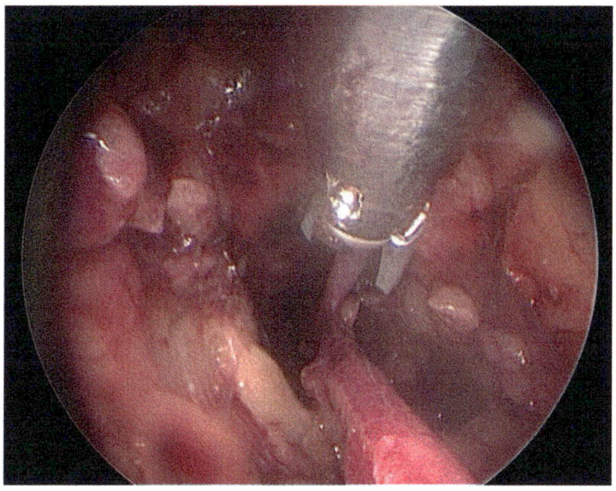

Fig. 6.6 Cauterization of branch during endoscopic vein harvest of the greater saphenous

is inferior to arterial conduits, it is still an accepted choice for non-LAD targets. Improvements in harvest techniques and technological advances with endoscopic vein harvesting have improved conduit quality, patency rates, and decreased wound complications. Demonstration of greater saphenous vein harvest utilizing the endoscopic technique is shown in Figs. 6.5 and 6.6. The finished product is demonstrated in Fig. 6.7. If the patient has known, or suspected, venous stasis or varicosities, vein mapping may be beneficial to assess quality and size of the saphenous vein prior to harvest.

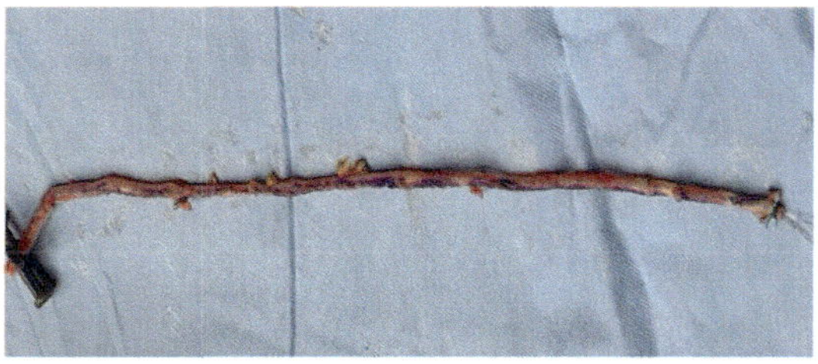

Fig. 6.7 Endoscopically harvested greater saphenous vein graft

The lesser saphenous vein is less frequently used in CABG surgery. Its role and patency are the same as the greater saphenous, however it is smaller in diameter and its anatomical position in the posterior lower leg make it difficult to harvest. The lesser saphenous vein terminates in the popliteal vein so the length of the lesser saphenous is also substantially shorter. It is most often utilized in redo operations where the greater saphenous has already been utilized, or if the patient has had vein ablation or stripping of the greater saphenous.

Gastroepiploic Artery

The gastroepiploic artery is the least utilized conduit in CABG. This is due to difficulty in exposure and harvest, short conduit length, and variation in size along the length of the artery [5]. This option is usually only considered when the other conduits have already been harvested in prior operations or are inadequate. Like the radial artery, the gastroepiploic artery is prone to spasm and is only recommended to be used on coronary arteries with a severe level of stenosis (>90%).

References

1. Lawton JS, Tamis-Holland JE, Bangalore S, Bates ER, Beckie TM, Mischoff JM, et al. ACC/AHA/SCAI guideline for coronary artery revascularization, a report of the American College of Cardiology/American Heart Association Joint Committee on clinical practice guidelines. J Am Coll Cardiol. 2021;2022:79.
2. The Society of Thoracic Surgeons; 2022. https://www.sts.org/resources/risk-calculator.

3. O'Brien SM, Feng L, He X, Xian Y, Jacobs JP, Badhwar V, et al. The Socieity of Thoracic Surgeons 2018 adult cardiac surgery risk models: part 2 - statistical methods and results. Ann Thorac Surg. 2018;105:1419–28.
4. Gharibeh L, Ferrari G, Ouimet M, Grau JB. Conduits' biology regulates the outcomes of coronary artery bypass grafting. JACC: basic to translational. Science. 2021;6(4):388–96.
5. Aldea GS, Bakaeen FG, Pal J, Thourani VH, Firestone S, Mitchell JD, et al. The Society of Thoracic Surgeons clinical practice guidelines on arterial conduits for coronary artery bypass grafting. Ann Thorac Surg. 2015;101(2):801–9.

Part III

Cardiac Electrophysiology

Satish Misra

The cardiac conduction system is a complex and highly regulated system including both specialized impulse generation regions, specialized conduction fibers, and the intrinsic properties of myocytes that facilitate propagation of electrical activity through the heart. The beat-to-beat properties of these components are dynamic, affected by intrinsic cardiac factors, such as ischemia or pressure overload, as well as extrinsic factors, like circulating inflammatory cytokines and the autonomic nervous system. Acquired and inherited disorders at each of these levels are associated with a wide range of pathology that will be encountered in the general cardiology practice. In this section, we will review these conditions as well as their management.

The cornerstone of management of arrhythmia disorders includes anti-arrhythmic therapy, cardiovascular implantable electronic devices (CIEDs), and catheter ablation. Management of relevant comorbid conditions is also critical. For example, for patients with atrial fibrillation, effective management of comorbidities such as diabetes mellitus and sleep apnea has been associated with reduced arrhythmia burden as have behavioral modification that leads to weight loss and increased aerobic exercise.

Anti-arrhythmic therapy will be reviewed in detail in this section. It is important to recognize that medical therapy is suppressive while catheter ablation, which will also be discussed, is potentially curative for many conditions including SVT, PVCs, and atrial flutter. For others, such as atrial fibrillation and ventricular tachycardia, it can often be more effective for arrhythmia suppression than medication therapy and help avoid associated toxicities, particularly with Class III agents. Procedural complication rates are low and with modern electro-anatomic mapping systems, can be completed without radiation exposure.

S. Misra
Atrium Health/Sanger Heart and Vascular Institute, Charlotte, NC, USA
e-mail: Satish.misra@atriumhealth.org

CIED therapy includes pacemakers and implantable cardioverter-defibrillators (ICDs) which can be single chamber, dual chamber, or biventricular. Pacemakers are used to manage the disorders of impulse generation and propagation that lead to symptomatic bradyarrhythmias such as heart block and sinus node dysfunction. In addition, biventricular systems, which include pacing leads for both the right and left ventricle, can help correct the abnormal mechanics associated with left bundle branch block which can contribute to systolic dysfunction. Finally, ICDs can help prevent sudden death associated with ventricular arrhythmias. Modern devices also include sophisticated heart failure monitoring algorithms which incorporate a range of physiologic data collected by these devices.

Electrophysiology as a field has seen rapid evolution over the past ten years, a trend that is likely to continue. In the catheter ablation arena, new modalities of ablation using different forms of energy to eliminate abnormal tissue are emerging such as pulsed field ablation. In addition, increases in computing power as well as advances in catheter/electrode design have enabled very high-density mapping of the heart's electrical activity, sometimes reaching thousands of measurements, and processing of that information to reflect information about underlying abnormalities in real-time. Novel CIEDs are also being developed including leadless pacing systems that can be implanted in both the atria and ventricles. In addition, there is a rapid evolution toward the use of conduction system pacing, whereby pacing leads are implanted in deep septal positions to recruit the native conduction system, thereby creating a more normal ventricular contraction with every heartbeat.

In this section, we will review the foundational knowledge that will help enable you to provide effective care for patients with arrhythmia disorders and collaborate with your electrophysiology colleagues to ensure the best outcomes for your patients.

Antiarrhythmic and Anticoagulant Agents

7

Craig J. Beavers

Anticoagulation Therapy

As outlined in the atrial fibrillation section (Chap. 9), one of the core goals in management is to prevent or reduce the risk of stroke and systemic embolism. The preferred strategy to decrease risk is systemic anticoagulation. The Atrial Arrhythmia chapter will provide the recommendations of when and to whom anticoagulation therapy should be prescribed. However, as with the antiarrhythmic agents, it is important to select the agent that optimizes efficacy and reduces risk of bleeding. Decisions should be made based on patient factors including renal function, liver function, weight, age, ability to adhere to regimen, cost, and other factors. In addition, the patient should have education provided about their anticoagulation at each encounter including benefits and risks (Tables 7.1 and 7.2).

C. J. Beavers (✉)
University of Kentucky College of Pharmacy,
Lexington, KY, USA
e-mail: cjbeav2@uky.edu

R. Musialowski, K. Allshouse (eds.), *Cardiovascular Manual for the Advanced Practice Provider*,
https://doi.org/10.1007/978-3-031-35819-7_7

Table 7.1 Antiarrhythmic agents

Pharmacological targets	Electrophysiological effects	Major clinical applications	Corresponding likely therapeutic mechanisms	Example drug(s)	Pharmacokinetic parameters	Common dose(s) in adults	Cardiovascular adverse events	Non-cardiovascular events
Class 0: Hyperpolarization-activated cyclic nucleotide-gated (HCN) channel blockers								
HCN channel mediated pacemaker current (I_f) block	Inhibition of I_f reducing the sino-atrial node (SAN) phase 4 pacemaker depolarization rate (decreased automaticity)	Potential new off label applications for tachyarrhythmias (e.g. inappropriate sinus tachycardia; not atrial fibrillation [AF])	Reduced in SAN automaticity	*Ivabradine*	*Half-life*: Distribution 2 h; effective ~6 h *Bioavailability*: ~40% *Metabolism*: Extensively intestinal and hepatic via CYP3A4 (CYP3A4 substrate) *Excretion*: Feces and urine (~4% has unchanged drug)	*Oral*: 5 mg twice daily; maintenance: 7.5 mg twice daily	Bradycardia, hypertension, atrial fibrillation	Phosphene (transient enhanced brightness in limited area of visual field, halos, image decompositions, colored bright lights, or multiple images; occurs in first 2 months and most cases resolve with discontinuation).

Class Ia: Voltage-gated Na + channel blockers								
Nav 1.5 open state, intermediate dissociation kinetics; often concomitant K+ channel block	Reduction in peak I_{Na}, action potential (AP) generation, with increased excitation threshold	Supraventricular tachyarrhythmias, particularly recurrent AF; ventricular tachycardia, ventricular fibrillation (including short QT syndrome [SQTS] and Brugada syndrome)	Reduction in ectopic ventricular/atrial automaticity; reduction in accessory pathway conduction; increase in refractory period, decrease reentrant tendency	*Quinidine*	*Half-life*: 4–10 h *Bioavailability*: >80% *Metabolism*: Substrate: CYP2C9 (minor), CYP2E1 (minor), CYP3A4 (major), P-glycoprotein (Pgp; minor) Inhibits: CYP2D6 (strong) CYP3A4 (weak), Pgp *Excretion*: Urine		QRS prolongation with toxic doses, torsades de pointes (not dose related) *Monitoring*: ECG as needed, at least every 6 months	Thrombocytopenia, cinchonism, pruritis, rash
				Disopyramide	*Half-life*: 4–10 h *Bioavailability*: >80% *Metabolism*: Extensively intestinal and hepatic via CYP3A4 (CYP3A4 substrate) *Excretion*: Urine	*Oral*: 100–200 mg every 6 h	Heart failure exacerbations; torsades de pointes *Monitoring*: ECG as needed, at least every 6 months	Anticholinergic (contraindicated in narrow-angle glaucoma); dry mouth; urinary retention; constipation, blurry vision
				Procainamide	*Half-life*: 3–4 h *Bioavailability*: Not applicable given intravenous administration *Metabolism*: Substrate: CYP2D6 (minor) *Excretion*: Urine	*IV*: 10–17 mg/kg (ideal body weight) at a rate of 20–50 mg/min or 100 mg every 5 min; maintenance infusion: 1–6 mg/min	Hypotension, cardiac arrhythmias, heart failure exacerbation *Monitoring*: Telemetry	Limited with intravenous use

(continued)

Table 7.1 (continued)

Pharmacological targets	Electrophysiological effects	Major clinical applications	Corresponding likely therapeutic mechanisms	Example drug(s)	Pharmacokinetic parameters	Common dose(s) in adults	Cardiovascular adverse events	Non-cardiovascular events
Class Ib: Voltage-gated Na+ channel blockers								
Nav 1.5 open state; rapid dissociation; I_{Na} window current	Reduction in peak I_{Na}, AP generation with increased excitation threshold	Ventricular tachyarrhythmias (ventricular tachycardia, ventricular fibrillation), particular after a myocardial infarction	Reduction in ectopic ventricular automaticity; reduction in delayed afterdepolarization (DAD) induced triggered activity; reduced reentrant tendency by converting unidirectional block, particularly in ischemic, partially depolarized myocardium	*Lidocaine*	*Half-life*: 120 min *Bioavailability*: Not applicable due intravenous administration *Metabolism*: Substrate: CYP1A2 (major), CYP2A6 (minor), CYP2B6 (minor); CYP2C9 (minor), CYP3A4 (major) *Excretion*: Urine	*Intravenous (IV)*: 1–1.5 mg/kg bolus, repeat at 0.5–0.75 mg/kg every 5–10 min (up to 3 mg/kg); follow with continuous infusion at 1–4 mg/min)	Bradycardia, cardiac arrhythmia *Monitoring*: Telemetry	Dizziness, nervousness, unsteady gait, gastrointestinal distress, nausea, vomiting, tremor
				Mexiletine	*Half-life*: 9–15 h *Bioavailability*: >80% *Metabolism*: Substrate: CYP1A2 (major), CYP2D6 (major) Inhibits: CYP1A2 (moderate) *Excretion*: Urine	*Oral*: 150–200 mg every 8–12 h; adjust dose as needed in 50–100mg increments no more frequently than every 2–3 days up to 300 mg every 8–12 h	Exacerbation of cardiac arrhythmia *Monitoring*: ECG as needed, at least every 6 months	Dizziness, nervousness, unsteady gait, gastrointestinal distress, nausea, vomiting, tremor

Class 1c: Voltage-gated Na+ channel blockers								
Nav 1.5 inactivated state; slow dissociation	Reduction in peak I_{Na} AP generation and with increase excitation threshold	Supraventricular tachyarrhythmias (atrial tachycardia, atrial flutter, atrial fibrillation, and tachycardias involving accessory pathways); ventricular tachyarrhythmias resistant to other treatment in the absence of structural heart disease, premature ventricular contraction, catecholaminergic polymorphic ventricular tachycardia	Reduction in ectopic ventricular/atrial automaticity; reduction in DAD-induced triggered activity; reduced reentrant tendency by converting unidirectional block to bidirectional block; slowed conduction and reduced of excitability particularly at rapid heart rates blocking reentrant pathways showing depressed conduction	*Propafenone*	*Half-life*: 9–15 h *Bioavailability*: >80% *Metabolism*: Substrate: CYP1A2 (minor), CYP2D6 (major), CYP3A4 (major) Inhibits: CYP1A2 (weak), CYP2D6 (weak); P-gp *Excretion*: Urine	*Oral*: Immediate release: 150 mg every 8 h with increase every 3–4 days up to 300 mg every 8 h; 450 mg once for pill in pocket dosing Extended release: 225 mg every 12 h; dose may increase every 5 days up to 425 mg every 12 h	Atrial flutter with 1:1 conduction, ventricular tachycardia, may unmask Brugada-type ST elevation, contraindicated with coronary disease *Monitoring*: ECG as needed, at least every 6 months	Metallic taste, dizziness
				Flecainide	*Half-life*: 10–18 h *Bioavailability*: >80% *Metabolism*: Substrate CYP1A2 (minor) and CYP2D6 (major) *Excretion*: Urine with some fecal	*Oral*: 50–300 mg/day in divided doses 8–12 h (can go up to 400 mg for ventricular arrhythmias management)	Atrial flutter with 1:1 conduction, ventricular tachycardia, may unmask Brugada-type ST elevation, contraindicated with coronary disease *Monitoring*: ECG as needed, at least every 6 months	Dizziness, headache, visual blurring

(continued)

Table 7.1 (continued)

Pharmacological targets	Electrophysiological effects	Major clinical applications	Corresponding likely therapeutic mechanisms	Example drug(s)	Pharmacokinetic parameters	Common dose(s) in adults	Cardiovascular adverse events	Non-cardiovascular events
Class 1d: Voltage-gated Na+ channel blockers								
Nav 1.5 late current	Reduction in late Na+ current (I_{Na}) affecting AP recovery, refrac4toriness, repolarization reserve, and QT interval	Ventricular tachycardia, as a potential new class of drugs for the management of tachyarrhythmias	Decrease AP recovery time; reduction in early afterdepolarization (EAD) induced triggered activity	*Ranolazine*	*Half-life*: 7 h *Bioavailability*: >76% *Metabolism*: Substrate: CYP2D6 (minor), CYP3A4 (major), P-gp (minor) Inhibits: CYP2D6 (weak), CYP3A4 (weak), P-gp *Excretion*: Urine	*Oral*: 500 to 1000 mg twice daily, may increase to 1000 ng twice daily as needed	Bradycardia, hypotension, prolonged QT *Monitoring*: ECG as needed, at least every 6 months, renal function	Dizziness, headache, constipation

Class II: Autonomic inhibitors and activators								
Class IIa								
Non-selective β- and selective β1-adrenergic receptor inhibitors	Inhibition of adrenergically induced G_s protein-mediated effects of increased adenylyl kinase activity and cyclic AMP with effects of including slowed SAN pacemaker rate	Sinus tachycardia or other types of tachycardic, including supraventricular (atrial fibrillation, atrial flutter, atrial tachycardia), arrhythmias; rate control of atrial fibrillation and ventricular tachyarrhythmias (ventricular tachycardia, premature ventricular contraction) Note: Atenolol, propranolol, and nadolol used in long QT syndrome; nadolol used in catecholaminergic polymorphic ventricular tachycardia	Reduction in SAN automaticity; reduction in AVN automaticity; reduction in ectopic ventricular/atrial automaticity; reduction in EAD-/DAD-induced triggered activity; reduced SAN reentry; reduction in AVN conduction terminating reentry	*Non-selective β inhibitors*: Carvedilol, propranolol, nadolol. Selective *β1-adrenergic inhibitors*: Atenolol, bisoprolol, betaxolol, esmolol, metoprolol (tartrate and succinate)	*Refer to drug reference/package insert for each agent's pharmacokinetic information* *Note: atenolol is cleared renally and should be avoided in patient with renal disease*	Refer to drug reference/package insert for each agent's dosing information	Bradycardia, hypotension *Monitoring*: Blood pressure and heart rate	Dizziness, fatigue

(continued)

Table 7.1 (continued)

Pharmacological targets	Electrophysiological effects	Major clinical applications	Corresponding likely therapeutic mechanisms	Example drug(s)	Pharmacokinetic parameters	Common dose(s) in adults	Cardiovascular adverse events	Non-cardiovascular events
Class IIb								
Non-selective β-adrenergic receptor activators	Activation of adrenergically induced G_s-protein effects of increasing adenylyl kinase activity and cAMP; decrease in RR and PR intervals	Accelerating rates of ventricular escape rhythm in cases of complete atrioventricular block before definitive pacemaker implantation; acquired, often-drug related, bradycardia-dependent torsades de pointes	Increase escape ventricular automaticity; suppression of Brady-cardia dependent EAD-related triggered activity	*Isoproterenol*	*Half-life*: 2.5–5 min *Bioavailability*: Not applicable due to intravenous administration *Metabolism*: None *Excretion*: Urine	*Intravenous*: 2–10 mcg/min IV; titrate to patient response	Cardiac arrhythmias, hypertension *Monitoring*: Heart rate, blood pressure, potassium	Flushing, dizziness, headache, hypokalemia
Class IIc								
Muscarinic M_2 receptor inhibitors	Inhibition of supraventricular (SAN, atrial, AVN) muscarinic M_2 cholinergic receptors; decrease RR and PR intervals	Mild or moderate symptomatic sinus bradycardia; supra-His, AVN, conduction block, elg. In vagal syncope or acute inferior myocardial infarction	Increase in SAN automaticity; increase in AVN conduction	*Atropine*	*Half-life*: 3–4 h *Bioavailability*: Not applicable due to intravenous administration *Metabolism*: None *Excretion*: Urine	*Intravenous, intramuscular*: 0.5–1 mg every 3–5 min; 1 mg preferred for severe bradyarrhythmia; maximum total dose 3 mg	Cardiac arrhythmias *Monitoring*: Heart rate, blood pressure, electrolytes, mental status	Hyperthermia, dizziness, confusion, electrolytes abnormalities

Class IId								
Muscarinic M_2 receptor activators	Activation of supraventricular (SAN, atrial, AVN) muscarinic M_2 cholinergic receptors activates K channels, hyperpolarizing the SAN and shortening APDs in atrial and AVN tissue	Sinus tachycardia or supraventricular tachyarrhythmias	Reduction in SAN automaticity; reduced SAN reentry; reduction in AVN conduction terminating reentry	*Digoxin*	*Half-life*: 38 h *Bioavailability*: 70–85% (formulation dependent) *Metabolism*: Substrate: CYP3A4 (minor), P-gp *Excretion*: Urine	*Oral*: 0.125–0.25 mg daily *Intravenous*: 0.25–0.5 mg over several min, with a repeat dose of 0.35 mg every 6 h to a maximum dose of 1.5 mg over 24 h	Cardiac arrhythmias *Monitoring*: Heart rate, blood pressure, electrolytes, digoxin level, serum creatinine	Digoxin toxicity (nausea, vomiting, visual disturbances [yellow, blurred vision, halos], lethargy, arrhythmias, worse with hypokalemia)
Class IIe								
Adenosine A_1 receptor activators	Activation of adenosine A_1 receptors in supraventricular tissue (SAN, atrial, AVN) activates G protein-coupled inward rectifying K^+ channels and I_{KAdo} current hyperpolarizing the SAN and shortening APDs in atrial and AVN tissue	Acute termination of AVN tachycardia and cAMP mediated triggered VTs; differentiation of sinus versus atrial tachycardia	Reduction in SAN automaticity; reduction in AVN conduction, terminating reentry; reduction in EAD-/DAD-induced triggered activity	*Adenosine*	*Half-life*: <10 s *Bioavailability*: Not applicable *Metabolism*: None	*Intravenous*: Initial 6 mg IV push (rapid, with 20 mL saline flush); if not effective within 1–2 min, 12 mg maybe given; may repeat 12 mg bolus if needed. Maximum single dose 12 mg. Note: Initial dose should be reduced to 3 mg if patient is currently receiving carbamazepine or dipyridamole, has a transplanted heart or if adenosine administered via central line	Cardiac arrhythmia, chest pressure *Monitoring*: ECG, heart rate, blood pressure	Headache, dizziness, facial flushing, gastrointestinal distress, neck discomfort, dyspnea

(continued)

Table 7.1 (continued)

Pharmacological targets	Electrophysiological effects	Major clinical applications	Corresponding likely therapeutic mechanisms	Example drug(s)	Pharmacokinetic parameters	Common dose(s) in adults	Cardiovascular adverse events	Non-cardiovascular events
Class III: K^+ channel blockers and openers (note this table will focus on class IIIa; IIB or IIc not highlighted due to lack of currently approved agents at time of publication)								
Class IIIa-voltage dependent K^+ channel blockers								
Nonselective K^+ channel blockers	Block of multiple K^+ channel targets resulting in prolonged atrial, Purkinje, and/or ventricular myocyte AP recovery, increased ERP, and reduced repolarization reserve; prolonged QT intervals	Ventricular tachycardia in patients without structural heart disease or with remote myocardial infarction (*amiodarone only*) tachyarrhyhtmias with Wolff-Parkinson white syndrome; atrial fibrillation with atrioventricular conduction via accessory pathway (*amiodarone only*); ventricular fibrillation and premature ventricular contraction (*amiodarone only*); Tachyarrhyhtmias associated with supraventricular arrhythmias and atrial fibrillation	*Increase in AP recovery time; increase in refractory period with decrease reentrant tendency; note: Amiodarone also slows sinus node rate and atrioventricular conduction (has class II and IV properties)*	*Amiodarone*	*Half-life*: 40–55 days *Bioavailability*: 35–65% *Metabolism*: Substrate: CYP1A2 (minor), CYP2C19 (minor), CYP2C8 (minor), CYP2D6 (minor), CYP3A4 (major), P-gp (minor) Inhibitor: CYP2C9 (weak), CYP2D6 (weak), CYP3A4 (weak), P-gp *Excretion*: Feces	*Supraventricular arrhythmias* *Intravenous*: 150 mg over 10 min, then 1 mg/min for 6 h, then 0,5 mg/min for 18 h. Continue for a total load up to 10 g; may finish load with oral dosing. *Oral*: 600–800 mg daily in divided doses for a total of 10 g load then maintenance of 200–400 mg once daily *Ventricular arrhythmias*: *Intravenous*: 150 mg over 10 min, then 1 mg/min for 6 h, then 0,5 mg/min for 18 h. Continue for a total load up to 10 g; may finish load with oral dosing. *Oral*: 400 mg every 8–12 h for 1–2 weeks, followed by 200–400 mg once	Sinus bradycardia, QTc prolongation, cardiac arrhythmias *Monitoring*: Blood pressure, heart rate, ECG, history and physical exam every 3–6 months, pulmonary function test, chest X-ray every 3–6 months, liver function test baseline and semiannually; electrolytes, thyroid function tests before treatment and periodically thereafter (3–6 months); regular ophthalmic exams	Pulmonary (acute hypersensitivity pneumonitis, chronic interstitial infiltrates); hepatitis; thyroid (hypothyroid or hyperthyroid): Photosensitivity; blue-grey skin discoloration with chronic high doses; nausea; ataxia; tremor; alopecia

				Dronedarone	*Half-life*: 13–19 h *Bioavailability*: Without food: 4%, with high fat meal 15% *Metabolism*: Substrate: CYP3A4 (major) Inhibits: CYP2D6 (weak), CYP3A4 (moderate),P-gp *Excretion*: Feces	*Oral*: 400 mg twice daily with meals	Bradycardia, new onset or worsening heart failure (death increased in patients with symptomatic heart failure), prolonged QTc/torsades de pointes *Monitoring*: ECG (at least every 3 months), heart rate, blood pressure, signs/symptoms of heart failure, signs of pulmonary toxicity, liver enzymes	Anorexia, nausea, hepatotoxicity, pulmonary toxicity

(continued)

Table 7.1 (continued)

Pharmacological targets	Electrophysiological effects	Major clinical applications	Corresponding likely therapeutic mechanisms	Example drug(s)	Pharmacokinetic parameters	Common dose(s) in adults	Cardiovascular adverse events	Non-cardiovascular events
Kv11.1 (HERG) channel-mediated rapid K^+ 1current (I_K) blockers	Prolonged atrial, Purkinje and ventricular myocyte AP recovery, increase ERP, and reduced repolarization reserve; prolonged QT intervals	Ventricular tachycardia in patients without structural heart disease or with remote myocardial infarction (*sotalol only*) tachyarrhyhtmias with Wolff-Parkinson white syndrome; atrial fibrillation with atrioventricular conduction via accessory pathway (*sotalol only*); ventricular fibrillation and premature ventricular contraction (*sotalol only*); Tachyarrhyhtmias associated with supraventricular arrhythmias1 and atrial fibrillation	*Increase in AP recovery time; increase in refractory period with decrease reentrant tendency*	*Dofetilide*	*Half-life*: ~ 10 h (extended with renal impairment) *Bioavailability*: >90% *Metabolism*: Substrate: CYP3A4 (major) *Excretion*: Renal	*Oral*: Note CrCl and QTc interval must be determined prior to first dose. If QTc > 440 ms (>500 ms in patients with ventricular conduction abnormalities), doffetilide is contraindicated. Adjust dose in those with CrCL <60 mL/min. Patient requires hospitalization for 3 days when starting Initial 500mcg twice daily (reduce dose based on QTc and CrCl; refer to package insert)	Torsades de pointes *Monitoring*: ECG monitoring, baseline and regular serum creatine, electrolytes	Headache, dizziness, nausea

			Ibutilide	*Half-life*: 2–12 h *Bioavailability*: Not applicable *Metabolism*: None *Excretion*: Urine	*Intravenous*: <60 kg: 0.01 mg/kg over 10 min ≥60 kg: 1 mg over 10 min	Torsades de pointes	Nausea
			Sotalol	*Half-life*: 12 h *Bioavailability*: Well absorbed; decreased by ~20% by meals compared to fasting *Metabolism*: None *Excretion*: Renal	Note CrCl and QTc interval must be determined prior to first dose. If CrCl ≤ 60 mL/min, dose adjustment warranted. Please see package insert. *Oral*: 80 mg twice daily *Intravenous*: 75 mg infused over 5 h twice daily	Bradycadia, torsades de pointes *Monitoring*: ECG monitoring, baseline and regular serum creatine, electrolytes, heart rate	Brochospasm

(continued)

Table 7.1 (continued)

Pharmacological targets	Electrophysiological effects	Major clinical applications	Corresponding likely therapeutic mechanisms	Example drug(s)	Pharmacokinetic parameters	Common dose(s) in adults	Cardiovascular adverse events	Non-cardiovascular events
Class IV: $Ca2^{+}$ (note this table will focus on class IVa; IVb, IVc,IVd, IVe not highlighted due to lack of currently approved agents at time of publication)								
Class IVa: Surface membrane Ca^{2+} channel blockers								
L-type Ca^{2+} current blockers	Block Ca^{2+} current (I_{Ca}), resulting in inhibition of SAN pacing, inhibition of AVN conduction, prolonged ERP, increased AP recovery time	Supraventricular arrhythmias and ventricular tachycardia without structural heart disease; rate control of atrial fibrillation	Reduction in AVN conduction, terminating reentry; reduction in EAD-/DAD-induced triggered activity	*Diltiazem*	*Half-life*: 3–9 h (depending on immediate or extended release) *Bioavailability*: ~40% *Metabolism*: Substrate: CYP2C9 (minor), CYP2D6 (minor), CYP3A4 (major), P-gp (minor) Inhibits: CYP2D6 (weak), CYP3A4 (moderate) *Excretion*: Urine	*Oral*: Immediate release: 30 mg four times daily; increase as needed to achieve rate control; usual doses 120–480 mg/day in 3–4 doses Extended release: Initial 120 mg once daily or in 2 divided doses; increase as needed; usual dose 120–480 mg/day *Intravenous*: Bolus dose: 0.25 mg/kg (actual body weight) over 2 min. If rate control insufficient after 15 min a repeat bolus dose of 0.35 mg/kg can be given Continuous infusion: Initial 5–10 mg/h; infusion rate maybe increased in 5 mg/h increments every 10–15 min up to maximum of	Bradycardia, hypotension, peripheral edema *Monitoring*: Blood pressure, heart rate	Headache

			Verapamil	*Half-life*: 2–12 h *Bioavailability*: 20–35% *Metabolism*: Substrate: CYP1A2 (minor), CYP2B6 (minor), CYP2C9 (minor), CYP3A4 (major), P-gp (minor) Inhibitor: CYP1A2 (weak), CYP3A4 (moderate), P-gp *Excretion: Urine*	*Oral*: Immediate release: Initial 40 mg three to four times daily; increase as needed to achieve rate control; maximum dose: 480 mg/day in 3–4 doses Extended release: 120–180 mg once daily; maximum daily dose 480 mg *Intravenous*: Bolus dose: 5–10 mg over 2 min if rate control insufficient after 15–30 min a repeat bolus dose of 0.35 mg/kg can be given Continuous infusion: Initial 5 mg/h; infusion rate maybe increased in 5 mg/h increments every 15–30 min up to maximum of 20 mg/h	Bradycardia, hypotension, peripheral edema *Monitoring*: Blood pressure, heart rate	Headache, constipation

AP-action potential; APD-action potential duration; AVN-atrioventricular node; CrCL- creatinine clearance; DAD-delayed afterdepolarization; EAD- early afterdepolarization; ERP- effective refractory period; P-gp-P-glycoprotein SAN- sino-atrial node

Adapted from the references [1–3]

Table 7.2 Oral anticoagulants used in stroke prevention for AF

Characteristic	Warfarin	Dabigatran	Apixaban	Edoxaban	Rivaroxaban
Mechanism of action	Vitamin K antagonist	Direct thrombin inhibitor	Factor Xa inhibition	Factor Xa inhibition	Factor Xa inhibition
Standard dosing	5 mg daily (avoid loading doses), adjust to achieve INR 2–3	150 mg twice daily	5 mg twice daily	60 mg daily	20 mg daily with evening meal
Renal impairment dosing	Consider starting doses of ≤2.5 mg daily if: • Age ≥65 • Weight ≤70 kg Poor nutritional status • Significant hepatic disease • Increase bleeding risk • Known warfarin sensitivity • Decompensated HF	75 mg twice daily (CrCL 15–30 mL/min)	2.5 mg twice daily If at least two of three criteria: • Age ≥80 • Weight ≤60 kg SCr ≥1.5 mg/dL	30 mg daily (CrCl 15–50 mL/min)	15 mg daily (CrCl 15–50 mL/min)
Hepatic impairment dosing	Consider starting doses of ≤ 2.5 mg daily if: • Age ≥65 • Weight ≤70 kg Poor nutritional status • Significant hepatic disease • Increase bleeding risk • Known warfarin sensitivity • Decompensated HF	No adjustment	Child-Pugh class B: Avoid or use with caution Child-Pugh class C: Avoid use	Child-Pugh class B: Avoid or use with caution Child-Pugh class C: Avoid use	Child-Pugh class B: Avoid or use with caution Child-Pugh class C: Avoid use
Time to peak	5–7 days	1–3 h	1–2 h	1–2 h	2–4 h
Half-life (h)	~40 h	8–15 h	12 h	10–14 h	7–11 h
Excretion	Hepatic, primarily through CYP2C9	80% renal	25% renal, 75% fecal	50% renal; also, bile, feces	66% renal (one-half as inactive form)
Metabolized	CYP2C9, CYP1A2, CYP3A4, CYP2C19	P-gp	P-gp and CYP3A4	P-gp	P-gp and CYP3A4
P-gp and/or strong CYP3A4 inducers	Consider higher starting dose, monitor INR closely	Avoid use	Avoid use	Avoid use	Avoid use
P-gp inhibitors	Not applicable	If CrCl <50 mL/min, avoid use or reduce dose	Not applicable	30 mg daily	Not applicable

Dual P-gp and strong CYP inhibitors	Consider lower starting dose, monitor INR closely	Not applicable	Avoid use • No dose change needed with concomitant clarithromycin	Not applicable	• Avoid use • No dose change needed with concomitant clarithromycin
Dual P-gp and moderate CYP3A4 inhibitors	Monitor INR closely	Not applicable	Use with caution	Not applicable	If CrCl <80 mL/min, avoid use unless benefit justifies potential risk
Reversal strategy	Vitamin K, prothrombin complex concentrate, or fresh frozen plasma	Idarucizumab	Andexanet alfa and prothrombin complex concentrate	Andexanet alfa and prothrombin complex concentrate	Andexanet alfa and prothrombin complex concentrate

Package inserts from https://www.nlm.nih.gov

References

1. Lei M, Lin W, Terrar D, Huang CL. Modernized classification of cardiac antiarrhythmic drugs. Circulation. 2018;138:1879–96.
2. Zimetbuam P. Antiarrhyhtmic drug therapy for atrial fibrillation. Circulation. 2012;125:381–9.
3. Package inserts from https://www.nlm.nih.gov.

Bradycardia

8

Hannah Kibler and Sharon Vannoy

Sinus Node Dysfunction

Sinus node dysfunction (SND) is often used to describe abnormalities of impulse conduction originating from the Sinoatrial (SA) node. Degenerative changes in sinus node tissue occur throughout the lifespan and can lead to alterations in the generation or conduction of impulses, such as a prolonged pauses or sinus bradycardic episodes. Sinus node dysfunction is most common in individuals over 70 years of age. Sick sinus syndrome (SSS) refers to the symptomatic expression of sinus node dysfunction in patients resulting in fatigue, presyncope, syncope, dizziness, dyspnea, and other outward signs of cardiac output.

Tachycardia- bradycardia syndrome refers to a condition, when an individual has a co-morbid conduction abnormality resulting in a rapid atrial rate, such as atrial fibrillation, atrial flutter, or other supraventricular tachycardia. Upon conversion from the tachycardia, the sinus node fails to efficiently create an impulse resulting in a pause or bradycardia. Patients may or may not be symptomatic with the conversion pause or bradycardia which results.

H. Kibler · S. Vannoy (✉)
Atrium Health Wake Forest Baptist, Winston-Salem, NC, USA
e-mail: hkibler@wakehealth.edu; svannoy@wakehealth.edu

Sinus Bradycardia

In some individuals, including trained athletes, a heart rate below 50 bpm is acceptable and a normal variant. Bradycardias can be noted as a manifestation of increased vagal tone, normal aging, and are common in the elderly population as a result of disease progression such as in hypothyroidism. Symptomatic bradycardia is due to reduced cardiac output, which is a function of stroke volume and heart rate. The need for intervention is determined by the presence of symptoms.

Sinus Pause

A sinus pause, or sinus arrest, is the failure of the sinus node to generate an atrial depolarization for a period of time, generally defined as 3 seconds or longer between atrial contractions. Pauses can result from a block of the normal impulse from the sinoatrial tissue or due to failure of the sinus node to depolarize. Nocturnal pauses are commonly related to obstructive sleep apnea, which should be considered in the differential for assessment and in the treatment plan. Pauses are also more common in patients with tachycardia-bradycardia syndrome occurring when the tachyarrhythmia terminates and the sinus node is in recovery. The presence of sinus pauses, in absence of symptoms, does not always warrant

R. Musialowski, K. Allshouse (eds.), *Cardiovascular Manual for the Advanced Practice Provider*,
https://doi.org/10.1007/978-3-031-35819-7_8

Table 8.1 Causes of bradycardia

Medications	Tissue disorders	Metabolic	Miscellaneous
Antiarrhythmics	Amyloidosis	Hyper/hypokalemia	Acute MI
Beta blockers	Cardiomyopathies	Hypocalcemia	Autonomic dysfunction
Calcium Channel blockers	Ischemic, non-ischemic,	Hypothermia	Cardiac surgery
(non-dihydropyridine)	infiltrative	Hypoxia	CABG, TAVR, maze,
Digoxin	Connective tissue disease	Ion channel	valve
Interferon	RA, SLE, scleroderma	dysfunction	Replacement, ablation
Lithium	Hemochromatosis		Hypothyroidism
Methyldopa	Sarcoidosis		Infection
Opioids	Degenerative fibrosis		Lyme disease, typhoid
Risperidone			fever
Psychotropic meds			Dengue fever, malaria
Sympatholytics			Guillain-Barre
Illicit drugs			Obstructive sleep apnea
Toxins			

Goldberger et al. [1], Kusumoto et al. [2], Semelka and Gera [3]

intervention and can be associated with various physiologic and pathologic conditions as well as extrinsic factors including medications, electrolyte imbalance, increased vagal tone, and others (*see* Table 8.1). Frequent sinus pauses lasting longer than 3 seconds and are symptomatic warrant consideration for pacing support.

Chronotropic Incompetence

Chronotropic incompetence is defined as the inability of the heart rate to adjust appropriately in concordance with increased physical activity or cardiovascular demand. Patients can present with fatigue, lightheadedness, dyspnea on exertion, or syncope associated with activity. Further criteria for diagnosis of chronotropic incompetence, which is well established, includes the failure of the individual to reach 80% of their maximum predicted heart rate at peak exercise. This can be evaluated with exercise stress testing on a treadmill or bicycle. It is important to thoroughly assess individuals in whom there is suspicion for chronotropic incompetence as the condition is also associated with increased risk of coronary artery disease and is seen in approximately one-third of individuals with congestive heart failure [4]. In these patients, pacemaker implantation can provide symptom relief through rate responsive pacing (see Chap. 13).

Atrioventricular Blocks

A disturbance of impulse conduction between the atria and ventricles is known as atrioventricular (AV) block or heart block. This can occur if there is delayed conduction, intermittent loss of conduction, or complete loss of conduction from the atria to the ventricles. AV block/heart block is categorized based on the severity of the impulse conduction disturbance. The types of AV block will be addressed separately below.

First Degree AV Block (See Figs. 8.1 and 8.2)

First-degree heart block is defined as prolonged conduction from the atria to the ventricles with a PR interval greater than 200 ms. This can be secondary to a conduction delay at the AV node and/or the His-Purkinje system. The site of delay can be difficult to differentiate, though one clue is response to exercise. Increased sympathetic tone can increase conduction velocity in AV node

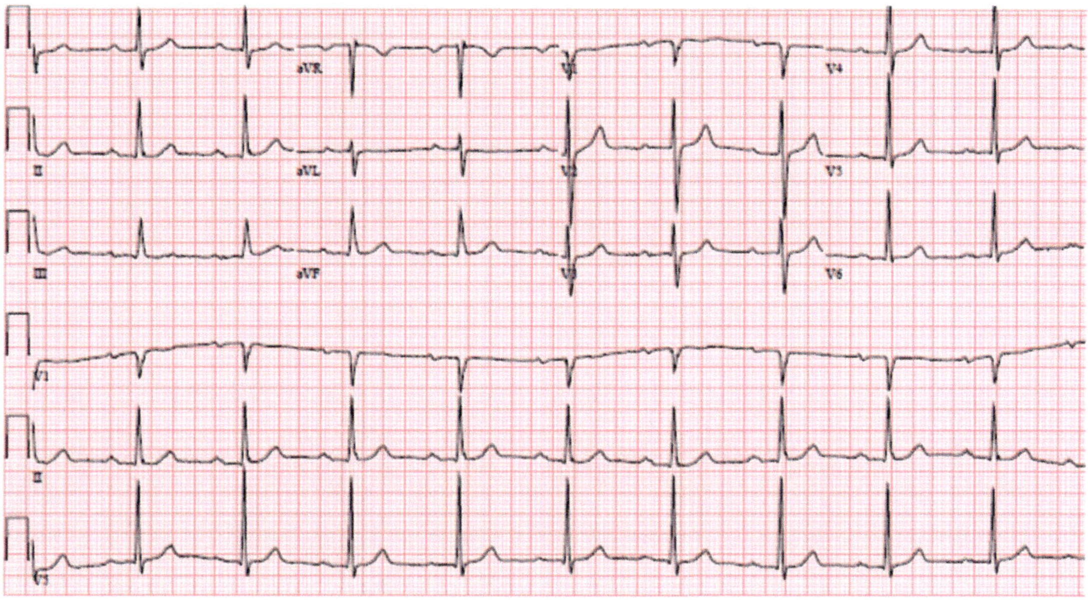

Fig. 8.1 Sinus rhythm with first-degree AV block. PR interval ~ 250 ms

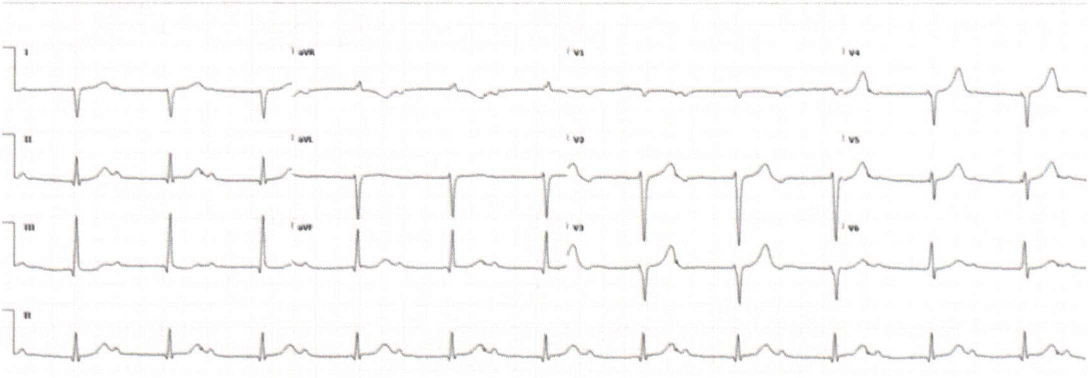

Fig. 8.2 Sinus rhythm with first-degree AV block. PR interval ~420 ms.

thereby shortening the PR interval if that is where the delay is occurring; absent PR shortening would suggest a lower level of delay.

Second-Degree AV Block (See Figs. 8.3 and 8.4)

Second-degree heart block is characterized by intermittent conduction from the atria to the ventricles. There are two separate types:

Mobitz Type I is also referred to as Wenckebach. This is noted on the ECG by progressive PR interval prolongation followed by a single non-conducted P wave.

Mobitz Type II appears on the ECG as a constant PR interval with intact conduction followed by a single non-conducted P wave.

Mobitz I and Mobitz II block refer to ECG patterns. Mobitz I block is more commonly at the level of the AV node and more responsive to changes in autonomic tone, occurring for example frequently with sleep in patients otherwise normal AV conduction. Mobitz II block, conversely, can be both in the AV node and His-Purkinje system, the latter to be suspected when

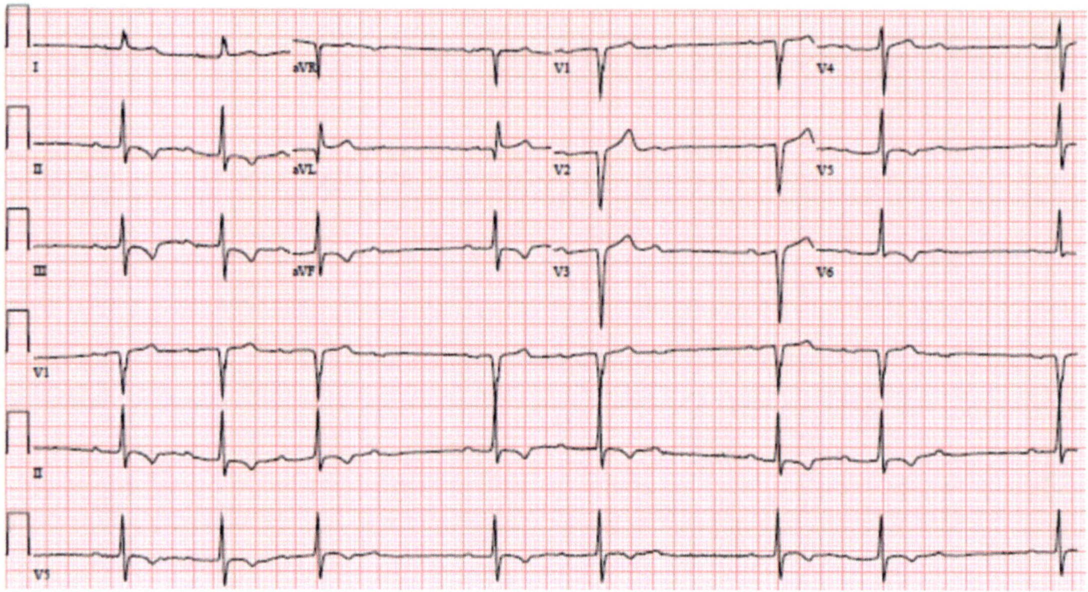

Fig. 8.3 Mobitz Type I (Wenckebach). PR interval gradually prolongs until a QRS is dropped and the next PR interval is shorter than the one prior to the drop

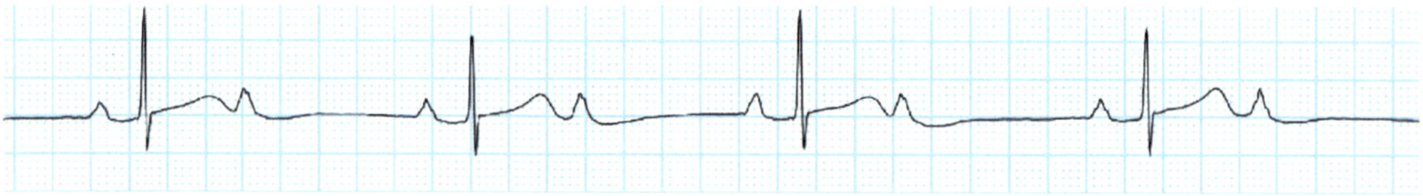

Fig. 8.4 Mobitz Type II. PR interval of conducted beats is stable, every other beat is dropped and QRS is narrow indicating block in the AV node

conduction disease (bundle branch or fascicular block) is present. This form of AV block is less responsive to changes in autonomic tone.

Advanced/High-Grade AV Block (Fig. 8.5)

High-grade AV block, which is differentiated from third-degree (complete) AV block, denotes intermittent conduction from the atria to the ventricles. When conducting from the atria to the ventricles, the PR interval is constant; however, there can be two or more consecutive non-conducted P waves (unlike second-degree heart block type II, where there is only a single non-conducted P wave). The mechanism of block is like Mobitz II AV block, though this finding is reflective of more advanced disease.

Third Degree/Complete Heart Block (Fig. 8.6)

Third-degree heart block is characterized by the absence of conduction between the atria to the ventricles. This is also frequently described as a complete dissociation between the atria and the ventricles. The ventricular rate is consequently driven by an escape rhythm. Portions of the conduction system have enhanced automaticity with impulse generation at rates that classically slow as the site of escape moves lower in the conduction system. Escape rhythms from the AV node below the level of block are often quite stable and

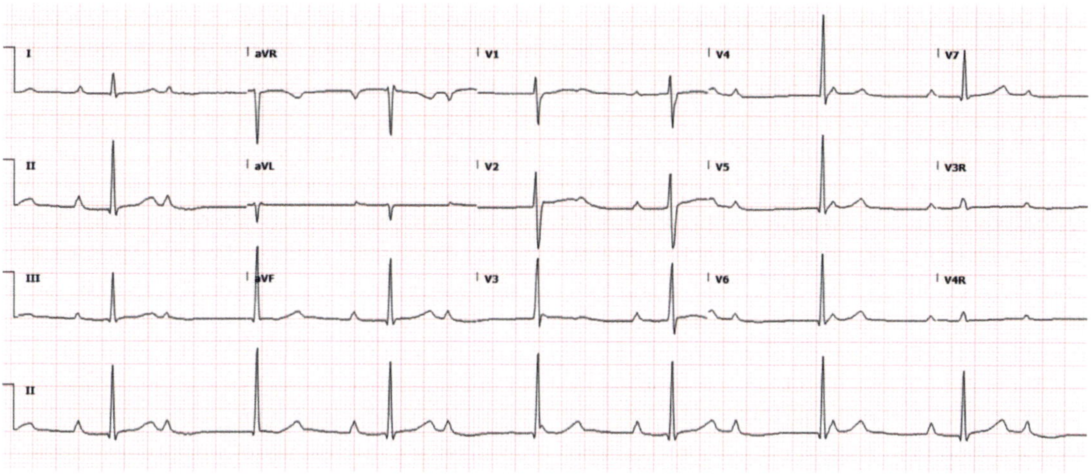

Fig. 8.5 Advanced or high-grade heart block

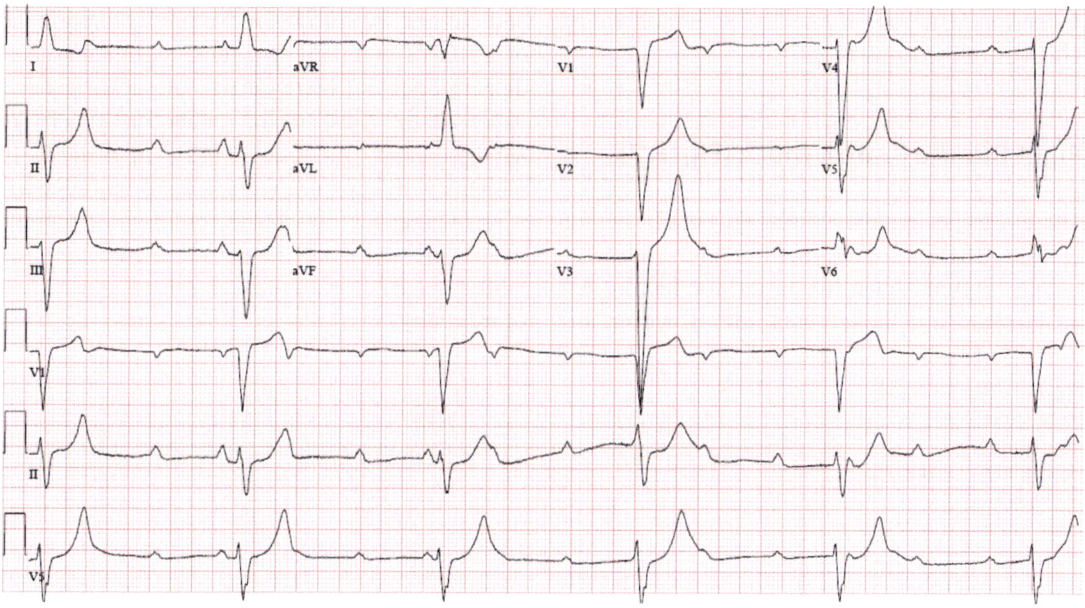

Fig. 8.6 Third-degree/complete heart block with LBBB escape rhythm

marked by a QRS complex nearly identical to baseline. Escape rhythms from the lower conduction system or ventricle, or wide complex escapes, are much less stable and high risk for hemodynamic instability. Placement of temporary pacemakers should be strongly considered in patients with wide escape rhythms, hemodynamically unstable heart rates, or presenting with syncope. Often, patients with complete heart block have compensatory hypertension due to increased SVR. Do not treat the hypertension. Vasodilating the patient may cause hemodynamic instability due to fixed cardiac output from the bradycardia.

Conduction System Abnormalities

Additional conduction abnormalities occur within the bundle branch system. The normal QRS interval ranges from 0.06–0.10 seconds; however, if a bundle branch block is present, the QRS duration is 0.12 seconds or longer. Despite the conduction delay associated with a bundle branch block, many patients remain asymptomatic. Changes in morphology related to bundle branch blocks can be best identified in various leads on the 12-lead ECG. In addition to the widened QRS interval, the QRS complex will have an abnormal shape. Furthermore, as depolarization is abnormal in a BBB, repolarization is also abnormal which results in T-wave inversion. Most commonly, this is noted in opposing deflection patterns of the QRS complex and T-waves of the same beat.

Right Bundle Branch Block (Fig. 8.7)

The electrical impulse of a right bundle branch block (RBBB) is conducted through the intraventricular septum down the faster conducting left bundle branch to the left ventricle. However, due to a block in conduction within the right bundle, the impulse reaches the RV through myocardial cell-to-cell conduction which is much slower. Electrocardiographic signs of RBBB include an initial small r wave in V_1 and V_2 (the right precordial leads) and a small q wave in leads I, aVL, V_5, and V_6 as septal depolarization from the left bundle is unaffected. Often the rSR' pattern that results in V_1 and V_2 is coined "rabbit ears" given the appearance of the two points on the R waves.

Right bundle branch blocks are the most common conduction disorder of the ventricular conduction system and can occur without any underlying cause or obvious pathology. Acutely, a RBBB can be seen in patients with ischemia or anterior MI and in additional associated conditions such as heart failure, valvular heart disease, and pulmonary embolism. Notably, the presence of a RBBB in a patient without significant heart disease does not increase risk of cardiovascular (CV) death; thus, if the patient is otherwise asymptomatic, no treatment is indicated. In patients with known CV disease, having a RBBB is an independent risk factor for all-cause mortality. In the setting of acute MI or the post MI period, a RBBB is associated with increased risk of mortality.

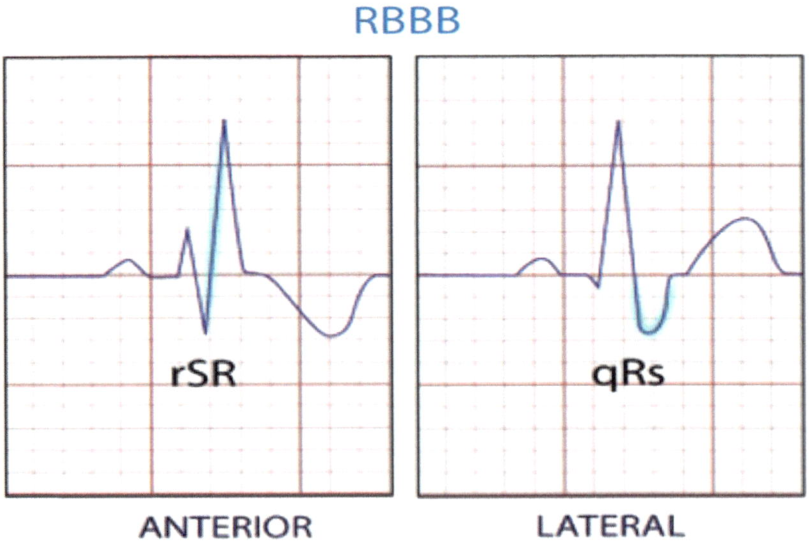

Fig. 8.7 Right bundle branch block morphology (Cardiology, Chang [5]: Springer)

Left Bundle Branch Block (Fig. 8.8)

In a left bundle branch block (LBBB), electricity moves quickly down the right bundle branch to depolarize the right ventricle. Next the impulse is carried more slowly across the interventricular septum and finally to the left ventricle, which is in opposition to normal depolarization. Electrocardiographic characteristics of a LBBB include a deep, wide QRS complex in lead V_1 and a large R wave in lead V_6, as well as a wide QRS complex with a T-wave in the opposite direction from the primary QRS deflection [6]. Often a left axis deviation is also present.

Conditions associated with LBBB include myocardial infarction (MI), hypertension, severe aortic stenosis (AS), Lenégre disease (a primary degenerative disease of the conduction system), and various cardiomyopathies. Cardiac surgery and trans-catheter aortic valve replacement as well as primary amyloidosis are all associated with increased risk of conduction disease. Left bundle branch blocks are more common in the elderly and in those with heart disease and should signal the need for further investigation as to causation such as echocardiography or stress testing. Of note, if a LBBB is found in the presence of acute MI, the patient has much greater risk of developing complete heart block leading to implantation of a pacemaker.

Due to the mechanism of the delayed conduction in a LBBB, the right ventricle receives the electric impulse before the left ventricle. In time, this can cause remodeling of the left ventricle due to alterations in left ventricular perfusion, mechanics, and workload. In the setting of heart failure, the presence of a LBBB is an independent predictor of mortality despite other risks associated with underlying disease, gender, or age. In comorbid heart failure with reduced ejection fraction, <35%, a QRS interval greater than 150 ms, and Class II or greater symptoms of heart failure, cardiac resynchronization therapy (CRT) is reasonable and may be recommended.

Left Anterior Fascicular Block (LAFB)

The left bundle branch further divides into the anterior and posterior fascicles. Conduction down the left bundle depolarizes the interventricular septum and causes a septal Q-wave in leads I, aVL, and V6. If the anterior fascicle is not conducting, the impulse proceeds from posterior to anterior resulting in a profound Left axis. The Q wave is present in the lateral leads as stated above. A small R wave is present with a very

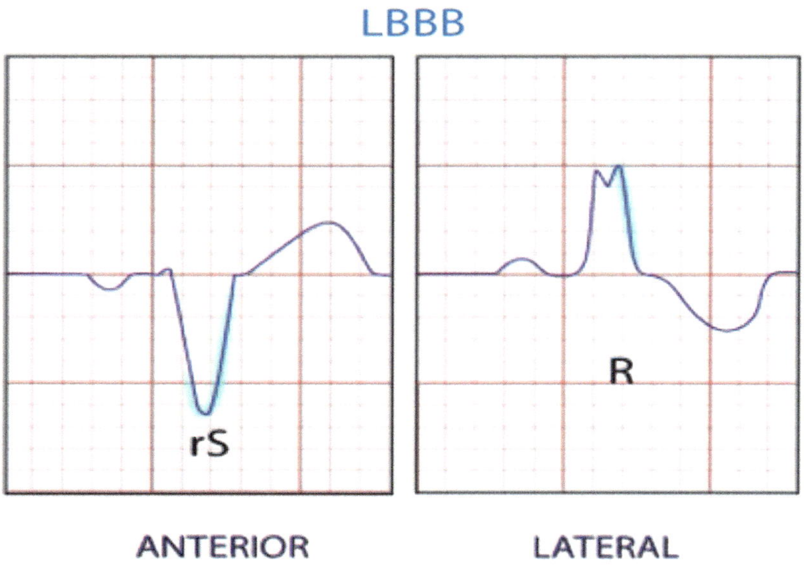

Fig. 8.8 Left bundle branch block morphology (Cardiology, Chang [5]: Springer)

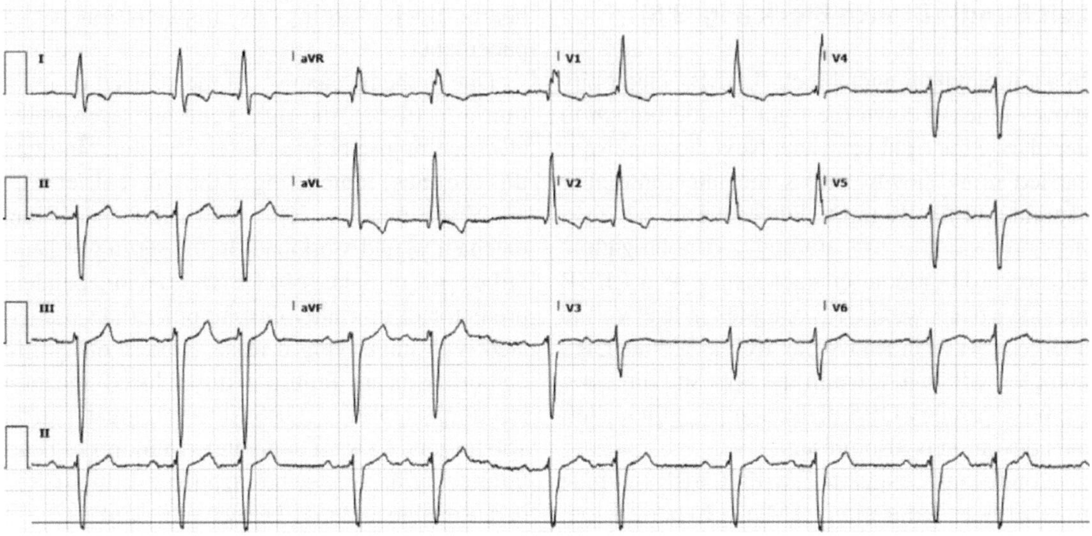

Fig. 8.9 First degree AV block with LAFB and RBBB

negative deflection in leads II and III as well. If a RBBB is present with a left axis, consider a LAFB which is called bifascicular block. If first degree block is also seen, it is called trifascicular block and has a higher risk of symptomatic bradycardia (*see* Fig. 8.9).

Evaluation and Management of Conduction Abnormalities

To evaluate causes of bradycardia, a thorough history and physical exam should be performed. When taking the history, emphasis should be placed on evaluation of the timing and relationship of symptoms to activity, meals, stress, position changes, and other triggers. A list of current medications, both prescription and non-prescription, are also vital to evaluating causation. Furthermore, the family history and complete cardiac history should be investigated. A comprehensive physical examination including carotid pulses and auscultation for bruits, peripheral pulses, heart sounds (to assess for structural/valvular disease), obtaining orthostatic vitals, and assessing for signs of systemic illness are of importance.

Following the history and physical exam, a 12-lead electrocardiogram (ECG) is the most helpful, initial test. Interpretation of the ECG rhythm with attention to interval lengths and waveforms and can further direct diagnosis and management. Based on the patient's history, symptoms, physical exam, and ECG findings, further evaluation with ambulatory cardiac monitoring may be completed. Home monitoring allows for a quantitative evaluation of arrhythmia as well as correlates the patient's symptoms with the timing and type of arrhythmia. The type of monitoring is dependent upon the frequency of symptoms. If the individual is experiencing daily symptoms, home monitoring through a wearable device is reasonable, noting more accurate diagnosis with longer recordings of 2–4 weeks as compared to a 24-to-48-hour monitoring window. For patients with less frequent symptoms of arrhythmia, or if syncope is the chief symptom, an implantable loop recording device should be considered. Furthermore, based on clinical history, if chronotropic incompetence is suspected, ambulatory heart monitoring and exercise stress testing is appropriate. As previously discussed, patients who have nocturnal sinus pauses should be evaluated for sleep apnea.

Laboratory studies to identify causes of bradycardia are directed by findings noted within the history and physical. Given potential underlying etiologies of thyroid disease, metabolic syndromes, electrolyte imbalance, and infectious processes, a metabolic panel including magnesium, a complete blood count, and thyroid function testing are reasonable to assess. Guidelines also support that individual with conduction disease be screened with Lyme titers, if they reside in endemic regions. For younger patients presenting with advanced blocks, further investigation for connective tissue diseases such as sarcoidosis and amyloidosis is warranted. Lastly, in patients with conduction disorders caused by genetic mutations including SCN5A sodium channel and LMNA (Lamin A/C) mutations, it is recommended that their first-degree relatives likewise undergo gene testing (Table 8.1).

For patients with incidentally diagnosed first-degree AV block and second-degree type I AV block, no immediate pacing intervention is required. Consideration of exercise stress testing, particularly with second-degree type I AV block is recommended to ensure adequate chronotropic competence. A transthoracic echocardiogram is recommended to evaluate for structural heart disease. If this is unrevealing for abnormality and the patient is asymptomatic, observation without further intervention can be considered. Ambulatory monitoring (2–4 weeks) is appropriate to ensure that there is no further underlying AV nodal disease such as second-degree type II AV block or high-degree AV block.

For patients with symptomatic second-degree type II AV block, high-degree AV block or third-degree AV block temporary pacing may need to be considered while further workup for reversible causes is performed. Furthermore, if no reversible cause is identified or if the patient will require AV nodal blocking agents for management of comorbidities, then permanent pacing is indicated. Temporary and permanent pacing will be discussed in Chap. 13.

Pearls

- Symptoms are the defining factors determining whether bradycardia needs treatment.
- Look for underlying causes of bradycardia before recommending permanent pacing.
- Type 1 and Type II Mobitz I do not need treatment.
- March out the P waves and then the R waves to determine their relationship.
- Normal PR is <200 ms.
- Normal QRS 0.6–0.10.

References

1. Goldberger A, Goldberger Z, Shvilkin A. Sinus and escape rhythms. In: Goldberger A, Goldberger Z, Shvilkin A, editors. Goldberger's clinical electrophysiology: a simplified approach. Philadelphia: Elsevier Inc; 2018. p. 122–9.
2. Kusumoto F, Schoenfeld M, Barrett C, Edjertons J, Ellenbogen K, Gold M, et al. 2018 guideline on the evaluation and Management of Patients with Bradycardia and Cardiac Conduction Delay: a report of the American College of Cardiology/American Heart Association task force on clinical practice guidelines and the Heart Rhythm Society. Circulation. 2019;140(8):e382–482. https://doi.org/10.1161/CIR.0000000000000628.
3. Semelka M, Gera J. Sick sinus syndrome: a review. Am Fam Physician. 2013;87(10):691–6.
4. Camm A, Fei L. Chronotropic incompetence-part II: clinical implications. Clin Cardiol. 1996;19:503–8.
5. Chang B. Cardiology. In: Lecker SC, editor. The ultimate medical school rotation guide. Cham: Springer; 2021. https://doi.org/10.1007/978-3-030-63560-2_16.
6. Geiter H. Understanding bundle branch blocks. Nurs Crit Care. 2010;5(6):5–8. https://doi.org/10.1097/01.CCN.0000389043.40866.b5.

9 Atrial Arrhythmias

Lora Raines

Introduction

According to the 2015 ACC/AHA/HRS Guidelines for the Management of Adult Patients with SVT, women have higher incidence of PSVT than men, and persons over age 65 have >5 times the risk of developing PSVT than younger persons [1].

SVTs typically have a narrow QRS complex on an ECG, but they may have a wide QRS complex if (1) there is a baseline bundle branch block present, (2) there is aberrancy, or (3) a bypass tract is present [1, 2]. SVTs typically occur due to enhanced automaticity of certain cells with pacemaker capabilities (automatic SVT) or the presence of a re-entry circuit that allows for rapid impulse conduction (re-entrant SVT). There are also triggered mechanisms for SVT.

- SVTs due to enhanced automaticity occur because of abnormalities in impulse initiation and typically exhibit spontaneous firing rates faster than the sinus node (though sinus tachycardia occurs due to enhanced automaticity of the sinus node) [1, 2].
- SVTs due to re-entry exhibit abnormal conduction of an electrical impulse due to the existence of two separate electrical pathways with different electrophysiologic properties and are dependent on these pathways [1, 2].

L. Raines (✉)
Wellstar Health System, Marietta, GA, USA
e-mail: Lora.Raines@wellstar.org

Inappropriate Sinus Tachycardia

Anatomy and Physiology

The sinus node is the heart's natural pacemaker. It is located in the superior lateral portion of the right atrium near its junction with the superior vena cava. It consists of pacemaker cells that can generate electrical impulses. The blood supply for the sinus node typically originates from the right coronary artery. The rate of electrical impulses that originate from the sinus node can vary, but normal sinus rhythm is typically 60–100 beats per minute. Sinus bradycardia is when the rate is less than 60 beats per minute. Sinus tachycardia is when sinus rates are greater than 100 beats per minute. There is also sinus arrhythmia, in which the impulses are still originating from the sinus node, but the timing of the impulses is irregular. This is a normal in healthy, young individuals and due to elevated vagal tone.

When the sinus node fires, the electrical activity travels through the right and left atrium down to the AV node. The initial indication of sinus node activity on the ECG is the P wave, although the P wave represents activation of the atria. Because the sinus node is in the high right atrium, the right atrium depolarizes before the left atrium.

R. Musialowski, K. Allshouse (eds.), *Cardiovascular Manual for the Advanced Practice Provider*,
https://doi.org/10.1007/978-3-031-35819-7_9

Therefore, the first half of the P wave is due to right atrial activation and the second half of the P wave is due to left atrial activation. On an ECG, normal sinus rhythm is indicated by a sinus P wave before every QRS with 1:1 conduction. A sinus P wave should be upright in lead II and will typically be upright in leads I, aVF, and V3-V6 [3]. Sinus rhythm will gradually increase and decrease on ECG or telemetry in response to exercise or increased metabolic needs (i.e., fever).

Pathology/Description

As mentioned, sinus tachycardia refers to sinus rhythm in which the rates are greater than 100 beats per minute. Impulse rates are governed by the sympathetic and parasympathetic divisions of the autonomic nervous system. Increases in parasympathetic activity decrease impulse rates and increases in sympathetic activity increase impulse rates. Heart rates up to 200–220 beats per minute can be observed with maximal sympathetic stimulation [3]. There are several factors that can result in sinus tachycardia including physiologic, pharmacologic, or pathologic factors. Some of these may be normal and appropriate, while others are pathologic. Some factors that can cause elevation in sinus rates include physical activity, emotional responses, hypovolemia/dehydration, anemia, hypoxia, hypotension, obstructive or restrictive conditions (such as acute PE, pericarditis, pericardial effusion, MI), heart failure, thyroid abnormalities, pain, fever, and treatment with beta agonists [2, 3]. Sinus Tachycardia is considered appropriate if there is an attributable underlying cause.

Inappropriate sinus tachycardia occurs when the rhythm occurs without any known or discernable cause. Rates are typically inappropriately elevated at rest as well. One of the main causes of inappropriate sinus tachycardia is enhanced automaticity of the pacemaker cells of the sinus node [2]. A clinical condition akin to inappropriate sinus tachycardia is postural orthostatic tachycardia syndrome (POTS). In this condition, patients will demonstrate sinus tachycardia while upright, and rates improve in the supine position.

Physical Exam Correlations

On exam, the rhythm will be regular, but tachycardic. Correlation with clinical conditions will help determine if the sinus tachycardia is an appropriate response to a particular stimulus, or inappropriate and pathologic. Signs of potential secondary causes should be considered during the exam, such as hyperthyroidism, hypercortisol state (Cushing's signs), heart failure, shock, or infection.

Diagnosis/Imaging

ECG findings associated with sinus tachycardia have already been discussed and should be combined with the patient's clinical condition to discern if the sinus tachycardia is appropriate or inappropriate. Another helpful diagnostic tool is continuous cardiac rhythm monitoring. In the outpatient setting, cardiac rhythm monitors provide data over several days (24 h to 30 days) to help determine average heart rate, minimal and maximal rates, and heart rate trends. In the inpatient setting, continuous telemetry is typically used for the same purposes.

Though not discussed in detail in this section, a tilt table test (or simply having the patient stand in the office) can be used to diagnose postural orthostatic tachycardia syndrome (POTS). An increase in heart rate $\geq$ 30 bpm beyond baseline that is sustained within 10 min of being in an upright position is diagnostic for POTS in an adult patient. Blood pressure usually remains stable in the POTS patient.

Management

If there is an underlying cause of the sinus tachycardia, rates will improve once the underlying condition is treated or stimulus is withdrawn.

There is usually no need for pharmacologic therapy in this setting.

For patients with inappropriate sinus tachycardia, prognosis is typically benign, and development of tachycardia induced cardiomyopathy is rare [1]. For this reason, treatment may not be necessary and is typically aimed at reducing any associated symptoms. According to the guidelines, pharmacologic treatment may include ivabradine, which can reduce sinus node rates (Class IIa), as well as beta blockers and non-dihydropyridine calcium channel blockers (diltiazem, verapamil), assuming there are no contraindications (Class IIb) [1]. Some patients may benefit from a combination of ivabradine and beta blockers (Class IIb) [1].

Sinus node ablation is not typically performed for inappropriate sinus tachycardia because risks can significantly outweigh benefits and include the potential for development of symptomatic bradycardia requiring pacemaker placement, phrenic nerve injury, and SVC syndrome due to narrowing of the SVC and RA junction [1].

Atrial Tachycardia

Anatomy/Physiology

Atrial tachycardia is an example of an SVT that originates somewhere in the atria other than in the sinus node, and usually occurs due to enhanced automaticity of the cells in that region (though there are some ATs that may occur due to an intra-atrial micro-reentrant mechanism or triggered activity) [1, 2].

Atrial tachycardias may be focal (arising from a single focus) or multifocal (arising from multiple foci). Common sites of origination include the annulus of the mitral or tricuspid valve, the right or left atrial free wall, the left atrial appendage, pulmonary veins, superior and inferior vena cava, coronary sinus, coronary cusps, and crista terminalis [1]. Focal AT occurs more frequently in the right atrium than the left atrium [1]. Atrial tachycardias are typically paroxysmal with abrupt onset and offset, though they can be incessant in some patients.

Pathology

Atrial tachycardias may be precipitated by other medical conditions or occur independently. Multifocal atrial tachycardia is commonly associated with other comorbid conditions. The most common associated condition is underlying pulmonary disease, but other associated conditions include pulmonary hypertension, coronary disease, and valvular disease [1, 2].

Imaging

Typical ECG findings in focal atrial tachycardia include a narrow complex tachycardia (unless baseline BBB present) with atrial rates between 100–250 bpm, ventricular rates >100 bpm, and P waves with a single morphology [1–3]. The P waves of a focal atrial tachycardia are different than sinus P waves, and characteristics of the P wave morphology can help an experienced provider narrow down the location of the focal AT (superior vs inferior, left atrium vs right atrium). However, the exact location of a focal AT is generally determined by mapping during an EP study [1]. In Fig. 9.1, the P wave axis is similar to the sinus node, and the focus is located in the RA. The prolonged PR interval and P wave location within the previous T wave suggests an ectopic atrial rhythm since the PR interval often shortens in sinus tachycardia. The AV node will determine the ventricular rate of atrial tachycardia. If there is abnormal conduction through the node, intermittent block will occur (Fig. 9.2). Figure 9.3 shows an example of sinus rhythm with a sudden onset of an atrial tachycardia. The axis of the P wave suddenly changes, and this morphology is sustained in the arrhythmia. The rhythm is not initiated by a PAC but begins with increased automaticity at a focus different from the sinus node.

Typical ECG findings for multifocal atrial tachycardia (MAT) include P waves with at least three different morphologies with atrial rates >100 bpm [1, 3] (Fig. 9.4) Because there are at least three different foci in different locations, there will be variability in the PR interval and R-R

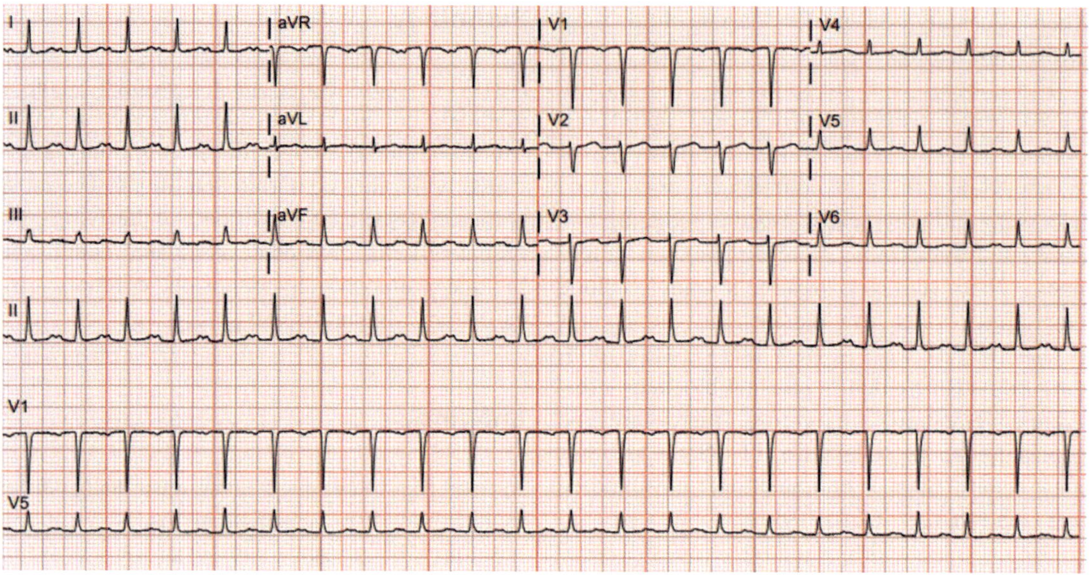

Fig. 9.1 EKG of atrial tachycardia

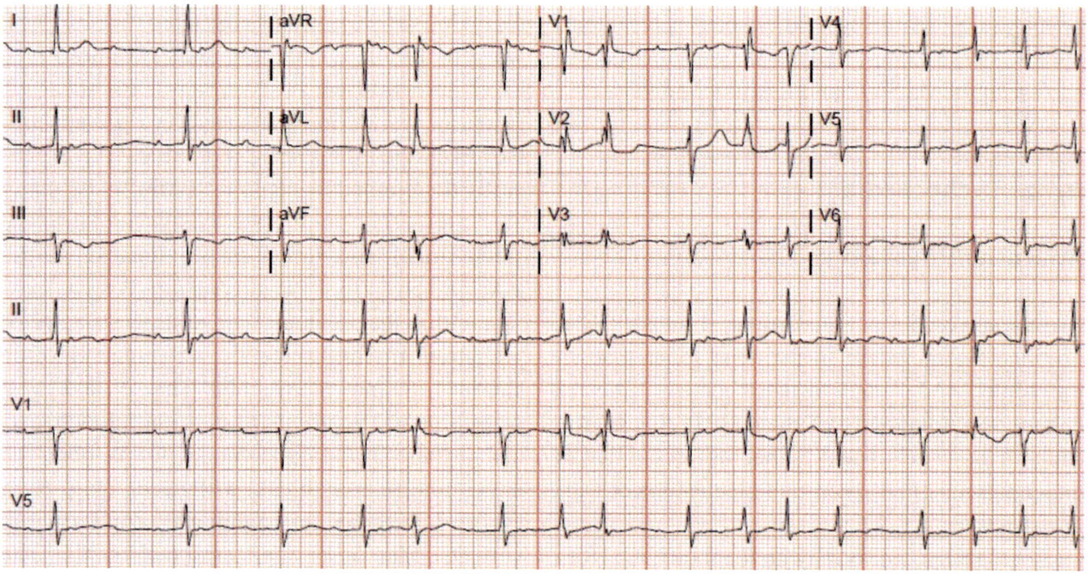

Fig. 9.2 Atrial tachycardia with variable conduction-flat baseline visible and P waves clearly visible

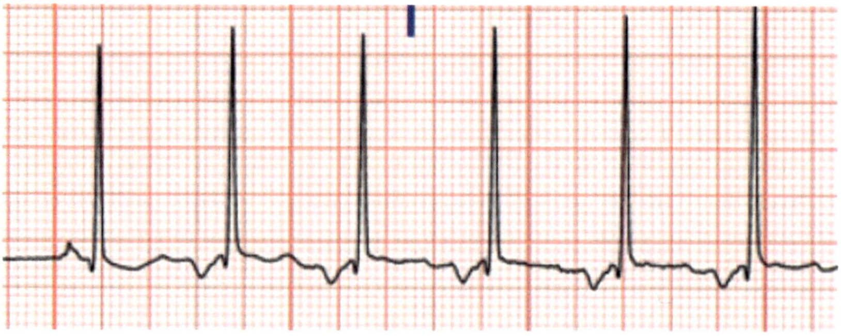

Fig. 9.3 Strip of atrial tach. The first beat being sinus, then change in P wave morphology during the tachycardia

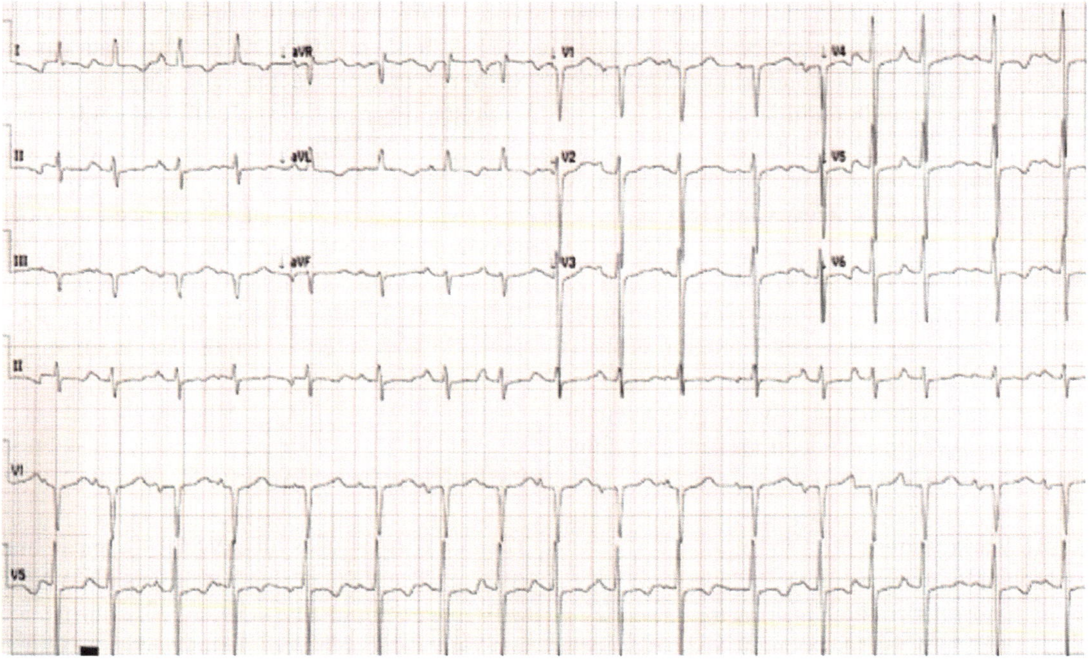

Fig. 9.4 EKG of multifocal atrial tachycardia (MAT). Note the 3+ morphologies of the P wave

interval, which can sometimes lead to an erroneous diagnosis of atrial fibrillation. However, unlike atrial fibrillation, an isoelectric line should be clearly visible between P waves [1, 3].

Management

As previously mentioned, atrial tachycardias may be precipitated by other medical conditions or occur independently. For some, treatment of an underlying condition or mechanism may result in termination of the arrhythmia. Otherwise, treatment for focal atrial tachycardia involves pharmacologic therapy or ablation.

Focal Atrial Tachycardia

Acute Management [1]

- IV beta blockers or non-dihydropyridine calcium channel blockers (diltiazem/verapamil) in hemodynamically stable patients (Class I).
- Synchronized cardioversion in hemodynamically unstable patients (Class I).
- Adenosine can be helpful to restore sinus rhythm or diagnose the mechanism of the tachycardia (Class IIa).
  - Automatic focal AT: may see transient suppression.
  - Triggered focal AT: adenosine can effectively terminate.
  - Re-entrant focal AT: adenosine will likely not be effective.
- IV amiodarone may be reasonable to restore sinus rhythm or slow ventricular rate in hemodynamically stable patients.
- IV Ibutilide may be reasonable to restore sinus rhythm in hemodynamically stable patients.

Ongoing management [1]

- Catheter ablation as alternative to pharmacologic therapy (Class I).
  - Success rates usually >90–95% with complication rate <1–2%.
- Oral beta blockers or non-dihydropyridine calcium channel blockers if no other contraindication exists (Class IIa).

- Flecainide or propafenone in patients without structural heart disease or ischemic heart disease (Class IIa) in combination with beta blocker, verapamil, or diltiazem.
- Oral sotalol or amiodarone may be reasonable, but due to risk of proarrhythmia, need to balance risk and benefits (Class IIb).

Multifocal Atrial Tachycardia

First-line treatment is typically aimed at managing the underlying associated condition if one is identified. However, if further treatment is needed, management typically includes attempts at slowing AV node conduction. Antiarrhythmic medications are not generally helpful [1].

Acute Management [1]

- IV metoprolol or verapamil (Class IIa).
  - If no other contraindication to its use exists, verapamil is likely preferred over beta blocker therapy since beta blockers can worsen underlying pulmonary disease, especially those with bronchospasm as the etiology of the rhythm.

Ongoing Management [1]

- Oral verapamil or diltiazem is reasonable for patients with recurrent, symptomatic MAT (Class IIa).
- Metoprolol is reasonable, but typically avoided in patients with pulmonary disease (Class IIa).

AV Node Reentry Tachycardia (AVNRT)

Anatomy and Physiology

AV Node Reentry Tachycardia (AVNRT) is the most common type of SVT, and the anatomic substrate is a re-entry circuit consisting of fast and slow pathways (dual pathways) within or around the AV node [1, 2]. The slow pathway has a shorter refractory period, while the fast pathway has a longer refractory period. AVNRT is typically triggered when a premature beat enters one of these pathways when that pathway is recovered and not in the refractory phase, but while the other pathway is still in the refractory phase, further details of which are reviewed below.

Clues that may help an experienced provider determine if an SVT is AVNRT, either typical or atypical, include: (1) characteristics of the start and end of the arrhythmia, (2) identifiable triggers, (3) R-P interval length/relation of the P wave to the QRS.

Pathology/Description

There are two types of AVNRT—typical and atypical. The EKG during both forms of AVNRT will appear minimally different. The difference can only be confirmed during an invasive EP study.

Typical AVNRT

Typical AVNRT is usually triggered by a premature atrial complex (PAC), which is blocked at the refractory fast pathway and travels down the fully recovered slow pathway to the ventricle (anterograde conduction) [2, 3]. Once the impulse reaches the end of the slow pathway, it exits and travels down the His bundle to activate the ventricles, while simultaneously traveling back up the fast pathway to the atria (retrograde conduction) [2, 3]. The atria are then reactivated, and the electrical impulse then re-enters the slow pathway and travels the same circuit repeatedly resulting in a re-entrant tachycardia [2, 3]. Typical AVNRT is also called "slow-fast" AVNRT for this reason. Atrial and ventricular activation is nearly simultaneous [2, 3].

Atypical AVNRT

In atypical AVNRT, anterograde conduction occurs via the fast pathway, and retrograde conduction occurs via the slow pathway, again resulting in a re-entrant tachycardia [2, 3]. This is also called "fast-slow" AVNRT.

Physical Exam Correlations

AVNRT is typically well tolerated in patients with structurally normal hearts. Symptoms may include palpitations, shortness of breath, feelings of anxiety, lightheadedness, and possibly chest pain. Syncope can occur if rates are fast enough. If the SVT occurs in patients with coronary disease, cardiomyopathy, or valvular stenosis, they may develop hypotension, ischemia, heart failure, or syncope. Prognosis in the absence of heart disease is usually quite good [1].

Imaging

ECGs and continuous cardiac rhythm monitoring are performed to help confirm the presence of an SVT suspected to be AVNRT. Ventricular rates are typically 180–200 bpm but may have a wider range. Both Holter monitors and continuous telemetry monitors are helpful for diagnosis.

Typical AVNRT

ECGs will show a narrow complex tachycardia with regular R-R intervals, and because of the nearly simultaneous atrial and ventricular activation, P waves may be buried in the QRS and not visible on the ECG. However, if activation of the atria and ventricles are not exactly in synch, a retrograde P wave may be observed on the ECG near the end of the QRS complex (Fig. 9.5) [3]. Since the P wave is located closer to the prior QRS complex than the subsequent QRS complex, typical AVNRT may be called a "short RP tachycardia." These retrograde P waves will be inverted in the inferior leads because of the retrograde activation of the atria [2, 3].

Atypical AVNRT

The ECG will usually show a narrow complex tachycardia with regular R-R intervals and a retrograde P wave in front of the next QRS [3]. Because of the location of the P wave, the RP interval is longer than the PR interval and may be termed as "long RP tachycardia" [1, 2].

Management

Acute Management [1]

- Vagal maneuvers should be first-line treatment/intervention (Class I). Examples:
  - Valsalva.
  - Carotid sinus massage after absence of bruit is confirmed.
  - Ice-cold wet towel to face.
- If vagal maneuvers are not effective, adenosine is the first-line drug choice (Class I).
  - Considered both therapeutic and diagnostic. Adenosine will be successful in converting AVNRT in ~95% of patients and

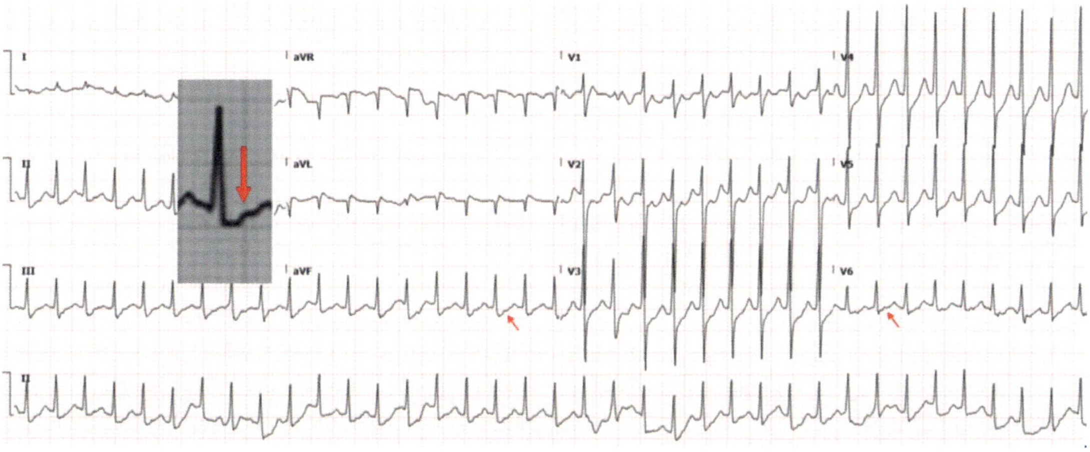

Fig. 9.5 EKG of typical AVNRT. Red arrows points to retrograde P wave immediately after QRS suggestive of AVNRT

may more clearly reveal atrial activity in arrhythmias such as atrial tachycardia or atrial flutter.
  - The initial dose is 6 mg given rapidly. If the first dose of adenosine does not convert the patient to sinus rhythm, up to two more doses of adenosine can be given at 12 mg each.
- Synchronized cardioversion in hemodynamically unstable patients if vagal maneuvers or adenosine do not convert the tachycardia or aren't feasible (Class I).
- Synchronized cardioversion (Class I) in hemodynamically stable patients when pharmacologic therapy isn't successful or is contraindicated (i.e., Bronchospasm).
- IV beta blockers or IV non-dihydropyridine calcium channel blockers are reasonable if no other contraindications exist in hemodynamically stable patients without pre-excitation (Class IIa).
- Oral beta blockers, diltiazem, or verapamil may be reasonable in hemodynamically stable patients assuming no other contraindications to their use (Class IIb).
- IV amiodarone can be considered in hemodynamically stable patients if other therapies are contraindicated or ineffective (Class IIb).

Ongoing Management [1]

If episodes are short, infrequent, and well tolerated, or if the patient can terminate episodes easily with vagal maneuvers, no prophylactic treatment may be needed. Some patients may respond well to as needed, "pill in the pocket" short acting beta blockers or calcium channel blockers. Another option is daily, longer acting beta blocker or calcium channel blocker therapy.

- Oral verapamil or diltiazem for patients who are not candidates for, or do not wish to undergo, catheter ablation if no other contraindication exists (Class I).
- Catheter ablation (Chap. 12) of the slow pathway (slow pathway modification) is first-line treatment (Class I).
  - Success rates typically >95%.
  - Risk of AV block is <1%.
  - Radiofrequency or cryoablation may be utilized—acute success rates are equivalent, however, with cryoablation, there is lower chance of AV block but higher rate of recurrence observed long term.
- Oral beta blockers are recommended in those who are not candidates for or prefer not to undergo ablation (Class I).
- Flecainide or propafenone—reasonable for patients who do not have structural or ischemic heart disease in those who are contraindicated or prefer not to undergo, catheter ablation and in whom rate control medications (BBs/CCBs) are ineffective or contraindicated (Class IIa).
- If minimally symptomatic, no pharmacologic therapy or ablation is reasonable (Class IIa).
- Oral sotalol or dofetilide may be reasonable in patients who are not candidates for, or prefer not to undergo, ablation (Class IIb).
  - These medications can be used in patients with structural heart disease or coronary artery disease, but initiation is done in the inpatient setting with continuous telemetry monitoring and serial ECGs due to potential for QT prolongation and torsades de pointes. Typically, these agents are reserved for patients who are not responsive to or are not candidates for treatments already outlined.
- Pill-in-the-pocket (self-administered) acute doses of as needed oral beta blockers or calcium channel blockers may be reasonable if AVNRT is infrequent and well-tolerated (Class IIB).

AV Re-entry Tachycardia (AVRT)

Anatomy and Physiology

AV Reentry tachycardia (AVRT) is the second most common type of SVT. The anatomic substrate for this type of SVT is a reentry circuit involving the AV node and a bypass tract, which directly connects the atrium and the ventricle [1]. Because of the direct connection between the atrium and ventricle, the normal conduction through the AV node and His-Purkinje system can be bypassed. These bypass tracts are also referred to as accessory pathways and can be manifest or concealed. They can conduct anterograde (A-V conduction), retrograde (V-A conduction), or both. [1, 2]

Pathways are manifest if they conduct in the anterograde direction and demonstrate pre-excitation with a short PR interval and a delta wave on the ECG [1–3]. Pre-excitation occurs when a specific area of ventricular myocardium is excited early due to the accessory pathway and starts to conduct prior to the impulse traveling down the His-Purkinje system to cause depolarization of the myocardium. This causes the PR interval to appear shorter as the ventricle starts contracting shortly after the P wave. The "delta" wave is the combination of the normal conduction down the AV node and early excitation of an area of myocardium caused by conduction down the accessory pathway. Manifest pathways can conduct in both the anterograde and retrograde direction but may only conduct in the anterograde direction. Experienced providers may be able to localize the bypass tract based on certain ECG characteristics.

Pathways are concealed if they only conduct retrograde and do not demonstrate pre-excitation on the ECG [1, 2].

Pathology/Description

When a bypass tract is present, an impulse can travel from the atrium to the ventricle via the AV node or via the bypass tract.

- Orthodromic AVRT—the impulse travels from the atrium to the ventricles in the anterograde direction through the AV node and returns to the atrium via the bypass tract in the retrograde direction [1, 2]. Orthodromic AVRT exhibits a narrow complex QRS because the ventricles are activated through the AV node, which is the normal activation pathway [3].
- Antidromic AVRT—the impulse travels from the atrium to the ventricles in the anterograde direction through the bypass tract and returns to the atrium via the AV node in the retrograde direct [1, 2]. Antidromic AVRT exhibits a wider complex QRS because the ventricles are activated outside of the normal conduction system through the bypass tract [3]. (In rare instances, an antidromic AVRT may consist of two bypass tracts instead of a bypass tract and the AV node.

In AVRT, the AV node is typically the slower pathway and the bypass tract is typically the faster pathway, though this is not always the case [2]. The reentry circuit in AVRT is known as a macro-reentry tachycardia because it involves a larger amount of cardiac tissue than that of AVNRT [2, 3]. Because of the size of the circuit, the atria and ventricles are not activated in synchrony, so P waves are typically seen on the ECG and not buried within the QRS if the QRS is narrow. As with AVNRT, there are typical and atypical forms of AVRT and P waves can occur after (typical) or before (atypical) the QRS [2]. It may not be possible to distinguish AVNRT and AVRT from the ECG alone, however, there may be higher suspicion for one or the other based on length of the RP interval (typically >80 ms in AVRT due to the larger tissue mass and time needed to traverse the re-entry circuit), and proximity of the retrograde P wave to the QRS for the same reason [2]. In AVNRT, the P wave is generally closer or connected to the QRS complex, but in AVRT, the P wave is likely separated from the QRS complex.

Management of Orthodromic AVRT (Narrow Complex AVRT)

Management of narrow complex AVRT is similar to the management of AVNRT described earlier, because the AVRT circuit is dependent on the AV node for conduction of the tachyarrhythmia. Thus, anything that interferes with conduction through the AV node can also inhibit an AVRT arrhythmia.

Acute management [1]

- Vagal maneuvers (Class I).
- Adenosine (Class I) can convert orthodromic AVRT in 90–95% of patients.
- Synchronized cardioversion in hemodynamically unstable patients if vagal maneuvers and adenosine ineffective or not feasible (Class I).
- Synchronized cardioversion in hemodynamically stable patients when pharmacologic therapy is ineffective or not feasible (Class I).
- Synchronized cardioversion in hemodynamically unstable patients with pre-excited atrial fibrillation (AF) (Class I).
- Ibutilide or IV procainamide in patients with pre-excited AF who are hemodynamically stable (Class I).
  - Both medications can decrease ventricular rate by slowing conduction over the accessory pathway and may possibly terminate AF.
- IV diltiazem, verapamil, or beta blockers can be effective for orthodromic AVRT who do not have pre-excitation on resting ECG during sinus rhythm (Class IIa).
- IV BB/CCB can be considered in patients with orthodromic AVRT who have pre-excitation on resting ECG and have not responded to other therapies (Class IIb), however, these therapies have a risk of enhancing conduction over the accessory pathway if the AVRT converts to AF and the ability of promptly perform electrical cardioversion must be available should this occur.
- IV digoxin, IV amiodarone, IV and oral BB/CCB are potentially harmful in patients with pre-excited AF (Class III) because these medications can enhance conduction over the accessory pathway, increase ventricular rate, and increase risk of ventricular arrhythmias.

Ongoing Management [1]

- Catheter ablation of accessory pathway (class I) in patients who have had AF and/or AVRT.
  - 93–95% success rate
- Oral BB/CCB in patients without pre-excitation on resting ECG (Class I).
- Oral flecainide or propafenone is reasonable in patients without structural heart disease or ischemic heart disease who have AVRT and/or pre-excited AF and are not candidates for, or prefer not to undergo, catheter ablation (Class IIa).
  - These agents slow or block conduction over the accessory pathway.
- Oral dofetilide or sotalol may be reasonable in patients with AVRT and/or pre-excited AF who are not candidates for, or prefer not to undergo, catheter ablation (Class IIa).
  - Can be used in patients with structural or ischemic heart disease but need to consider risk of QT prolongation/torsades/medication interactions, and other possible contraindications.
- Oral amiodarone may be considered with AVRT and/or pre-excited AF patients who are not candidates for, or prefer not to undergo, catheter ablation in whom BB/CCB/flecainide/propafenone are ineffective or contraindicated (Class IIb).
  - Need to consider possible toxicities associated with long-term amiodarone use.
- Oral BB/CCB may be reasonable for patients with orthodromic AVRT and pre-excitation on resting ECG who are not candidates for, or prefer not to undergo, catheter ablation (class IIb), however, these patients may develop AF during an episode of AVRT and be at increased risk of rapid conduction over the accessory pathway, so need to exercise caution with these agents.
- Oral digoxin may be reasonable in orthodromic AVRT without pre-excitation if not a candidate for, or prefer not to undergo, catheter ablation (Class IIb).
- Oral digoxin potential harmful in patients with AVRT or AF and pre-excitation on resting ECG (Class III) because digoxin shortens the refractory period of the accessory pathway.

Wolff-Parkinson-White

WPW Pattern Vs WPW Syndrome

The distinguishing factor here is the presence or absence of arrhythmia. Patients with WPW pattern have pre-excitation that is manifest on the ECG in the absence of symptomatic arrhythmia. Patients with WPW syndrome have pre-excitation that is manifest on the ECG associated with symptomatic arrhythmias.

As previously outlined, impulse conduction through the AV node is delayed, but this same delay does not occur in the bypass tract. Therefore, the impulse travels faster down the bypass tract, resulting in premature activation of the ventricles [1, 2]. Because of the earlier ventricular activation, the characteristic ECG findings of WPW include a short PR interval and a slurring of the initial portion of the QRS complex, known as a delta wave [1]. The delta wave may be more or less prominent depending on a couple of factors: (1) the proximity of the bypass tract to the sinus node and (2) how much of the myocardium is activated via the bypass tract [1, 2] (see Fig. 9.6a, b).

One of the primary concerns with WPW is the risk of sudden cardiac death. This is because of the absence of the delay in impulse conduction down the accessory pathway. This is of particular concern, for example, if a patient with WPW also develops atrial fibrillation. With atrial fibrillation,

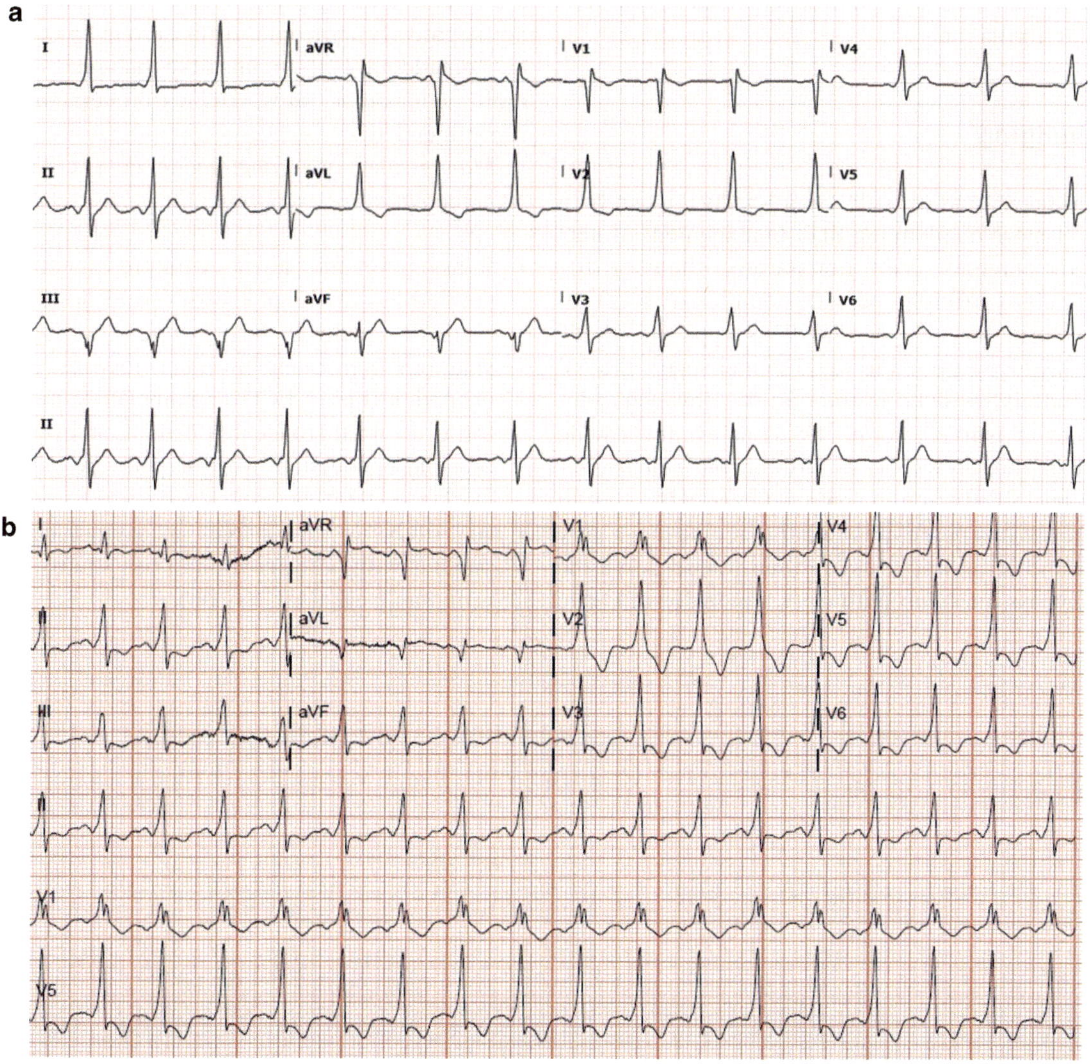

Fig. 9.6 (**a**) EKG of WPW. A delta wave is visible at the beginning of the QRS complex. (**b**) Another EKG of WPW

the atrial rate can range from 300–600 beats per minute. In patients without an accessory pathway, the AV node acts as a gatekeeper between the atria and the ventricles, and, though it may allow for some degree of rapid conduction to the ventricle, it will not allow all the atrial impulses to conduct through. Thus, the ventricular rate will generally only be allowed to increase to a rate around 200 bpm or so (though this upper rate can vary) when the AV node/His-Purkinje system is utilized. Accessory pathways do not have the same gatekeeping properties of the AV node. Therefore, the hundreds of impulses generated from atrial fibrillation conducting ungoverned down an accessory pathway can lead to ventricular fibrillation.

Imaging

Management of wide complex AVRT can be a bit more challenging than management of narrow complex AVRT. For starters, it may be difficult to differentiate wide complex AVRT from ventricular tachycardia. This type of AVRT may also respond to vagal maneuvers if the AV node is involved in the circuit. However, adenosine is likely not the first-line agent for wide complex AVRT [1, 2]. Adenosine can trigger atrial fibrillation in some patients, which could result in a potentially lethal outcome if the very rapid atrial impulses are then forced down the bypass tract (fast pathway), which doesn't have the slowing properties and governance that the AV node has [2] (see Fig. 9.7). In some patients, atrial fibrillation could degenerate to ventricular fibrillation. For this reason, AV nodal agents should also be avoided [1, 2]. Another reason adenosine and AV nodal agents may not be preferred is that the circuit may include two bypass tracts instead of the AV node and a bypass tract. If the AV node is not involved, then agents directed at slowing AV node conduction will not be effective. First-line agents for the acute management of wide complex AVRT include the antiarrhythmics procainamide and ibutilide [2]. These antiarrhythmics are effective at blocking bypass tracts and are not negatively inotropic. Amiodarone can also be considered [2]. In unstable patients with rapid ventricular rates, DC cardioversion is recommended.

Management of Asymptomatic Patients with Asymptomatic Pre-excitation [1]*:*

- In asymptomatic patients with pre-excitation, the findings of abrupt loss of conduction over a manifest pathway during exercise testing in sinus rhythm or intermittent loss of pre-excitation during ECG or ambulatory monitoring are useful to identify patients at low risk of rapid conduction over the pathway (Class I).
- EP study is reasonable in asymptomatic patients with pre-excitation to risk stratify for arrhythmic events (Class IIa).

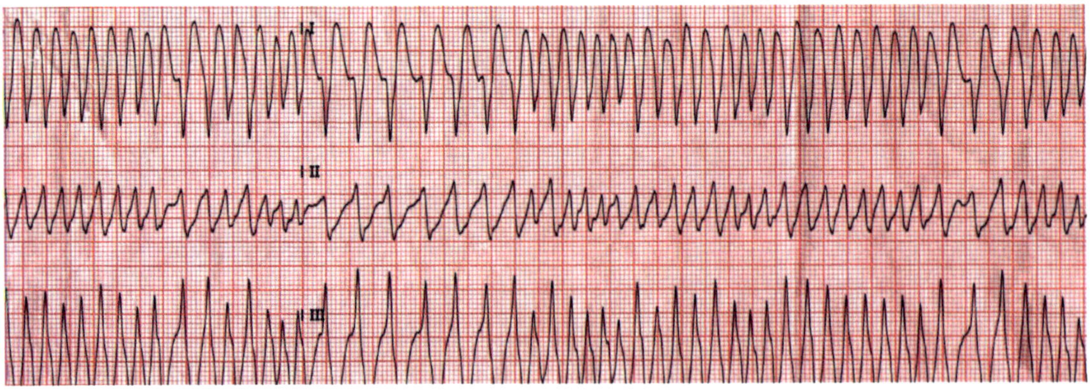

Fig. 9.7 Pre-excited atrial fibrillation

- Catheter ablation of an accessory pathway is reasonable in asymptomatic patients with pre-excitation in an EP study that identifies a high risk of arrhythmic events, including rapidly conduction pre-excited AF (Class IIa).
- Catheter ablation of the accessory pathway is reasonable in asymptomatic patients if the presence of pre-excitation precludes specific employment (such as with pilots) (Class IIA).
- Observation, without further evaluation or treatment, is reasonable in asymptomatic patients with pre-excitation (Class IIa).

Management of Symptomatic Patients with Manifest Accessory Pathways [1]:

- In symptomatic patients with pre-excitation, the findings of abrupt loss of conduction over the pathway during exercise testing in sinus rhythm or intermittent loss of pre-excitation during ECG or ambulatory monitoring are useful for identifying patients at low risk of developing rapid conduction over the pathway (Class I).
- An EP study is useful in symptomatic patients with pre-excitation to risk stratify for life-threatening arrhythmic events (Class I).

Atrial Flutter

Anatomy and Physiology

Atrial flutter is a type of macro-re-entrant SVT, and the re-entry circuit occurs within the right atrium. The atrial rate is usually about 250–350 beats per minute, and the classic ECG pattern of atrial flutter is the characteristic *regular* "sawtooth" appearance of the flutter waves [3]. The circuit can be counterclockwise or clockwise [1, 2].

Typical atrial flutter, or counter-clockwise atrial flutter, is the most common type of atrial flutter. In typical atrial flutter, an impulse travels down the lateral free wall of the right atrium and back up the septum in a counter-clockwise direction [1]. In reverse typical flutter, or clockwise flutter, the re-entry circuit is the same, but the direction the impulse travels is opposite—that is, the impulse travels down the septum and back up the lateral free wall of the right atrium in a clockwise direction [1]. Part of this circuit involves an area in the right atrium between the ostium of the tricuspid valve and the inferior vena cava, known as the cavotricuspid isthmus (CTI) [1, 2]. Therefore, typical and reverse typical atrial flutters are also known as CTI-dependent atrial flutters.

Atrial flutters can also occur in the left atrium near the pulmonary veins or around scar or surgical lesions. Other circuits include paths around the mitral annulus and re-entry involving the LA roof. This type of flutter is termed atypical flutter (or non-isthmus dependent) and circuits are categorized as either macro-re-entrant or micro-re-entrant [1, 2] (Fig. 9.8).

Patients with atrial flutter are at increased risk of having concomitant atrial fibrillation or of developing atrial fibrillation in the future. According to the 2015 AHA/ACC/HRS SVT guidelines, 22–50% of patients developed AF after CTI ablation after mean follow-up of 14–30 months and risk factors for developing AF included LV dysfunction, presence of structural or ischemic heart disease, inducible AF, and increased left atrial size [1].

Patients with atrial flutter are at the same risk of thromboembolism as patients with atrial fibrillation, and recommendations for anticoagulation are the same for atrial flutter as for atrial fibrillation [1].

Imaging

ECG

- The classic ECG pattern of atrial flutter is the characteristic *regular* "sawtooth" appearance of the atrial flutter waves; the atrial rate is typically 250–350 bpm and the ventricular rate can be variable [3]. QRS will usually be narrow unless there is a pre-existing bundle branch block or aberrancy.
- *Typical atrial flutter*: flutter waves are usually inverted in leads II, III, and AVF and upright in V1 [2, 3] (Fig. 9.9).

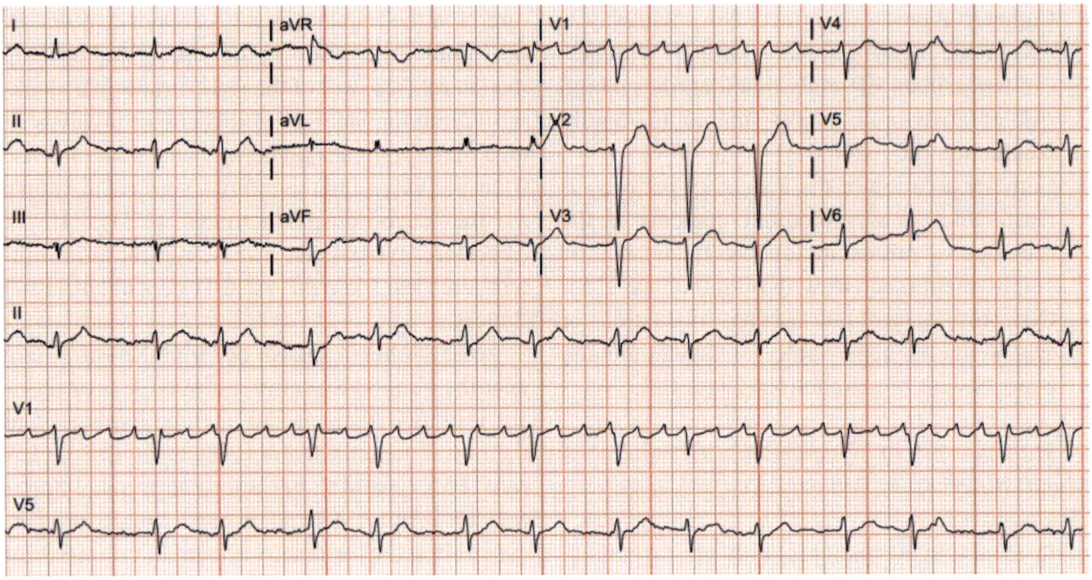

Fig. 9.8 EKG of atypical atrial flutter. The flutter waves are less sawtooth in appearance, narrow, and organized as seen in lead V1

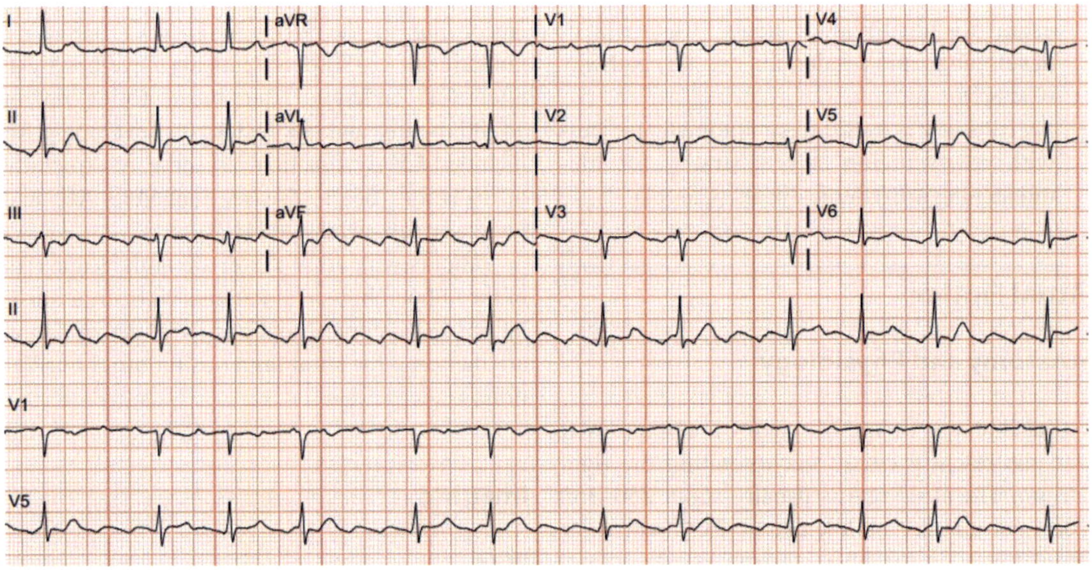

Fig. 9.9 EKG of typical atrial flutter. Note the negative flutter waves in the inferior leads

- *Reverse typical flutter*: flutter waves are usually upright in leads II, III, and AVF and inverted in V1 [2, 3].

For some, differentiating atrial flutter and atrial tachycardia can be difficult. Some helpful tips for ECG differentiation include the following:

- Atrial rate: the atrial rate with atrial flutter is typically 250–350 bpm. Atrial rate with atrial tachycardia is typically 150–250 bpm [2, 3].
- P wave morphology: in atrial flutter the P wave is usually inverted in leads II, III, AVF. Atrial tachycardia usually shows upright P wave in lead II, III, AVF [2, 3].

Management

Acute management of atrial flutter is typically focused on patient stability, anticoagulation for stroke prevention, rate control, and conversion to sinus rhythm. Atrial flutter can be more difficult to rate control than atrial fibrillation.

Acute Management

- In unstable patients in whom atrial flutter is poorly tolerated, direct current cardioversion is a Class I recommendation [1].
- If a patient is stable and not in decompensated heart failure or hypotensive, rate control with AV nodal agents, such as the nondihydropyridine calcium channel blockers or beta blockers, can be attempted and have a class I recommendation [1].
- IV amiodarone can be useful for rate control in the absence of pre-excitation in patients with flutter and CHF when BB are contraindicated or ineffective (Class IIa) [1].
  - Amiodarone has less negative inotropic effect than BB/CCB and may produce less hypotension [1].
  - Though unlikely to convert a patient to sinus rhythm, the potential to do so exists, so potential risks and benefits should be considered for patients with flutter ≥48 h duration who are not adequately anticoagulated [1].
- In stable patients, conversion to sinus rhythm can be achieved electrically with direct current cardioversion, or pharmacologically, with an antiarrhythmic drug. Prior to proceeding with cardioversion (either electric or pharmacologic), if arrhythmia onset is >48 h or unknown, the presence of a left atrial appendage thrombus will need to be ruled out, either by TEE or CT [1]. The most common antiarrhythmic agents (Chap. 7) used for converting a patient to sinus rhythm include procainamide (1A antiarrhythmic), flecainide or propafenone (1C antiarrhythmics), and amiodarone or Ibutilide (Class III antiarrhythmics). Factors to consider when choosing an agent for pharmacologic cardioversion include the presence of structural heart disease, presence of coronary artery disease, renal function, and presence of ECG abnormalities such as IVCD/bundle branch block, QRS duration, QT duration [2, 4]. In patients with a pacemaker or defibrillator with the presence of an atrial pacing wire, rapid atrial pacing is useful for acute conversion of atrial flutter (Class I)—this is known as pace termination and recommendations for anticoagulation are the same as that for pharmacologic and electrical cardioversion [1].

Anticoagulation

Anticoagulation should be considered in all patients, especially if the onset of arrhythmia duration is greater than 48 hours or unknown. The CHA2DS2VASc score is used to calculate stroke risk and components include CHF/LV dysfunction, hypertension, age, diabetes, prior stroke/TIA, presence of vascular disease, and gender. In the acute setting, if not contraindicated, IV heparin can be utilized with subsequent transition to a direct oral anticoagulant (apixaban, rivaroxaban, or dabigatran) or warfarin (once INR therapeutic). Anticoagulation should be continued uninterrupted for at least 1 month post cardioversion, but possibly longer depending on the CHA2DS2VASC score [1, 5].

Ongoing Management

Long-term treatment for right-sided (typical and reverse typical) atrial flutter includes consideration of EP study and flutter ablation (Class I recommendation) [1]. Because the re-entry circuit involves the cavotricuspid isthmus, that area is usually the target site for ablation. Ablation has a very high success rate for treatment and elimination of right-sided atrial flutter and should be considered for most patients who are otherwise not contraindicated for ablation. Patients will need to be able to tolerate anticoagulation for up to 1 month prior to ablation and 4–6 weeks post flutter ablation [1, 5].

For patients who are hemodynamically stable, but otherwise contraindicated or do not wish to undergo catheter ablation, beta blockers/calcium channel blockers are useful with Class I recommendation [1].

As previously mentioned, patients with atrial flutter are at increased risk of developing or having concomitant atrial fibrillation. Up to 80% or more of patients who undergo typical flutter ablation will develop AF within 5 years [1]. For this reason, even if atrial flutter is treated with ablation, ongoing surveillance for development of atrial fibrillation should be considered, as well as addressing risk factors. One method for ongoing monitoring includes placement of an ambulatory monitor to look for atrial fibrillation. Other methods emerging include wearables or patient-centered monitoring devices including watches with ECG capabilities (e.g., Apple Watch®) and the FDA-approved KardiaMobile® EKG monitor.

Atrial Fibrillation

Atrial fibrillation is a relatively common arrhythmia and prevalence increases with age (Table 9.1). Symptoms associated with atrial fibrillation have a wide distribution and range from completely asymptomatic to severe. It is typically associated with underlying structural heart disease (CAD, CHF, valvular heart disease) and other chronic conditions, such as hypertension and diabetes [2, 5]. Atrial fibrillation is a progressive condition in which episodes generally increase in frequency and duration over time and may become persistent if left untreated. Similar to atrial flutter, atrial fibrillation is associated with increased risk of stroke and CHF.

Table 9.1 Definitions of atrial fibrillation

- Paroxysmal AF—self-terminating or intermittent; resolves spontaneously or within 7 days of onset [5]
- Persistent AF—rhythm is sustained greater than 7 days. Fails to self-terminate but can be terminated with pharmacologic or electric cardioversion [5]
- Long-standing persistent AF—continuous AF of greater than 12 months duration [5]
- Permanent AF—this term is used when the decision has been made to stop attempts at restoring sinus rhythm [5]
- Nonvalvular AF—AF that occurs in the absence of moderate to severe mitral stenosis or a mechanical heart valve [6]
- Valvular AF—generally refers to AF that occurs in the setting of moderate to severe mitral stenosis or in the presence of an artificial (mechanical) heart valve [6]

Anatomy and Physiology

Atrial fibrillation is a supraventricular arrhythmia that is characterized by uncoordinated atrial activity, with atrial rates >350 bpm [2, 4, 5]. As a result, there is a decrease in the atrial mechanical function with an associated irregular ventricular response. The uncoordinated atrial activity results in the loss of effective atrial contraction, also known as "atrial kick", and can decrease ventricular filling and cardiac output [4, 5]. The mechanisms that underlie AF are likely multifactorial and involve multiple independent reentrant wavelets that exist within the atria, and are primarily initiated by focal triggers that originate at or near the pulmonary veins in the left atrium [2, 4, 5]. Structural and electrophysiologic abnormalities can alter the properties of atrial tissue and allow for abnormal impulse initiation or conduction. Some precipitants include alcohol, drugs, caffeine, exercise, stress/emotion, sleep apnea, obesity, and hyperthyroidism [4, 5].

Physical Exam Correlation

Symptoms can be variable and range from no symptoms to fatigue, shortness of breath, palpitations/cardiac awareness, weakness, dizziness, lightheadedness, hypotension, heart failure, and even syncope. Some patients who are initially asymptomatic may develop heart failure symptoms if tachycardia-induced cardiomyopathy occurs. Some patients present with TIA or stroke symptoms. If associated with valvular heart disease, a murmur may be present on exam. Pulse rate will be irregularly irregular.

Imaging

- ECG/telemetry monitoring:
  - Characteristic ECG findings include irregular R-R intervals, absence of discrete P waves, and irregular atrial activity (which may be fine or coarse) [2, 5] (see Fig. 9.10).
  - There are several types of wearable devices available as well, that have ECG recording capabilities. One such device is the Apple Watch™. Another device is the KardiaMobile® device (or AliveCor® monitor).
- Transthoracic echocardiogram:
  - All patients with AF should have an echocardiogram performed. This is helpful in determining LVEF, evaluation of the LA and RA sizes, and determine if there is any concomitant valve disease.
- Transesophageal echocardiogram:
  - A transesophageal echo is more sensitive for evaluating possible left atrial appendage (LAA) thrombus and should be performed in patients being considered for either pharmacologic or electric cardioversion if duration of AF is > 48 h or unknown [5] (see Fig. 9.11).
- Cardiac CT:
  - A structural cardiac CT can also evaluate the LAA for thrombus reliably.
- Ischemic evaluation in those without previously diagnosed CAD is helpful in guiding pharmacotherapy since some antiarrhythmics are contraindicated in patients with underlying CAD. Options for ischemic evaluation include stress testing, CT of the coronaries, cardiac MRI with stress, or cardiac catheterization. Decision on which type of test is pursued is typically guided by associated symptoms, history, and if any possible contraindication to a particular test exists (ex. renal dysfunction for CT/catheterization, etc.).
- Thyroid testing to evaluate for clinical or subclinical hyperthyroidism.

Management

- *Rate control* (Chap. 7).
  - Beta blockers.
    - Metoprolol.
    - Atenolol.
    - Carvedilol.

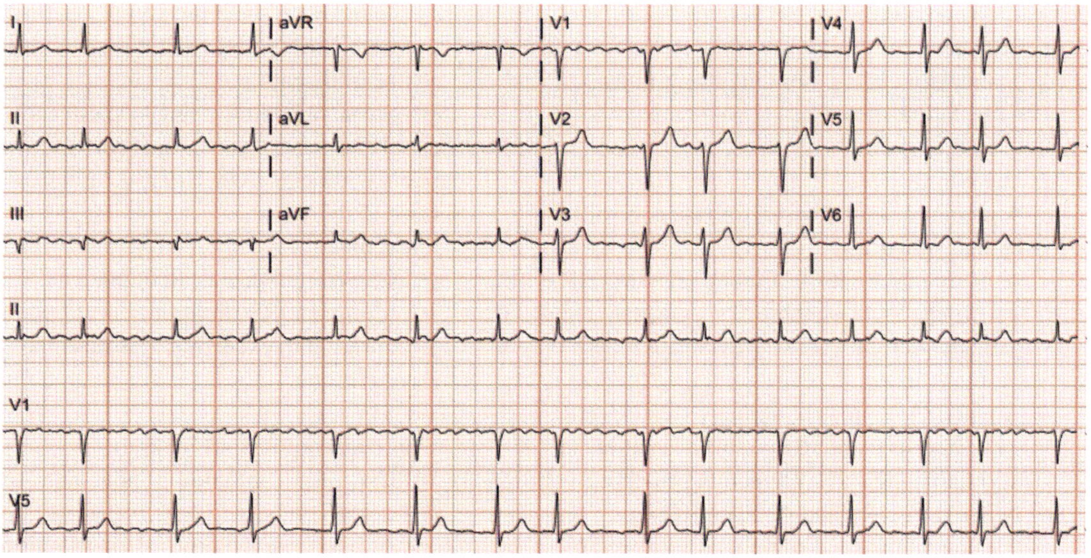

Fig. 9.10 EKG of atrial fibrillation with irregular R-R intervals. No discernible P waves or PR interval confirms the diagnosis of AF. Irregular R to R intervals can be rhythms other than AF: NSR with PAC's, wandering atrial pacemaker, MAT are often misdiagnosed as AF

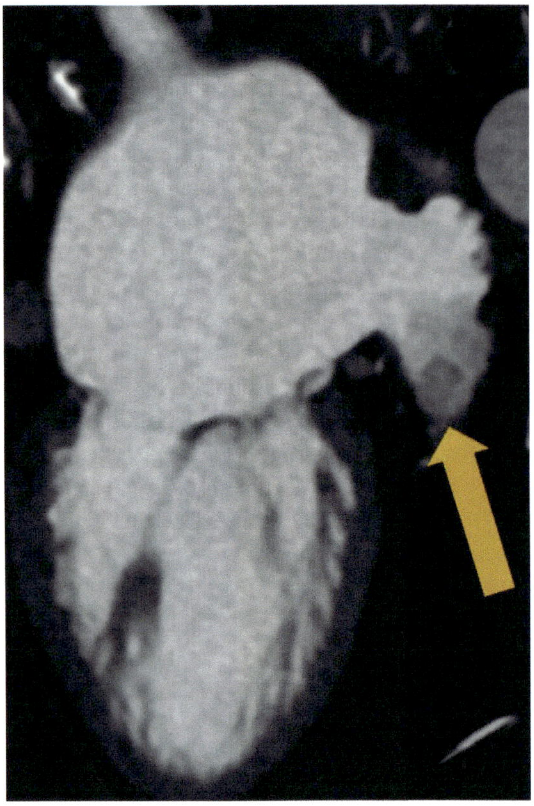

Fig. 9.11 Image of clot seen in left atrial appendage

Esmolol.
Propranolol.

- Calcium channel blockers—nondihydropyridine.
  - Diltiazem.
  - Verapamil.
- Digoxin.
- Amiodarone can be used for rate control in certain situations.
- A heart rate control strategy (resting HR <80 bpm) is reasonable for symptomatic patients. – ACC/AHA/HRS and AFFIRM [5, 6].
- A lenient rate control strategy (resting HR <110 bpm) may be reasonable if a patient is asymptomatic and LV function preserved. – ACC/AHA/HRS and AFFIRM [5, 6].
- Permanent pacemaker implant followed by AV nodal ablation can be one method for rate control if the arrhythmia is refractory to pharmacologic therapy. However, this method is irreversible and results in pacemaker dependency, so is usually reserved as a last option [5, 6].

- *Rhythm control.*
- There are multiple considerations when choosing an appropriate antiarrhythmic agent, including presence/absence of CAD, left ventricular function, LV wall thickness, renal function, liver function, ECG characteristics such as QT interval, presence of IVCD/BBB, AV block, and other medications that can be relative or absolute contraindications if used alongside a particular antiarrhythmic [5, 6]. Drug selection is mainly guided by safety, rather than efficacy [5]. Risks of initiating an antiarrhythmic should be considered, including that of proarrhythmia. Antiarrhythmic drugs can prolong the QT interval and risk causing torsades de pointes [4–6]. We want to avoid precipitating ventricular arrhythmias in an attempt to suppress atrial arrhythmias.
- Antiarrhythmic drugs for the treatment of atrial fibrillation (Chap. 7):
  - Class IA [5, 6].

    Disopyramide.
    - Negative inotrope.
    - May be desirable in patients with hypertrophic cardiomyopathy associated with dynamic LVOT obstruction. Otherwise avoided in structural heart disease.
    - Strong anticholinergic side effects.
  - Class IC—these agents are for use in patients without CAD/CHF/structural heart disease [5, 6].

    Flecainide.
    - Can be initiated as an outpatient.
    - Monitor QRS duration: do not want duration to exceed > 15% baseline.

    Propafenone.
  - Class III.

    Amiodarone [2, 4–6].
    - Can be initiated inpatient or outpatient.
    - Has a large volume of distribution and long half-life, so typically loaded at higher doses with subsequent taper over several weeks.

- Probably the most effective antiarrhythmic for maintenance of sinus rhythm for patients with AF.
- Can be used in patients with or without CHF or structural heart disease.
- Potential toxicities include liver, thyroid, lung, eye, skin among others and need surveillance with LFTs/TFTs every 6 months and yearly PFTs/CXR and eye exams.

Dofetilide (Tikosyn®) [5, 7].

- Must be initiated in the inpatient setting with continuous telemetry and serial ECG monitoring. Want QT prolongation no more than 15% baseline.
- Concern for QT prolongation and torsades.
- MULTIPLE drug interactions and contraindications.
- Dose adjusted based on QT interval, renal function. Contraindicated if baseline QT > 440 sec.

Dronedarone [5].

- A structural analogue of amiodarone, but without the iodine component of amiodarone. Lower incidence of adverse events compared to amiodarone, but also not as effective.
- For use in patients who do not have CHF.
- Monitor LFTs.
- Used less frequently due to contraindications.

Sotalol [5].

- Renally cleared, so caution/contraindication in patients with CKD.
- Typically initiated inpatient, but some experts may consider outpatient initiation in certain patients with close surveillance.

Can worsen CHF.

Options for rhythm control other than antiarrhythmic therapy include:

- Cardioversion.
- Atrial fibrillation ablation [2, 4–6].

AF is often triggered by ectopic focal discharges, which most commonly arise from the left atrial myocardial cells that extend into the pulmonary veins. Because of this, atrial fibrillation ablation involves pulmonary vein isolation as the primary target for ablation. However, triggers can also arise from the posterior wall of the left atrium, ligament of Marshall, SVC/IVC, coronary sinus, and LA appendage, so these areas can also be ablated.

Though somewhat newer over the past few years, hybrid atrial fibrillation ablation is becoming more common. This type of ablation involves both electrophysiology and cardiac surgery, and patients undergo both catheter-based endocardial ablation, as well as surgical epicardial ablation.

Catheter ablation has been shown to be an effective treatment for patients who previously failed antiarrhythmic medications, however recent studies have shown ablation to be an appropriate *first line* treatment without first needing to trial and/or fail antiarrhythmic therapy. Therefore, early referral to electrophysiology should be considered, especially in younger patients.

- *Anticoagulation.*
- Anticoagulation should be considered in all patients, especially if the onset of arrhythmia duration is greater than 48 h or unknown [5]. The CHA2DS2VASc score is used to calculate stroke risk and components include: CHF/LV dysfunction, hypertension, age, diabetes, prior stroke/TIA, presence of vascular disease, and gender [6]. According to the most recent ACC/AHA/HRS guidelines (2019), for patients with a CHA2DS2VASc score of 2 or greater in men, and 3 or greater in women, oral anticoagulants are recommended [6].
  - IV heparin.

    In the acute setting, if not contraindicated, IV heparin can be utilized with subsequent transition to a direct oral anticoagulant (apixaban, rivaroxaban, or dabigatran) or warfarin (once INR therapeutic).
  - Apixaban (Eliquis®) [5, 6].

    Direct Factor Xa Inhibitor.

Dose based on weight (60 kg), serum creatinine (1.5 mg/dL), and age (80 years).

Doses: 5 mg BID; otherwise, 2.5 mg BID if meets 2 of the above criteria.

Able to be used in patients with ESRD on dialysis.

Notable trial: ARISTOTLE.

- Rivaroxaban (Xarelto®) [5, 6].

  Direct Factor Xa Inhibitor.

  Dose based on renal function due to predominant renal clearance.

  Administered once daily with the evening meal to ensure adequate absorption.

  Doses: 20 mg daily; 15 mg daily for creatinine clearance 30–49 mL/min.

  Notable trial: ROCKET AF.

- Dabigatran (Pradaxa) [5, 6].

  Direct thrombin inhibitor.

  Renally cleared, dose based on renal function.

  Doses: 150 mg BID; 75 mg BID for creatinine clearance 15–30 mL/min.

  Notable trial: RE-LY.

- Edoxaban [6].

  Doses: 60 mg daily for creatinine clearance 50–95 mL/min; 30 mg daily for creatinine clearance 15–50 mL/min.

  Direct Factor Xa inhibitor.

  Notable trial: ENGAGE-AF.

- Warfarin [5, 6].

  A vitamin K antagonist with multiple action sites along the coagulation cascade.

  Requires regular PT/INR monitoring with goal 2–3 for AF in the absence of a mechanical heart valve.

  Warfarin is the recommended oral anticoagulant for those with mechanical heart valves and target INR is based on the type and location of the prosthetic valve. (Supported by results from the RE-ALIGN trial).

  Bridging is required for patients with AF and a mechanical heart valve if the procedure requires warfarin interruption. For patients with AF and without a mechanical heart valve, decisions on bridging should balance risk of stroke and risk of bleeding, as well as the duration of time off anticoagulation.

  Reversal agent: vitamin K.

Notable points regarding the newer direct oral anticoagulants (DOACs). More information can be found by referencing the trials noted above, as well as specific drug packaging inserts

Fewer drug interactions than warfarin
More rapid onset/offset
Less risk of intracranial bleeding when compared with warfarin
Bridging with heparin should be individualized and may not be needed
DOACs are not to be utilized in patients with valvular AF or mechanical valve prosthesis.
Twice daily dosing (apixaban, dabigatran) vs daily dosing (rivaroxaban, edoxaban)
Rivaroxaban should be taken with food
Consideration and dose adjustment in patients with CKD and ESRD

Left Atrial Appendage Occlusion

For patients with contraindication to long-term anticoagulation, exclusion of the left atrial appendage via a percutaneous strategy can be considered [5, 6]. One such device for left atrial appendage occlusion is the Watchman® device. Another device is the Amplatzer Amulet®. These devices are typically placed in the cardiac catheterization lab or EP lab via a femoral catheter approach. Patients will require short-term anticoagulation after device placement but will not require long-term anticoagulation.

Cryptogenic Stroke

If a person has a stroke with unknown cause or etiology, and if external ambulatory monitoring is unrevealing, placement of an implantable loop recorder is reasonable to identify silent atrial fibrillation.

Clinical Pearls

- DOACs have quicker onset, fewer drug interactions and lower bleeding risk than Warfarin.

- Warfarin is the drug of choice for valvular atrial fibrillation.
- First-line treatment of SVT is always dependent on patient stability.
- Short RP tachycardias: typical AVNRT, orthodromic AVRT, junctional tachycardia.
- Long RP tachycardias: atypical AVNRT, atrial tachycardia, sinus tachycardia.
- Avoid AV nodal blocking agents with WPW (or pre-excited atrial fibrillation).
- Typical flutter is counterclockwise, around the CTI, with negative appearance of the flutter wave.
- The earlier, the better for atrial fibrillation ablation.

References

1. Page RL, Joglar JA, Caldwell MA, Calkins H, Conti JB, Deal BJ, Estes NAM 3rd, Field ME, Goldberger ZD, Hammill SC, Indik JH, Lindsay BD, Olshansky B, Russo AM, Shen WK, Tracy CM, Al-Khatib SM. 2015 ACC/AHA/HRS guideline for the Management of Adult Patients with supraventricular tachycardia. J Am Coll Cardiol. 2016;67(13):e27–e115.
2. Baltazar RF. Basic and bedside electrocardiography. Philadelphia: Wolters Kluwer; 2009.
3. Wagner GS. Marriott's practical electrocardiography. 10th ed. Philadelphia: Lippincott, Williams & Wilkins; 2001.
4. Mann DL, Zipes DP, Libby P, Bonow RO, Braunwald E, editors. Braunwald's heart disease. A textbook of cardiovascular medicine, vol. 1. 10th ed. Philadelphia, PA: Elsevier; 2015.
5. January CT, Wann LS, Alpert JS, Calkins H, Cigarroa JE, Cleveland JC Jr, Conti JB, Ellinor PT, Ezekowitz MD, Field ME, Murray KT, Sacco RL, Stevenson WG, Tchou PJ, Tracy CM, Yancy CW, American College of Cardiology/American Heart Association Task Force on Practice Guidelines. 2014 AHA/ACC/HRS guideline for the management of patients with atrial fibrillation. J Am Coll Cardiol. 2014;64(21):e1–76.
6. January CT, Wann LS, Calkins H, Chen LY, Cigarroa JE, Cleveland JC Jr, Ellinor PT, Ezekowitz MD, Field ME, Furie KL, Heidenreich PA, Murray KT, Shea JB, Tracy CM, Yancy CW. 2019 AHA/ACC/HRS focused update of the 2014 AHA/ACC/HRS guideline for the management of patients with atrial fibrillation. J Am Coll Cardiol. 2019;74(1):104–32.
7. Tikosyn treatment guidelines.

Ventricular Tachycardia

10

Robert Hipp

Introduction

Ventricular tachycardia (VT) is wide complex tachyarrhythmia with a QRS duration greater than 120 ms and a heart rate greater than 100 bpm [1]. It is defined as 3 or more premature ventricular contractions with a heart rate greater than 120% of the underlying rate. It can be nonsustained (greater than 3 beats) or sustained (greater than 30 seconds or with hemodynamic compromise). In acute presentations, any wide-complex tachycardia should be treated as VT until proven otherwise.

VT can be described based on QRS morphology to include monomorphic, polymorphic, and ventricular fibrillation. Monomorphic VT has a consistent QRS morphology from beat to beat [2]. Polymorphic VT has a consistent deviation in QRS morphology between beats [2]. Ventricular fibrillation (VF) is a disorganized tachyarrhythmia with no clear QRS complexes and leads to sudden hemodynamic compromise given failure of relevant cardiac contraction.

In some cases, VT is caused by the presence of chronic ventricular scar which leads to abnormal impulse formation and propagation. These presentations often have regular R-R intervals and monomorphic morphology. VT can also occur acutely in the presence of ischemia. Arrhythmias secondary to acute ischemia are often faster and more irregular than ones caused by chronic scar or structural heart disease.

R. Hipp (✉)
Cardiac Electrophysiology, Hospital of the University of Pennsylvania, Philadelphia, PA, USA
e-mail: Robert.Hipp@pennmedicine.upenn.edu

Pathophysiology

The mechanism for initiation of VT is either abnormal automaticity, triggered activity, or re-entry. In the case of re-entry, there must be an early stimulus such as a PVC as well as a substrate to sustain the arrythmia. Re-entry is the most common mechanism of ventricular arrhythmias and often occurs in the presence of structural heart disease [3]. Triggered and automatic ventricular arrythmias are less common and are caused by changes to the cardiac action potential resulting in abnormal impulse formation [1].

Re-entry

Ventricular Tachycardia is most caused by a re-entrant circuit in the ventricle due to a direct insult (such as an MI) leading to remodeling (scar formation) [3]. Re-entrant circuits often cause monomorphic VT with regular R-R intervals. Scar-related re-entry is commonly seen in patients with heart disease from infarction and fibrosis, but can also occur with other types of cardiomyopathies. Other causative conditions

R. Musialowski, K. Allshouse (eds.), *Cardiovascular Manual for the Advanced Practice Provider*,
https://doi.org/10.1007/978-3-031-35819-7_10

include cardiac sarcoidosis, arrhythmogenic right ventricular cardiomyopathy (ARVC), surgical correction of congenital heart disease, and myocarditis [2].

Re-entry circuits form in the area or zone between myocardial scar and healthy tissue. Circuits can be subendocardial, epicardial, or extend through the entire thickness of the myocardium [3]. These regions blending live myocytes with fibrotic areas allow for abnormal impulse propagation and areas of slow conduction. When an appropriately timed premature ventricular beat occurs, re-entry is triggered. A single large scar can have several VT circuits (with different QRS morphologies) arising from it using different exit sites.

Automaticity

Abnormal automaticity leading to ventricular arrhythmia is caused by changes in phase 4 of the cardiac action potential where the myocardial cells are spontaneously depolarizing at a considerably faster rate than normal [4]. Abnormal automaticity is associated with acute, reversible conditions such as electrolyte abnormalities, hypoxemia, and acute MI [3]. Some VT may not be associated with underlying heart disease and has characteristic locations and EKG appearance (i.e., RVOT-VT).

Triggered Activity

Electrolyte imbalance, sympathomimetic drugs, catecholaminergic polymorphic ventricular tachycardia (CPVT), pause dependence, and QT offending medications are also causes of VT independent of scar or fibrotic changes [3]. Low potassium, magnesium, and calcium levels are all known to change action potentials, while congenital or medication acquired QT prolongation impacts repolarization allowing for the development of VT, or more commonly torsade de pointes.

QT prolongation occurs with lengthening of the action potential duration (phase 3) and allows for PVC to fall on the T wave, initiating polymorphic VT. Hypokalemia and a prolonged QT interval (either genetic Long QT syndrome or taking QT offending medications) can increase the possibility of this arrhythmia [1]. Ion channel dysfunction (inherited or otherwise) may also lengthen repolarization leading to the development of early after depolarizations (EADs) and triggered extrasystoles [3].

Catecholaminergic polymorphic ventricular tachycardia (CPVT) is a VT occurring with increased catecholamine release (such as with exertion) or during a severe emotional disturbance. This occurs in the setting of a structurally normal heart without the fibrotic changes associated with reentry [3]. Bidirectional VT is a hallmark of CPVT but may also be seen with digoxin toxicity.

Symptoms

Most patients are highly symptomatic when experiencing ventricular tachycardias. Common symptoms include dizziness, lightheadedness, palpitations, or shortness of breath. In some cases, particularly in the setting of fast VTs, the patient can become hemodynamically unstable and develop syncope or have a cardiac arrest. Rarely, patients may have minimal symptoms besides a generalized feeling of fatigue, especially if the VT has a slow rate.

Physical Exam

The patient in VT will have a tachycardic rate with potential jugular venous pulsation "cannon A waves" due to A-V dissociation. These waves are caused by atrial contraction against a closed tricuspid valve during the ventricular arrhythmia. Blood pressure may be low, and patients may be tachypneic. There may also be signs of compromised cardiac output including poor peripheral perfusion, mental status changes, signs of heart failure.

Diagnostics

Making a diagnosis of VT is based on several ECG findings including heart rate greater than 100 bpm, QRS duration greater than 120 ms, and a grossly regular R to R interval although there may be subtle variation from beat to beat during initiation (Fig. 10.1) [1, 3].

AV dissociation (Fig. 10.2) is seen with the arrows illustrating P waves superimposed within the ventricular complexes. There is concordance through the precordial leads (Figs. 10.1 and 10.3), and r-S > 100 ms in any single precordial lead [5]. Figure 10.4 is also consistent with a diagnosis of VT. These findings are critical in the differentiation of VT from supraventricular tachycardia (SVT), however, if there is any uncertainty, always assume it is VT until proven otherwise. Figure 10.5 reveals a regular, wide complex tachycardia (WCT), but upon review the r-S ratio is <80 ms, thus ruling out VT and confirming SVT. Always compare EKG in VT to EKG in sinus!

EKG features favoring VT
wide QRS (>140 ms)
AV dissociation
fusion beats
capture beats
extreme axis deviation
chest lead concordance
R-S > 100 ms

Confirmation of a ventricular tachycardia diagnosis can be definitively ascertained through electrophysiologic testing. In the electrophysiology lab, catheters are positioned in the right ventricle via the femoral or jugular vein. Programmed electrical stimulation (PES) is delivered via these catheters to simulate various sequences of PVCs with the intention of inducing the clinical arrhythmia. In patients with an internal cardioverter defibrillator (ICD), PES can be performed noninvasively via the device. Whether performed invasively or noninvasively, an external defibrillator should be nearby and prepared to defibrillate the patient should they become

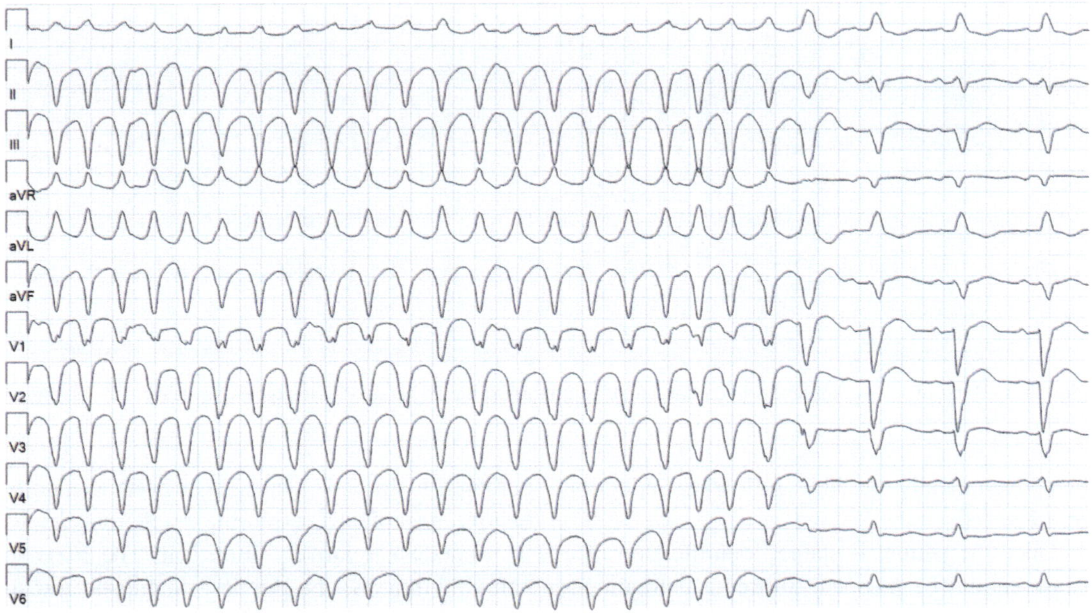

Fig. 10.1 Wide complex tachycardia converting to sinus rhythm with different QRS morphology suggestive of VT

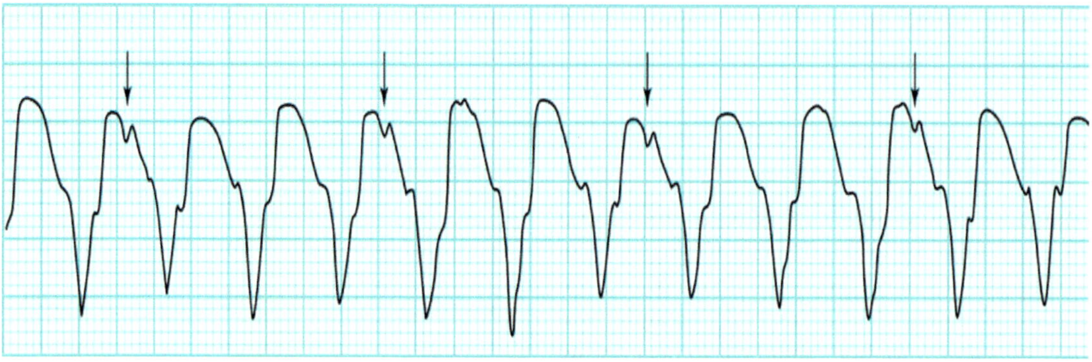

Fig. 10.2 Wide complex tachycardia with arrows demonstrating P waves and atrioventricular (AV) disassociation

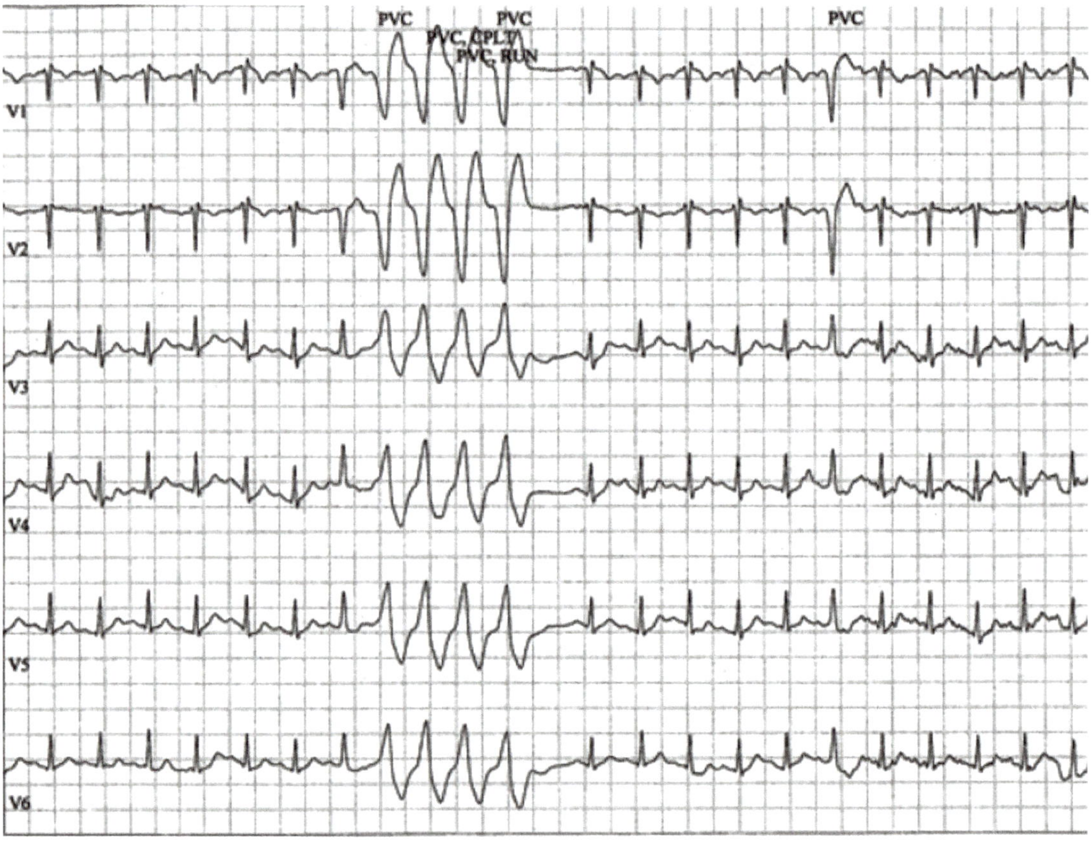

Fig. 10.3 Burst of wide complex tachycardia which is monomorphic and concordant suggestive of VT

hemodynamically unstable following induction of VT or VF.

Once the patient is stable, identification of a cause should be pursued. Subsequent treatment can then be tailored to the patient-specific disease process. A complete history, closely assessing for personal history of syncope, as well as family history, specifically exploring premature deaths in immediate relatives, is critical. The ECG in sinus rhythm will be the first diagnostic test to potentially shed light on the etiology of the VT. Cardiac ischemia or scar, hypertrophic cardiomy-

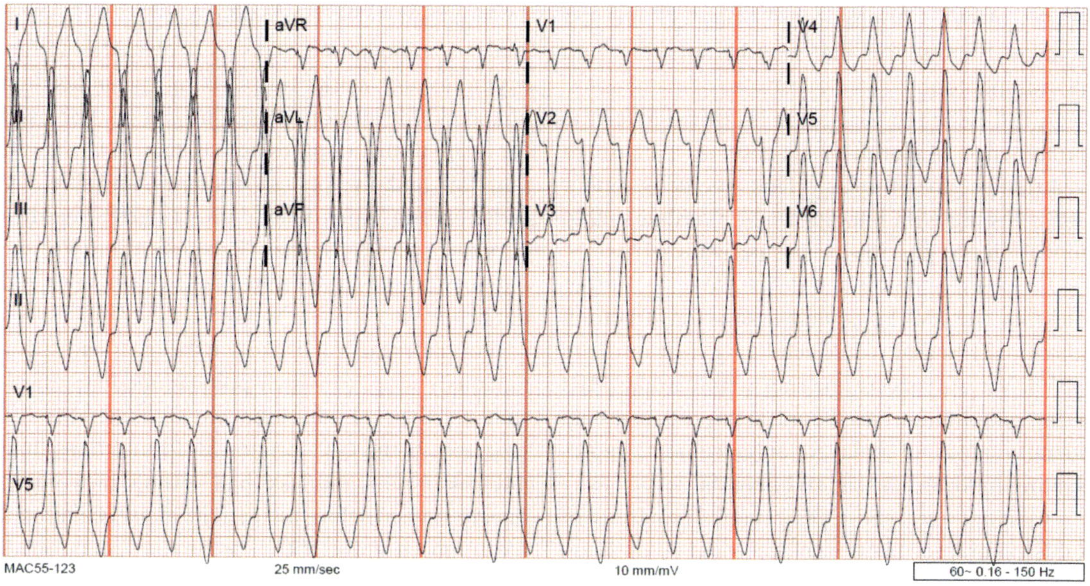

Fig. 10.4 A r-s interval of >100 ms suggestive of VT

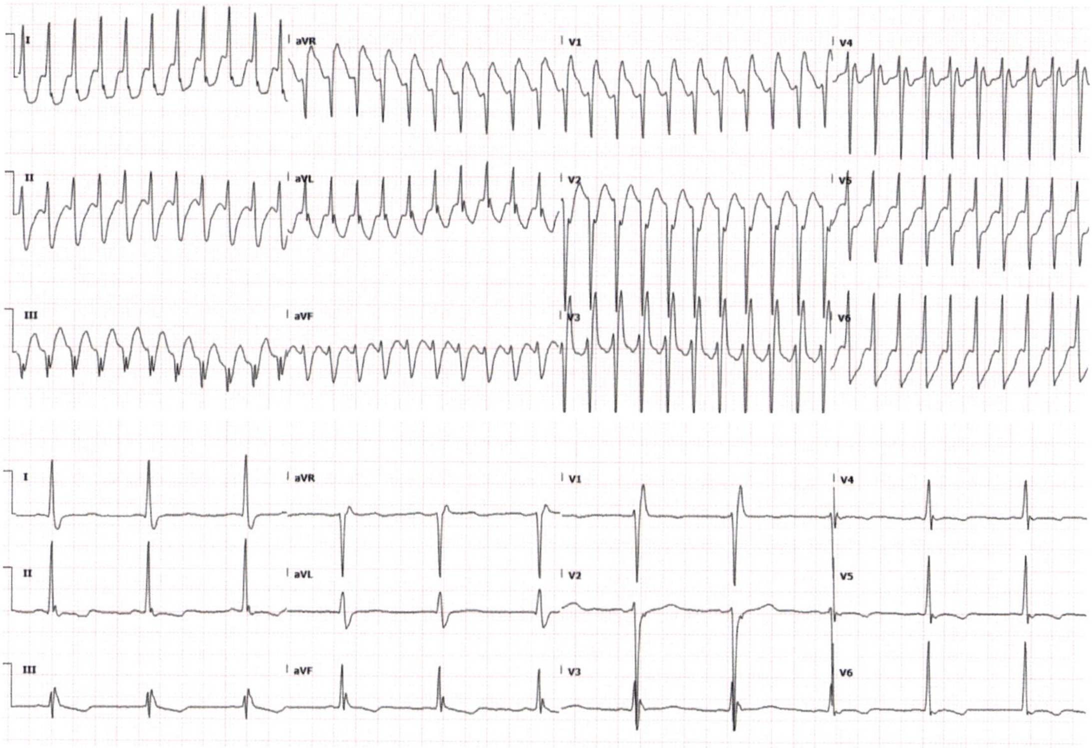

Fig. 10.5 A wide complex tachycardia (WCT) and a QRS interval <100 ms is suggestive of SVT. Also, compare to EKG in sinus rhythm below-the complexes are similar

opathy, ARVC, Brugada, and Long QT are just some of the diseases that may be apparent with this simple tool.

A full ischemic evaluation is critical given the prominence of coronary disease as a cause of ventricular arrhythmias. This includes either stress testing with imaging and/or cardiac catheterization and possible revascularization [6].

Echocardiography should be done to further quantify the LVEF, as well assess for structural abnormalities that would lead to a clear etiology of VT/VF. Advanced imaging with cardiac MRI using gadolinium-based contrast agents can help identify areas of delayed enhancement, representing myocardial scar and fibrosis.

A signal averaged ECG reviews hundreds of QRS complexes from surface tracings and can identify late potentials following the QRS complex that may not be identified on a traditional ECG. These late potentials can represent slow conduction secondary to fibrotic changes of a re-entry circuit [1].

Finally, genetic testing should be arranged if there is no identifiable cause of the arrhythmia, to further confirm the diagnosis or for planning for cascade family testing [2].

Acute Management

Upon presentation, all wide complex tachycardias should be treated as ventricular tachycardia until proven otherwise [1]. The acute treatment of VT/VF revolves around the hemodynamics of the patient. Any patient that is in monomorphic VT with hemodynamic collapse requires *synchronized* direct current cardioversion to restore sinus mechanism. Synchronization is a setting on the defibrillation device that tracks the QRS to avoid decompensation to VF by a shock on the T wave (R on T). If they are in sustained polymorphic VT or VF, they will need immediate defibrillation due to either rapidly changing, or unstable QRS complexes.

If a patient presents in stable monomorphic VT with adequate organ perfusion, an attempt at restoring sinus rhythm with antiarrhythmic drug (AAD) therapy is reasonable using a medication such as amiodarone. This is a class III antiarrhythmic and works by blocking the potassium channels. Intravenous lidocaine can also be used for arrhythmia suppression (Chap. 7). Should that fail and the patient becomes unstable, IV sedation and *synchronized* direct current cardioversion is needed. If the VT degrades into VF, the patient should have immediate unsynchronized defibrillation.

Polymorphic VT is likely to be brief and spontaneously stop, at which point immediate attention to the QT duration in sinus rhythm is required. If the QT duration is normal (less than 440 ms in men and less than 460 ms in women) during sinus rhythm, the patient should be treated like monomorphic VT as previously mentioned. However, if, during sinus rhythm, they have a prolonged QT interval they should be treated with magnesium to suppress or reduce the amplitude of EADs and isoproterenol to increase the heart rate. Of note, a QTc greater than 500 ms in both men and women is associated with malignant arrhythmias, specifically torsade de pointes.

Patients should be quickly assessed for electrolyte disturbances and treatment should be started to stabilize the ion channels. The possibility of acute myocardial ischemia should be assessed. If this is thought to be the cause of the arrhythmia, the patient will require cardiac catheterization and prompt revascularization [1].

Again, it is paramount to always rule on the side of any WCT being VT over SVT. Intravenous adenosine can be given to the hemodynamically stable patient in a WCT to potentially confirm SVT diagnosis.

Long-Term Treatment

Chronic treatment, baring side effects or contraindications, will more than likely include beta blockade and possible antiarrhythmic therapy for ongoing malignant arrhythmia suppression [3]. Beta blockade has been proven to increase survival, but the combination of beta blockade and amiodarone leads to improved outcomes and less

VT recurrence. The use of antiarrhythmic therapy does not increase survival but controls arrhythmias and improves symptoms [3]. For an episode of VT lasting greater than 30 s and not in the setting of a reversible cause such as acute myocardial infarction including cardiac arrest or VT in the setting of low EF, placement of a secondary prevention implantable cardiac defibrillator is necessary [7]. Furthermore, catheter ablation of VT can be considered if medications are ineffective or not tolerated for monomorphic VT [6]. Areas of live cells within the scar or areas of slow conduction may be targeted. Most originate close to the subendocardium. Some ablations require epicardial access. In the case of polymorphic VT, the PVC focus can be targeted.

Conclusion

Ventricular tachycardia is a potentially life-threatening arrhythmia that affects hundreds of thousands of Americans every year with varying presentation and etiology. Acute treatment is centered around maintaining hemodynamic stability and restoring normal sinus rhythm. The patient should then undergo a thorough workup to determine the underlying cause which will inform the long-term treatment plan. This plan can include any combination of chronic antiarrhythmic therapy, implantable cardioverter defibrillator, and ablation.

Pearls

- Wide complex tachycardia should be treated as VT until proven otherwise.
- Can try adenosine if patient stable to help in diagnosis of VT vs. SVT.
- VT is common with underlying structural or cardiovascular heart disease.
- VT may be due to re-entry, triggered, or automatic substrates.
- Acute treatment is maintaining hemodynamic stability and restoration of sinus rhythm.
- Chronic treatment may include antiarrhythmics, ablation, or ICD placement.

References

1. Abedin Z. Essential cardiac electrophysiology: with self-assessment. 1st ed. Wiley-Blackwell; 2006.
2. Foth C, Gangwani MK, Alvey H. Ventricular tachycardia. [Updated 2021 Aug 11]. In: StatPearls [Internet]. Treasure Island, FL: StatPearls Publishing; 2022. https://www.ncbi.nlm.nih.gov/books/NBK532954/.
3. Fogoros R. Electrophysiologic testing. 5th ed. Wiley-Blackwell; 2012.
4. Antzelevitch C, Burashnikov A. Overview of basic mechanisms of cardiac arrhythmia. Card Electrophysiol Clin. 2011;3(1):23–45. https://doi.org/10.1016/j.ccep.2010.10.012.
5. Brugada P, Brugada J, Monts L, Smeets J, Andries E. A new approach to the differential diagnosis of a regular tachycardia with a wide QRS complex. Circulation. 1991;83(5):1649–59. https://doi.org/10.1161/01.cir.83.5.1649.
6. Cronin EM, Bogun FM, Maury P, Peichl P, Chen M, Namboodiri N, Aguinaga L, Leite LR, Al-Khatib SM, Anter E, Berruezo A, Callans DJ, Chung MK, Cuculich P, D'Avila A, Deal BJ, Della Bella P, Deneke T, Dickfeld TM, et al. 2019 HRS/EHRA/APHRS/LAHRS expert consensus statement on catheter ablation of ventricular arrhythmias. Europace. 2019;21(8):1143–4. https://doi.org/10.1093/europace/euz132.
7. 2017 AHA/ACC/HRS ventricular arrhythmia and prevention of sudden cardiac death guidelines. Circulation. 2018;138(13):e210–71.

Cardiac Channelopathies

11

Krista Allshouse

Introduction

Primary inherited arrhythmia syndromes or "channelopathies" are a set of disorders in which one or more of the cardiac ion channels functions abnormally. Mutations in genes encoding critical ion channels, most commonly sodium, calcium, and potassium channels, are the cause of the cardiac pathology. This has various implications on cardiac conduction including resultant Long or Short QT Syndrome, Brugada Syndrome, and Catecholaminergic Polymorphic Ventricular Tachycardia (CPVT), all of which are considered channelopathies.

Channelopathies may be identified after an individual cardiac arrest, family history of sudden cardiac death (SCD), or clinical suspicion based on evaluation after a syncopal event. Patients with channelopathies generally have structurally normal hearts. The more recent widespread use of genetic testing has allowed providers to better identify patients at risk and initiate treatment. This may, in turn, lower the overall risk to the patient and immediate family members.

The Guidelines for Sudden Cardiac Death and Arrhythmia Evaluation recommend genetic testing as a part of diagnosis, depending on specific channelopathy suspected. Genetic testing is not only important to obtain a specific diagnosis with high clinical suspicion, but to risk stratify, guide therapy, and provide screening for relatives. Recently, it has been more common to use multigene or whole exome sequencing using a blood or buccal swab. These tests have high sensitivity, can identify multiple gene mutations simultaneously, and can identify "modifier" genes which affect expression or intensity of expression in the patient. Interpretation is complicated and testing should only be completed by providers versed in counseling on the implications of the results. There are often "variants of unknown significance" identified. These are genetic variants but the specific location on the gene is not specifically associated with a disease.

Long QT Syndrome

The first identified and most common channelopathy is the Long QT Syndrome (LQTS). This syndrome occurs when the QT interval on the EKG is prolonged due to either a congenital mutation or acquired due to medications, electrolyte abnormalities, metabolic disorders, ischemia, or intracranial pathology. The most common QT-prolonging medications are listed on the Crediblemeds.org website. Important offending medications to know would be specific antiemetics, PPIs, SSRIs, antipsychotics, and some antibi-

K. Allshouse (✉)
Atrium Health, Levine Childrens' Congenital Heart Center, Charlotte, NC, USA
e-mail: Krista.Allshouse@atriumhealth.org

R. Musialowski, K. Allshouse (eds.), *Cardiovascular Manual for the Advanced Practice Provider*,
https://doi.org/10.1007/978-3-031-35819-7_11

otics/antifungals. Many frequently used medications including Zofran, Benadryl, Pepcid, Protonix, Celexa, Paxil, Imodium, Zithromax, and antiarrhythmics are on the list. The most commonly associated electrolyte abnormalities associated with QT prolongation are hypokalemia, hypomagnesemia, and hypocalcemia.

The QT interval is the total electrical sum of ventricular depolarization and repolarization. It is measured from the beginning of the QRS complex to the end of the T wave on a 12-lead EKG. A normal QT interval is <440 ms in a male or <460 ms in a female. It should shorten with higher heart rates and lengthen with slower heart rates. The corrected QT interval (QTc) is calculated by measuring the intervals on EKG and using a formula to correct for the heart rate. There are various correction formulas that can be used including Bazett, Framingham, Hodges, and Fredericia to adjust for heart rate. The Bazett (most common) formula for the corrected QT (QTc) interval is QT/ $\sqrt{}$ R-R (see below) and should be directly measured rather than relying on the computer read, which is often inaccurate. The QT interval should be measured in leads V5 or II. The limb lead with the sharpest end of the T wave can also be used. The R-R interval should be measured immediately preceding the beat where QT was measured. In atrial fibrillation, the average of 5 consecutive QT intervals should be measured and then averaged, due to the potential irregularity of the R-R interval (Figs. 11.1 and 11.2).

When the QT prolongs, it predisposes the patient to R-on-T phenomenon which is where a PVC occurs during a vulnerable period of repolarization of the ventricule (during the T wave). This triggers polymorphic ventricular tachycardia, or Torsades de Pointes (TdP). Torsades can be preceded by a long-short R-R interval or bradycardia causing "pause-dependent" ventricular tachycardia (VT).

The prevalence of the genetic type of LQTS occurs in about 1/2000 individuals. The risk of death in untreated LQTS is 21% in the year after a first syncopal event but decreases to ~1% over 15 years if treated [7]. SCD can be the initial presentation of this syndrome. Arrhythmias are more common in younger patients and can occur around menses or childbirth.

The congenital form of LQTS can be caused by multiple gene mutations with 13 types now identified. Approximately 15–20% of patients with a prolonged QT are gene positive and less than 5–10% are de novo mutations. The most common types are Long QT I, II, and III. Romano-

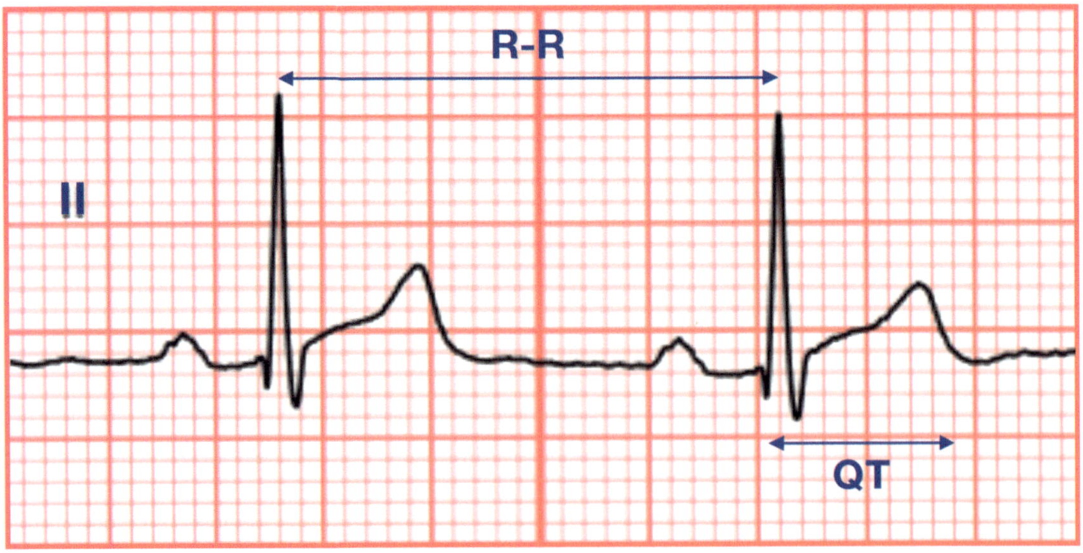

Fig. 11.1 Measure QT and previous R-R. Then calculate QTc with formula: measured QT/$\sqrt{\text{R-R}}$

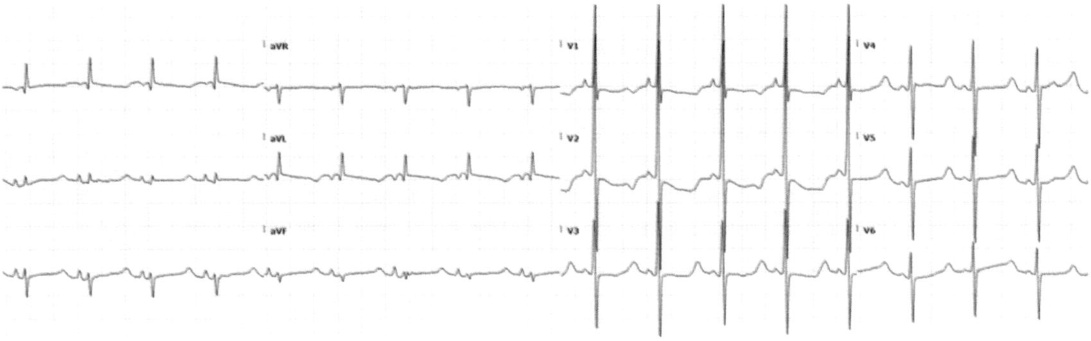

Fig. 11.2 Long QT interval on EKG

Ward syndrome is the autosomal-dominant form and Jervell-Lange Nielson syndrome is autosomal recessive and associated with congenital deafness. LQTS1 is associated with a gene mutation in KCNQ1 and described as an event occurring during exertion, especially during swimming. LQTSII has a gene mutation in KCNH2 and is classically associated with ventricular arrhythmia triggered by a startle or by emotional stress. LQTS3 is a defect in SCN5A and is associated classically with ventricular arrhythmia and cardiac arrest during sleep.

Treatment of all types of Long QT Syndrome includes a reduction in adrenergic tone and prevention of ventricular arrhythmias. Beta blockers are indicated in all diagnosed patients, with nadolol being the preferred agent and propranolol as the second-line agent due to therapeutic characteristics including being non-cardioselective. Beta blockers are most effective in patients with LQTS1 as it blocks the epinephrine released during exertion. Mexiletine, flecainide, or ranolazine may also be added for LQTS3 patients. Implantable cardioverter defibrillators (ICDs) are recommended in patients with resuscitated SCD, syncope, ventricular arrhythmia, or other high-risk features such as significantly prolonged QT or significant family history. Left cervicothoracic stellectomy/gangliectomy (sympathetic denervation) is also an option for non-responders to therapy or if therapy cannot be tolerated. This procedure is accomplished with a video-assisted thoracoscopic technique (VATS procedure) where the left stellate ganglion and a few left thoracic ganglion are removed, blocking sympathetic signals to the heart.

Short QT Syndrome

This condition is due to an accelerated repolarization phase of cardiac conduction. Short QT is defined as a QTc ≤340 ms or ≤360 ms with a pathogenic gene mutation or family history. Associated genes are inherited in an autosomal-dominant fashion in KCNH2, KCNQ1, and KCNJ2. EKG may also show peaked T waves. This is an uncommon disorder but is associated with 40% of patients having a cardiac arrest by age 40. Other arrhythmias are common, especially atrial fibrillation, and diagnosis may be elicited by a stress test or electrophysiology study. No risk factors for SCD have been identified other than syncope. Treatment consists of ICD implantation, hydroquinidine, or other antiarrhythmics depending on specific gene mutation (Fig. 11.3).

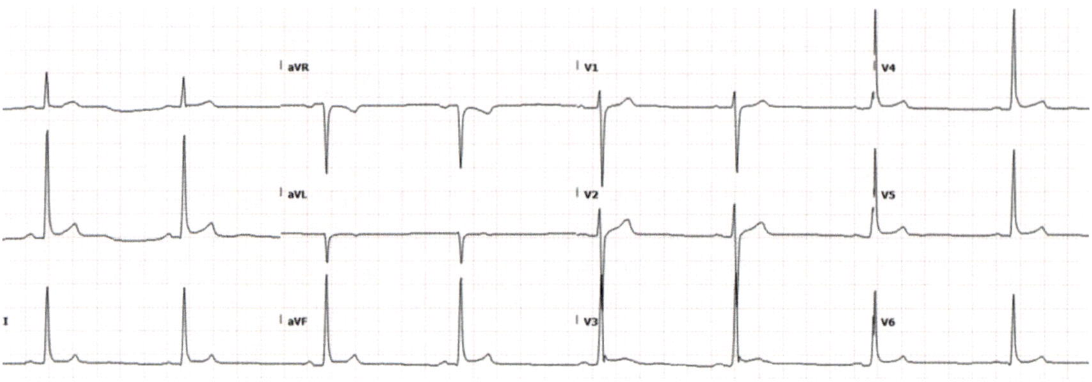

Fig. 11.3 Short QT interval on EKG

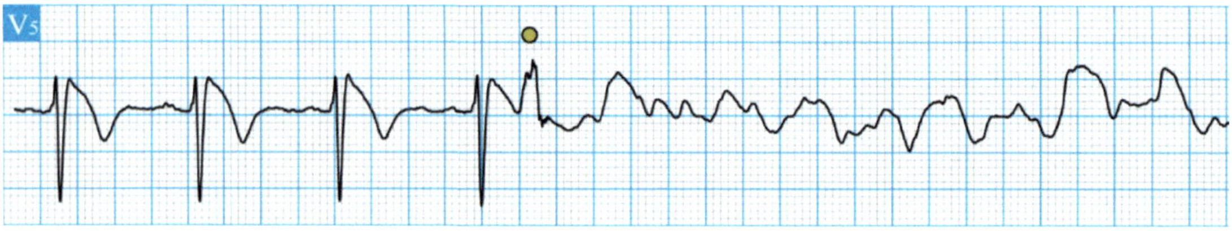

Fig. 11.4 Brugada pattern with PVC falling on a T wave, initiating polymorphic VT

Brugada Syndrome

Brugada syndrome (BrS) is a disorder characterized by right precordial ST elevation on EKG with or without right bundle branch block, predisposing to SCD. SCD risk is due to polymorphic VT degenerating to ventricular fibrillation (VF) (*see* Fig. 11.4). It usually presents in males in the 3rd or 4th decade of life as syncope or SCD. The prevalence is about 1/5–10,000, more commonly in Southeast Asia (where it is known as the Widow Ghost who comes in the night to carry off the souls of their young males). Diagnosis can be made based on symptoms and emergence of Type I pattern in leads V1 or V2 (Fig. 11.5). The sensitivity may be increased with these leads moved to the second intercostal space. The pattern may emerge during fever or with provocative testing. There are three patterns associated with Brugada syndrome, Type I, II, and

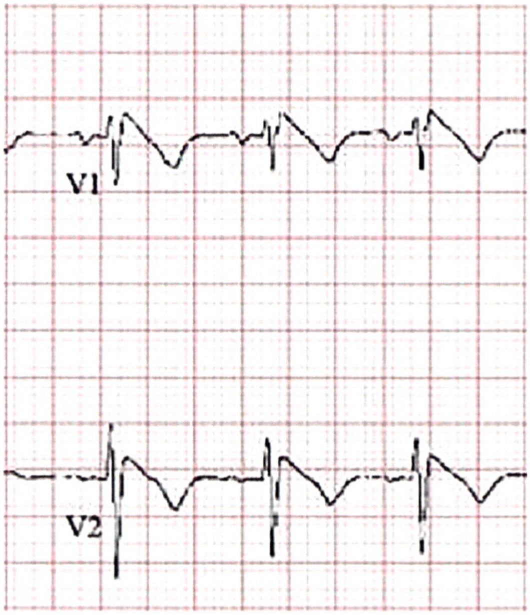

Fig. 11.5 Type I Brugada pattern Type 1

III. Diagnosis can only be made in the setting of Type I pattern but Type II and III may manifest Type I pattern in the setting of fevers or provocative testing. Type I pattern is associated with increased risk of SCA (see below).

The most common gene mutation is in SCN5A with genetics being positive in only about 25% of patients. Brugada syndrome is inherited in an autosomal-dominant fashion. Management consists of avoiding certain drugs (BrugadaDrugs.org) and aggressively treating fever. ICDs are reserved for high-risk patients (syncope or SCD). While often used, beta blockers are of more limited efficacy in patients with Brugada syndrome. Quinidine has been shown to be effective in prevention of recurrent ventricular arrhythmias in patients with this syndrome. More recently, catheter ablation has shown favorable outcomes as well, targeting abnormal tissue on the epicardial RVOT surface that has been implicated as the initiating substrate for ventricular arrhythmia in these patients.

CPVT

Catecholaminergic Polymorphic Ventricular Tachycardia (CPVT) is a condition of adrenergically mediated ventricular arrhythmia that causes syncope, cardiac arrest, or SCD with a structurally normal heart. Exertion or emotional stress precedes the event and baseline EKG is normal or shows resting bradycardia. Patient may have Premature Ventricular Contractions (PVCs), bidirectional VT (Fig. 11.6), or TdP during exercise test (Fig. 11.7). This condition can coexist with LQTS, BrS, or hypertrophic cardiomyopathy. Mean age of symptom onset is 8 years old but the potential for a first syncopal event may not occur until adulthood. The more common gene defect is an autosomal-dominant mutation in RYR2 but less commonly CPVT may be due to a recessive mutation in CASQ2. Genetics are positive in 65% of CPVT patients and 30% of patients have SCD as their first presentation. Treatment consists of a beta blocker. Flecainide has also shown to be effective in patients with symptoms despite beta blocker therapy. ICD implantation is indicated in patients with recurrent ventricular arrhythmia (VA) despite beta blocker therapy although they must be used with caution as ICDs shocks can increase adrenergic tone which can further promote VA in these patients. Specific risks versus benefits must be weighed due to possible VT storm with ICD shocks. Left cardiac sympathetic denervation is also a potential added therapy.

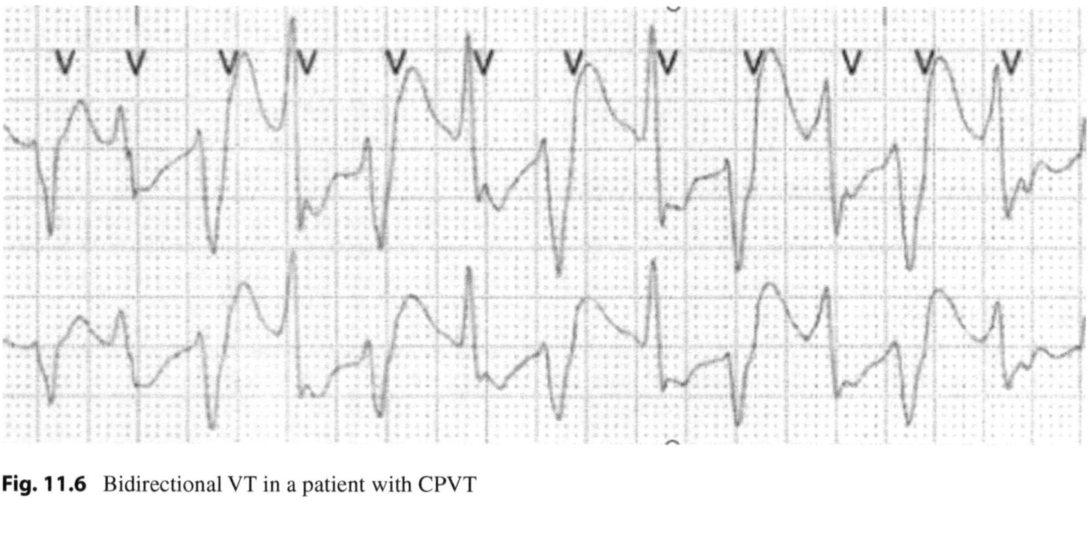

Fig. 11.6 Bidirectional VT in a patient with CPVT

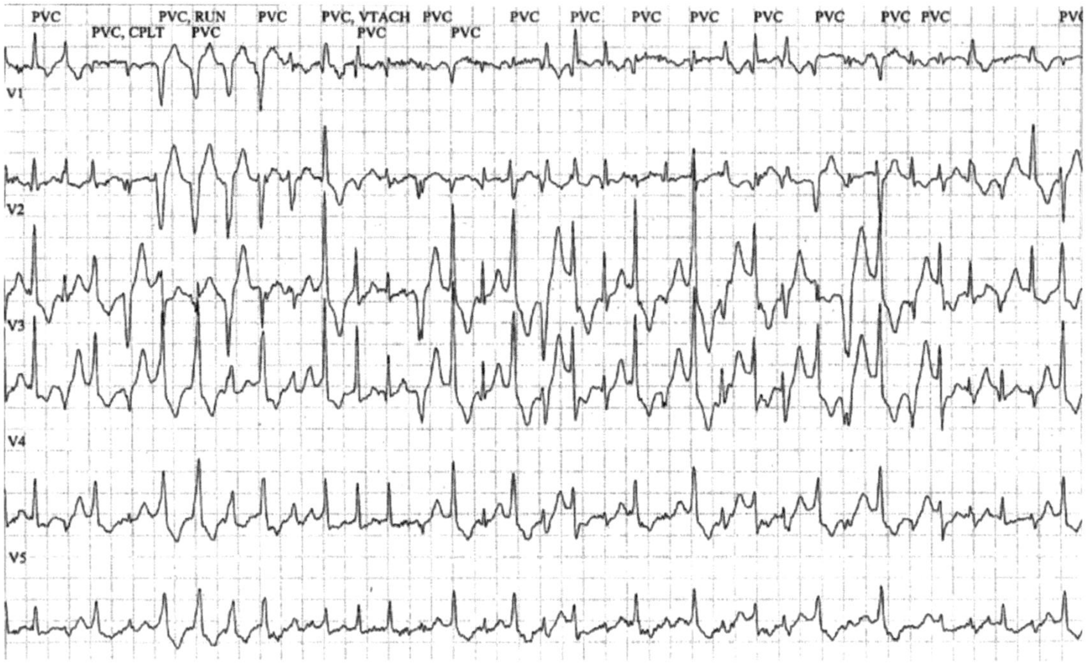

Fig. 11.7 Rhythm on a stress test of a patient with CPVT

Pearls

- QTc = QT/√R-R.
- LQTS1 = KCNQ1 gene mutation, events with exertion.
- LQTS2 = KCNH2 gene mutation, events with startle.
- LQTS3 = SCN5A gene mutation, events with sleep.
- Beta blockers for all Long QT-Nadolol or Propranolol are best.
- Brugada-Type 1 pattern in V1, V2-3rd or 4th decade of life, more in males.
- CPVT-VT with adrenaline-RYR2 or CASQ2.

Further Reading

1. Moss AJ, Adams FH. Cardiac channelopathies, syncope and SCD (Chapter 20). In: Heart disease in infants, children and adolescents. Philadelphia: Wolters Kluwer; 2022. p. 534–50.
2. Wilde AAM, Ackerman MJ. Beta blockers in the treatment of congenital LQT syndrome: is one beta-blocker superior to another. JACC. 2014;64(13):1359–61.
3. Ackerman MJ. Genetic purgatory and the cardiac channelopathies: exposing the variants of uncertain/unknown significance issue. Heart Rhythm. 2015;12(11):2325–31.
4. Ackerman MJ, et al. HRS/EHRA expert consensus statement on the state of genetic testing for the channelopathies and cardiomyopathies. Europace. 2011;13(8):1077–109.
5. HRS/EHRA/APHRS expect consensus statement on the diagnosis and management of patient with inherited primary arrhythmia syndromes. 2013.
6. Cho Y. Left cardiac sympathetic denervation: an important treatment option for patients with hereditary ventricular arrhythmias. J Arrhythm. 2016;32(5):340–3. Published online 2015 Oct. 29. https://doi.org/10.1016/j.joa.2015.08.002.
7. Schwartz PJ, Crotti L, Insolia R. Long-QT syndrome: from genetics to management. Circ Arrhythm Electrophysiol. 2012;5(4):868–77. https://doi.org/10.1161/CIRCEP.111.962019.

Introduction to Cardiac Ablation 12

Krista Allshouse

An electrophysiology study (EPS) is a cardiac procedure performed in a specialized lab by a cardiac electrophysiologist to diagnose and treat arrhythmias. Prior to the procedure, patients are sedated using conscious sedation or general anesthesia, access sites are sterilely prepped, and catheters are placed via the left and right femoral veins (and potentially other veins such as the internal jugular vein) into specific areas of the heart. These may include the high right atrium, HIS bundle area, coronary sinus, right ventricle, and may also be placed into the left heart via a puncture of the atrial septum for left-sided arrhythmias (transseptal puncture) (Fig. 12.2). An arterial line may also be placed for blood pressure monitoring. Systemic heparin is used for anticoagulation during the procedure while catheters are in the body. Fluoroscopy is sometimes used for catheter placement as well. These catheters are attached to the recording systems for signal analyzation (Fig. 12.1). Most procedures are also performed with electroanatomic mapping systems which use a combination of magnetic sensors and impedance measurements within intracardiac catheters. External references to triangulate catheter position within the heart are used to generate three-dimensional cardiac models. Electrical measurements are tracked based on catheter position to define impulse propagation in the heart.

Baseline recordings of the intracardiac electrical signals are taken in sinus rhythm (Fig. 12.1). Normal cardiac conduction properties are measured such as the conduction through the AV node and His bundle. Diagnostic pacing maneuvers are then carried out to test the conduction system and induce arrhythmias. These can identify the presence of conduction pathways that may mediate arrhythmias, such as a slow pathway within the AV node or an accessory atrioventricular pathway in WPW. Sympathomimetic drugs such as isoproterenol or dobutamine can also be used to support blood pressure and help with arrhythmia induction. Additionally, mapping catheters can be used to measure the electrical potentials of specific areas of myocardium to identify signals or scar tissue which may form an arrhythmic substrate. This mapping can be done endocardially in the right heart, via trans-atrial septal puncture or retrograde aortic access in the left heart, and epicardially via subxiphoid access. A hybrid procedure involving all the mapping options may be needed as well. These may help define the mechanism of arrhythmia and guide treatment.

Once a specific arrhythmia is found, ablation may be undertaken with radiofrequency (heat energy) or cryoablation (freezing energy). The choice of modality used depends on the specific arrhythmia and where the ablation site is anatom-

K. Allshouse (✉)
Atrium Health, Levine Childrens' Congenital Heart Center, Charlotte, NC, USA
e-mail: Krista.Allshouse@atriumhealth.org

R. Musialowski, K. Allshouse (eds.), *Cardiovascular Manual for the Advanced Practice Provider*,
https://doi.org/10.1007/978-3-031-35819-7_12

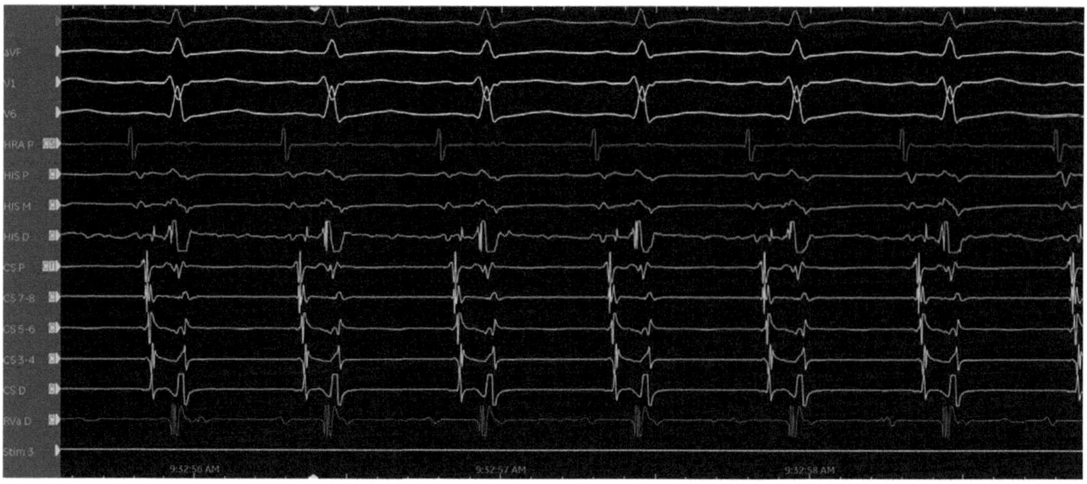

Fig. 12.1 EP recording system screen with surface EKG leads on top (white), coronary sinus catheter recordings in green, HIS bundle recording in yellow, and right ventricle recordings in red

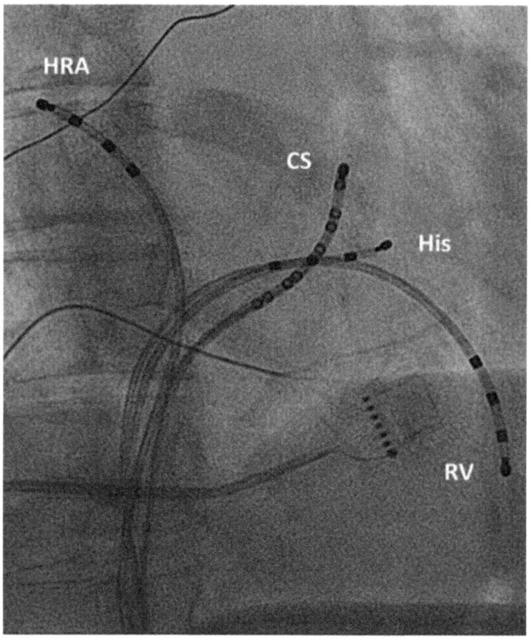

Fig. 12.2 Fluoroscopy image of catheter placement in the heart: high right atrium (HRA), coronary sinus (CS), His bundle (His), and right ventricle (RV) [1]

ically located. Post-ablation testing is then completed to make sure the conduction system remains unaffected, rule out additional arrhythmias, and to make sure the ablated arrhythmia is terminated.

Post-procedurally, catheters are removed, and hemostasis is obtained using a variety of methods including manual compression, temporary skin sutures, and closure devices. A period of bedrest is generally required. Depending on the procedure type and duration, the patient may be discharged the same day or the following morning. Immediately post-procedure, the patient will be closely monitored including evaluation of peripheral pulses in the legs, access site assessments, vital signs, and neurologic evaluations to make sure there are no complications. Post procedure labs may be ordered per physician protocol and patient should be monitored on telemetry and have a post procedure EKG completed.

The risks of these procedures may include groin bleeding/hematoma formation, pseudoaneurysm, retroperitoneal bleeding, stroke, cardiac perforation, arrhythmia requiring cardioversion, or death. Specific types of ablation procedures may also carry unique risks. For example, atrial fibrillation ablation is associated, rarely, with atrio-esophageal fistula (AE) in which esophageal injury during ablation leads to an esophageal-left atrial fistula. Generally presenting 2–4 weeks post-ablation, aorto-enteric fistulas are life-threatening and prompt recognition increases survival Right phrenic nerve injury is possible with atrial fibrillation ablation as well as right atrial ablation in specific areas. Epicardial ablation can be associated with abdominal organ injury due to subxiphoid access. Ablation of AV nodal re-entrant tachycardia and WPW can be associated with heart block requiring permanent pacemaker.

References

1. Wenzl FA, Manninger M, Wunsch S, et al. Post-cardiac injury syndrome triggered by radiofrequency ablation for AVNRT. BMC Cardiovasc Disord. 2021;21:611. https://doi.org/10.1186/s12872-021-02436-1.

Further Reading

Dick M. Clinical cardiac electrophysiology in the young. 2nd ed. New York: Springer; 2015.

Fogoros RN, Mandrola JM. Fogoros' electrophysiologic testing. 6th ed. Wiley; 2018.

Steinberg JS, Mittal S. Electrophysiology, the basics. A companion guide for the cardiology fellow during the EP rotation. Philadelphia, PA: Lippincott, Williams, and WIlkins; 2010.

Introduction to Electrophysiology Devices

13

Jamie A. Dietrich

Basics of Pacemakers

The components of a permanent pacemaker are the pulse generator on the chest and the leads. The leads are insulated wires that deliver electrical impulses from the generator to the myocardium and can sense cardiac depolarization. The leads are most commonly transvenous, which means they go through the vein to the cardiac chambers. Leads are usually placed through the subclavian vein. Leads can be placed in the right atrium, right ventricle, or the epicardial surface of the left ventricle via the coronary sinus. In the right ventricle, leads can be placed in the RV myocardium or targeted to the conduction system. In the latter setting, leads are positioned at either the His bundle or deeply embedded in the interventricular septum to engage the left bundle with a goal of engaging the conduction system to generate more physiologic pacing. When there is a right and left ventricular lead in place, the device is referred to as a biventricular or cardiac resynchronization therapy (CRT) device. A CRT-P is a biventricular pacemaker, and a CRT-D is a biventricular pacemaker with defibrillator. When patients frequently pace in the right ventricle, it can result in loss synchrony between the left and right ventricles and result in worsening left ventricular function and clinical heart failure. In fact, RV apical pacing produces a LBBB on EKG. This is especially important since patients with left bundle branch block and QRS duration of >150 ms with HFrEF have indication for CRT. Leads can also be placed on the epicardium surgically if pacing is indicated and there is difficulty anatomically accessing the appropriate cardiac chambers.

Leadless pacemakers are a newer type of pacemakers which are placed into the right ventricle. These devices only provide single chamber pacing support with some capability to track and pace according to atrial activity. These are typically indicated in patients with permanent atrial fibrillation, tachycardia bradycardia syndrome with low pacing requirements or patients with intermittent heart block with limited life expectancy. These devices can also be considered in patients who have higher than normal infectious risks or recurrent device infections [1]. Clinical trials are now ongoing with dual chamber leadless pacing systems Fig. 13.1.

Sensing is the term used to describe the detection of electrical activity in a particular cardiac chamber. The leads detect the depolarization of the local myocardium where they are implanted and transmit this data to the pulse generator. The magnitude of the signal is measured in millivolts (mV). Sensitivity is a device setting defining the threshold, in mV, at which the device will recognize that depolarization of the cardiac chamber in

J. A. Dietrich (✉)
Atrium Health Wake Forest Baptist,
Winston-Salem, NC, USA
e-mail: jadietri@wakehealth.edu

R. Musialowski, K. Allshouse (eds.), *Cardiovascular Manual for the Advanced Practice Provider*,
https://doi.org/10.1007/978-3-031-35819-7_13

which the lead is positioned has occurred. For example, suppose for a lead in the right atrium that during atrial depolarization, a signal measuring 2 mV is measured. If the sensitivity of the device is 1 mV, the device will recognize that the atrium has depolarized; if set to 3 mV, it will not.

If the pacemaker senses the atrial or ventricular depolarization it was looking for, then it will not pace (inhibit). If it does not sense the atrial or ventricular depolarization it was looking for, then it will pace the heart. A common analogy used to describe the sensitivity settings is that of a fence. If a tall fence or higher sensitivity setting is in place, the pacemaker cannot see a lot of electrical activity over the fence, so it is less sensitive. If a short fence or low sensitivity setting is in place, the pacemaker can see electrical impulses over the fence, so it is more sensitive. Oversensing leads to under pacing; undersensing leads to overpacing [2].

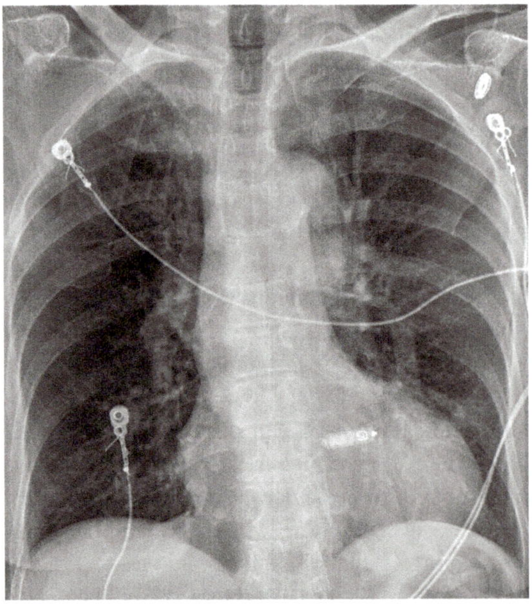

Fig. 13.1 Leadless pacemaker is seen within the heart. No evidence of pacemaker pulse generator or traditional leads are seen on the CXR

The pacing threshold is the minimum amount of energy, measured in voltage delivered over time, needed to depolarize enough local myocardium to drive full depolarization of the cardiac chamber. The parameters above are determined at the time of pacemaker implant and are monitored over time [2]. They can sometimes vary in the setting of certain medications or marked metabolic derangements [2].

The current is defined as the electricity flow, which can be in either direction from the heart to the pacemaker or from the pacemaker to the heart. Impedance is anything that opposes the normal flow of current. Ohm's law is defined as voltage (V) = current (I) × resistance (R) Resistance is another term for impedance. This is a measurement by the device to track the functionality. If there are abnormalities in the impedance, it usually indicates a problem with the leads (either lead fracture or insulation break).

The pacemaker code consists of four letters which conveys the mode in which the pacemaker is operating. The letters describe in order the chamber paced, chamber sensed, function, or pacing response to a sensed beat and rate responsiveness. This code is used when describing single and dual chamber pacemakers (see Table 13.1).

For example, the most common type of pacemaker setting is DDDR. This means that the pacemaker can pace in both the right atrium and right ventricle, sense the intrinsic electrical activity in both chambers, track the atrial activity with inhibition of ventricular pacing, and pacing that is rate adaptive. VVI is another common setting that might be seen with patients in permanent atrial fibrillation who need pacing support. This means that the pacemaker will pace in the right ventricle, sense in the right ventricle, and then not deliver a stimulus if intrinsic beat is sensed in

Table 13.1 Pacemaker code [3]

Chamber paced	Chamber sensed	Function	Rate responsive
O = none	O = none	O = none	O = none
A = atrium	A = atrium	I = inhibition	R = rate adaptive
V = ventricle	V = ventricle	T = tracking	
D = dual	D = dual	D = dual	

the ventricle. If the patient will remain in atrial fibrillation, there is no need to provide pacing support to the atrium. The mode depends on the indication for which the pacemaker is placed. In a patient with sinus node dysfunction who has a problem with conduction in the right atrium, it would be reasonable to program AAI or AAIR but it is more common in the United States to place a dual chamber device and program DDD. In a patient with problems through the AV node, the mode is typically DDD or DDDR. Rate responsiveness means that the pacemaker can increase the heart rate during exertion to meet the metabolic demands of the body. Pacemakers typically have an accelerometer in the generator which can sense movement and respond with increase in heart rate. Application of a magnet to a pacemaker results in asynchronous pacing modes, AOO, VOO, or DOO meaning the device does not sense intrinsic impulses [3].

Another important function of dual chamber pacemakers is the ability for mode switching. Tracking is a normal pacemaker behavior where the device senses activity in one chamber (atrium) and then delivers a stimulus in another chamber (ventricle). The reason for mode switching is that one would not want to pace the ventricle at the atrial rate during atrial fibrillation or flutter, which could be as high as 300 bpm [3]. This means that if the atrial rate is high as occurs in atrial fibrillation or atrial flutter, the pacemaker will automatically switch to a mode where it does not track.

Temporary Pacemakers

There are several types of temporary pacemakers including transcutaneous pacing and temporary transvenous pacemakers.

Transcutaneous pacing is using external pacing pads as well as an external cardiac monitor/defibrillator to pace the patient. The indication for transcutaneous pacing is in patients with second- or third-degree heart block with hemodynamic compromise refractory to medical therapy such as atropine or dopamine until the bradyarrhythmia resolves or a transvenous temporary or permanent pacemaker can be placed. It can be uncomfortable for the patient, and sedation is typically required. It also can be limited by high capture thresholds since the pacemaker is external. Once the pacing pads have been applied to the patient, the heart rate should be set at 60–80 bpm. Energy output in a temporary pacemaker is measured in current (mA) rather than voltage. Typically, output should be programmed at 10 mA and then turned up until capture is achieved, which is usually 50–100 mA. Capture is always verified by assessing the pulse of the patient, not only looking at the monitors.

Transvenous pacing is using a temporary pacemaker wire placed through either the internal jugular or femoral vein and then into the right ventricle to provide pacing support. This can be a floating temporary pacing wire, sometimes with a balloon at the tip for stability, or an active fixation lead with a helix that can be used to fixate the lead into the myocardium. The patient is also bedbound in this case with limited mobility. Complications such as infection or lead migration (perforation) arise more frequently if these are left in place for longer than 48 h.

Indications for Pacemakers

Current class I recommendations for pacemakers include:

1. Symptomatic sinus node dysfunction that leads to symptomatic bradycardia. This is the most common indication for pacemaker placement. This indication also includes patient with tachycardia-bradycardia syndrome and chronotropic incompetence.
2. Second-degree Mobitz type II atrioventricular (AV) block with symptoms, with wide QRS escape or with block during exercise without ischemia present.
3. Complete heart block/advanced second-degree HB with symptoms, pauses >3 s, escape <40 bpm, wide escape, ablation of AV node, AF with brady and pauses >5 s while awake.

4. Fascicular block with intermittent CHB with symptoms or second degree with or without symptoms.

It is important to remember that the above are indications for permanent pacemakers regardless of symptoms and not attributable to reversible or physiologic causes. If patients develop symptomatic AV block because of GDMT for which there is not alternative treatment, permanent pacing is also recommended [4].

Another important patient population to keep in mind are those patients with neuromuscular diseases associated with conduction disorders. These include myotonic dystrophy or Kearns-Sayre syndrome. These patients may develop second- or third-degree AV block. In the presence of these blocks or if the His bundle to ventricular myocardium time is greater than 70 ms (noted on intracardiac electrograms during EP study), then permanent pacemaker is indicated with defibrillator capability if needed and meaningful survival of greater than 1 year is expected [4].

Interpreting Device Interrogations

There are several important data points to review with each device interrogation. The device reports will have varying formats depending on the manufacturer, but most of the important information will be on the first page of the report. Six key things to note are:

1. Battery life (estimated in years): If a device has reached elective replacement interval or ERI, it is approaching time for a generator change. Typically, the devices have 3 months from the date of ERI to safely replace the battery without compromising the device function.
2. Settings: The pacemaker code will be put on this, and it is important to know if it is DDDR, VVIR, etc.
3. Events: If any high atrial rates, ventricular rates or mode switches have occurred, these will be contained in this summary. The EGMs for the events should appear on the following pages.
4. Lead impedance: An abrupt or greater than 30% change in lead impedance can signal a lead fracture or insulation break.
5. Atrial arrhythmia burden or mode switches: Some devices will report AT/AF burden in terms of percentage. You can also get information about how many episodes of mode switching occurred. This can give you important diagnostic information about atrial fibrillation burden.
6. Pacing percentages: If a patient is pacing more than 40% in the right ventricle (LBBB), this could lead to a pacemaker-induced cardiomyopathy due to loss of synchrony between the ventricles. An echocardiogram would be the next step to assess, especially if the patient is symptomatic or the pacing percentages have increased from prior device reports. In patients with LVEF <50% and high burden of ventricular pacing, upgrade to biventricular pacing (CRT-P) can be considered.

Implantable Cardioverter Defibrillators (ICDs)

Basic Principles of Defibrillators

An ICD can both pace and defibrillate the heart. The pacemaker functions apply to the ICD as well. In addition, the ICD technology can recognize lethal arrhythmias such as ventricular tachycardia (VT) and ventricular fibrillation (VF). The device can either pace the patient out of the rhythm (for ventricular tachycardia) or deliver synchronized or unsynchronized shocks. This pacing is called antitachycardia pacing or ATP.

The ICD uses the heart rate to decide if a rhythm should be treated. The settings are called "zones." Different zones can be used for VT and VF. Commonly, patients who are on an antiarrhythmic such as amiodarone can have a slower VT, so it can be necessary to make the zone lower in order to sense the VT and treat it appropriately [5]. Modern ICDs also have algorithms to try to recognize SVT and avoid shock delivery. These algorithms are based on the morphology of the signal detected in reference to regular rhythm, relationship of atrial and ventricular activity, and characteristics at onset of the rapid rhythm.

It is important to remember that an ICD can provide therapy inappropriately for a tachycardia. This can occur when a patient has atrial fibrillation with rapid ventricular response among other SVTs. Reviewing a device interrogation and EGMs for a patient with a shock is important to ensure that the shock was appropriate [5].

Institutions have various shock protocols if a patient receives an ICD shock. If a patient receives one shock, it is important to review device interrogation as well as to ask about symptoms that could have precipitated the shock including ischemia or worsening heart failure. Typically, the patient does not need to come to clinic or the emergency room for this. If multiple shocks are delivered in a short period of time, the patient should go to the closest emergency room. VT storm is defined as three or more ICD shocks in a 24 h period and is a medical emergency [5].

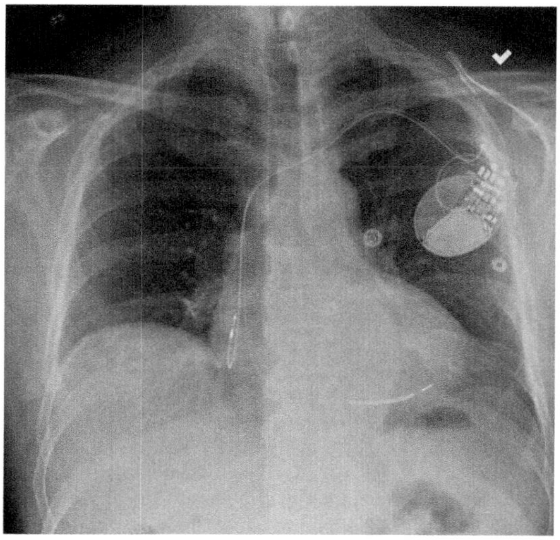

Fig. 13.2 Dual chamber ICD with a lead in the RV and one in the RA

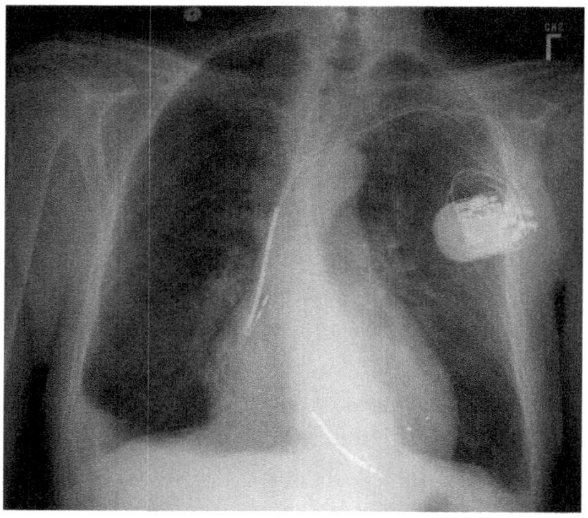

Fig. 13.3 Biventricular ICD with a wire in the RV, RA, and a LV lead at the 5 o'clock position

Temporary Defibrillators

There are temporary defibrillators called wearable cardioverter defibrillator (WCD). WCD is a class IIb recommendation after acute myocardial infarction in patients with an LVEF of less than or equal to 35%. It may be used if a patient has an infection necessitating removal of a device as a stop gap measure until a new device can be placed [5].

Permanent Defibrillators

ICDs can be single chamber with one lead in the right ventricle, dual chamber with one lead in the right atrium and one in the right ventricle (see Fig. 13.2) or biventricular (Fig. 13.3). A CRT-D is an ICD with one lead in the right ventricle and one lead in the left ventricle via the coronary sinus. Subcutaneous ICDs are devices that are implanted in the upper left abdominal area and have no part of the device in the vasculature [5]. Subcutaneous ICDs are devices that are implanted in the left axillary region with a lead that courses from there to the parasternal region (Fig. 13.4). These devices are fully extravascular and offer the advantage of reduced infection risk, avoiding vascular compromise and comfort in some patients. It is not capable of pacing.

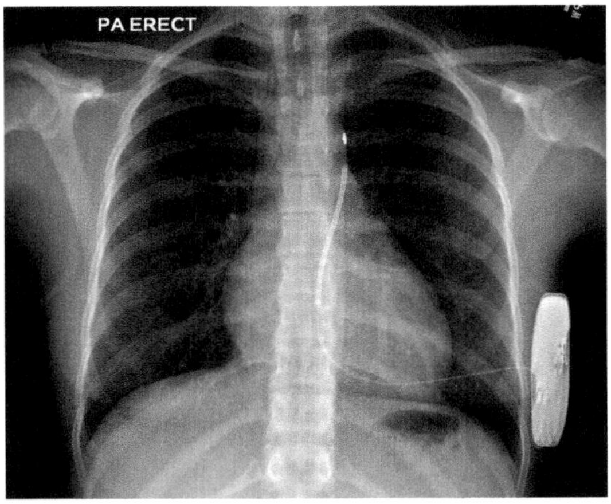

Fig. 13.4 Sub-cutaneous ICD generator in place on left lateral chest with lead running along the sternum tunneled under the skin

Indications for Defibrillators

Primary prevention ICD means that the patient has not had sustained VT or cardiac arrest. Secondary prevention means that the patient has had sustained VT or cardiac arrest. Sustained VT is defined as at least 30 s of VT [5].

Class I indications for ICDs include:

1. For primary prevention in patients with ischemic heart disease who are greater than 40 days from MI and/or more than 90 days from revascularization despite maximally tolerated GMDT with an EF ≤ 35% with at least class II NYHA symptoms or with an EF ≤ 30% with NYHA class I symptoms. Patients need to have a life expectancy of greater than 1 year.
2. For secondary prevention in patients with ischemic heart disease regardless of LVEF or have syncope thought to be cardiac in etiology with LVEF less or equal to 35%. Patients need to have life expectancy of greater than 1 year.
3. For primary prevention in patients with non-ischemic cardiomyopathy with HF NYHA class II-III symptoms and LVEF less than or equal to 35% despite maximally tolerated GDMT. Patients need to have life expectancy of greater than 1 year.
4. For secondary prevention in patients with nonischemic cardiomyopathy if they have had sudden cardiac arrest or sustained VT [5].

Patients with hypertrophic cardiomyopathy have increased risk of sudden death. There are numerous risk factors, risk modifiers, as well as high risk substrates. Risk stratification should be performed every 1–3 years in these patients to determine the need for an ICD [5]. Indications for subcutaneous defibrillators are typically patients without any need for a pacemaker function or in patients with high infectious risk or recurrent device infections. Many young patients with hypertrophic cardiomyopathy receive subcutaneous defibrillators if indicated as the patients are younger and likely to live longer than a transvenous system would last [6]. Other indications for subcutaneous defibrillators include having cardiac anatomy that is difficult to access or in patients with active lifestyles.

Interpreting Device Interrogations

The same principles as with pacemaker interrogations apply here. The important differences include any tachycardia events, ICD therapies which include antitachycardia pacing (ATP) or shocks. The EGMs on the device interrogation are important to review as well to get a sense if the shock was appropriate or not.

Common Problems and Troubleshooting Pacemakers and ICDs

Cardiac device manufacturers provide a great deal of support for devices. It is important to remember that a call can be placed to the cardiac device company for an interrogation or troubleshooting. Often, the representatives can assist in programming changes. Most device clinics also employ cardiac device technicians to check and monitor devices in the clinic. These individuals can be invaluable in terms of knowledge and troubleshooting devices.

One of the most common problems with a permanent pacemaker or ICD is either a lead fracture or a break in the insulation of the wire. The lead impedance (measured in ohms) will provide information on the integrity of a lead. An abrupt or greater than 30% change in the lead impedance is concerning. If a lead itself fractures, the impedance or resistance will go up. If the insulation is broken, the impedance or resistance will go down. This also can result in premature battery depletion and oversensing. If a lead problem is suspected based on the device interrogation, the next step is to obtain a chest x-ray, both anterior posterior and lateral [4]. If there is an abrupt rise or fall in the impedance on the RV lead in patient with history of complete heart block or who is dependent on their device, the patient may need to be hospitalized to manage this issue. Lead fractures can also manifest themselves as loss of capture, oversensing, and undersensing.

Loss of capture means that a pacemaker spike can be seen on the monitor, but no depolarization of the heart occurs (Fig. 13.5). If you are evaluating a patient with a temporary transvenous pacemaker, the first step is to check all the connections. Then you can turn the milliamps on the device console slowly to see if this changes. Consider ordering a chest x-ray at this point to check lead position. Acute causes of failure to capture include lead dislodgement or malposition, which can be more common with temporary pacemakers or in the immediate post-operative period after implantation of a permanent device. Premature battery depletion is another cause of loss of capture. Depending on the indication for the device, the patient may need to be admitted for expedited generator change. Other causes include battery at end of life of device, lead fracture, insulation breach, fibrosis where the lead is implanted, as well as metabolic derangements [7].

Undersensing means there is a failure to sense the intrinsic activity. Pacing spikes will be seen where they should not be present on telemetry or an EKG. Commonly, pacemaker spikes may be seen within intrinsic QRS complexes. To correct this, the fence or sensitivity needs to be lowered so that the device appropriately senses chamber depolarization. The lead may need to be replaced if programming changes do not correct the problem.

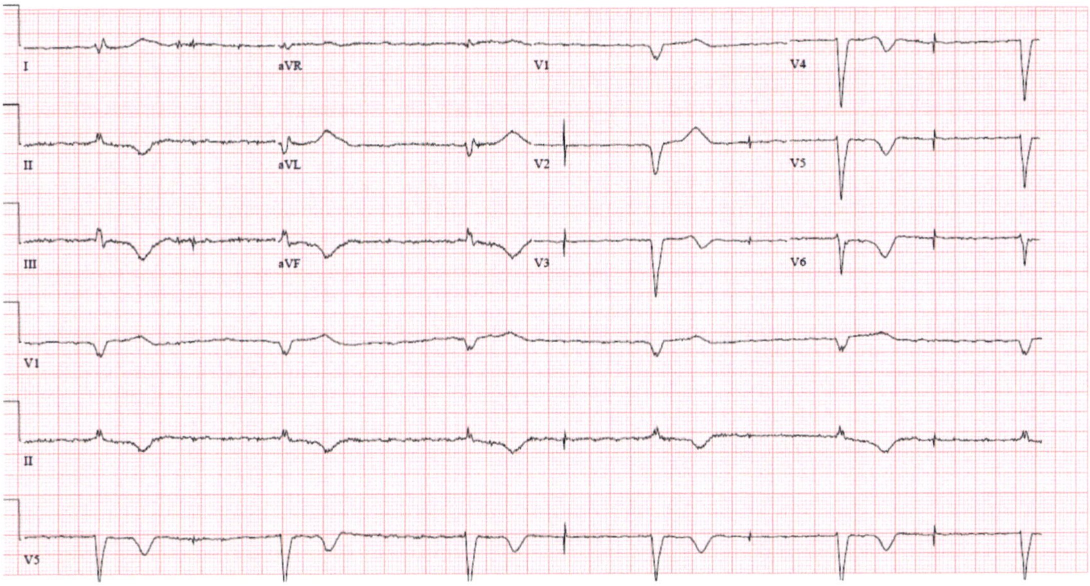

Fig. 13.5 Loss of capture in a dual chamber pacemaker secondary to end of life. There are no QRS waveforms seen after any pacemaker spikes

Oversensing means there is inappropriate detection of a signal that is not intrinsic activity. There is a lack of pacing activity when there should be spikes on telemetry or EKG. To correct this, the fence needs to be raised so that background noise is not detected by the device as chamber depolarization. In emergency settings, the device sensitivity can be set to least sensitive (highest mV level) or asynchronous, where pacing occurs at a fixed rate and sensing is disabled by utilizing the magnet. The lead may need to be replaced if programming changings do not correct the problem.

One of the other issues encountered on a device interrogation maybe called lead noise. This essentially means there is an issue interfering with the device's ability to sense the intrinsic activity. This can be due to lead fracture or insulation breach, oversensing, interactions between leads, or electromagnetic interference from external source. If the noise is on a RV lead in an ICD, there would be concern that the device could provide inappropriate shocks to the patient as it thinks the noise is VF. There are some algorithms on ICDs which can differentiate lead noise from VT/VF and withhold detection if there is lead noise noted on the RV lead.

There may be times when the defibrillator function of an ICD should be turned off urgently or a programmer is not available. This could occur if a patient is having recurrent inappropriate shocks or if a patient is at end of life. Placing a magnet overtop of the ICD will suspend any arrhythmia therapies but will not interfere with the pacing programing of a defibrillator if it is needed [5].

Clinical Pearls

- CRT has leads in right and left ventricle to resynchronize the "squeeze".
- CRT should have a high percentage of biventricular pacing to get maximal benefit.
- RV apical pacing appears as LBBB on EKG, while biventricular pacing may have a more RBBB morphology.
- Magnet over a pacemaker asynchronously paces at a preprogrammed rate.
- Magnet over an ICD suspends any arrhythmia therapies but does not affect the pacing function.
- Oversensing = underpacing; undersensing = overpacing.

References

1. Weachter R. Leadless cardiac pacemaker therapy. An overview for the hospitalist. Am J Hosp Med. 2018;2(3):2018.016. https://doi.org/10.24150/ajhm/2018.016.
2. Kenny T. The nuts and bolts of cardiac pacing. Wiley-Blackwell; 2005.
3. Wang P. Pacemakers. 2022. American College of Cardiology Self-Assessment Program. www.acc.org.
4. Kusumoto F, Schoenfeld M, Barrett C, Edgerton J, Ellenbogen K, Gold M, Goldschlager N, Hamilton R, Joglar J, Kim R, Lee R, Marine J, McLeod C, Oken K, Patton K, Pellegrini C, Selzman K, Thompson A, Varosy P. 2018 ACC/AHA/HRS guideline on the evaluation and management of patients with bradycardia and cardiac conduction delay. J Am Coll Cardiol. 2019;74(7):e51–e156. https://doi.org/10.1016/j.jacc.2018.10.044.
5. Chen J. Implantable cardioverter-defibrillator. 2022. American College of Cardiology Self-Assessment Program. www.acc.org.
6. Al-Khatib S, Stevenson W, Ackerman M, Bryant W, Callans D, Curtis A, Deal B, Dickfield T, Field M, Fonarow G, Gillis A, Granger C, Hammill S, Hlatky M, Joglar J, Kay G, Matlock D, Myerburg R, Page R. 2017 AHA/ACC/HRS guideline for management of patient with ventricular arrhythmias and the prevention of sudden cardiac death. J Am Coll Cardiol. 2018;72(14):e91–e220. https://doi.org/10.1016/j.jacc.2017.10.054.
7. Sabbagh E, Abdelfattah T, Karim M, Farah A, Grubb B, Karim S. Causes of failure to capture in pacemakers and implantable cardioverter-defibrillators. J Innov Card Rhythm Manag. 2020;11(2):4013–7.

14 Cardioversion

Lora Raines

Cardioversion refers to the restoration of sinus rhythm, either by electrical cardioversion (DCCV) or pharmacologic cardioversion. Direct current cardioversion is performed by delivering an electrical shock that is synchronized with the QRS to avoid inducing ventricular fibrillation. Pharmacologic cardioversion is performed by administering an antiarrhythmic agent for the purpose of restoring sinus rhythm. Patients should be adequately anticoagulated prior to proceeding with either electric or pharmacologic cardioversion and should continue oral anticoagulation (OAC) for at least 4 weeks post cardioversion [1].

Electrical Cardioversion

For patients undergoing electrical cardioversion, electrodes are placed in an anteroposterior location. The patient is then sedated, and once they are no longer conscious, a synchronized electrical shock is delivered in an attempt to restore normal sinus rhythm. The primary risk associated with a cardioversion is stroke. Depending on whether or not a patient has been adequately anticoagulated, a TEE may be performed just prior to the cardioversion to rule out a LAA thrombus. In some cases, a CT scan may be performed to rule out LAA thrombus.

Pharmacologic Cardioversion

Certain antiarrhythmics may be used to try to convert a patient to sinus rhythm. Some of the most common drugs used are high dose flecainide or propafenone and ibutilide [1, 2]. Pharmacologic cardioversion should be performed in the hospital during continuous telemetry monitoring [1].

For patients receiving Ibutilide, the major risk is QT prolongation and development of polymorphic VT. ECG monitoring should be continuous and should be continued for ≥4 hours after administration [2].

An oral dose of flecainide or propafenone can be used to try to restore sinus rhythm. Because conversion to sinus rhythm may be associated with bradycardia due to sinus node or AV node dysfunction, the initial conversion trial should be performed in a monitored setting with continuous ECG/telemetry [1, 2].

Recommendation for Prevention of Thromboembolism [3]

- For patients with AF or Aflutter of 48 hours duration or longer (or if duration unknown), anticoagulation with warfarin (INR 2–3), a

L. Raines (✉)
Wellstar Health System, Marietta, GA, USA
e-mail: Lora.Raines@wellstar.org

R. Musialowski, K. Allshouse (eds.), *Cardiovascular Manual for the Advanced Practice Provider*, https://doi.org/10.1007/978-3-031-35819-7_14

factor Xa inhibitor, or a direct thrombin inhibitor is recommended for at least 3 weeks before and at least 4 weeks after cardioversion, regardless of CHA2DS2VASc score or method (electrical or pharmacologic) (Class I).
- For patients with AF or Aflutter of more than 48 hours duration (or unknown duration) that requires immediate cardioversion due to hemodynamic instability, anticoagulation should be started as soon as possible and continued for at least 4 weeks after DCCV unless contraindicated (Class I).
- After DCCV for AF of any duration, decision on long-term OAC should be based on risk of both thromboembolism and bleeding (Class I).
- If AF/Aflutter duration less than 48 hours with CHA2DS2VASc ≥ 2 in men and ≥ 3 in women, administration of heparin, factor Xa inhibitor, or direct thrombin inhibitor is reasonable as soon as possible before cardioversion, followed by long-term therapy (Class IIa).
- For patients with AF/AFL duration 48 hours or longer (or unknown) who have not been anticoagulated for the preceding 3 weeks, it is reasonable to perform a TEE before cardioversion and proceed with cardioversion if no LA/LAA thrombus is identified, provided that anticoagulation is started before the TEE and maintained for at least 4 weeks after cardioversion (Class IIa).
- In patients with AF/AFL of less than 48 hours duration with CHA2DS2VASc = 0 in men and 1 in women, initiation of IV heparin, factor Xa inhibitor, or direct thrombin inhibitor vs no anticoagulation therapy may be considered before DCCV, without need for post-cardioversion anticoagulation.

Clinical Pearls

- Patients can be converted with electricity or medications.
- If a patient is in an atrial arrhythmia > 48 hours, they should have an atrial thrombus ruled out prior to elective cardioversion of any kind.
- Any patient post cardioversion should be anticoagulated for at least 4 weeks after conversion.
- CHA2DS2VASc score is used to evaluate patient's stroke risk.

References

1. January CT, Wann LS, Alpert JS, Calkins H, Cigarroa JE, Cleveland JC Jr, Conti JB, Ellinor PT, Ezekowitz MD, Field ME, Murray KT, Sacco RL, Stevenson WG, Tchou PJ, Tracy CM, Yancy CW, American College of Cardiology/American Heart Association Task Force on Practice Guidelines. 2014 AHA/ACC/HRS guideline for the management of patients with atrial fibrillation. J Am Coll Cardiol. 2014;64(21):e1.
2. Baltazar RF. Basic and bedside electrocardiography. Philadelphia: Wolters Kluwer; 2009.
3. January CT, Wann LS, Calkins H, Chen LY, Cigarroa JE, Cleveland JC Jr, Ellinor PT, Ezekowitz MD, Field ME, Furie KL, Heidenreich PA, Murray KT, Shea JB, Tracy CM, Yancy CW. 2019 AHA/ACC/HRS focused update of the 2014 AHA/ACC/HRS guideline for the management of patients with atrial fibrillation. J Am Coll Cardiol. 2019;74(1):104–32.

Cardiac Syncope

15

Krista Allshouse and Richard Musialowski

Introduction and Pathophysiology

Cardiovascular syncope is described as a sudden loss of consciousness with loss of postural tone. This clinical presentation may be caused by tachycardia, bradycardia, and hypotension. Syncopal events are common, occurring 3% in men and 3.5% in women over a lifetime according to the Cleveland Clinic [1]. These events become more common as individuals age. There are many causes, some of which are more concerning. Cardiac syncope is the most concerning etiology as it carries a 1-year mortality rate of 20–40%. The high risk of patient mortality occurs within 1–6 months after an event especially in patients with structural heart disease. Thorough evaluation for the underlying cause of a syncopal event is essential for risk stratification and prognosis. Cardiac etiologies may be divided into electrical and obstructive. Electrical causes include bradycardic or tachycardic arrhythmias. Obstructive causes include HCM, valvular disease, tamponade, and pulmonary embolus (PE) (see Table 15.1).

K. Allshouse (✉)
Atrium Health, Levine Childrens' Congenital Heart Center, Charlotte, NC, USA
e-mail: Krista.Allshouse@atriumhealth.org

R. Musialowski
Sanger Heart and Vascular Institute, Atrium Health, Charlotte, NC, USA
e-mail: Richard.Musialowski@atriumhealth.org

Table 15.1 Cardiac causes of syncope

Electrical	Structural
VT/Torsades	HCM
VF	AS
Bradycardia: SSS-sinus arrest, conversion pause, marked sinus brady	MS
Heart block	Atrial myxoma
Tachycardia: SVT, WPW with atrial fib	Tamponade
Inherited channelopathy-LQTS, Brugada, CPVT	Pulmonary HTN
	PE

Adapted from chart Recognizing Life-Threatening Causes of Syncope. Cardiology Clinics. Vol. 31, Issue 1, P51–66. Feb. 1, 2013

Symptoms

Cardiac syncope often occurs suddenly, without preceding symptoms. It is often associated with true loss of consciousness, and the patient often incurs traumatic injury from the loss of postural tone. Some patients may experience chest pain, shortness of breath, palpitations, or dizziness before a syncopal episode. Syncope often has prodromal symptoms including sweating, nausea, or near loss of consciousness. Symptoms prior to the event are important to ascertain, as cardioinhibitory syncope allows the patient to sit or lay down before they lose consciousness (see cardioinhibitory below). The presence of these prodromal symptoms often suggests an etiology other than high risk cardiac syncope.

Most acute syncope evaluations are completed on an inpatient basis if the patient has underlying

R. Musialowski, K. Allshouse (eds.), *Cardiovascular Manual for the Advanced Practice Provider*,
https://doi.org/10.1007/978-3-031-35819-7_15

cardiac disease or if the event appears to be high risk (i.e., resulting in injury). The etiology of more than half of syncopal events may be discerned from the history alone. Detailed history-taking is critical to guide additional testing. It is imperative to be aware of "red flags" indicating more concerning symptoms including syncope related to exercise (either during or after), syncope without preceding symptoms or with resultant significant injury. Traumatic facial injuries are highly suggestive of cardiac syncope. Seizure-like activity and loss of bowl or bladder control are also concerning but less common with cardiac syncope. These symptoms more commonly lead to a diagnosis of seizure disorder. Seizures may occur in severe syncope of any etiology due to hypoperfusion of the brain.

It is critical to obtain a specific, detailed history regarding the syncopal episode. The events preceding the syncopal event should be discussed. This includes symptoms, relation to activity, how the patient looked to others, any resultant injury, and how quickly the patient recovered. The patient's last conscious recollection before the event and the first memory afterward is very important to determining the diagnosis. Ask about any similar symptoms in the past.

The patient's medical history should be reviewed including medical problems, daily medications, over the counter meds/supplements, and any new medications recently started. Exercise habits and tolerance should be ascertained. Social history is important regarding smoking, vaping, or use of illicit or synthetic drugs. Family history should be obtained including any history of sudden cardiac death (SCD) before age 50, unexplained motor vehicle accidents, SIDS deaths or drownings, ICDs/PPMs, and seizure disorders.

Physical Exam

A full cardiovascular exam is warranted to evaluate potential causes of syncope. Patients with a cardiac etiology of syncope may have structural findings such as a systolic murmur of valvular dysfunction or hypertrophic cardiomyopathy (HCM). Vital signs including BP and HR may show abnormalities, including orthostatic changes. Abnormal extra heart sounds (S3, S4) or displaced impulses may be noted.

Diagnostics

EKG is the first test that should be performed with syncope. This may show evidence of ischemia, abnormalities in conduction, including signs of block, arrhythmia, or QT interval prolongation.

Transthoracic echocardiography should be completed to assess for structural disease if any abnormalities are found on physical exam. Echocardiography can assess for valvular abnormalities, HCM, abnormal coronary origins in young adults, and evaluate for decreased LV function. Risk of death with low EF and syncope is high (see Ventricular Tachycardia, VT). If the etiology of syncope appears to be non-cardiac by history, echocardiography is not required.

Other tests may be done based upon the findings of the initial workup. If no structural disease is found, a patient can have ambulatory monitoring such as event or looping monitors. Subcutaneous loop recorders may be implanted for suspicious or recurrent events.

Syncope can occur in a patient with a previously implanted pacemaker. Interrogation of the device is important to determine the potential cause including device malfunction and exact rhythm during the syncopal event. Think of an implanted pacemaker as a continuous monitor of the cardiac rhythm. Representatives of the device manufacturers are always available for assistance.

Stress testing may be done to rule out exercise-induced arrhythmias and ischemia if the event occurred with activity. If underlying coronary artery disease or congestive heart failure is suspected, a cardiac catheterization may be warranted. An electrophysiology study may be needed to test the patient's conduction system and evaluate for ventricular arrhythmias.

Management

If patient has structural disease, management will be guided by specific disease type. Referral to a cardiac specialist should be considered. A patient with significant HCM and syncope will likely need medical treatment and potential ICD. Syncope with a reduced EF and structural heart disease must be treated as potential VT and EP evaluation and ICD should be considered. If a valvular or coronary anomaly is found, surgery may be the treatment recommendation. If the patient has ischemia on EKG or stress testing, cardiac catheterization may be needed for evaluation and ultimate treatment. Symptomatic bradycardia is a common cause of sudden, unprovoked syncope. If the EKG shows conduction abnormalities, pacemaker implantation may be needed (see bradycardia). If the EKG shows QT segment abnormalities suggestive of a channelopathy, further testing may be needed (see Chap. 11). There are other unusual etiologies that may require specialized management including pulmonary hypertension, cardiac tamponade, and PE.

Another common type of syncope is neurocardiogenic. This is an umbrella term describing various types of syncope including reflex syncope, vasodepressor syncope, postural syncope, and autonomic dysfunction. This may be described as the "common faint" and occurs in a patient with a normal heart. Prodromal symptoms occur more slowly with preceding symptoms of lightheadedness, blurry/blackened vision, muffled hearing, sweating, and nausea. Patients tend to be pale, bradycardic, and sweaty immediately prior to and after an episode. Recovery of mentation is usually quick when supine. The mechanism is not well understood but is thought to involve dysfunction of the autonomic nervous system, orthostatic intolerance, and intravascular volume depletion.

Patients may complain of dizziness while upright, tingling of the ears, nose, fingers, nausea, headaches, fatigue, atypical sharp stabbing chest pain, and palpitations. It can be worse in the heat, during menses or with febrile illness. Postural Orthostatic Tachycardia Syndrome, POTS, is a subset of this condition where the heart rate increases 30 beats per minute within 10 minutes of upright posture during a TILT table test without the blood pressure drop of orthostatic hypotension. TILT table testing has limited utility and should be considered only if the history of POTS is unclear.

Management of this constellation of symptoms consists of intense oral hydration, salt supplementation, lower extremity exercises (the Dallas protocol), and compression sleeves for the calves. Some patient symptoms improve with medications such as fludrocortisone, a mineralocorticoid or midodrine, a vasoconstrictor (alpha adrenergic agonist). Some patients may also have improvement with taking selective serotonin reuptake inhibitors, regulating their menstrual cycle (OCPs), and other therapies. Many centers now have multidisciplinary Dysautonomia Clinics for difficult cases. Difficult to manage patients may have concomitant collagen vascular disease or significant spinal injury.

Patients with high risk and unexplained syncopal events may not be allowed to drive for 6 months (state dependent) following the event unless underlying cause is corrected.

Clinical Pearls

- Facial or other severe trauma after syncope is suggestive of a cardiac cause.
- Syncope with structural heart disease or cardiomyopathy is high risk and ventricular tachycardia must be considered.
- Prodromal symptoms often suggest a noncardiac cause of syncope.
- The clinical history is important to determine the etiology of syncope.

Further Reading

1. Dick M. Clinical cardiac electrophysiology in the young. 2nd ed. New York: Springer; 2006/2015.
2. Eagle KA, Balinga RR. Practical cardiology. Evaluation and treatment of common cardiovascular disorders. Philadelphia, PA: Lippincott, Williams and Wilkins; 2013.

Part IV

Structural/Valvular Heart Disease

Anne Booke Michael Rinaldi
Elisabeth A. Powell Larry Watts
Rick Musialowski

Introduction

The heart valves have very important and specific functions which will be further discussed in this chapter. These valves are instrumental in creating cardiac output as described in Chap. 2. The bedside description of the cardiac cycle is defined by the opening and closing of the valves during ventricular systole and diastole. The heart sounds (S1 and S2) heard during physical examination are the closure of the atrioventricular and semilunar valves, respectively. This synchronized series of valve open and closure allows proper movement of blood oxygenating the tissues with each cardiac contraction.

Pathologic changes of the valves result in very specific disease states with corresponding physical examination findings. These pathologies may be described as stenotic or regurgitant. As the leaflets degenerate due to age and other etiologies, the structure of the leaflets and/or supportive apparatus will change. Depending on the valve and underlying etiology of the changes, the leaflets will develop reduced mobility (stenosis) and restrict the forward movement of blood. The leaflets may become incompetent and allow blood to reverse course back to the cardiac chamber just exited (regurgitant). Often, there is a combination of both pathologies.

A. Booke · M. Rinaldi
Interventional and Structural Heart Cardiology, Atrium Health/Sanger Heart and Vascular Institute, Charlotte, NC, USA
e-mail: Anne.Booke@atriumhealth.org

L. Watts · R. Musialowski
Atrium Health/Sanger Heart and Vascular Institute, Charlotte, NC, USA
e-mail: Michael.Rinaldi@atriumhealth.org; Larry.Watts@atriumhealth.org; Richard.musialowski@atriumhealth.org

E. A. Powell
Banner University Medical Center, Tucson, AZ, USA
e-mail: elisabeth.powell@bannerhealth.com

These different disease states cause a diverse spectrum of symptoms and physical findings. Stenotic pathology of the aortic and pulmonic valves produces a crescendo/decrescendo murmur due to rapidly changing pressure and volume of blood flow during ventricular systole. This murmur will radiate according to the path of blood flow after passing over the stenotic valve leaflets. Incompetence of mitral and tricuspid valves results in a holosystolic blowing murmur as blood flows back into the atria at a fixed pressure and volume. Radiation of these murmurs also follows the direction of the turbulent blood flow. These systolic murmurs are noted between S1 and S2. Incompetence of the aortic and pulmonic valves produces diastolic murmurs as the high pressure of the great vessels pushes blood back in the ventricles during ventricular diastole. These sounds occur after the second heart sound (S2) and are decrescendo in nature due to a runoff of great vessel pressure. Diastolic sounds of the mitral and tricuspid valves are rare and difficult to auscultate.

The management of valve disease is dependent on the valve and specific pathology. This chapter will review the cardiac valves with relevant examples of regurgitant and stenotic physiology. This is a rapidly advancing field with changes in management of valvular heart disease ever evolving. Surgical intervention with replacement and repair has an important role. Catheter based interventions are rapidly developing with less associated morbidity and mortality. Collaborative patient management using structural heart teams, advanced cardiovascular imaging, and therapeutic discussions are critical for best practice management.

General Information About Valve Disease

In evaluating patients with known or suspected valvular disease, transthoracic echocardiography (TTE) is the primary test for assessment of the valve anatomy, etiology, concurrent valve disease, ventricular function, and associated abnormalities such as aortic dilatation. For stenotic valves, key measurements include the maximum velocity, mean gradient, and valve area. For regurgitant valves, key measurements include the regurgitant orifice area, regurgitant volume, and regurgitant fraction as determined by Doppler readings. Assessment of pulmonary systolic pressures along with RV size and function is also important. When indicated, additional testing is obtained, including but not limited to chest X-ray, stress testing, transesophageal echocardiography TEE, CT heart, cardiac MRI, and cardiac catheterization for measurement of hemodynamics.

The American College of Cardiology (ACC) and American Heart Association (AHA) Indications for surveillance echocardiogram vary depending on stage of valvular disease and patient symptomatology. At a minimum, patients should be seen for yearly examination. Additionally, patients should report changes in their symptoms and a physical exam should be performed at each visit with echo performed if there are changes in exam. The purpose of follow-up is to prevent consequences of valvular heart disease, including alterations of ventricular function and pulmonary circulation, and to determine when referral is indicated for consideration of intervention (Fig. 1).

Stage	Aortic Stenosis	Aortic Regurgitation	Mitral Stenosis	Mitral Regurgitation
Progressive (Stage B)	Every 3-5 y (mild severity; V_{max} 2.0-2.9 m/s)	Every 3-5 y (mild severity)	Every 3-5 y (MV area >1.5 cm^2)	Every 1-2 y (moderate severity)
	Every 1-2 y (moderate severity; V_{max} 3.0-3.9 m/s)	Every 1-2 y (moderate severity)		Every 3-5 y (mild severity)
Severe asymptomatic (Stage C1)	Every 6-12 mo (V_{max} ≥4 m/s)	Every 6-12 mo Dilating LV: more frequently	Every 1-2 y (MV area 1.0-1.5 cm^2)	Every 6-12 mo Dilating LV: more frequently
			Every year (MV area <1.0 cm^2)	

Adapted from (6)

Fig. 1 Type of valve lesion. (Adapted from Otto CM, Nishimura RA, Bonow RO, Carabello BA, Erwin JP III, Gentile F. 2020 ACC/AHA Guideline for the management of patients with valvular heart disease: a report of the American College of Cardiology/American Heart Association Joint Committee on clinical practice guidelines. J Am Coll Cardiol. 2021;77(4):e25–e197)

16 Aortic Valve Disease

Anne Booke, Michael Rinaldi, Elisabeth A. Powell, Larry Watts, and Richard Musialowski

Bicuspid Aortic Valve (BAV)

BAV is the most common congenital cardiac anomaly (see Chap. 29), affecting 0.5–2.0% of adults, with males more commonly than females at about 3:1 predominance (Fig. 16.1) [1, 2]. The pathology can occur as an incomplete separation of the cusps during fetal development or when only two leaflets develop as seen in Fig. 16.2. Patients with BAV are at risk for developing isolated AI, AS, a combination of AS and AI, along with infective endocarditis. 20–40% of patients with BAV develop an aortopathy involving the aortic root, ascending aorta, or less frequently aortic coarctation [1]. Aortopathy may also occur independently of valvular disease and consists of dilation of aortic sinuses, ascending aorta, or aortic arch placing these patients at increased risk for aortic dissection. The prevalence of BAV in first degree relatives is 20–30% [1]. A specific genetic cause has not been identified and it is reasonable to screen first degree relatives with TTE to look for the presence of BAV or asymptomatic dilation of ascending aortic and aortic sinuses.

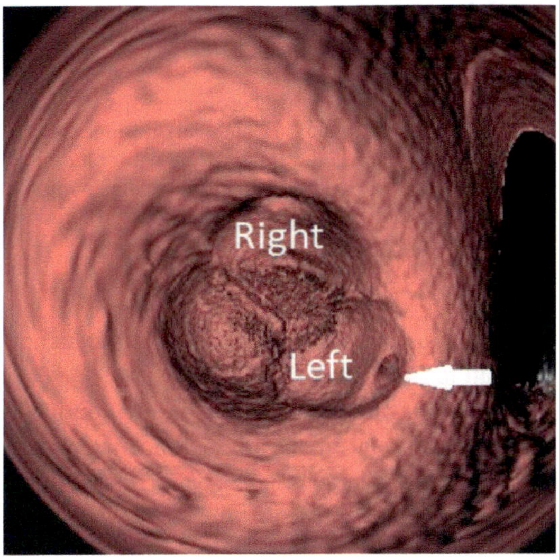

Fig. 16.1 CT Image of normal aortic cusps and origin of coronary arteries. The circular structure at the white arrow is the Left Main coronary artery arising above the left coronary cusp (LCC). The RCA origin arises above the right cusp but is in a different plane and not seen in this image

TTE is indicated in patients with BAV to evaluate valve morphology, severity of AS and AI, the Sinuses of Valsalva, the sinotubular junction (STJ), and the ascending aorta. When morphology cannot be fully assessed by TTE, Cardiac CT or CMR angiography is indicated for better assessment. Annual aortic imaging is recom-

A. Booke (✉) · M. Rinaldi · L. Watts
R. Musialowski
Sanger Heart and Vascular Institute, Atrium Health, Charlotte, NC, USA
e-mail: Anne.Booke@atriumhealth.org; Michael.Rinaldi@atriumhealth.org; Larry.Watts@atriumhealth.org; Richard.musialowski@atriumhealth.org

E. A. Powell
Banner University Medical Center, Tucson, AZ, USA
e-mail: elisabeth.powell@bannerhealth.com

R. Musialowski, K. Allshouse (eds.), *Cardiovascular Manual for the Advanced Practice Provider*, https://doi.org/10.1007/978-3-031-35819-7_16

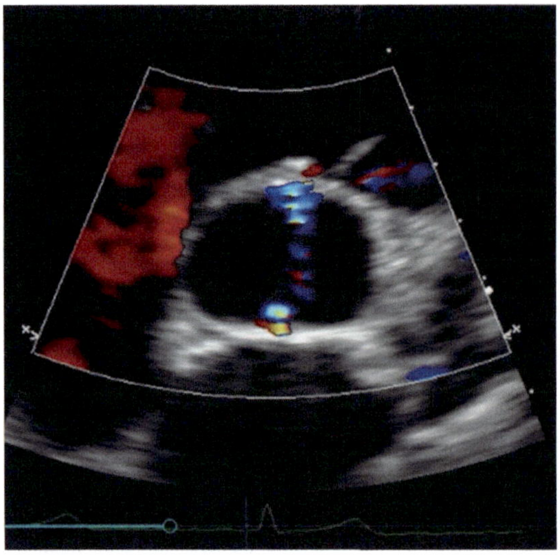

Fig. 16.2 Two closed aortic coronary cusps (right and left) seen with regurgitation (blue jet) during diastole. EKG at the bottom of the image shows the blue circle before the QRS and confirms ventricular diastole and a closed aortic valve. The closure is eccentric when compared to a trileaflet valve

mended in patients with BAV and significant aortic dilation (>4.0 cm).

The timing and type of surgical intervention in aortic valve replacement are dependent on anatomy, patient characteristics, and institutional expertise (see Fig. 6 from the 2020 AHA/ACC Valve Guidelines) [1]. (See further discussion in surgical AS section).

The timing and type of intervention for patients with BAV with AS or AI are like those for trileaflet valves, although most interventions commonly occur about a decade before those patients with trileaflet valves.

Aortic Stenosis (AS)

Etiology/Pathophysiology of Aortic Stenosis

The three main causes of aortic stenosis are (1) degeneration of the trileaflet valve, (2) calcification of a congenital bicuspid aortic valve (BAV), (3) rheumatic heart disease affecting the aortic valve [1, 2]. Mediastinal radiation has also been associated with scarring, fibrosis, and calcification of aortic leaflets [2].

- Degeneration occurs due to vascular atherosclerosis, endothelial dysfunction, lipid accumulation, inflammatory cell activation, and cytokine release with eventual deposition of calcium hydroxyapatite [3]. Patients typically develop symptoms in the 6th- 8th decades of life.
- Patients with BAV typically have larger aortas and are at increased risk for associated aortopathy and usually will develop symptoms one decade before patients with tricuspid aortic valve.
- Rheumatic changes result in commissural fusion, sometimes resulting in a bicuspid-appearing valve. Rheumatic heart disease is much less common in developed countries. Rheumatic AS is almost always associated with involvement of the mitral valve (mitral stenosis) and aortic insufficiency [1, 2].
- Currently, there is no medical therapy that remarkably slows or reverses the aging process of the aortic valve.

As the aortic valve narrows, the left ventricle (LV) must overcome the impedance to blood flow, resulting in increased LV systolic and diastolic pressures with concentric hypertrophy. Over time this reduces ventricular compliance resulting in increasing LV end diastolic pressures (LVEDP), or preload, and subsequent remodeling of the left atrium. Due to increasing afterload the LV contractile function declines over time. The cardiac output along with the LV aortic pressure gradient decline, and there is a rise in the mean left atrial pressure, pulmonary artery pressures, and right ventricular pressures [2]. In advanced stages of AS, patients may develop severe pulmonary hypertension resulting in RV dysfunction, secondary tricuspid regurgitation, and pulmonary venous hypertension [2].

Aortic stenosis is a progressive disease. The average rate of progression per year in Moderate

AS (peak aortic velocity 3–3.9 m/s on echocardiography) is an increase in velocity of 0.3 m/s, increase in mean pressure gradient by 7 mmHg, and decrease in AVA by 0.1 cm [4]. Severe AS (aortic velocity >/=4.0 m/s), rapidly progresses to symptoms with an event-free survival rate of 30–50% at 2 years [1]. See Table 16.1 for stages of progressive aortic valve disease.

Patients with severe AS may have concomitant degrees of MR that may improve with replacement of the aortic valve. In patients with concomitant rheumatic AS and MS, the decreased cardiac output induced by the MS lowers the pressure gradient across the aortic valve, masking the severity of the AS [2].

Cardiac Amyloidosis is also frequently associated with AS in elderly patients with a 9–15% incidence [1]. As amyloid will persist post valve intervention, it is associated with poor long-term prognosis for the patient despite valvular intervention. When cardiac amyloidosis is clinically suspected, amyloid labs and CMR should be considered prior to valvular intervention [1].

Symptoms

AS is an insidious disease with a long latency period with the most common reported symptom being dyspnea or decreased exercise tolerance. The classic triad of severe AS includes congestive heart failure (CHF), syncope, and angina. The progression of symptoms and severity of aortic valve disease is associated with a high rate of death (~ 50% in the first 2 years after symptoms appear) [1, 6].

Dyspnea results from narrowing of the aortic valve orifice along with elevated pulmonary pressures due to elevated LV diastolic pressures (LVEDP) in the setting of impaired relaxation and reduced LV compliance [2].

Angina occurs given the imbalance between oxygen supply and demand. Exertional syncope occurs because the LV cannot increase stroke volume (SV), and thus cardiac output (CO) during exercise given the narrowed aortic orifice in combination with vasodilation of peripheral muscle beds with exercise (decreased systemic vascular resistance, or SVR).

Table 16.1 Stages of aortic stenosis

Stage	Definition	Symptoms	Valve anatomy	Valve hemodynamics
A	At risk of AS	None	BAV (or other congenital valve anomaly) Aortic valve sclerosis	Aortic V_{max} <2 m/s with normal leaflet motion
B	Progressive AS	None	Mild to moderate leaflet calcification/fibrosis of a bicuspid or trileaflet valve with some reduction in systole motion [or] Rheumatic valve changes with commissural fusion	Mild AS: Aortic V_{max} 2.0–2.9 m/s or mean ΔP <20 mm Hg Moderate AS: Aortic V_{max} 3.0–3.9 m/s or mean ΔP 20–39 mm Hg
C: Asymptomatic severe AS				
C1	Asymptomatic severe AS	None Exercise testing is reasonable to confirm symptom status	Severe leaflet calcification/fibrosis or congenital stenosis with severely reduced leaflet opening	Aortic $V_{max} \geq 4$ m/s or mean $\Delta P \geq 40$ mm Hg AVA typically is ≤ 1.0 cm^2 (or AVAi 0.6 cm^2/m^2) but not required to define severe AS Very severe AS is an aortic $V_{max} \geq 5$ m/s or mean $\Delta P \geq 60$ mm Hg

Adapted from [5]

Patients may also exhibit symptoms of volume overload such as orthopnea, lower extremity edema, or paroxysmal nocturnal dyspnea.

Physical Exam/Cardiac Studies

The AS murmur is a mid to late peaking systolic murmur, commonly low-pitched and rough, heard at the second right intercostal space/the base of the heart. The AS murmur often radiates to the carotid arteries and to the apex of the heart where it may be confused with the MR murmur, and this is known as the Gallavardin effect [2]. The intensity of the murmur does not directly correlate with the severity of stenosis. The murmur may even become softer with increasing severity. The absence of the second heart sound suggests critical stenosis.

ECG. There is no close correlation between AS and ECG findings, although LVH is often present.

Labs: There are no labs that correlate with AS, but an elevated serum BNP may be a marker of subclinical HF and LV decompensation.

Echocardiogram. TTE assesses thickening and calcification of aortic valve leaflets, along with mean aortic gradient, calculated valve area, LV/RV function, concomitant valve disease, visualization of proximal aorta, and estimation of pulmonary pressures (Table 16.2 and Fig. 16.3). The improvement in echocardiographic technology and its ability to accurately define valve dynamics help determine the timing of intervention. Patients with poorly controlled hypertension (high SVR) should be optimized prior to undergoing echo to avoid flow effects of increased afterload which may result in falsely low aortic valve gradients [1].

Dobutamine Stress Echo (DSE). May be used to evaluate the asymptomatic patient or those with low flow, low gradient (LFLG) AS (see below). This is a class 2a indication in asymptomatic patients to assess for angina, dizziness, or abnormal BP response [1]. DSE increases the CO and helps determine if the AVA is truly less than severe. If the gradients and AVA worsen in severity with the increased flow from dobutamine, the stenosis is severe. DSE should be avoided in symptomatic patients given high risk of complications including syncope, VT/VF, and death. Asymptomatic patients with symptoms provoked by DSE should be considered symptomatic.

CT imaging. CT is used to further evaluate the degree of aortic calcification, valve area, aortic annulus, and concomitant cardiac disease. Aortic valve calcification is a strong predictor of clinical outcomes and Agatston units are a measurement of calcification. Per 2020 ACC/AHA guidelines, the sex-specific Agatston unit thresholds for severe AS are 1300 in women and 2000 in men (Fig. 16.4) [1]. The ESC guidelines further break it down as men >3000 Agaston units and women >1600 have a high likelihood, men >2000 and women >1200 are likely, and men <1600 and women <800 are unlikely [5].

Cardiac Catheterization. Cardiac catheterization is used for further hemodynamic assessment of the aortic valve. Those that are undergoing evaluation for aortic valve intervention often require cardiac catheterization to assess the degree of coronary artery disease prior to treatment of AS. With improvement in imaging technology, direct hemodynamic assessments with catheterization are less common.

Table 16.2 Echocardiographic parameters assessing aortic stenosis severity

	Normal	Mild	Moderate	Severe
Mean gradient (mmHg)	~5	≤20	20–39	≥40
Calculated valve area (cm^2)	2.5–4.5	>1.5	1.0–1.5	≤1.0
Peak V_{max} (m/s)		2.0–2.9	3.0–3.0	≥4.0

Evaluation/Management

As clinicians it is important to assess patient symptomatology. When reported symptoms worsen or murmur intensity on exam changes, repeat TTE is indicated. TTE monitors the degree of severity and concomitant valve disease along with ventricular remodeling. Routine surveil-

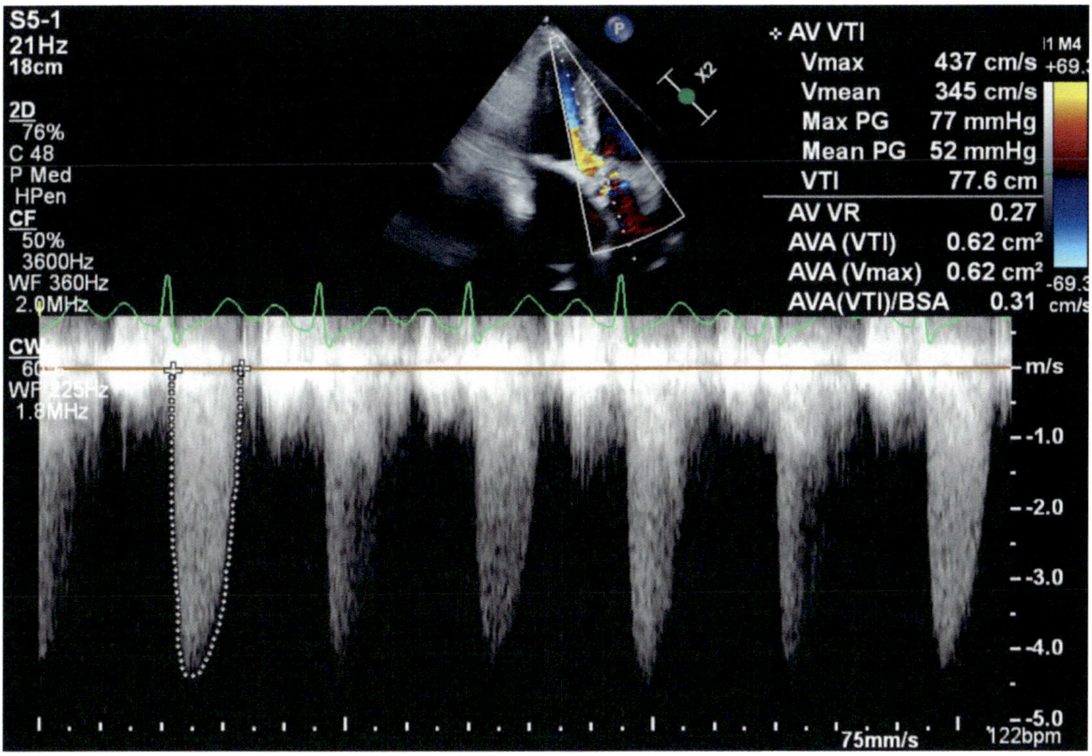

Fig. 16.3 Doppler of severe Aortic Stenosis. Mean gradient 52 mmHg, Peak velocity max >4 cm/s and aortic valve area (AVA) 0.62 cm^2 suggestive of severe AS

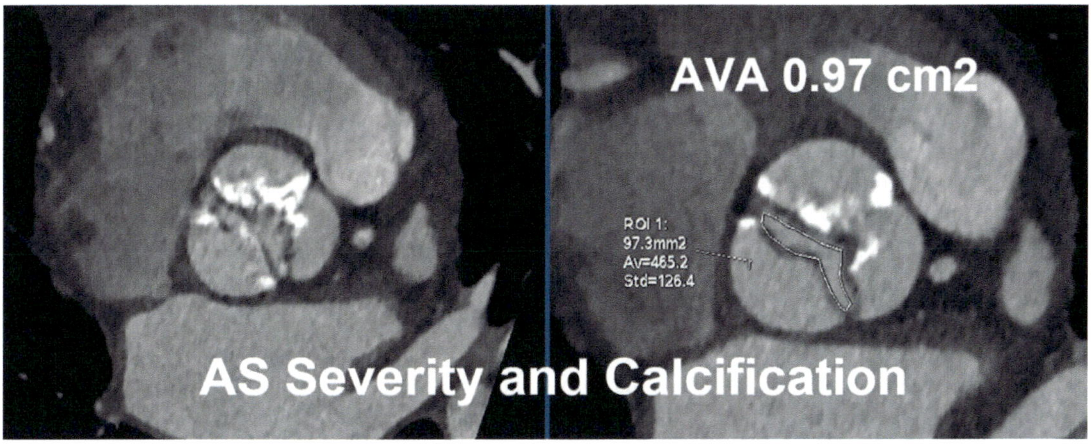

Fig. 16.4 CT images of severe calcific aortic stenosis. Left image during ventricular diastole with closed trileaflet valve. Right image shows reduced opening and a severely reduced area of <1 cm^2

lance every 6–12 months is indicated in patients with AS to time intervention on the valve.

It is important to remember that degree and severity of aortic stenosis by TTE and symptomatology may change in various clinical scenarios and hemodynamic states. Examples include but are not limited to anemia, GI bleed, surgery, pregnancy, and acute illness.

Low-flow-low-gradient (LFLG) AS is a diagnostic and therapeutic challenge. This occurs in the setting of decreased systolic dysfunction or in the setting of significantly hypertrophied LV with a small LV cavity despite a normal left ventricular ejection fraction (LVEF) [2]. Patients with AS with low EF (<50%) may present with decreased aortic valve area, but low mean gradient or velocity and may have low flow low gradient aortic stenosis. Severe AS with LV systolic dysfunction attributable to afterload mismatch must be distinguished from primary myocardial dysfunction with only moderate AS.

Low flow is arbitrarily defined by a stroke volume index (SVi) ≤ 35 mL/m2 - a threshold that is under current debate. The ESC defines four broad categories of AS:

1. High gradient AS (mean gradient ≥40 mmHg, peak velocity ≥ 4.0 m/s, valve area ≤ 1 cm^2). Severe AS assumed irrespective of LV function and flow conditions [7].
2. Low-flow, low-gradient AS with reduced LVEF (mean gradient <40 mmHg, valve area ≤ 1 cm^2, LVEF <50%, SVi ≤ 35 mL/m^2). Low dose DSE is recommended to distinguish between true severe and pseudo-severe aortic stenosis (increase in valve area to >1.0 cm2 with increased flow) and identify patients with no flow or contractile reserve [7].
3. Low-flow, low-gradient AS with preserved LVEF (mean gradient <40 mmHg, valve area ≤ 1 cm^2, LVEF ≥50%, SVi ≤ 35 mL/m^2). Typically encountered in hypertensive elderly patients with small LV size and marked hypertrophy. May also result from conditions associated with low stroke volume such as moderate/severe MR, severe TR, severe MS, large VSD, and severe RV dysfunction [7].
4. Normal-flow, low-gradient aortic stenosis with preserved LVEF (mean gradient <40 mmHg, valve area ≤ 1 cm^2, LVEF ≥50%, SVi >35 mL/m^2). These patients usually have only moderate AS although in a symptomatic patient without other explanation for symptoms a low index of suspicion should be maintained [7].

Standard Guideline Directed Medical Therapy (GDMT) drug therapy for LV function should be continued including diuretics, ACE-I/ARB/ARNI, Aldactone, beta-blockers, and biventricular pacing as hemodynamics allow (see sect. 5). Clinicians should avoid abruptly lowering blood pressure in AS patients and use caution with the addition of betablockers in uncompensated patients [1]. Caution with over-diuresis as the preload reduction will reduce stroke volume, especially if LV cavity is small [1]. Nitrates should also be used cautiously, or avoided, in AS as they will cause vasodilatation and decreased preload resulting in hypotension.

Intervention

Symptomatic AS has a dismal prognosis and early intervention is recommended. Caveats to this are those with severe comorbidities and unlikeliness of improving quality of life, malignancy, or expected survival of <1 year. Once severe AS is confirmed, or concern for severe AS is suspected, patients should be referred to a valve center for evaluation for aortic valve replacement (AVR) either surgically or by a transcatheter approach.

Eligibility for AVR depends on the presence of symptoms, the preservation of left ventricular ejection fraction (LVEF), and the degree of stenosis. According to the 2020 ACC/AHA guidelines, recommendations for intervention are categorized into classes ranging from recommended to may/might be reasonable. Recommendations are based on surgical benefit to risk ratios [1]. The indications for SAVR, as defined by the ACC/AHA guidelines, are outlined in Table 16.3.

Without intervention, symptomatic AS has a poor prognosis of 50% mortality within 2 years, reducing to less than 1 year with the development of symptomatic left heart failure [8]. Surgical intervention is still recommended in asymptomatic patients, but the prognosis is better with the risk of sudden death less than 1% per year [8]. Timing of intervention for asymptomatic patients depends on physiological factors indicating heart strain. Reduction of LVEF, elevated BNP >3x normal, and rapid progression of disease on TTE are all indications.

Current data is limited regarding progression of aortic dilation and risk of dissection after AVR in patients with a bicuspid aortic valve (BAV) [1].

Table 16.3 Indications for surgical aortic valve replacement (SAVR)

Class 1 (Recommended)	
Symptomatic AS	*Severe*, high-grade AS ($V_{max} \geq 4$ m/s or ΔP mean ≥ 40 mm Hg)
	Severe Low-flow, Low-gradient AS with LVEF < 50% ($V_{max} < 4$ m/s and AVA ≤ 1.0 cm^2 at rest and $V_{max} \geq 4$ m/s and AVA ≤ 1.0 cm^2 at any flow rate with dobutamine stress echocardiogram
	Severe low-gradient AS with LVEF > 50% and AS most common cause of symptoms (AVA ≤ 0.6 cm^2 and stroke volume index < 35 mL/m^2)
Asymptomatic AS	*Severe* AS with LVEF < 50%
	Severe AS when patient undergoing another cardiac surgery (i.e. CABG)
Class 2a (Reasonable)	
Asymptomatic AS	Exercise treadmill test with ↓ BP or exercise capacity
	$V_{max} \geq 5$ m/s and low surgical risk
	BNP > 3x normal and low surgical risk
	Rapid disease progression and low surgical risk
Class 2b (may/might be reasonable)	
Asymptomatic AS	*Severe* AS with reduction of LVEF to <60% on 3 serial studies
Asymptomatic AS	*Moderate* AS and patient undergoing another cardiac surgery

Adapted from [5]

Current guidelines recommend aortic root and/or ascending aorta replacement at the time of SAVR due to severe AS if the diameter is >4.5 cm [1]. Refer to section on BAV intervention and chapter on aortic aneurysms for further discussion and guidelines.

Evaluation for AVR includes assessment by a cardiac surgeon and interventional cardiologist and often includes advanced imagers, physician assistants, nurse practitioners, and nurse navigators as part of the care team. The team will evaluate the patient and review all clinical imaging to determine if the patient is best served by surgical aortic valve replacement (SAVR) or transcatheter aortic valve replacement (TAVR). Risk assessment is a foundational element of preprocedural evaluation of patients with valvular heart disease (VHD). The Society of Thoracic Surgeons (STS) score and other technical, clinical, and anatomic factors are considered for the best therapeutic option (see below).

As part of the decision between TAVR vs SAVR, the multidisciplinary team will look at age (< 65 years), comorbidities, predicted life expectancy, implantation risk, prosthesis durability, potential need for sequential procedures (valve in valve vs redo operation) to determine what is the best option for an AVR patient. Lifetime management for valve disease is a critically important concept in younger patients undergoing AVR who will likely outlive the first valve. TAVR valves appear harder to remove than SAVR and may require full root replacement.

Aortic Valve Pre-Intervention Testing

As discussed under surgical management for coronary artery disease (Chap. 6), surgical work-up begins with establishing patient's baseline condition with a full history, physical, and diagnostic work up. Refer to Tables 6.1 and 6.2 in Chap. 6 for discussion on preoperative assessment.

Along with the standard preoperative testing, all patients undergoing cardiac surgery should have a cardiac catheterization to assess for coronary artery disease. With the use of coronary CT, certain patients may have coronary arteries cleared by CT, thus avoiding cardiac catheterization. This is especially important in patients with AS since concurrent CAD is common [1]. If obstructive coronary disease is present, CABG should be completed at the time of the SAVR or PCI should be considered prior to TAVR.

Cardiac CTA is essential to determine aortic valve anatomy, annular size and shape, extent and distribution of valve and vascular calcification, risk of coronary ostial obstruction, aortic root dimensions, optimal fluoroscopic projections for valve deployment, and feasibility of vascular access for TAVR (femoral, subclavian, axillary, carotid, transcaval, or transapical). While CTA may be able to ascertain patency of coronary arteries, coronary angiography is generally recommended to establish severity of CAD.

While studies have shown that CABG at the time of SAVR improves outcomes in patients with significant coronary obstruction, revascularization prior to TAVR remains controversial and is the subject of an ongoing randomized trial. Generally, most operators will revascularize proximal severe disease supplying significant myocardial territory particularly if angina is a prominent component of the patients' symptoms.

When indicated, patients may also undergo cardiac MRI, carotid ultrasound, pulmonary function testing, and if they have other comorbidities may be referred to other specialties or undergo further testing prior to AVR.

In patients undergoing valve surgery, it is imperative to take a dental health history and note any prominent dental caries, abscesses, or poor dental hygiene. If there are issues of concern, the patient should be evaluated and cleared by a dental professional preoperatively to decrease the risk of endocarditis after the placement of a prosthetic valve.

Preoperative work up is both patient and surgeon specific. Surgical and medical decision making is multifactorial and should include a multidisciplinary team.

The STS risk calculator may be utilized to aid in decision making and risk mitigation prior to SAVR. Further discussion on the STS risk calculator can be reviewed in Chap. 6: Surgical management for coronary artery disease. For risk categories covered with the STS calculator, refer to Table 6.3 in that chapter. In general, the overall operative mortality for an isolated SAVR in patients under 70 years old is considered low at 1–3%, with a slight rise to 4–8% in older populations [8]. Currently, the STS calculator does not calculate the risk for aortic valve repair.

Transcatheter Aortic Valve Replacement (TAVR)

TAVR is a less invasive method for AVR than traditional surgery. It has been shown to improve survival, reduce HF hospitalization, reduce symptoms in nonsurgical candidates, and has been shown to be an alternative to surgery with lower stroke, death, and major complications compared to surgery in both intermediate and low risk surgical candidates over age 65. TAVR was first performed in 2002 and has undergone several multicenter trials known as the Placement of Aortic Transcatheter Valves (PARTNER) Trials.

Valve selection in TAVR is based on several measurements obtained from cardiac CT imaging. Sizing of the valve is important to avoid aortic rupture during valve deployment, valve dislocation with embolization, or resultant perivalvular leak if the valve is undersized. Patient prosthetic mismatch (as determined by patient body surface area to valve size) is to be avoided because symptoms may not improve after the valve intervention.

TAVR is performed under mild sedative or general anesthesia (Fig. 16.5). Once sedated, vascular arterial access is obtained, most commonly femoral access but those with unfavorable femoral anatomy may require alternative access such as subclavian, axillary, carotid, transcaval, or transapical. In the procedural lab, a clear view of the aortic annulus is established on fluoroscopy, balloon aortic valvuloplasty is performed in select patients with aortic stenosis, and then the heart is rapidly paced to produce ventricular standstill while the bioprosthetic aortic valve is deployed. Procedural risks include vascular complications, electrical conduction disturbance, bleeding, stroke, MI, renal dysfunction, and death.

TAVR Procedural Conduction Management

All TAVR patients require rapid ventricular pacing during deployment in order to produce ventricular standstill and accurate positioning of the prosthesis. Patients at increased risk of requiring permanent pacemaker have preexisting LBBB, RBBB, atrial fibrillation with innately slow ventricular response, and those with short membranous septum lengths. This cohort of patients may receive a temporary pacing wire (often an active fixation lead via the right internal jugular vein) for at least 48 hours.

For patients with new LBBB at discharge or RBBB that was present pre-procedure that did not progress to advanced heart block requiring

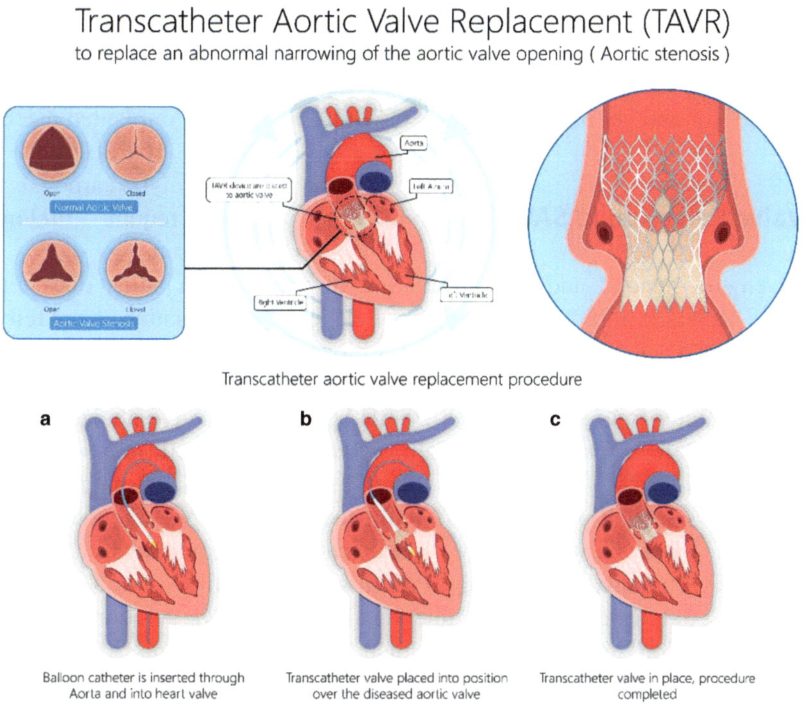

Fig. 16.5 TAVR for aortic stenosis

pacemaker implant during their hospital stay, a 2-week monitor is typically placed at discharge to monitor for progression of heart block.

Post TAVR Valve Implant Management

Post procedure patients are placed on aspirin 81 mg indefinitely and Plavix 75 mg for 3 months; aspirin monotherapy is used in patient with high bleeding risk (HBR). Of note that regimen may change if patients have an indication for systemic oral anticoagulation (OAC), recent coronary stenting with longer indication for dual antiplatelet therapy (DAPT), increased risk for bleeding, or other factors.

If the patient has an indication for OAC, it is recommended that OAC is continued for life with optional addition of aspirin which can be withheld in patients with HBR. For patients undergoing surgical procedures requiring cessation of antiplatelet and anticoagulation agents, it is safe to briefly withhold all agents without the need for bridging. Patients are typically seen at 1 week, 1 month, and 1 year following discharge with an ECG and TTE at 1 month and 1 year.

There are no guidelines for echocardiographic follow up of TAVR patients, but many practices advocate yearly TTE given the uncertainties around durability and the higher rates of development of hypo attenuated leaflet thickening (HALT) and partial valve thrombosis (see bioprosthetic valve dysfunction section below).

Surgical Management of Aortic Stenosis

Aortic valve replacement (AVR) is the treatment of choice for AS and the most common reason for surgical intervention on the aortic valve [8]. During surgical aortic valve replacement (SAVR), the heart is placed on cardiopulmonary bypass, the heart is arrested, and the patient's native valve is removed. After debridement of any residual calcification is complete, a prosthetic valve is sewn in, ensuring not to block the left and right coronary ostium which sits right above the aortic valve. Replacement of the AV is recommended in severe AS and considered reasonable in moderate AS when patient is already undergoing cardiac surgery for another purpose, such as CABG.

Valve Selection in SAVR

Given the stenotic and calcified nature of the valve leaflets in aortic stenosis, repair of the leaflets is not justified. AVR with either a bioprosthetic valve or mechanical valve is the standard of care. Refer to Fig. 11 in the 2020 AHA/ACC Valve Guidelines for current prosthetic valve recommendations [1].

Valve selection is a serious, multi-faceted decision made between surgeon and patient which is continually evolving. Patient's age, medical compliance, ability to tolerate lifelong anticoagulation, and patient's individual desires must all be considered. The 2020 ACC/AHA Guidelines recommend mechanical valves in patients younger than 50 years old and bioprosthetic valves for patients greater than 65 years old. This requires consideration of the patient's life expectancy and potential need for a reoperation if the patient's lifespan exceeds the longevity of the selected valve. Mechanical valves are the valve of choice in younger patients (<50 years old), as they are extremely durable and will not degenerate over time. With mechanical valves, strict life-long anticoagulation with warfarin is required to prevent thrombus formation. Thrombus on a mechanical valve may lead to thromboembolic events such as stroke, or thrombose the physical valve leaflets, preventing leaflets from opening or closing. When implanting a mechanical valve, the patient must fully understand the risks associated with chronic anticoagulation and the implications of subtherapeutic INRs or medical noncompliance. Another important consideration in the placement of a mechanical valve is the chance of pregnancy in young women (Chap. 34). In the case of pregnancy, there are multiple anticoagulation alternatives during each trimester; however, no therapy is consistently safe for both mother and fetus. Given the anticoagulation requirement, there is a serious complication to either the mother or the fetus during pregnancy in one-third of the women with mechanical valves [1].

An implanted mechanical AV is demonstrated in Fig. 16.6. Here the On-X™ valve, constructed of pyrolytic carbon, is demonstrated. This patient will require lifelong anticoagulation with Warfarin.

If a patient does not want to take lifelong anticoagulation, is not felt to be an appropriate candidate for vitamin K antagonists (VKA), or is elderly, then a bioprosthetic valve is an appropriate valve choice. These "tissue valves" are constructed from bovine or porcine conduit and have decreased longevity and valve durability when compared to the mechanical valve. Deterioration of the valve occurs sooner in younger vs older patients (> 65 years old). In general, the risk of valve deterioration requiring reoperation is 22% in patients 50 years old, 30% in patients 40 years old, and 50% in patients 20 years old [1]. Although tissue valves do not require long-term anticoagulation, 3–6 months of VKA anticoagulation is reasonable if the patient is at low risk for bleeding. This decreases stroke risk until the bioprosthetic valve is endothelialized [1]. Replacement of a patient's native aortic valve with a bioprosthetic tissue valve is demonstrated in Fig. 16.7 and post-operative CT imaging is seen in Fig. 16.8.

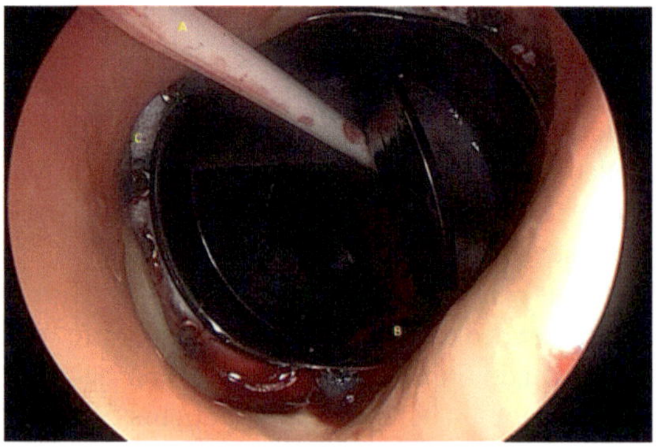

Fig. 16.6 Aortic valve replacement with a mechanical valve. Viewed from the ascending aorta down into the left ventricle. (**a**) valve tester demonstrating functional opening leaflets. (**b**) prosthetic valve leaflets. (**c**) Valve sewing ring

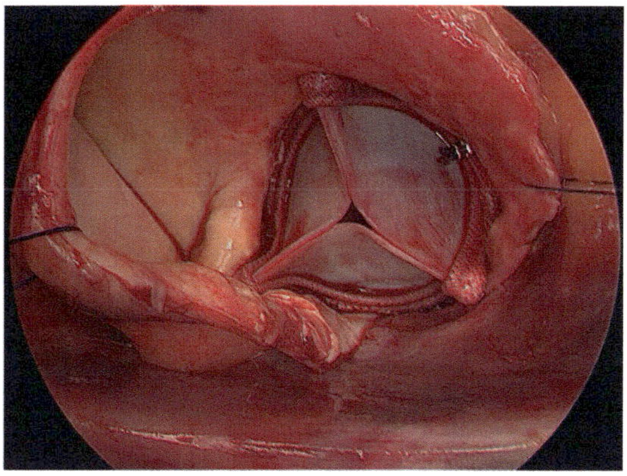

Fig. 16.7 Aortic valve replacement with bioprosthetic valve

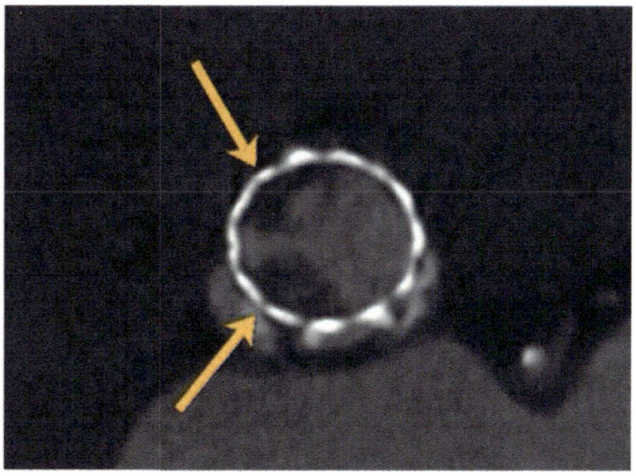

Fig. 16.9 Bioprosthetic aortic valve with thrombus (HALT) and restricted leaflet mobility on CT as shown by arrows

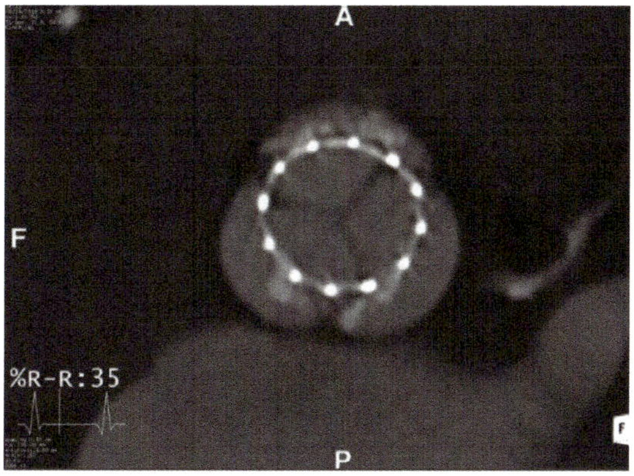

Fig. 16.8 Normal appear bioprosthetic valve on cardiac CT

With advancements in the durability of bioprosthetic valves and the introduction of the TAVR, potentially negating the need for a re-sternotomy at the time of valve replacement, bioprosthetic valves have been justified in a younger population. At the same time, advancements with the mechanical valves are leading to lower anticoagulation recommendations, creating a safer and more tolerated valve. These advancements and the role of the TAVR have created a gray area in the guidelines for patients between the ages of 50 and 65 years old. This is a situation where surgeon-patient discussions, critical thinking, and judgment are crucial in medical decision making. Current guidelines for anticoagulation management for valve replacement are outlined in Fig. 12 in the 2020 AHA/ACC Valve Guidelines [1].

Aortic Bioprosthetic or Mechanical Valve Dysfunction

Bioprosthetic aortic valves may thrombose or degenerate overtime. Thrombosis most commonly occurs in the first 3 months following implantation but has also been described years later [1]. While bioprosthetic valves are less thrombogenic than mechanical valves, the diagnosis of subclinical thrombosis has increased with the use of CT imaging.

Bioprosthetic thrombosis appears more common with transcatheter valves versus with surgical valves and leaflet thrombosis should be suspected with increased transvalvular gradients by TTE imaging. When transvalvular gradients are increased, then cardiac CT should be obtained to evaluate. Early hypoattenuated leaflet thickening (HALT) occurs in at least 10% of TAVR patient and prognostic information is uncertain [9]. While HALT is not associated with mortality or cerebrovascular events, it is associated with symptomatic valve deterioration and patients are placed on systemic anticoagulation [9] (Fig. 16.9).

Bioprosthetic aortic stenosis can occur with both mechanical and bioprosthetic valves and may be due to thrombus formation leading to abnormal leaflet mobility, pannus ingrowth, or structural valve deterioration due to degeneration by leaflet thickening or calcification [1]. Patients with symptomatic bioprosthetic stenosis should be referred to Valve Centers for consideration of valve replacement, either with redo surgery or transcatheter valve in valve therapy.

Bioprosthetic insufficiency may occur in the setting of leaflet tear or infective endocarditis destroying the valve leaflet resulting in heart failure and is an indication for patients to be referred to a Valve Center for replacement. These are patients that should be rapidly referred for assessment. See Fig. 14 in the 2020 AHA/ACC Valve guidelines for recommendations [1].

Aortic Insufficiency (AI) or Aortic Regurgitation (AR)

Acute Aortic Insufficiency

Etiology

Acute AI most commonly occurs in the setting of endocarditis, trauma, and/or aortic dissection. In endocarditis, vegetation causes direct disruption of the valve coaptation, or physical perforation of the leaflets (see Chap. 19). In aortic dissection, aortic valve insufficiency is secondary to the dilation of the aortic root, stretching the valves so they do not coapt, or dissection of the valve commissure (see Chap. 28).

Acute AI results in a sudden increase of volume in the LV at the end of diastole (preload), due to valve incompetence, leading to rapid hemodynamic instability and flash pulmonary edema.

Physical Exam

Acute AI may have no murmur due to rapid equalization of pressure. There will be a wide pulse pressure and low diastolic pressure. When the murmur is better appreciated on the right sternal border, concern should be raised for aortic dissection [3]. The murmur may be a high-pitched, blowing decrescendo diastolic murmur heard best at the third intercostal space of the left sternal border. The closure of the aortic valve (A2) is usually absent.

Intervention/Management of Acute AI

Medical therapy, including IV diuretics or vasodilators, can help reduce LV afterload to allow for temporary stabilization, although surgery should not be delayed, especially in setting of hypotension, pulmonary edema, or end-organ hypoperfusion. In patients with hypertension, blood pressure can be controlled with initiation of ACE/ARB or dihydropyridine CCBs. Beta-blockers, while they can help in patients if indicated in acute aortic dissection, should be avoided in acute AI as they will block compensatory tachycardia necessary for cardiac output, resulting in hypotension and shock. Intra-aortic balloon pumps are also contraindicated.

Acute severe AI is a surgical emergency. Surgical intervention of acute is dependent on the acuity of the deficiency and development of symptoms. A sudden change in hemodynamics requires urgent surgical intervention.

Chronic Aortic Insufficiency

Etiology

Chronic AI may be caused by primary valve disease, primary root disease, or secondary causes. The most common cause for AI in high income countries is BAV and in low to middle income countries is rheumatic heart disease [1]. Membranous subaortic stenosis may lead to thickening and scarring of aortic leaflets resulting in AI and in ~15% of patients with a VSD, there is prolapse of the aortic cusp resulting in AI [2]. Marked aortic annular dilatation, retrograde aortic dissection involving the annulus, or medical degeneration of the ascending aortic in conditions such as Marfan's, idiopathic aortic dilation, osteogenesis imperfecta, and severe chronic hypertension may also result in AI. AI is less commonly seen secondary to syphilis and ankylosing spondylitis. AI commonly occurs with infective endocarditis.

In patients with chronic AI, the LV stroke volume increases resulting in an increase in LVEDP (preload). The LV hypertrophies and dilates resulting in increased preload and afterload, and once LV adaptive measures fail, the LV function deteriorates [2]. In chronic AI, there is commonly elevation in LA, PA wedge, PA, and RV pressures. Patients with AI may experience myocardial ischemia secondary to increased myocardial oxygen requirements from LV dilation or hypertrophy.

Since the development of AI is slow, the left ventricle (LV) has time to compensate for the gradual increase in preload. The LV diameter slowly dilates resulting in eccentric hypertrophy. As the LV compensates for the increased volume, the onset of symptoms and need for surgery are delayed. Patients will complain of dyspnea first, with progression to orthopnea, PND, diaphoresis, angina, and lower extremity edema.

Physical Exam

An AI murmur is a high-pitched, blowing decrescendo diastolic murmur heard best at the third ICS of the LSB and the closure of the aortic valve (A2) is usually absent. When the murmur is better appreciated on the right, sternal border concern should be raised for aortic dissection [3]. Severe AI is associated with a wide pulse pressure and low diastolic pressure.

Evaluation/Management

ECG. ECG may demonstrate LVH, lateral (I, aVL, V5, V6) ST-depressions of T-wave inversions, left axis deviation, QRS widening.

Imaging Studies. TTE provides diagnostic information about the etiology and mechanism of AI and evaluates degree of LVEF and LV chamber remodeling. TTE is useful in the evaluation of a dilated aortic annulus and root, aortic dissection, and primary leaflet morphology.

When TTE measurements are discordant with clinical findings, Cardiac MRI (CMR) can be used. CMR accurately quantifies the regurgitation severity and LV remodeling. In asymptomatic patients, CMR is predictive of those who will require surgery and who will have incomplete reverse modeling, and those with late gadolinium enhancement having worse outcomes. TEE can further assess the aortic valve, cardiac catheterization with aortic angiography and CT scan can further assess the aorta. Six months to yearly echocardiographic surveillance is indicated to optimize timing surgical intervention (Fig. 16.10).

In asymptomatic patients with chronic AI, medical therapy should be initiated for hypertension, heart failure, or other comorbidities. In asymptomatic patients, treatment of systolic BP to <140 mmHg is recommended. Patients with severe AI with or without LV dysfunction, who are prohibitive surgical risks, GDMT with ACE/ARB, sacubitril/valsartan, or dihydropyridine CCBs is recommended [1].

TAVR for AI is technically challenging given dilation of aortic annulus or root and lack of aortic valve calcification to act as scaffolding for the aortic valve. The aortic bioprosthesis can migrate, creating a significant paravalvular leak. In patients who are surgical candidates, TAVR should not be performed.

Surgical intervention for chronic AI is dependent on the presence of symptoms. If a patient's severe AI becomes symptomatic, surgery is warranted regardless of LV function [1]. If a patient with severe AI remains asymptomatic, the timing of surgery becomes dependent on the presence of decreased LV function. These parameters are a left ventricular ejection fraction (LVEF) below 55% or increase of left ventricular end-systolic dimension of >50 mm seen on cardiac imaging [1]. If the patient requires another cardiac operation, such as a CABG, the aortic valve should be repaired/replaced simultaneously if moderate or severe AI is present at the time of the index operation [1]. (See Fig. 4 in the 2020 AHA/ACC Valve Guidelines [1]).

AI is surgically corrected by performing an aortic valve replacement (SAVR) or an aortic valve repair (SAVr). A SAVR entails removing the patient's aortic valve and replacing the entire apparatus with either a bioprosthetic valve or a mechanical valve. Aortic valve replacement remains the gold standard treatment of aortic valve disease when the cause of AI stems primarily from the valve leaflets. Insufficiency from

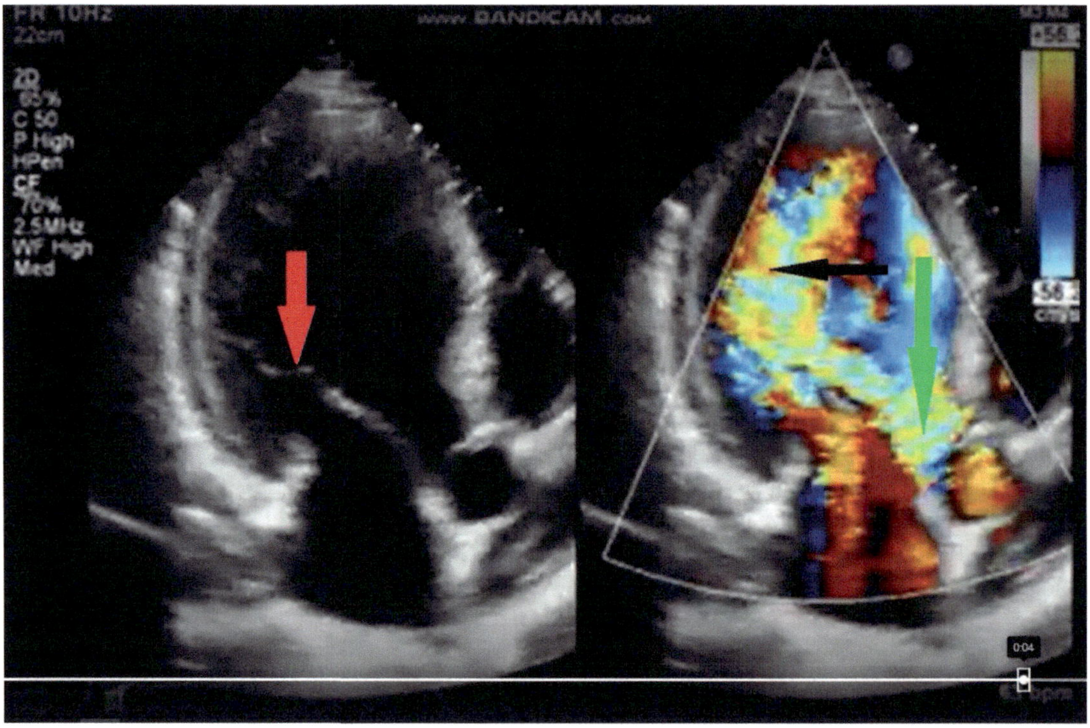

Fig. 16.10 TTE Image of severe AI with ventricular dilatation. The left panel of Fig. 16.10 shows the mitral valve is open (red arrow) confirming ventricular diastole. The right panel shows a green arrow pointing at the regurgitant jet filling the LVOT, and this AI jet swirls into the LV (black arrow) suggestive of severe and acute AI

a bicuspid valve, endocarditis, or annular dilation warrants valve replacement. A valve repair involves maintaining the native valve and repairing the defect that is causing the valve to leak. SAVr is gaining popularity with numerous advances in techniques and reproducible results. Aortic valve repair or "valve-sparing" operations are becoming commonplace when the regurgitation is secondary to coaptation from a dilated aortic root or aortic aneurysm. In these scenarios, the aortic leaflets otherwise appear functional. This type of repair is demonstrated in Fig. 16.11. Here the patient's aneurysmal root was replaced with a tube graft and the native valve was resuspended within. This technique re-establishes coaptation of the native leaflets with no residual aortic insufficiency. As understanding of the mechanics and geometry of the aortic valve expand, surgical repair techniques continue to improve. With time, the durability of the AV repair may become more apparent and may become a more prominent treatment for aortic valve insufficiency.

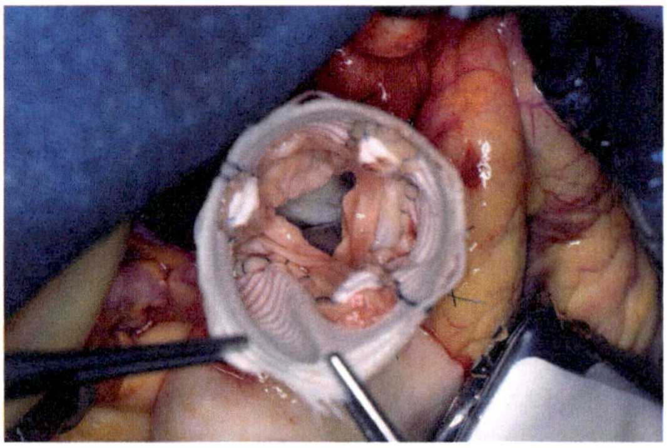

Fig. 16.11 Aortic root replacement with a native valve-sparing repair due to aortic aneurysm and insufficiency. Photo Credit: Bob Hooker, MD

Current data is limited regarding progression of aortic dilation and risk of dissection after AVR in patients with a bicuspid aortic valve (BAV). Current guidelines recommend aortic root and/or ascending aorta replacement at the time of SAVR due to severe AI if the diameter is >4.5 cm [1]. Refer to section on BAV intervention and chapter on aortic aneurysms for further discussion and guidelines.

Preoperative Assessment and Calculating Risk

Preoperative assessment and risk stratification are the same for aortic valve intervention regardless of etiology. Preoperative work-up includes a detailed history and physical exam including dental history, and also basic lab and imaging modalities. Preoperative cardiac catheterization should be completed to assess for coronary artery disease. Refer to similar section under Surgical Management of CAD Tables 6.1, 6.2, and 6.3. Again, the overall operative mortality for an isolated AVR in patients under 70 years old is considered low at 1–3% and increases to a risk of 4–8% in older populations [8].

Valve Selection

As with AS, if the aortic valve is unrepairable, the next step is valve selection between a mechanical or a bioprosthetic valve. This decision is multifactorial and is based on age, medical compliance, risk of lifelong anticoagulation, and the patient's individual desires. Valve selection is a serious, multi-faceted decision made between surgeon and patient which is continually evolving. Recent advancements in technology for both types of valves have made them more acceptable to outlying patients. Bioprosthetic valves are becoming more durable while mechanical valves require lower levels of anticoagulation. Refer to the section on AS for further discussion.

References

1. Otto CM, Nishimura RA, Bonow RO, Carabello BA, Erwin JP III, Gentile F. 2020 ACC/AHA guideline for the management of patients with valvular heart disease: a report of the American College of Cardiology/American Heart Association Joint Committee on clinical practice guidelines. J Am Coll Cardiol. 2021;77(4):e25–e197.
2. Loscalzo J, Fauci A, et al. Harrison's principles of internal medicine. 21st. ed, Volume 1 and Volume 2. New York: McGraw Hill; 2022.
3. Lawton JS, Tamis-Holland JE, Bangalore S, Bates ER, Beckie TM, Mischoff JM, et al. 2021 ACC/AHA/SCAI guideline for coronary artery revascularization, a report of the American College of Cardiology/American Heart Association Joint Committee on clinical practice guidelines. J Am Coll Cardiol. 2022, 79:e21–e129.
4. The Society of Thoracic Surgeons. 2022. https://www.sts.org/resources/risk-calculator.
5. O'Brien SM, Feng L, He X, Xian Y, Jacobs JP, Badhwar V, et al. The Society of Thoracic Surgeons 2018 adult cardiac surgery risk models: part 2 - statistical methods and results. Ann Thorac Surg. 2018, 105:1419–28.
6. Taramassa M, et al. Tricuspid regurgitation, predicting the need for intervention, procedural success, and recurrence of disease. JACC Cardiovasc Imaging. 2019;12(4):605–21. https://doi.org/10.1016/j.jcmg.2018.11.034.
7. Vahanian A, Beyersdorf F, Praz F, Milojevic M, Baldus S, Bauersachs J, Capodanno D, Conradi L, De Bonis M, De Paulis R, Delgado V, Freemantle N, Gilard M, Haugaa KH, Jeppsson A, Jüni P, Pierard L, Prendergast BD, Sádaba JR, Tribouilloy C, Wojakowski W, ESC/EACTS Scientific Document Group, ESC National Cardiac Societies. 2021 ESC/EACTS Guidelines for the management of valvular heart disease: Developed by the Task Force for the management of valvular heart disease of the European Society of Cardiology (ESC) and the European Association for Cardio-Thoracic Surgery (EACTS). Eur Heart J. 2022;43(7):561–632.
8. Chung J, Shum-Tim D. The current indications and options for aortic valve surgery. J Surg. 2014;2(1).
9. Hein M, Schoechlin S, Schulz U, Minners J, Breitbart P, Lehane C, Neumann F-J, Ruile P. Long-term follow-up of hypoattenuated leaflet thickening after transcatheter aortic valve replacement. JACC Cardiovasc Interv. 2022;15(11):1113–22.

Mitral Valve Disease

17

Anne Booke, Michael Rinaldi, Elisabeth A. Powell, Larry Watts, and Richard Musialowski

Mitral Insufficiency/Mitral Regurgitation (MR)

Acute Mitral Insufficiency

Acute MR is related to primary valve pathology affecting the leaflets, chords, papillary muscle, or mitral anulus. Infective endocarditis may cause leaflet tears or chordal rupture. Myxomatous mitral valves degenerate over time which may result in spontaneous chordal rupture. Papillary muscle rupture, most commonly the posteromedial papillary muscle, may occur as a complication of inferior STEMI resulting in acute MR. Acute MR may also be seen in transient ischemia and in patients with blunt chest wall trauma. Acute MR results in acute volume overload resulting in pulmonary congestion and a low forward cardiac output. Rapid diagnosis is essential as these patients are at elevated risk for hemodynamic compromise (Figs. 17.1 and 17.2) [1].

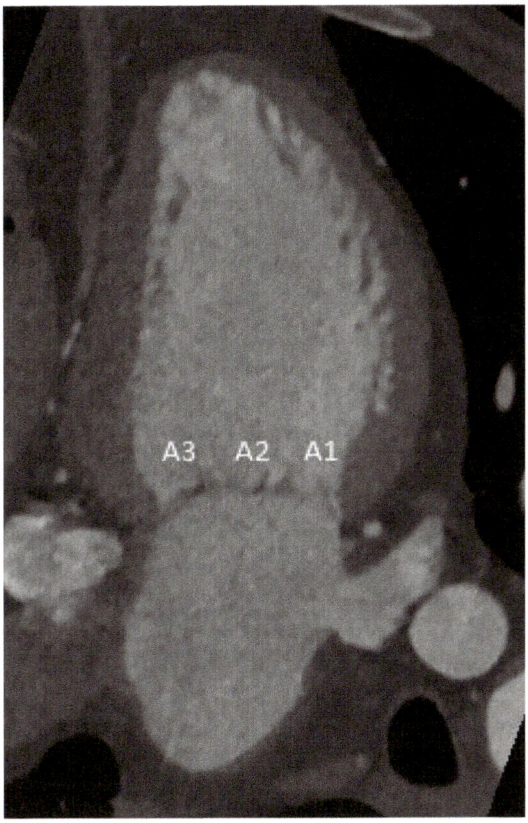

Fig. 17.1 Long axis view on CT showing the cusps starting at lateral A1 under the left atrial appendage to medial A3

Acute MR may not have a murmur but can still be the etiology of cardiogenic shock. The MR jet on TTE may be unimpressive but in the

A. Booke · M. Rinaldi · L. Watts · R. Musialowski
Sanger Heart and Vascular Institute, Atrium Health, Charlotte, NC, USA
e-mail: Anne.Booke@atriumhealth.org; Michael.Rinaldi@atriumhealth.org; Larry.Watts@atriumhealth.org; Richard.musialowski@atriumhealth.org

E. A. Powell (✉)
Banner University Medical Center, Tucson, AZ, USA
e-mail: elisabeth.powell@bannerhealth.com

R. Musialowski, K. Allshouse (eds.), *Cardiovascular Manual for the Advanced Practice Provider*, https://doi.org/10.1007/978-3-031-35819-7_17

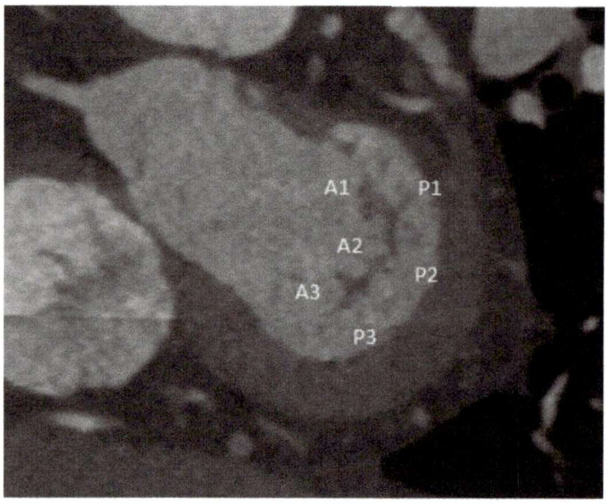

Fig. 17.2 Short axis view on CT showing the coaptation of the anterior and posterior leaflets and cusps. The location of pathology is communicated using this cusp nomenclature

setting of hemodynamic compromise with no other cause for deterioration, TEE is especially helpful for further evaluation.

Vasodilatory therapy, including nitroprusside or nicardipine, may help improve hemodynamic compensation, although use of medications may be limited in the setting of hypotension. An intra-aortic balloon pump (IABP) can be used to help stabilize the patient by decreasing LV afterload, increasing forward output, and decreasing the regurgitant volume.

Prompt recognition, management, and urgent mitral valve repair is lifesaving in acute severe primary MR. Multidisciplinary team-based discussions are essential in this high-risk group. Urgent surgical intervention may be required. In patients with prohibitive surgical risk and favorable anatomy, emergent transcatheter end-to-end repair (TEER) could be considered.

Surgical Intervention for Acute MR

Urgent mitral valve intervention is warranted to re-establish hemodynamics, reduce strain on the heart, and alleviate symptoms. This could require repair or replacement depending on the etiology of the acute decompensation. A team-based approach is essential in this high-risk cohort of patients.

Chronic Mitral Insufficiency

Etiology and Pathophysiology

MR results from an abnormality or disease process affecting one of the components of the mitral valve apparatus. To assess and manage chronic mitral insufficiency, it is important to distinguish between primary (degenerative, disease of the mitral valve apparatus) and secondary (functional, disease of the ventricle or atria) MR (Table 17.1). Primary MR is related to disease of the mitral apparatus, one or more components of the mitral valve (leaflets, chordae tendineae, papillary muscles, annulus, adjacent myocardium) which causes valve incompetence with resultant systolic regurgitation. Cord rupture with flail segment is a common cause of many etiologies (Fig. 17.3). Secondary MR occurs in a structurally normal mitral valve, where disease or enlargement of the atria or ventricles may cause annular enlargement, papillary muscle displacement, leaflet tethering, or malcoaptation. MR in the setting of hypertrophic cardiomyopathy occurs secondary to anterior papillary muscle displacement and systolic anterior motion (SAM) of the anterior mitral valve leaflet into the LV outflow tract (see Chap. 20).

With MR, the LV emptying (afterload) is reduced and consequently the LV is decompressed into the left atrium. As LV volume increases overtime, the severity of the MR and the LV contractile reserve diminishes, and increased LA volume with

Table 17.1 Classification of mitral regurgitation

Primary: Leaflet Pathology	Secondary: Myopathic Abnormality
Mitral valve prolapse (MVP)	Dilated cardiomyopathy
Rheumatic valve disease	Papillary muscle ischemia
Cleft mitral valve	Regional wall motion abnormality causing leaflet tethering
Endocarditis with leaflet destruction	Mitral annular calcification
Radiation valvopathy	Dilated atria causing atrial MR
Connective tissue disorders	

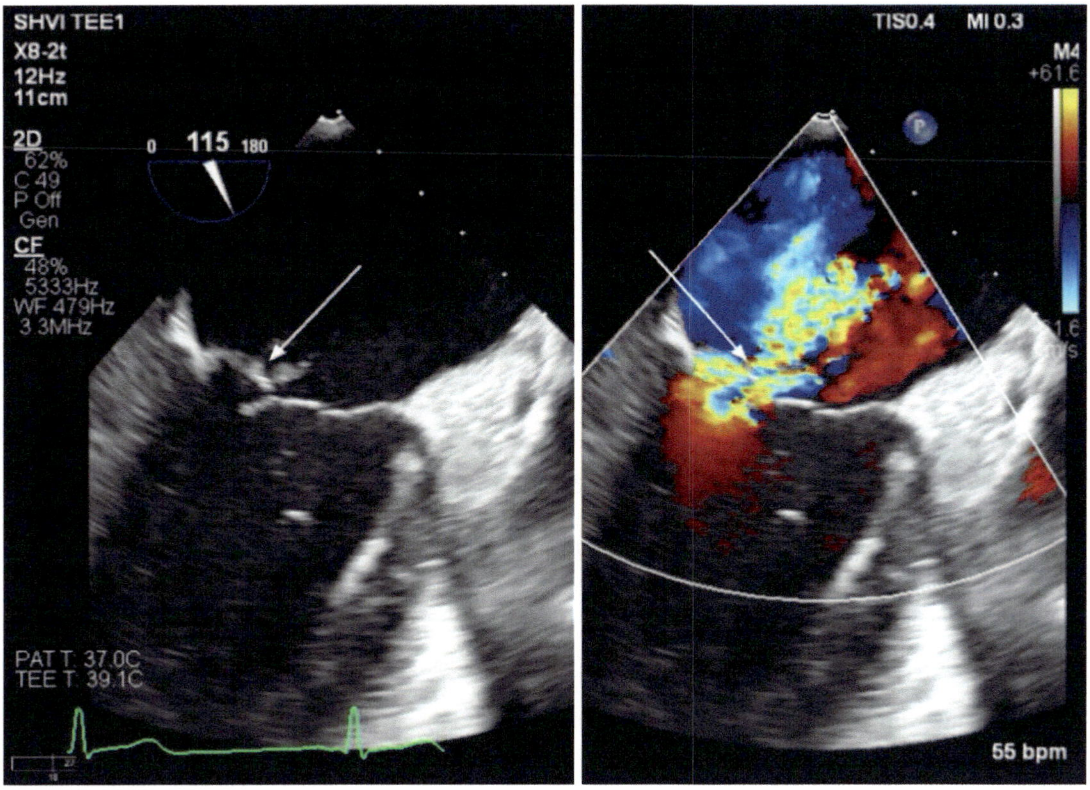

Fig. 17.3 Flail P2 segment left arrow. The ruptured cord and leaflet tip is pointing back into atria which is the hallmark of a flail leaflet. Severe 4 + primary MR on color doppler is shown by the arrow in the right panel

progressive LA enlargement is associated with decreased cardiac output [1]. Chronic MR is often progressive as LA enlargement places increased tension on the posterior mitral leaflet, worsening the degree of MR, causing progressive dilation of the LA and LV [1]. This may lead to a perpetuating cycle of worsening MR with increasing LV volume. The unloading of the LV with flow back into the LA increases the LVEF thus a "normal" LVEF in significant MR is ~70%. When the LVEF declines toward 60% and the LVESD is <40 mm, LV dysfunction is present. With severe chronic MR, patients begin to develop pulmonary hypertension and may develop secondary TR along with right heart failure.

Symptoms

Severe chronic MR can be asymptomatic for extended periods of time but inevitably is associated with the development of exertional dyspnea, fatigue, and eventually clinical heart failure including lower extremity edema, orthopnea, and ascites. Patients in acute heart failure may present with acute pulmonary edema. Once the LA dilates enough, patients will develop atrial fibrillation as well.

Physical Exam/Cardiac Studies

The traditional murmur of secondary MR is a holosystolic blowing murmur originating at the apex and directed toward the axilla. The primary MR murmur is often harsher in quality and may radiate anteriorly from apex to the lower left sternal border and is often confused with aortic stenosis. This MR murmur will not change with respiration nor radiate to the carotids, confirming the diagnosis.

Imaging Modalities

EKG

In patients with severe MR, the ECG may show evidence of atrial or ventricular enlargement. Atrial fibrillation is a common finding as well.

Echocardiography

TTE is an excellent screening study for the detection of mitral insufficiency. Its severity is graded as 1+ (mild), 2+ (moderate), 3+ (moderately severe), and 4+ (severe) with 3–4+ considered clinically relevant and can be associated with symptoms. When patients develop change in symptomatology, repeat TTE is indicated.

For patients with less than severe MR but exertion symtoms, exercise treadmill echocardiography can be helpful to demonstrate more severe MR with activity. This includes assessment to pulmonary artery pressures. Cardiopulmonary exercises testing (CPET) may also determine the hemodynamic significance of MR.

TEE, given its high degree temporal resolution, is primarily used to determine the mechanism of MR and is used to guide both surgical and transcatheter therapies (Fig. 17.3). While TEE can be used to quantify the severity of MR, TEE can underestimate the severity due to procedural sedation, which decreases SVR and afterload. Blood pressure challenge with pressors can be used to better assess severity during TEE.

Because TTE can have diagnostic limitations, the quantification of MR can be challenging. Cardiac MRI can be used for quantification of MR severity and is the gold standard for severity assessment.

Imaging modalities are used to assess the pathology of MR to determine methodology for repair or replacement. Alain Carpentier MD, the father of mitral valve repair, developed a complete classification system to describe the pathologies of MR and the associated approaches to valve repair [2]. The Carpentier classifications are listed in Table 17.2. The Carpentier systematic approach to repair involves quadrangular leaflet resection of prolapse, placement of normal chords to the prolapsing leaflet tissue if needed for support, and placement of a ring prosthesis to remodel the annulus for stability and improved coaptation of the leaflets [2]. Although techniques and technology have evolved with time, these same concepts are utilized today.

Table 17.2 Carpentier classifications

Type 1 (normal leaflet motion)	• The leaflets are normal but flattened with lack of central coaptation resulting in a central jet • Caused from annular dilation from progressive atrial or ventricular dilation (e.g., atrial dilation secondary to chronic AF) or leaflet perforation • This is a less common form of secondary MR
Type 2 (increased leaflet motion)	• Primary leaflet pathology with prolapse or flail of one or both leaflets • *The most common form of primary MR*
Type 3a (restricted leaflet motion—systole of diastole)	• Restricted leaflets relatively immobile in both systole and diastole • Seen in rheumatic disease • In contrast to rheumatic mitral stenosis, the leaflets are partially fixed open • Always some degree of mixed stenosis present • This is a less common form of primary MR
Type 3b (restricted leaflet motion—systole)	• Restricted leaflets during systole only • Related to chronic LV failure with wall motion abnormality of the inferoposterior wall and associated tethering of the posterior leaflet leading to a posteriorly directed jet • *The most common form of secondary MR*

Management of Primary MR

Patients with primary MR should be treated with GDMT for hypertension, volume overload, and LV dysfunction.

Patients with severe primary MR should be referred to a surgeon for evaluation. Refer to Fig. 8 from the guidelines [1]. For patients who are poor surgical candidates with primary MR, transcatheter edge-to-edge repair (TEER) can be considered as an alternative. Clinical trials of surgery vs TEER have shown lower complications and quicker recovery with TEER but better procedural success with surgery. Surgical repair is associated with a 95% ≤1+ residual regurgitation, while TEER can be associated with an 80% ≤1+ residual leak in contemporary studies. In patients with rheumatic mitral valve disease, with thickened or calcified leaflets and subvalvular involvement surgical repair is less suitable and TEER is likely not feasible.

Management Secondary MR

When secondary MR exists with systolic LV dysfunction, the primary therapy is guideline directed medical therapy for systolic heart failure including beta blockers, ACE-I/ARB/ ARNI, mineralocorticoid receptor antagonists, SGLT-2 inhibitors, hydralazine nitrates, and diuretics (Class 1). For patients with EF ≤35% and LBBB, CRT can also reduce MR severity (Class 1). In patients with obstructive CAD, revascularization can also improve LV function and reduce MR. Patients with systolic CHF should have medications uptitrated at regular intervals with contact every 1–2 weeks until maximum-tolerated dosing is achieved and once GDMT is maximized TTE should be repeated to reassess MR degree. An example of this would be secondary MR related to inferoposterior wall motion abnormality with chronic systolic CHF (Carpentier 3b) which is a disease of the left ventricle.

If persistent severe 3–4+ MR remains present, and EF is between 25 and 50% with LVEDV <7 cm, transcatheter edge-to-edge mitral valve repair (TEER) can be considered based on data from the COAPT trial (Class 2a). TEE is performed to assess anatomic feasibility. Surgical repair or replacement can be considered in patients without suitable anatomy for TEER who are surgical candidates although the data for benefit is less robust (Class 2b). For both TEER and surgical MVR, patients will respond less favorably if they have concomitant severe TR, severe RV failure, pulmonary hypertension, and less severe MR in proportion to LV systolic dysfunction. For example, patients with an EF 15–20% and 2–3+ MR are less likely to respond favorably to TEER and should be considered for advanced heart failure therapies such as VAD or transplant if appropriate.

Atrial functional MR (AF MR) is another category of secondary MR (Carpentier 1) where LVEF may be preserved and annular dilation from progressive LA enlargement can result in lack of coaptation of the leaflets. Maintenance of SR appears to reduce progression of MR and should be achieved if possible. Diuretics and adequate BP management may reduce MR severity. For patients with persistent severe symptomatic MR, surgical mitral valve repair or replacement or TEER could be considered but is less well studied (See Fig. 9 in 2020 AHA/ACC Valve Guidelines) [1].

Transcatheter Edge-to-Edge Mitral Valve Repair (mTEER)

TEER improves quality of life, hospitalization rate, and survival for patients with systolic heart failure despite maximally tolerated GDMT, as studied in the COAPT trial. During mTEER, a patient is placed under general anesthesia and TEE guidance is used to guide the positioning of mitral clip and assess the reduction of MR. Right femoral venous access is obtained and with transseptal puncture, the implanting physician gains direct access to the mitral valve. The clip grasps the diseased cusp of the anterior leaflet and simultaneously grasps the posterior leaflet, causing reduction in leaflet mobility and will result in a degree of mitral stenosis. It is important for physicians to monitor the degree of MS prior to release of the clip as if resultant MS is too high the patient will not receive symptomatic relief. Utilization of the intraoperative TEE helps determine if additional clip placement is indicated and the degree of resultant MS with clip placement. Post-procedure providers may increase beta blockade to slow heart rate and decrease any degree of MS. Figure 17.4 demonstrates what mitral clip implantation looks post deployment.

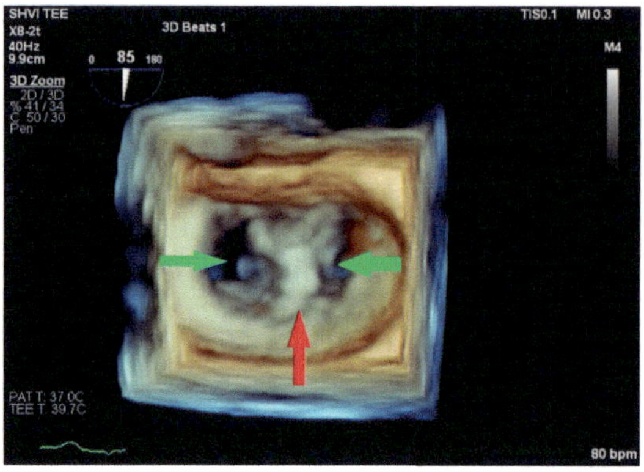

Fig. 17.4 Red arrow is a deployed TEER clip to the A2P2 segments of the mitral valve for a flail segment with resultant two channels during ventricular diastole (green arrows)

Antithrombotic therapy following TEER is studied to be aspirin 81 mg indefinitely and Plavix 75 mg for 2 months post procedure. In patients with atrial fibrillation or other indications for systemic oral anticoagulation, the regimen is adjusted.

Surgical Management of Mitral Regurgitation

The timing of surgical intervention for MR depends on the acuity of the MR (acute vs chronic) and the cause of the MR (primary vs secondary). Mortality rates for primary MR decrease with early surgical intervention before symptoms and LV systolic dysfunction (LVEF ≤60% or ESD ≥ 40 mm) occur [1]. Once a patient develops symptoms and LVEF ≤60, the prognosis is poor [1]. This was confirmed by a recent data analysis completed by the STS demonstrating reduced survival associated with late referral for surgical intervention [3]. Close monitoring of MR progression with imaging surveillance, despite presence of symptoms, is vital in planning surgery before LV dysfunction deteriorates [1].

In MR, surgical correction can be accomplished by either mitral valve repair (MVr) or mitral valve replacement (MVR). Mitral valve repair is preferred over mitral valve replacement and should be attempted if leaflets are salvageable. Valve repair is shown to have superior durability, lower rates of thromboembolism, resistance to endocarditis, and does not require anticoagulation therapy in most patients [2]. Techniques and concepts regarding MV repair are continually evolving and range from simple to comprehensive. Simple repairs may only involve placement of an annular ring to support the valve while complicated repairs involve both the anterior and posterior leaflet, as well as the chordae. The goal of the repair is to re-establish the integrity of the valve, improve coaptation of the leaflets, and decrease annulus size if dilation exists.

In the operating room, MV repairs are immediately assessed by a certified advanced imaging physician via TEE. If the MV repair is inadequate, immediate MV replacement should be considered while still in the OR.

Mitral valve replacement is warranted when the leaflets are not salvageable due to presence of calcification, perforation, infection, or the presence of rheumatic disease. If repair is attempted in rheumatic disease, the risk of reoperation is 50–60% of patients within 20 years [1].

Surgical Intervention for Chronic Primary MR

The timing of surgery depends on the severity of the disease and LV function. Unlike surgical treatment of the aortic valve or mitral stenosis, the lack of symptoms should not delay the timing of intervention for primary MR. In mitral valve prolapse affecting only half of the posterior leaflet, mitral valve repair is the gold standard of care with outcomes superior to both biological and mechanical valve replacement [1]. Studies demonstrate that patients who undergo mitral valve repair for primary MR have a life expectancy equal to that of the general population after surgery, regardless of age [4]. When mitral valve repair is successful, operative mortality rate is <1%, with 95% freedom from reoperation and 80% freedom from recurrent moderate or severe MR at 15–20 years postoperatively [1]. In accordance with the ACC/AHA guidelines, if severe primary MR is isolated to less than half of the posterior leaflet and only simple repair to the posterior leaflet is necessary, MV replacement is considered harmful and should not be completed unless MV repair has been attempted and failed [1].

Surgical Intervention for Chronic Secondary MR

In chronic secondary MR, the role of surgical intervention is controversial. MR is multifactorial and restoration of MV competence does not mitigate the underlying cardiac pathology. Although it has not been shown to directly improve survival, surgical intervention has been shown to improve functional outcomes and reduce symptoms [5].

According to the ACC/AHA guidelines, MV surgery for chronic secondary MR is warranted: [1]

- In the presence of severe symptoms when the valve is not favorable to TEER.
- When patient is undergoing CABG with severe MR and LV dysfunction secondary to CAD.
- When severe MR is isolated from annular dilation related to atrial fibrillation, MV surgery with MAZE procedure may be reasonable.

With surgical intervention of chronic secondary MR, MV replacement should be considered in cases with ischemic or dilated cardiomyopathy. The durability of a mitral repair depends on the regression of the underlying dilation, and if the dilation progresses postoperatively, the repair will not be durable and survival is limited [1].

Preoperative Assessment and Calculating Risk

As with other cardiac surgeries, a detailed history, physical, and a myriad of diagnostic testing is completed to determine patient's baseline status and operative risk. A cardiac catheterization should be completed to assess for any coronary artery disease that may need to be addressed during the operation. A thorough dental history should also be obtained to rule out a disease process which may put patient at increased risk for developing endocarditis postoperatively. Refer to previous chapters regarding preoperative assessment for further discussion and Tables 6.1 and 6.2 in Chap. 6.

Risk stratification for MV repair and MV replacement can be calculated on the STS website. Refer to Chap. 6 for further discussion and Table 6.3 for a list of categories assessed with the risk calculator.

Surgical Approach and Valve Selection

As discussed above, MV repair is preferred to MV replacement in the setting of MR. Surgical approach begins with visual assessment of the mitral valve apparatus to determine if repair is feasible. Figure 17.5 depicts visualization of the mitral valve via the left atrium during surgery. This mitral valve has a flail posterior leaflet resulting in severe MR.

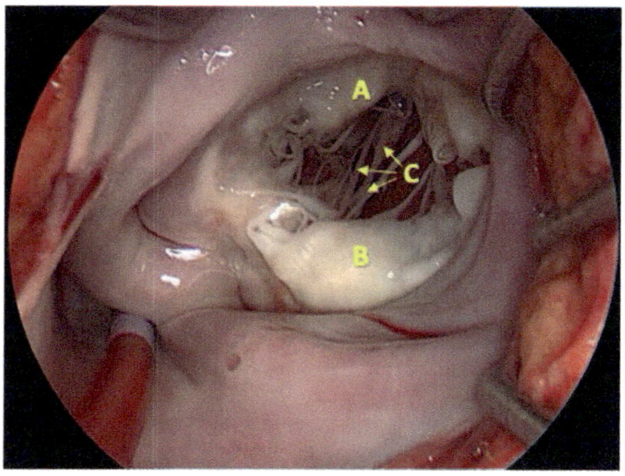

Fig. 17.5 Mitral valve with flail posterior leaflet. (**a**) Anterior leaflet. (**b**) Posterior leaflet. (**c**) Chordae Tendinae

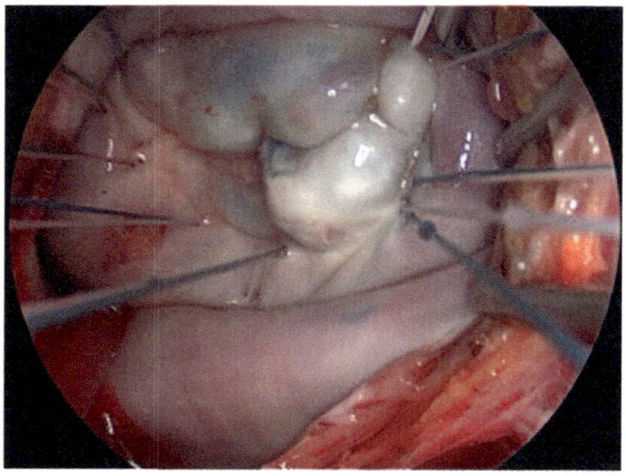

Fig. 17.6 Insertion of valve sutures to implant an annuloplasty ring into mitral position for mitral repair

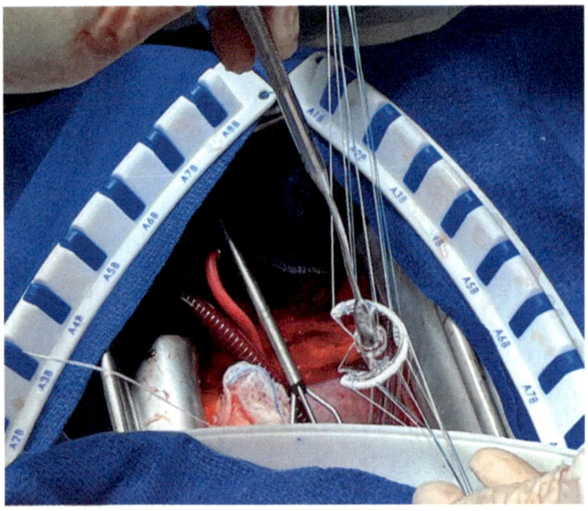

Fig. 17.7 Insertion of an annuloplasty ring for mitral repair utilizing sutures from Fig. 17.6

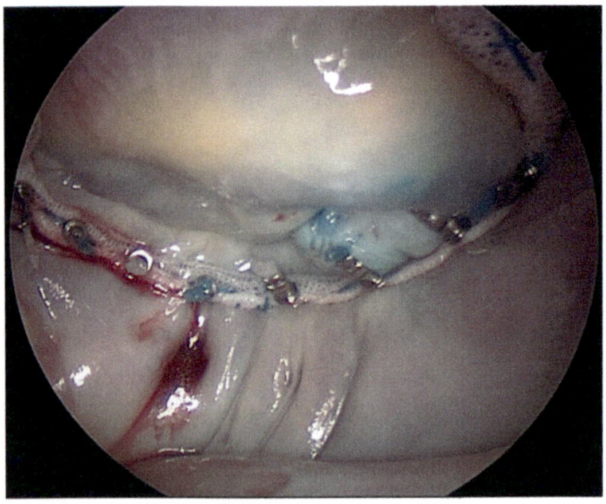

Fig. 17.8 Mitral valve repair of Fig. 17.5 with triangular resection of P2 and placement of ring

With MV repairs, an annuloplasty ring is always placed to support the annulus and provide structure, regardless of the type or complexity of repair. Sutures are first placed along the annulus (Fig. 17.6) and then the annuloplasty ring is parachuted down into the correct position (Fig. 17.7). Once the repair is complete, the valve is assessed intra-operatively for residual valvular leak prior to closure. Successful mitral valve repair with competent valvular coaptation is demonstrated in Fig. 17.8.

If the mitral valve is unable to be repaired and replacement is necessary, the type of prosthesis needs to be addressed. This discussion must be completed with the patient preoperatively, even if a MV repair is planned. Refer to the chapters on valve selection under surgical management of aortic valve disease for further discussion.

Mitral Stenosis

The etiology of mitral stenosis is most commonly rheumatic or degenerative (Table 17.3). Rheumatic fever is the leading cause of mitral valve disease worldwide and rheumatic MS is more common in women (80% case) compared to men [1]. Clinical presentation can vary, and patients may present earlier in life, even in their teens. Patients presenting at a younger age, often have commissural fusion but pliable, noncalcified mitral valve leaflets [1]. Patients presenting later in life more commonly have calcified fibrotic mitral leaflets in addition to commissural fusion and subvalvular involvement [1]. Degenerative mitral stenosis is seen in elderly patients with significant mitral annular calcification.

The normal mitral valve orifice is 4–6 cm^2 and when the mitral orifice is <2 cm^2 the left atrial pressure rises to generate blood flow across the narrowed orifice into the LV. To compensate for increased left atrial pressure, both pulmonary

Table 17.3 Causes of mitral stenosis

Rheumatic fever worldwide
Degenerative from age
Congenital
Chest radiation
Systemic lupus
Rheumatoid arthritis
Carcinoid heart disease

venous and arterial wedge pressures rise, which contributes to exertional dyspnea. Untreated, longstanding MS causes passive backward transmission of the elevated left atrial pressure triggering pulmonary arterial constriction, resulting in pulmonary changes and subsequent pulmonary hypertension, RV enlargement with tricuspid regurgitation, and right heart failure [1]. In patients with severe MS, cardiac output is near normal at rest but fails to rise substantially with exertion.

Patients with mitral stenosis are at increased risk of developing atrial fibrillation and thrombi in the left atrium (valvular atrial fibrillation).

Symptoms

The most common presenting symptom is exertional dyspnea or cough, followed by exercise intolerance. Patients may also present with symptoms of right heart failure. Symptoms from MS are exacerbated by physical exertion, tachycardia, volume shifts, fever, severe anemia, pregnancy, and thyrotoxicosis.

Physical Exam/Cardiac Studies

The mitral stenosis murmur is best heard at the apex and described as an opening snap with a low pitched, rumbling, diastolic murmur. It is very difficult to appreciate.

ECG. If there is left atrial enlargement, it may be reflected by the p wave. In patients with pulmonary hypertensions, the ECG may show right axis deviation and RV hypertrophy [6].

Echocardiogram. TTE is used to evaluate mitral leaflets along with extent of valvular calcification into the mitral apparatus, the transvalvular gradient, degree of chamber enlargement and function, concomitant tricuspid valve disease, and pulmonary pressures. TEE may be used to obtain superior images of the mitral valve for planning of intervention (see Fig. 17.9).

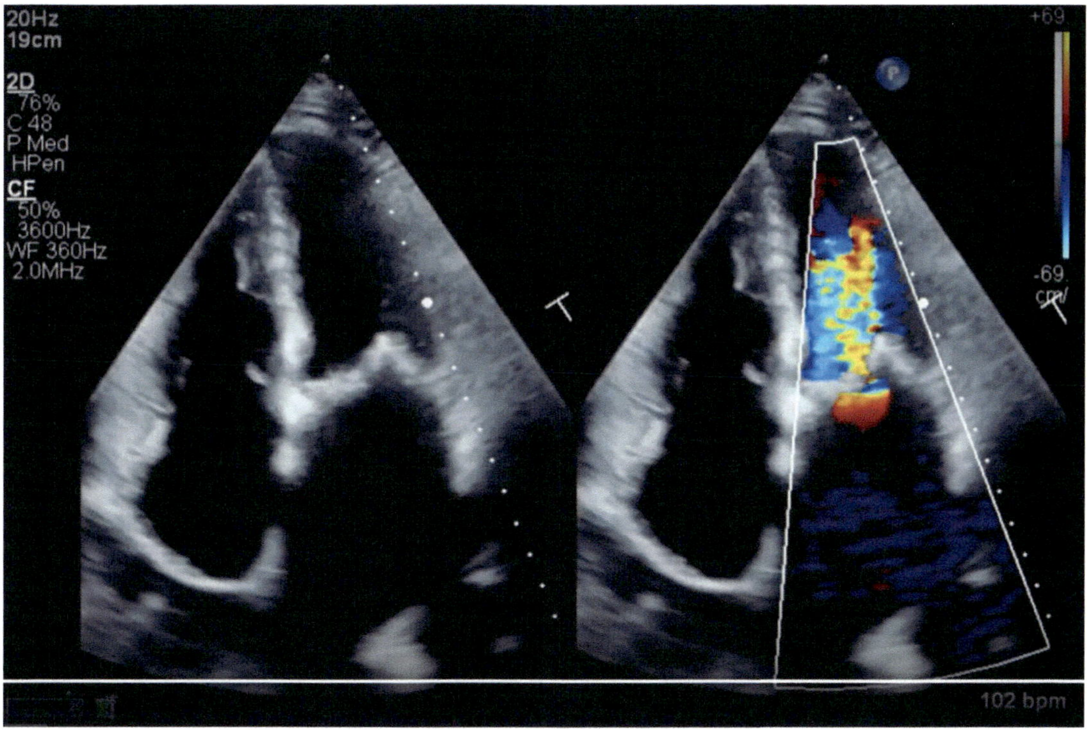

Fig. 17.9 Echo showing mitral stenosis. Heavily calcified and reduced mobility of the mitral leaflets in the left panel with restricted diastolic mitral flow in the right panel suggestive of severe mitral stenosis. Note the tricuspid valve is open confirming diastole

Table 17.4 Stages of mitral stenosis

Stage	Definition	Symptoms	Valve Anatomy	Valve Hemodynamics
A	At risk of MS	None	Mild valve doming during diastole	Normal transmitral flow velocity
B	Progressive MS	None	Rheumatic valve changes with commissural fusion and diastolic doming of the mitral valve leaflets Planimetered mitral valve area >1.5 cm^2	Increased transmitral flow velocities Mitral valve area >1.5 cm^2 Diastolic pressure half-time <150 ms
C	Asymptomatic severe MS	None	Rheumatic valve changes with commissural fusion and diastolic doming of the mitral valve leaflets Planimetered mitral valve area ≤1.5 cm^2	Mitral valve area ≤1.5 cm^2 Diastolic pressure half-time ≥150 ms
D	Symptomatic severe MS	Decreased exercise tolerance Extertional dyspnea	Rheumatic valve changes with commissural fusion and diastolic doming of the mitral valve leaflets Planimetered mitral valve area ≤1.5 cm^2	Mitral valve area ≤1.5 cm^2 Diastolic pressure half-time ≥150 ms

Adapted from (6)

Cardiac Catheterization. Left and right heart catheterization is helpful for hemodynamic assessment and to assess concomitant disease.

Staging of MS requires the combination of patient symptomatology, valve anatomy and hemodynamics, along with assessment of cardiac consequences from MS, as seen in Table 17.4.

Mitral Stenosis Management

Patients with rheumatic mitral stenosis and valvular atrial fibrillation, prior embolic event, or LAA thrombus should be initiated on warfarin (INR goal 2–3). There is no evidence to support DOACs in atrial fibrillation secondary to MS. Control or lowering of heart rate with beta blockers or calcium channel blockers are useful as it lengthens the diastolic filling period, lowers the LA pressure, and decreases symptoms. Cardioversion may be performed but does not durably restore sinus rhythm. Amiodarone is most effective in maintaining sinus rhythm post cardioversion [7]. Diuretics, digoxin, and ivabradine may also help improve symptoms.

Patients with clinically significant rheumatic MS (mitral valve area ≤ 1.5 cm^2 and diastolic mitral gradient ≥5–10 mmHg) should be followed annually with TTE. TTE helps determine the severity of stenosis and when severe MS is present will help determine the suitability for Percutaneous Mitral Balloon Commissurotomy (PMBC) versus surgery. TEE will further evaluate the mitral valve anatomy, presence of MR, and left atrial appendage thrombus (Fig. 17.10).

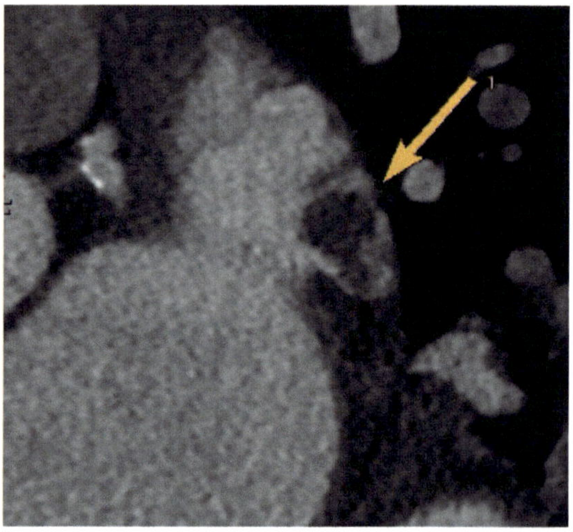

Fig. 17.10 Yellow arrow shows a markedly enlarged left atrial appendage (LAA) with the organized thrombus on CT imaging. DOACs are contraindicated for treatment of thrombus associated with mitral stenosis

Degenerative, Nonrheumatic Calcific MS

Calcific MS is the result of calcification of the mitral annulus that extends into the leaflets bases resulting in narrowing of the annulus and progressive leaflet rigidity [1, 8]. There is usually no commissural fusion and typically the leaflet tips are unaffected [1, 8]. Degenerative MS is usually observed in the elderly population and progression of MS is variable and may range from 1 to 9 mmHg annually (Fig. 17.9). The prognosis for patients with this type of MS is extremely poor with a 50% mortality within 5 years [1]. These patients are typically at high risk for any intervention given the extent of calcification, advanced age, and comorbidities.

Medical management is the same as for rheumatic MS. Degenerative MS is not amenable to PMBC and severe mitral annular calcification (MAC) limits surgical options given the difficulty in attaching a prosthetic mitral valve and risk of narrowing the mitral orifice. MV repair is usually not feasible and MV replacement is the treatment of choice. Due to the risk, current guidelines recommend surgical intervention only once the MS becomes severe, patient become extremely symptomatic, and medical therapy is no longer effective [1]. The evaluation of transcatheter therapies (TMVR) in the mitral position is ongoing. A multidisciplinary team approach is essential in these complex patients.

Rheumatic Mitral Stenosis Intervention

The optimal treatment of patients with rheumatic MS is either percutaneously mitral balloon commissurotomy (PMBC) or surgery (Fig. 7 in 2020 AHA/ACC Valve Guidelines [1]). PMBC is performed by advancing balloon catheters across the mitral valve and expanding them to split the mitral commissures. Long-term follow-up demonstrated that at 10 years 70–80% of patients with a good initial PMBC result were free of symptoms, and 30–40% remained free of symptoms out to 20 years [9]. In symptomatic patients with severe rheumatic MS (valve area ≤ 1.5 cm^2), < 2+ moderate MR, and absence of LA thrombus, PMBC is recommended [9]. Contraindications to PMBC are listed in Table 17.5.

Table 17.5 Contraindications for percutaneous mitral balloon commissurotomy in rheumatic MS

- Mitral valve area > 1.5 cm^2
- Left atrial thrombus
- More than mild MR
- Severe or bicommissural calcification
- Absence of commissural fusion
- Concomitant CAD requiring surgery
- Severe concomitant aortic or tricuspid valve disease requiring surgery

An anatomic mitral morphology score can be used to determine the suitability of PMBC and to evaluate the appearance of the commissures and degree of calcification. Clinical factors such as age, NHYA class, presence/absence of atrial fibrillation, and Wilkins score assist in predicting outcome.

The *Wilkins* score uses echocardiographic parameters to grade rheumatic MS for possible PMBV using characteristics of (1) leaflet mobility, (2) leaflet thickening, (3) leaflet calcification, and (4) sub valvular thickening. Each characteristic can have four points if the disease is more severe for a maximum of 16. A score of <8–9 are considered candidates for PMBV depending on degree of mitral insufficiency and a score of >9–10, especially with moderate MR should be considered for surgery.

Mitral valve repair or replacement are both utilized in the surgical treatment of MS. The surgical approach to MS depends on the pathology of the disease, the involvement of the valve leaflets, and the extent of calcification present. As stated above, PMBC is the first-line therapy for Rheumatic MS unless contraindicated. According to the ACC/AHA, MV surgery for rheumatic MS is warranted in the following patients [1]:

- Severe MS (mitral valve area ≤ 1.8 cm^2),
- MS with severe limiting symptoms,
- Who are not a candidate for PMBC given unfavorable valve morphology or presence of left atrial thrombus,
- Previous failure of PMBC, and
- Already undergoing cardiac surgery for another reason.

Like PMBC, the preferred approach to surgical management is mitral valve repair with commissurotomy. During surgical commissurotomy, a sternotomy is completed, the heart is placed on cardiopulmonary bypass, and under direct visualization the fissure between the mitral leaflets is separated. This technique is not routinely performed by surgeons in the United States and should only be completed at experienced centers [1]. If neither a PMBC repair nor open commissurotomy can be completed, then a mitral valve replacement may be considered in rheumatic stenosis.

As with other cardiac surgeries, a detailed history, physical, and a myriad of diagnostic testing are completed to determine patient's baseline status and operative risk. As with any valve surgery, a thorough dental history should be obtained to rule out a disease process which may put patient at risk for endocarditis postoperatively. Risk stratification for MV repair and MV replacement can be calculated on the STS website. Refer to Chap. 6, Table 6.3 for a list of categories assessed with the risk calculator.

Mitral Valve Selection

Provider and patient must jointly decide between a bioprosthetic and mechanical valve conduit in case a valve replacement is warranted. This decision is multifactorial and is based on patient age, life expectancy, medical compliance, and ability to tolerate long-term systemic anticoagulation. Refer to the section on valve selection under surgical management of aortic stenosis for further discussion.

The ACC/AHA guidelines for mitral valve replacement recommend mechanical valves in patients <65 years old and tissue valves in patients ≥65 years old [1]. A mechanical valve in the mitral position for mitral stenosis has the highest long-term embolic risk and requires strict therapeutic INR levels postoperatively. Refer to Figs. 11 and 12 for the 2020 AHA/ACC Valve Guidelines [1]. Figure 17.11 demonstrates a mitral valve replacement with a bioprosthetic valved conduit viewed from the left atrium. The mitral bioprosthetic conduits are manufactured as a trileaflet valve for structural support.

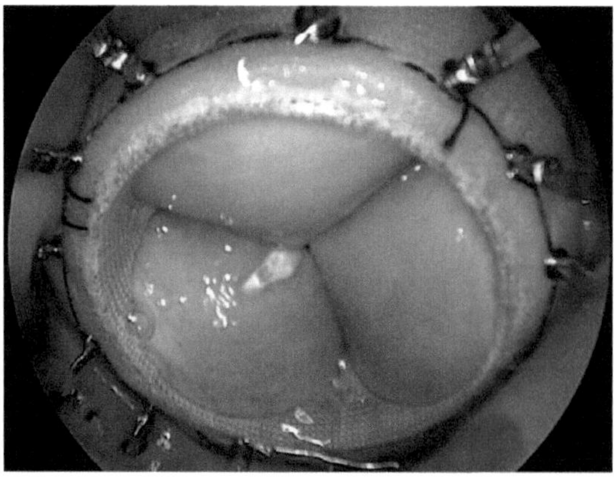

Fig. 17.11 Mitral valve replacement with a bioprosthetic valve

References

1. Otto CM, Nishimura RA, Bonow RO, Carabello BA, Erwin JP III, Gentile F. 2020 ACC/AHA Guideline for the management of patients with valvular heart disease: a report of the American College of Cardiology/American Heart Association Joint Committee on clinical practice guidelines. J Am Coll Cardiol. 2021;77(4):e25–e197.
2. Fedak PWM, McCarthy PM, Bonow RO. Evolving concepts and technologies in mitral valve repair. Circulation. 2008;117(7):963–74.
3. Gammie JS, Chikwe J, Badhwar V, Thibauld DP, Vemulapalli S, Thourani VH. Isolated mitral valve surgery: The Society of Thoracic Surgeons adult cardiac surgery database analysis. Ann Thorac Surg. 2018;106(3):716–27.
4. Watts TMF, Brescia AA, Murray SL, Burn DA, Wisniewski A, Romano MA, Bolling SF, Michigan Mitral Research Group (MMRG). Degenerative mitral valve repair restores life expectancy. Ann Thorac Surg. 2020;109(3):494–801.
5. Bonow RO, O'Gara PT, Adams DH, Badhwar V, Bavaria JE, Elmariah S, et al. 2019 AATS/ACC/SCAI/STS expert consensus systems of care document: operator and institutional recommendations and requirements for transcatheter mitral valve intervention. J Am Coll Cardiol. 2020;76(1):96–117.
6. Hein M, Schoechlin S, Schulz U, Minners J, Breitbart P, Lehane C, Neumann F-J, Ruile P. Long-term follow-up of hypoattenuated leaflet thickening after transcatheter aortic valve replacement. JACC Cardiovasc Interv. 2022;15(11):1113–22.
7. O'Brien SM, Feng L, He X, Xian Y, Jacobs JP, Badhwar V, et al. The Society of Thoracic Surgeons 2018 adult cardiac surgery risk models: part 2 - statistical methods and results. Ann Thorac Surg. 2018;105:1419–28.
8. Vahanian A, Beyersdorf F, Praz F, Milojevic M, Baldus S, Bauersachs J, Capodanno D, Conradi L, De Bonis M, De Paulis R, Delgado V, Freemantle N, Gilard M, Haugaa KH, Jeppsson A, Jüni P, Pierard L, Prendergast BD, Sádaba JR, Tribouilloy C, Wojakowski W, ESC/EACTS Scientific Document Group, ESC National Cardiac Societies. 2021 ESC/EACTS Guidelines for the management of valvular heart disease: developed by the task force for the management of valvular heart disease of the European Society of Cardiology (ESC) and the European Association for Cardio-Thoracic Surgery (EACTS). Eur Heart J. 2022;43(7):561–632.
9. The Society of Thoracic Surgeons. 2022. https://www.sts.org/resources/risk-calculator.

18 Tricuspid Valve Disease

Anne Booke, Michael Rinaldi, Elisabeth A. Powell, Larry Watts, and Richard Musialowski

Tricuspid Insufficiency/ Regurgitation (TI/TR)

Etiology

TR is categorized as primary or secondary. Secondary is more common, occurring in >90% of patients with TR (Table 18.1). At least 70% of adults have some degree of TR [1]. Most primary TR is related to implantable devices. Functional TR is secondary to dilation of the RA/RV annulus with leaflet tethering and is associated with pulmonary hypertension, atrial fibrillation, cardiomyopathy, and mitral disease. Functional TR is associated with pulmonary hypertension, RV dilation, RV infarction, or cardiomyopathy. Importantly, TR is an independent predictor of mortality.

In early TR, right atrial dilation occurs, resulting in annular dilatation. This process causes reduction in leaflet coaptation and with progression of TR, adaptive RV dilation occurs with RV remodeling to maintain cardiac output [2]. This cycle progresses until clinical signs of right heart failure develop (see Chap. 22). Severe, refractory TR is associated with hepatic and renal failure due to venous hypertension.

A. Booke · M. Rinaldi · L. Watts · R. Musialowski
Sanger Heart and Vascular Institute, Atrium Health, Charlotte, NC, USA
e-mail: Anne.Booke@atriumhealth.org; Michael.Rinaldi@atriumhealth.org; Larry.Watts@atriumhealth.org; Richard.musialowski@atriumhealth.org

E. A. Powell (✉)
Banner University Medical Center, Tucson, AZ, USA
e-mail: elisabeth.powell@bannerhealth.com

Symptoms

Symptoms of TR are due to two pathologic mechanisms: pulmonary congestion and central venous congestion. Patients develop fatigue, exertional dyspnea, and also symptoms associated with right heart failure including orthopnea, abdominal bloating or right upper abdominal discomfort, PND, and peripheral edema.

Physical exam findings with TR include systolic murmur that increases in intensity

Table 18.1 Etiology of tricuspid regurgitation

Primary (abnormal leaflets)	Secondary (normal leaflets)
Rheumatic disease	LV dysfunction
Congenital heart disease-Ebstein's anomaly	RV infarction
Myxomatous changes	Pulmonary hypertension
Carcinoid heart disease	Infiltrative disease of the RV
Iatrogenic - device entrapment, biopsy injury	Atrial annular dilation
Radiation	Left sided valve disease
	Chronic RV pacing

R. Musialowski, K. Allshouse (eds.), *Cardiovascular Manual for the Advanced Practice Provider*, https://doi.org/10.1007/978-3-031-35819-7_18

with inspiration, prominent JVD, peripheral edema, hepatomegaly, ascites, and a third heart sound that also increases with inspiration (RV S3).

Evaluation

ECG. Usually non-diagnostic, although may see signs of RA or RV enlargement, bizarre RBBB pattern, evidence of prior inferior MI, or atrial fibrillation [3].

Imaging. The etiology and severity of TR are assessed by TTE (Fig. 18.1). When indicated, TEE, MRI, or CT scan may be used to provide additional information about the tricuspid valve and RV function. Particular attention should be paid to TR grade/regurgitant jet, valve morphology (annular dimension, leaflet coaptation/tethering), enlargement of RA/RV/IVC to properly stage TR, pulmonary systolic pressure, and degree of hepatic vein reversal [4].

Trace to mild degrees of TR are commonly detected on TTE in patients with normal valves and are of no physiological consequence [3].

Management

Medical therapy is limited and attention should be focused on reversing any underlying causes of TR. Management of heart failure is the first approach to management of TR, with the use of diuretics to treat volume overload and medical therapy for patients who have pulmonary arterial hypertension (PAH), particularly WHO type II (see Chap. 22). Patient with volume overload and hepatic congestion are more responsive to torsemide over furosemide. Use of loop diuretics can be limited as RV function worsens or in those with low output syndrome. Patients with reduced LVEF contributing to TR should be initiated on GDMT to offload the LV. In patients with TR secondary to annular dilation from atrial fibrillation

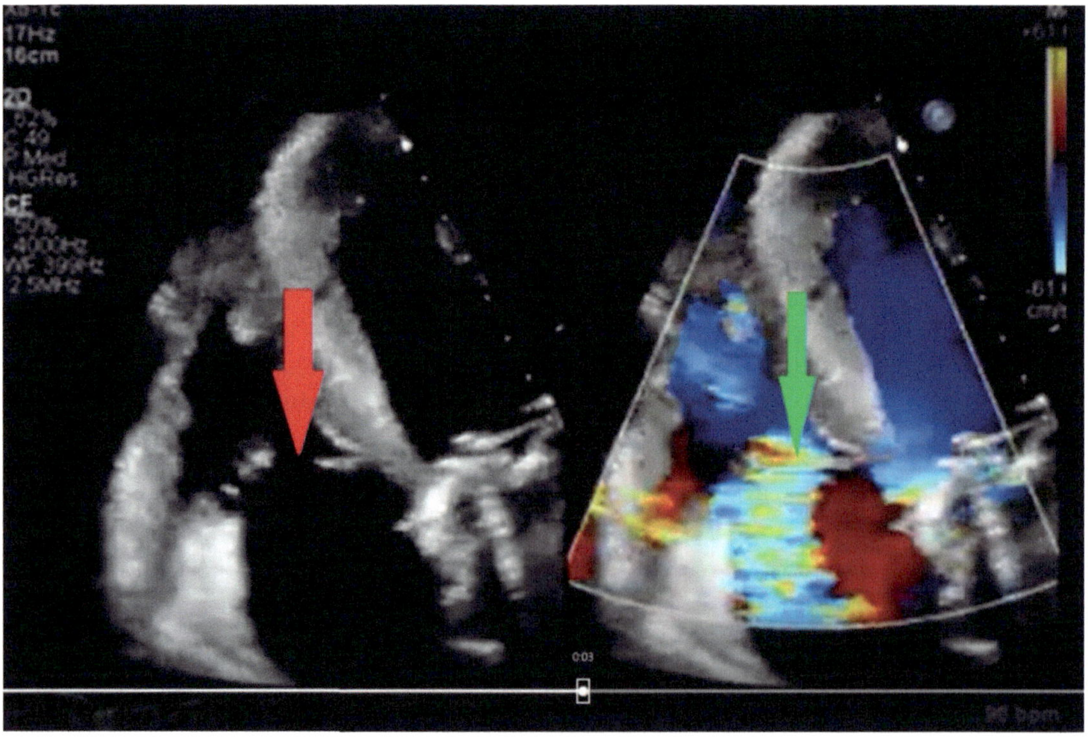

Fig. 18.1 The left panel shows a closed tricuspid valve with defect and annular dilatation. The right panel shows a green arrow indicating severe secondary tricuspid regurgitation

it is beneficial to restore sinus rhythm. There are limited options for patients who have advanced TR with end-stage heart failure and low cardiac output [3, 4].

Timing of intervention upon the tricuspid valve is tricky as the disease can progress quickly, is often associated with concomitant pulmonary hypertension or permanent atrial fibrillation, and also a poor prognosis.

Surgical treatment is performed for select patients with valvular disease. Surgical intervention should be completed with the presence of moderate to severe TR at the time of a left-sided valve operation. Once the left-sided valve lesion is corrected and there is reduction of the right ventricular afterload, TR may not improve. If the TV is not intervened upon at the time of the left-sided valve surgery, there is a 25% chance that there is progression of the TR if certain risk factors are present [3]. These risk factors include dilated annulus >4.0 cm, history of right-sided HF, and atrial fibrillation [3]. If the TR is not corrected at the time of the initial operation, and does not improve postoperatively, reoperation for severe isolated TR is associated with a perioperative mortality of 10–25% [3]. Even in cases where only mild to moderate secondary TR exists, tricuspid valve (TV) intervention should still be considered.

Transcatheter tricuspid valve interventions are emerging as an alternative for highly symptomatic patients who are felt to be too high risk for conventional open-heart surgery and research is ongoing in determining effectiveness. There are currently no guidelines addressing transcatheter tricuspid valve therapies. Novel transcatheter therapies are evolving and include "leafletplasty" with clip therapy, valve replacement, percutaneous repair, and annuloplasty.

Surgical Management of Tricuspid Regurgitation

Surgical treatment of moderate to severe TR can be accomplished by either tricuspid valve repair (TVr) or tricuspid valve replacement (TVR). As the primary cause for TR stems from left-sided heart disease, the number one indication for surgical intervention is the presence of severe TR at the time of a left-sided valve operation [3]. When possible, a repair should be attempted prior to replacement. Repairs are preferred to replacement in TR as they do not require long-term anticoagulation, have greater durability, and are resistant to endocarditis. Repair of the tricuspid valve usually only requires an annuloplasty ring or band to decrease annular dilation, create support, and improve coaptation of the leaflets. A TVr with an annuloplasty ring is demonstrated in Fig. 18.2.

Replacement of the tricuspid valve is reasonable when the valve is unrepairable or in select secondary forms of TR. Valves should undergo replacement when the TR is a primary defect in the valve leaflet such as with injury from device leads, endocardial biopsy, trauma, or in infectious endocarditis. TV replacement should also be completed if a TV repair has failed. A TVR with a bioprosthetic valve is demonstrated in Fig. 18.3 Guidelines for surgical intervention of TR are outlined in Fig. 10 in the 2020 AHA/ACC Valve Guidelines [3].

Isolated TR intervention is rare and perioperative mortality risk is considered high. Intervention is more dependent on the presence of right-sided heart failure, progressive RV dilation, and dysfunction. According to the ACC/AHA guidelines, isolated TV surgery is considered reasonable in

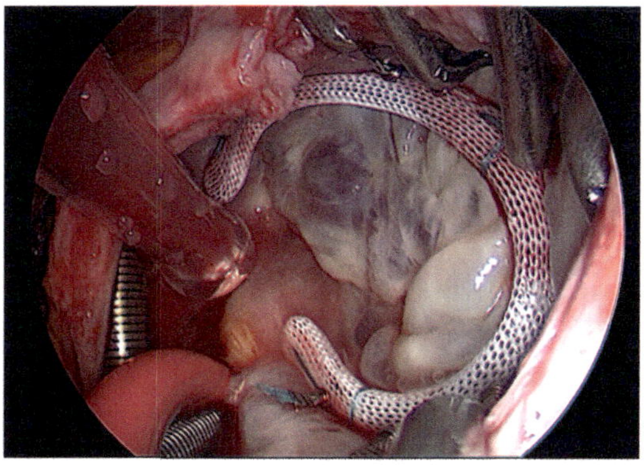

Fig. 18.2 Tricuspid valve repair with placement of an annuloplasty ring

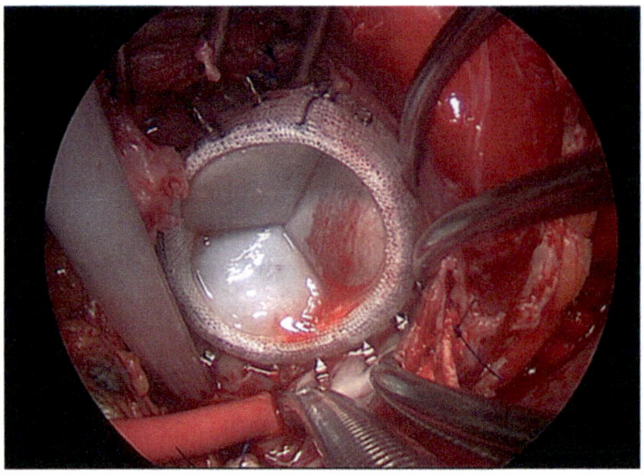

Fig. 18.3 Tricuspid valve replacement with a bioprosthetic valve

patients with severe primary TR if symptomatic or severe secondary TR which has responded poorly to medical therapy [3]. Surgery is also deemed reasonable in asymptomatic patients with severe primary TR and progressive RV dilation or systolic dysfunction [3].

The timing of surgical intervention is preferrable before the onset of significant RV dysfunction or end-organ damage. Once these are present, surgery has a significantly increased risk with mortality rates of 8–20% and the additional risk of RV failure [3]. In specific cases where patients develop acute severe primary TR, TV surgery should be considered urgent and completed prior to the onset of RV dysfunction [3]. Acute TR may develop from injury to the valve apparatus, and survival is directly related to RV function.

Preoperative Assessment and Surgical Risk

Preoperative assessment for tricuspid valve surgery begins with a history, physical, and baseline diagnostic testing. Dental evaluation is recommended preoperatively to decrease the risk of endocarditis following the placement of a prosthetic valve. Refer to previous chapters regarding preoperative assessment for further discussion and Chap. 6: Tables 6.1 and 6.2.

Along with the standard preoperative testing and transesophageal echo (TEE), all patient's undergoing cardiac surgery should have a cardiac catheterization to assess for coronary artery disease. If cardiac disease is present, CABG should be completed at the time of the valve surgery.

The STS does not include tricuspid valve repair/replacement as part of their STS risk calculator. However, patient statistics and outcomes may be viewed in the database to aid in the surgeon's justification for risk assessment. In the cases involving tricuspid valve surgery, a provider must account for physical assessment, frailty, clinical judgment, and multidisciplinary team discussions to determine if patient is an appropriate surgical candidate.

Valve Selection

With tricuspid regurgitation, valve repair is the preferred surgical approach. In tricuspid valve repair, an annuloplasty ring is placed to correct dilation, improve coaptation, and provide support to the valvular apparatus. If repair is not feasible, tricuspid valve replacement is warranted. The surgical decision-making regarding valve selection is complex, multifactorial, and based on patient age, life expectancy, medical compliance, and ability to tolerate long-term anticoagulation. Refer to the section on valve selection under surgical management of aortic insufficiency in Chap. 16 for further discussion.

Currently, there is no superiority between bioprosthetic and mechanical valves in TV replacement [5]. This may change as transcatheter TVR modalities evolve and percutaneous valve-in-valve replacements gain popularity.

Tricuspid Stenosis

Tricuspid stenosis is most frequently rheumatic in origin and often coexists with TR. Given that TS is primarily rheumatic in origin, it is often associated with rheumatic MS. Rare causes of tricuspid stenosis are congenital, carcinoid, drug induced, endocarditis, and right atrial tumors. As diastolic pressures rise, systemic venous congestion occurs, resulting in right-sided heart failure. Cardiac output falls and fails to rise with exertion.

Symptoms

Patients will experience exertional dyspnea that is out of proportion to the hepatomegaly, ascites, and edema they experience [6]. Severe TS is associated with hepatic congestion resulting in cirrhosis, jaundice, malnutrition, anasarca, and ascites.

Evaluation

Often the murmur of TS is missed given that usually there is concomitant MS. If the provider can auscultate the TS murmur, one might hear an opening snap with a diastolic murmur along the left lower sternal border that worsens with inspiration [6].

TTE will provide the most useful information, although tricuspid stenosis is most often overlooked. One should evaluate valve anatomy and assess the subvalvular apparatus. Stenosis is significant when the mean transvalvular gradient is ≥5 mmHg [2].

Management/Intervention

Patients with TS also often have TR and exhibit marked systemic venous congestion. Diuretics are the mainstay of management but have limited long-term efficacy [6]. Intervention is usually performed concomitantly with left-sided valve disease in symptomatic patients despite optimal medical therapy.

Percutaneous tricuspid balloon valvuloplasty frequently induces significant tricuspid insufficiency and long-term results are lacking [2].

Surgical Management of Tricuspid Stenosis

Tricuspid valve replacement is the surgical treatment of choice for tricuspid stenosis (TS). Given the calcific nature of the leaflets in stenotic disease, the native leaflets are not amenable to repair. Refer to the chapter on aortic stenosis for further discussion on valve selection.

During tricuspid valve surgery, there are multiple areas to be mindful of during suture placement. The right coronary artery (RCA) lies in the AV groove with close approximation to the posterior leaflet of the tricuspid valve. Placement of valve sutures may result in functional stenosis or direct suturing of the coronary artery [5]. Care should also be taken at the level of the AV node. The AV node lies along the anteroseptal commissure at the base of the septal leaflet. Injuring the AV node during repair or replacement with valve stitches may result in AV nodal blockade [5].

Indication and timing of surgical intervention for TS is dependent on severity of disease and timing of concomitant left-sided valve interventions. Isolated tricuspid valve disease is rare. Rheumatic disease is the primary cause of TS and occurs concurrent with rheumatic mitral valve disease. Once surgical intervention of the mitral valve is undertaken, the tricuspid valve is simultaneously addressed. Both the ACC/AHA guidelines and the European Society of Cardiology (ESC) recommend tricuspid valve surgery on (1) patients with severe TS at the time of operation for left-sided valves and (2) on isolated TV with symptomatic, severe TS [5].

Overall, tricuspid stenosis is rare in the given population and is infrequently seen as an isolated procedure in the operating room.

References

1. Zoghabi WA, et al. Recommendations for evaluation of the severity of native valvular regurgitation with two-dimensional and Doppler echocardiography. J Am Soc Echocardiogr. 2003;16(7):777–802.
2. Vahanian A, Beyersdorf F, Praz F, Milojevic M, Baldus S, Bauersachs J, Capodanno D, Conradi L, De Bonis M, De Paulis R, Delgado V, Freemantle N, Gilard M, Haugaa KH, Jeppsson A, Jüni P, Pierard L, Prendergast BD, Sádaba JR, Tribouilloy C, Wojakowski W, ESC/EACTS Scientific Document Group, ESC National Cardiac Societies. 2021 ESC/EACTS Guidelines for the management of valvular heart disease: developed by the Task Force for the management of valvular heart disease of the European Society of Cardiology (ESC) and the European

Association for Cardio-Thoracic Surgery (EACTS). Eur Heart J. 2022;43(7):561–632.
3. Otto CM, Nishimura RA, Bonow RO, Carabello BA, Erwin JP III, Gentile F. 2020 ACC/AHA guideline for the management of patients with valvular heart disease: a report of the American College of Cardiology/American Heart Association Joint Committee on clinical practice guidelines. J Am Coll Cardiol. 2021;77(4):e25–e197.
4. Taramassa M, et al. Tricuspid regurgitation, predicting the need for intervention, procedural success, and recurrence of disease. JACC Cardiovasc Imaging. 2019;12(4):605–21. https://doi.org/10.1016/j.jcmg.2018.11.034.
5. Cevasco M, Shekar PS. Surgical management of tricuspid stenosis. Ann Cardiothorac Surg. 2017;6(3):275–82.
6. Loscalzo J, Fauci A, et al. Harrison's principles of internal medicine. 21st. ed, Volume 1 and Volume 2. New York: McGraw Hill; 2022.

Infective Endocarditis 19

Allen Stephens, Todd McVeigh, Cary Ward, Elisabeth A. Powell, and Larry Watts

Symptoms

Symptoms of infective endocarditis are diverse and often nonspecific. The most common presenting symptoms are fever, chills, weakness, and malaise. Patients may also present with dyspnea which can be indicative of a severe lesion causing onset of heart failure. See Table 19.1 for presenting symptoms [1].

The diagnosis of IE based upon physical examination findings alone can be difficult and is often missed due to the variability of disease presentation [2]. Patients can present with nonspecific primary symptoms over a course of weeks to months [3]. IE should be on the differential diagnosis in patients presenting with sepsis without an obvious cause, as well as in patients who present with a fever of unknown origin and have IE risk factors (*see* Table 19.3). Acute presentations of IE can progress rapidly, as patients can present with sudden onset of heart failure, stroke, systemic or pulmonary embolization, severe sepsis with fevers, rigors, or septic shock.

Table 19.1 Symptoms in infective endocarditis

Symptom	Patients affected (%)
Fever	80–95
Chills	40–70
Weakness	40–50
Malaise	20–40
Sweats	20–40
Anorexia	20–40
Headache	20–40
Dyspnea	20–40
Cough	20–30
Weight loss	20–30
Myalgia/arthralgia	10–30
Stroke	10–20
Confusion/delirium	10–20
Nausea/vomiting	10–20
Edema	5–15
Chest pain	5–15
Abdominal pain	5–15
Hemoptysis	5–10
Back pain	5–10

Adapted from Braunwald's Heart Disease Textbook (10th Edition) Page 1527

A. Stephens (✉) · T. McVeigh · C. Ward
Duke University Health System, Durham, NC, USA
e-mail: Allen.stephens@duke.edu; Todd.mcveigh@duke.edu; c.ward@duke.edu

E. A. Powell
Banner University Medical Center, Tucson, AZ, USA
e-mail: elisabeth.powell@bannerhealth.com

L. Watts
Atrium Health/Sanger Heart and Vascular Institute, Charlotte, NC, USA
e-mail: Larry.Watts@atriumhealth.org

R. Musialowski, K. Allshouse (eds.), *Cardiovascular Manual for the Advanced Practice Provider*, https://doi.org/10.1007/978-3-031-35819-7_19

Physical Exam

The most common physical examination findings are shown in Table 19.2 with fever (present in 80–90% of patients) and a cardiac murmur (present in 75–85% of patients) being the two most prevalent. Although IE is commonly associated with a heart murmur (typically due to valvular regurgitation), new murmurs are present in less than 50% of cases [4]. A worsening of a pre-existing heart murmur accounts for the remainder of murmurs found on physical exam in IE. A central neurologic abnormality, such as focal deficits consistent with a cerebrovascular accident, can be identified in 20–40% of IE patients [5]. An abdominal exam can elicit nonspecific findings of tenderness, which can be suggestive of splenic embolization and infarction when in the left upper quadrant [1]. The spleen was found to be the second-most common site of septic embolization after the brain in one study [1].

The classic diagnostic findings of Janeway lesions (painless hemorrhagic macules on the soles and palms), Osler nodes (painful, erythematous nodular lesions on the pads of the fingers and toes), and Roth spots (retinal hemorrhages) are vascular and immunologic phenomena (Fig. 19.1). Acute IE can often evolve too quickly for the development of these phenomena [6]. These classically described findings are more characteristic of later stages of subacute, untreated IE. Approximately 75% of patients with IE are now diagnosed within 30 days of the onset of infection, so these long-term findings are less commonly seen [2].

The diagnosis of IE cannot be excluded on history and physical exam findings alone. Given the variety of patient presentations and varying physical exam findings, misdiagnosis and delays in diagnosis are common. These delays can postpone definitive management and contribute to increased mortality due to progressive structural heart damage that can eventually become irreparable [2].

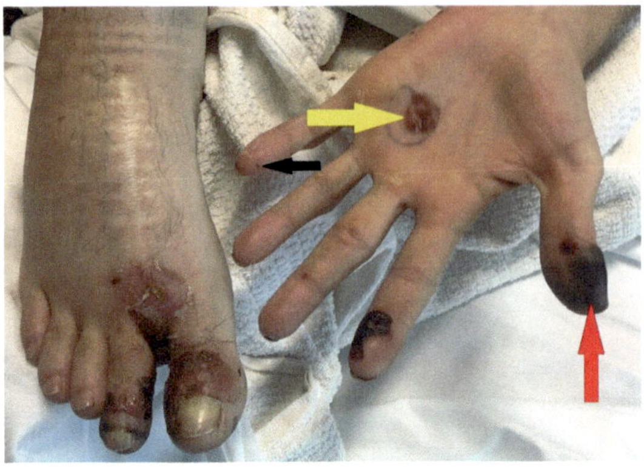

Fig. 19.1 Ischemic digit from emboli (red), Osler's node (black), and Janeway spots (yellow) in a patient with MSSA endocarditis

Table 19.2 Physical findings in infective endocarditis

Physical Findings	Patients affected (%)
Fever	80–90
Heart murmur	75–85
New murmur	10–50
Changing murmur	5–20
Central neurologic abnormality	20–40
Splenomegaly	10–40
Petechiae/conjunctival hemorrhage	10–40
Splinter hemorrhages	5–15
Janeway lesions	5–10
Osler nodes	3–10
Retinal lesion or Roth spot	2–10

Risk Factors

The incidence of IE is influenced by a variety of risk factors, both cardiac and non-cardiac (Table 19.3). In less developed countries, rheumatic degenerative heart disease remains the most common risk factor. In developed countries, the most common risk factors include intrinsic cardiac factors (history of prior infective endocarditis, congenital heart disease), followed by pre-existing valve disease, such as mitral or aortic regurgitation, and the presence of implanted devices. Non-cardiac risk factors include IV drug use, immunocompromising conditions, such as cancer or diabetes, and recent dental or surgical procedures [7].

Table 19.3 Endocarditis risk factors

Age >60 years old
IV drug use
History of prior endocarditis
Poor dentition or recent dental procedure
Presence of intracardiac device or prosthetic valve
History of valvular heart disease (rheumatic disease, congenital heart disease such as aortic stenosis or bicuspid aortic valve)
Indwelling intravenous catheter
Immunosuppression
Hemodialysis patients

Pathology/Description

Infective endocarditis occurs when an underlying valvular or nonvalvular structural abnormality results in turbulent blood flow leading to endothelial injury [1]. This injury results in an inflammatory response releasing cytokines and tissue factors causing platelets and thrombin to adhere to the sub endothelium. This ultimately forms a microthrombotic lesion and bacteria in the blood stream then adhere to the microthrombus. This colonization leads to additional bacterial replication and formation of an infective vegetation. These vegetations have high bacterial density and are poorly infiltrated by neutrophils, allowing them to easily grow and fragment into the blood stream [5].

Microbiology

Positive blood cultures are a hallmark of endocarditis. Gram positive bacteria account for 80% of cases of native infective endocarditis. This includes Staphylococcus aureus (35–40%), streptococci (30–40%), and enterococci (10%) (Table 19.6). Coagulase negative staphylococci are more common in prosthetic-valve infective endocarditis [5]. The HACEK organisms (*see* Table 19.4) are fastidious gram-negative bacilli that are difficult to grow in culture and are less common causes of subacute IE. If these organisms are considered, discussion with the ID specialist and microbiology laboratory is important for appropriate testing to be performed. Fungi are extremely rare as cause of IE. Unfortunately, some patients with endocarditis can have negative blood cultures, most commonly because of recent antimicrobial exposure [1].

Table 19.4 HACEK organisms

Hemophilic parainfluenzae
Aggregatibacter actinomycetemcomitans
Cardiobacterium hominis
Eikenella corrodens
Kingella kingae

Imaging

Echocardiography is a key modality in the diagnosis of endocarditis and is a major component of the Duke criteria (see below). Traditional transthoracic echocardiography (TTE) has a sensitivity for vegetation detection between 50–60% while transesophageal echocardiography (TEE) has a sensitivity close to 90%. Both modalities have specificities close to 95% [5]. TEE has increased sensitivity because it circumvents impediments such as body habitus, pulmonary disease, and other acoustic interference between the chest wall and heart [1]. With improved spatial resolution in TTE technology, some newer studies have shown sensitivity for TTE as high as 89% (Fig. 19.6) [1]. Other imaging studies such as cardiac CT (Fig. 19.2) can also be useful in the diagnosis of perivalvular extension and embolic complications. Echocardiography demonstrates the hemodynamic significance of the leaflet destruction and regurgitant lesions in real time (Figs. 19.3 and 19.7.

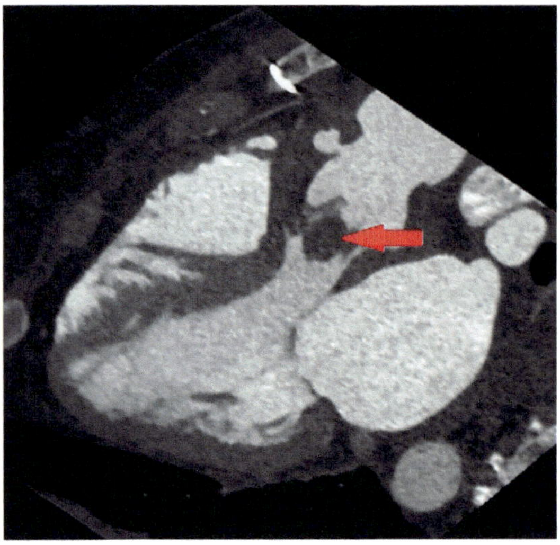

Fig. 19.2 Cardiac CT showing vegetation of infective endocarditis of the native aortic valve (red arrow)

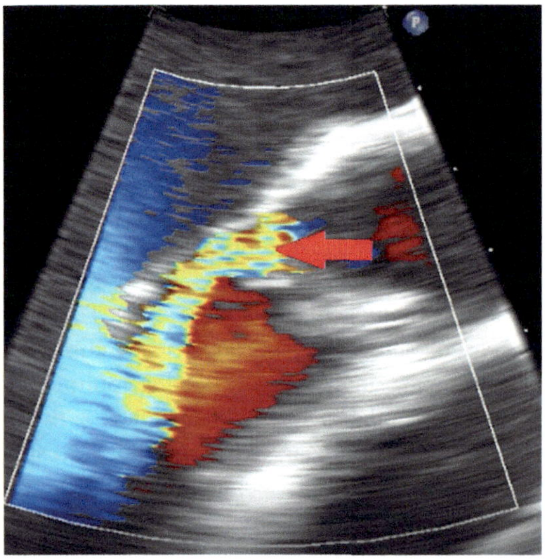

Fig. 19.3 Destruction of the aortic valve leads to severe eccentric insufficiency (red arrow) seen on echocardiography

EKG

12-lead EKG is less useful in diagnosis of IE and is usually associated with nonspecific findings. Perivalvular extension of infection at the aortic root can cause new atrioventricular block (AVB) or bundle branch block (BBB) because of proximity to the AV node and proximal intraventricular conduction system. Specifically, a lesion involving the right and non-coronary cusps is at risk of impacting the conduction system. A less common presentation is a perivalvular extension or vegetation embolization which affects coronary artery patency resulting in ischemic ECG changes (ST depression, T wave inversion, or ST elevation) [1].

Diagnostic Criteria

The Duke Criteria for endocarditis were created in 1994 to establish the definite or possible diagnosis of IE as well as reject the diagnosis. Multiple clinical trials have reported sensitivity of Duke Criteria to be around 80% with specificity and negative predictive value of approximately 90% [1]. The Duke criteria incorporate clinical findings, microbiologic analysis, and imaging results. Criteria are weighted as major or minor (*see* Table 19.5).

Table 19.5 Duke major and minor criteria for IE

Major criteria	Minor criteria
Blood culture positivity with an organism associated with IE on two separate blood cultures sets (Tables 19.4 and 19.6)	Fever >38 °C
Evidence of endocardial involvement seen on imaging to include mobile vegetation, abscess, and/or dehiscence of a prosthetic valve	Predisposing heart condition (implanted prosthetic material, recent or unrepaired CHD, previous IE), or IV drug use
	Vascular phenomena and evidence of embolic disease (Janeway spots), Intercranial hemorrhage
	Microbiological evidence not meeting major criteria (organism not associated with IE, single positive blood culture)
	Immunologic phenomena Rheumatoid F, Osler's nodes, glomerulonephritis

Definite diagnosis requires (a) two major criteria, (b) one major with three minor, or (c) five minor criteria.

P*ossible* diagnosis requires (a) one major and one minor or (b) three minor criteria.

Diagnosis is rejected with (a) no clinical criteria are met or (b) complete resolution of ID syndrome or absence of anatomic evidence for IE on antibiotic therapy for no more than 4 days or (c) an alternative diagnosis explains the patient presentation [8].

Management

In general, randomized controlled trials to guide IE are minimal, and none of the recommendations in international guidelines on IE are backed by Level A evidence [8]. The management of infective endocarditis (IE) includes prompt diagnosis, treatment with antimicrobial therapy, and in some cases of complicated IE, surgical management [9]. Given its ability to cause complications both at the cardiac site and at extracardiac locations, management of IE requires a team approach. In all cases, decisions on intervention should be multifactorial and include a discussion involving multidisciplinary teams including cardiothoracic surgery, cardiology, and infectious disease. If a patient has endured an embolic stroke from their IE, neurology should be consulted to make recommendations regarding the timing of surgery. Stroke is an independent risk factor for postoperative death, especially if the stroke is hemorrhagic. Consultation with addiction medicine and discussion with an ethics team should also be considered in cases regarding IV drug abuse associated IE, especially for recurrent IE. These cases are complicated with longer hospital stays, higher readmission rates, medical non-compliance, and re-infection from continued IV drug abuse. Addiction medicine therapy has shown to reduce mortality and morbidity rates in this patient population postoperatively [10]. It is best practice for patients with IE to be managed in a medical center that offers these different specialists [5].

Antimicrobial Therapy

The American Heart Association, American College of Cardiology, and American Association for Thoracic Surgery have each published guidelines on the management of IE. While these guidelines are generally concordant, there are minor differences in their recommendations about antimicrobial therapy [2]. Because there are continuous changes in antimicrobial sensitivity over time, as well as regional and site-specific differences in antimicrobial susceptibility profiles, consultation with infectious disease is imperative for treatment [2]. The infectious disease team is also essential as resistance to many antibiotics is rising and has become one of the greatest threats to modern health care [8].

The primary goal of antibiotic treatment is to stabilize vegetations and eventually eradicate infections [6]. The penetration of antibiotics is a significant challenge in the treatment of IE because cardiac vegetations, which are composed of fibrin and platelets, pose a considerable mechanical barrier between the antibiotic and the embedded targeted microorganisms [6]. These vegetations create a protective micro-environment that is poorly accessible to neutrophils and host defense molecules. Vegetations are loaded with bacteria at very high densities [5].

In treating IE, determination of the causative pathogen is of prime importance, allowing clinicians to narrow and target therapy specifically to the pathogen (Table 19.6) [4]. Empiric antibiotic therapy should be initiated and continued after blood cultures (ideally 3 sets) are obtained [2].

Table 19.6 Common organism and antibiotic regimens for IE

Common causes of IE	Example of common antibiotic regimen
Staphylococcus aureus 35–40%	
MRSA	Daptomycin or vancomycin
MSSA	Anti-staphylococcal PCN (ex: Nafcillin)
Streptococci 30–40%	Gentamicin plus penicillin or ceftriaxone
Enterococci 10%	Ampicillin plus gentamicin or ceftriaxone

Once these cultures have been obtained, therapy should be started very quickly [8]. The choice of empiric therapy should take into consideration the most likely pathogens. Gram positive bacteria account for approximately 80% of cases of native valve IE. These bacteria include methicillin-sensitive Staphylococcus Aureus (MSSA) and methicillin-resistant Staphylococcus Aureus (MRSA) (35–40% of cases), streptococci (30–40% of cases), and enterococci (10% of cases). S. aureus is the leading cause of IE (both native and prosthetic valve) in the United States. More rare species include other gram-positive pathogens, fungi, polymicrobial infection, and finally gram-negative bacilli [5]. Though fungal IE is rare, it has well-recognized associated risk factors including IV drug use, immunocompromised state, and indwelling devices [6]. After initial blood cultures have been obtained and empiric antibiotic therapy started, adjustments in antimicrobial selection depend on the blood culture isolate and its antimicrobial susceptibility [5]. The expectation is that this empirical therapy will be revised once the susceptibility results are obtained, as optimal treatment of IE is based on antimicrobial therapy that is effective against the specific infective organism identified [6].

Rarely, IE can occur without associated positive blood cultures. Most often this is caused by recent administration of antibiotics prior to blood culture collection or by organisms that grow poorly or not at all in standard blood culture media [5]. Empiric treatment of patients with culture negative IE should cover both gram positive and gram-negative organisms, and infectious disease involvement is imperative in these cases. PCR assays are now available for a variety of these less-common microorganisms. Karius Testing™ can also identify pathogen DNA in plasma even when blood cultures are negative, which can lead to more prompt antibiotic therapy.

Because pathogen-specific recommendations for antibiotics are often changing and vary geographically, organism-specific treatment regimens are outlined in consensus guidelines [9]. In general, for patients with native valve IE, vancomycin plus ceftriaxone is a reasonable choice for empirical therapy to cover likely pathogens while blood cultures are pending [5]. It should be noted that recommendations for antimicrobial therapy for IE are based almost entirely on observational studies rather than on randomized controlled trials [5]. Common antibiotic regimens for specific organisms are seen in Table 19.6.

As mentioned, S. aureus is the most common cause of IE (both native valve and prosthetic valve). The rates of S. aureus IE have increased over the years and are primarily a consequence of healthcare contact (intravascular catheters, surgical wounds, indwelling prosthetic devices, and hemodialysis) [6]. Antibiotic treatment decisions for S. aureus IE hinge on the presence or absence of antibiotic resistance [4]. Single antibiotic therapy is usually enough for native valve IE. However, for S. aureus-infected prosthetic valves, combination therapy from multiple antibiotic classes is recommended [4]. Daptomycin or vancomycin monotherapy is recommended for treatment of native-valve IE caused by MRSA. An anti-staphylococcal penicillin (nafcillin) is the drug of choice for IE caused by MSSA, as these agents have shown higher cure rates for MSSA than vancomycin [7]. Despite early diagnosis and appropriate therapy, IE after S. aureus bacteremia is frequently associated with disabling and life-threatening sequelae [2].

For streptococcal IE, treatment regimens vary widely based on the microorganism. Two common regimens for streptococcal IE are penicillin and gentamicin or ceftriaxone and gentamicin. Single antibiotic therapy (penicillin, ceftriaxone, or vancomycin) alone is also a common treatment strategy for streptococcal IE.

For enterococcal IE, combination therapy is recommended. Two common combination regimens involve ampicillin and ceftriaxone or ampicillin and gentamicin. The use of single-drug vs combination drug therapy can vary according to the specific pathogen, potential presence of antibiotic resistance, and whether the infection involves a native or prosthetic valve [4].

Serial blood cultures should be obtained to confirm clearance of bacteria with therapy. While undergoing treatment, these cultures are typically obtained every 24–48 h until bloodstream infection is cleared [6]. Antibiotics should generally be continued for 4–6 weeks after blood cultures convert to negative [5]. Antimicrobial therapy duration must be sufficient to ensure complete eradication of microorganisms within vegetations [6]. The duration of antibiotics for native-valve endocarditis typically ranges from 4–6 weeks. Factors that compel the extended 6-week antibiotic course include: left-sided vegetations (which tend to have higher bacterial densities), the presence of drug-resistant organisms, and the use of slowly bactericidal antibiotics such as vancomycin [9].

Most patients with IE become afebrile 3 to 5 days after initiation of appropriate antimicrobial therapy. Patients with S. aureus IE may respond somewhat more slowly, remaining febrile for up to 5–7 days after initiation of therapy [11]. Patients with right-sided IE and septic pulmonary emboli may remain febrile for an even longer duration of time, given the recurrent embolic events.

Careful serial examinations should be performed to evaluate for heart failure (new or worsening), emboli, or other complications. Patients who develop new complications while on appropriate antimicrobial therapy should have an urgent repeat echocardiogram [11].

The first year after implantation is a vulnerable period for prosthetic valve endocarditis because of a greater exposure to healthcare contact along with incomplete endothelialization of the prosthetic valve early after implantation. Mortality with antibiotics alone with the presence of a prosthetic valve is high (26–75%) [3]. There are some indications for antibiotic therapy alone in prosthetic valve IE, including hemodynamically stable patients, improvement on antibiotic therapy, early diagnosis of prosthetic valve IE, and right-sided endocarditis [3]. Treatment of prosthetic valve IE is typically more difficult than treatment of native-valve endocarditis and often requires surgical replacement of the prosthesis in addition to antibiotic therapy. The typical duration of therapy in prosthetic valve IE is the full 6 weeks.

Surgical Management

In many patients with IE, despite antimicrobial treatment, surgery is needed for effective treatment. Surgical treatment is typically undertaken in 40–50% of patients with IE [12]. Infection causes destructive mobile vegetations on the valve leaflets (Figs. 19.4, and 19.5). These vegetations prevent hemostatic coaptation of the leaflets and can produce detrimental tears or perforations within the valve leaflet (Figs. 19.2, 19.3, 19.6, and 19.7). These changes can lead to acute regurgitation requiring urgent surgical intervention. Paravalvular infection may also occur including annular or aortic abscesses which are considered life threatening and has a ≥40% mortality rate and increased risk of heart block (Fig. 19.8) [10]. The main goal of surgical inter-

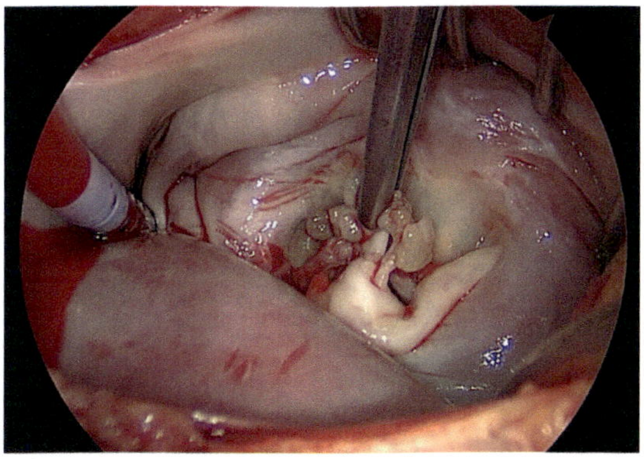

Fig. 19.4 Mitral valve endocarditis with multiple vegetations

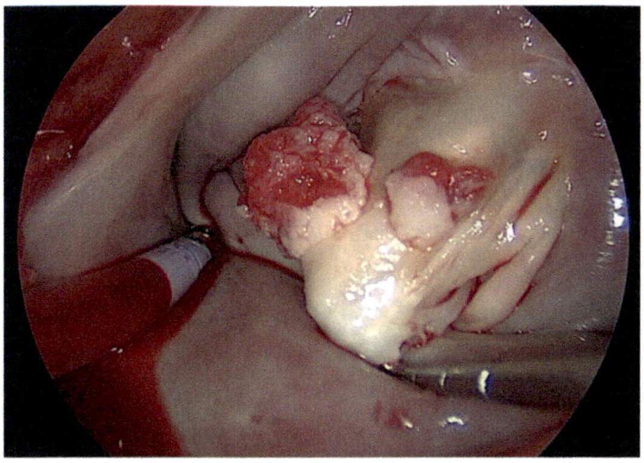

Fig. 19.5 Mitral valve endocarditis with large vegetation

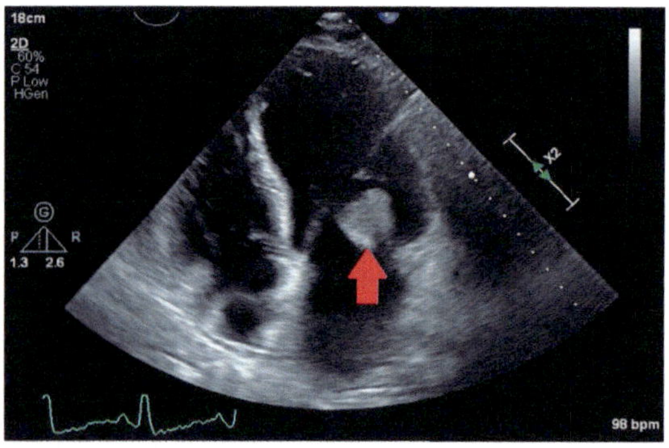

Fig. 19.6 Vegetation on the posterior of the mitral valve (red arrow)

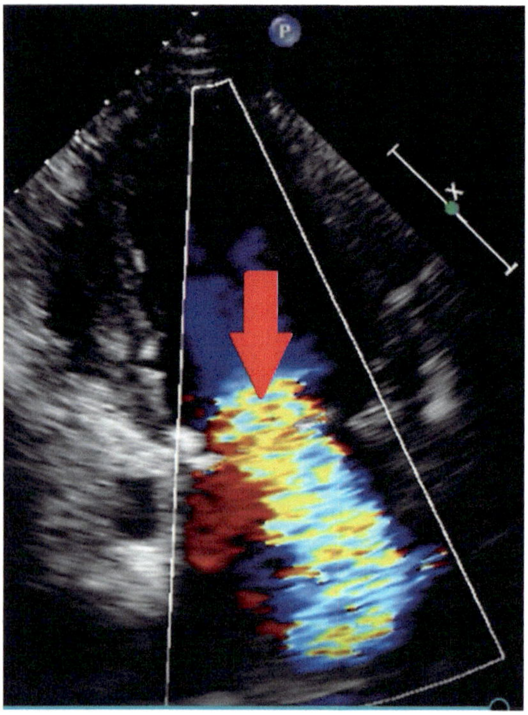

Fig. 19.7 Severe mitral regurgitation due to destruction of the valve leaflet by vegetation

vention is to remove all damaged and infected tissue by debridement and restore valve integrity. If salvageable, valve repair is always preferred over replacement to avoid placement of prosthetic material into an infected space. This is especially important with right-sided endocarditis associated with IV drug users (IVDU) as repair is associated with better late survival and longer freedom from recurrent IE [13]. If the valve is unrepair-

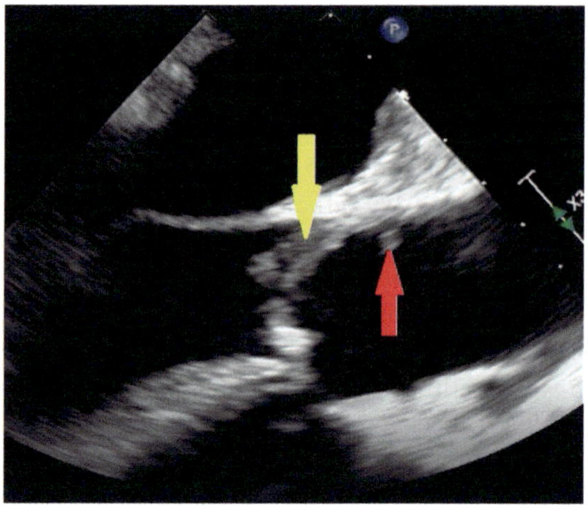

Fig. 19.8 Aortic valve endocarditis complicated by annular abscess. Vegetation in the ascending aorta (red arrow) in communication with leaflet and hypodense abscess formation in the aortic annulus (yellow arrow). Management requires urgent surgical intervention

able, infection is unable to be effectively debrided, or an abscess is present, valve replacement is warranted. Valve selection is challenging in IE with the decision between bioprosthetic and mechanical valve being critical. Prosthetic valves are at risk for reinfection if active infection persists. However, in the setting of IE secondary to IVDU, medical compliance is questionable and mechanical valve placement is not advised. Refer to Chap. 16 on aortic stenosis for further discussion on valve selection. Homograft or freestyle aortic valves are utilized when the endocarditis involves an aortic root abscess and root extraction is warranted. In patients with relapsing prosthetic valve endocarditis after a full course antibiotic therapy, the prosthetic valve is presumed to be the source and should be removed [10].

The timing of valve surgery is not well defined and is a highly individualized decision that is best made by an experienced multidisciplinary team [14]. The timing of surgery, criteria for potentially delaying surgery, and predictors of surgical mortality and poor outcomes need to be better defined. However, intervention is recommended during the initial hospitalization and prior to the completion of the recommended course of antibiotics when the below listed indications for early

Table 19.7 Indications for early intervention valve surgery for the treatment of IE

• Patients who present with valve dysfunction resulting in symptoms of HF
• Patients with left-sided IE caused by *S. aureus*, a fungal organism, or another highly resistant organism
• Patients with IE complicated by heart block, annular or aortic abscess, or destructive penetrating lesions
• Patients with IE and evidence of persistent infection as manifested by persistent bacteremia or fevers lasting >5 days after initiation of antimicrobial therapy
• For patients with IE and an implanted cardiac electronic device, complete removal of the pacemaker, or defibrillator system is indicated
• Patients with prosthetic valve endocarditis and relapsing infection (defined as bacteremia recurrence after antibiotic course completion and negative blood culture results)
• Patients with IE present with recurrent emboli and persistent vegetations despite appropriate antibiotic therapy

Adapted from the American College of Cardiology/American Heart Association 2020 Guideline for the Management of Valvular Heart Disease

surgery are present (see Table 19.7). In this population, early intervention has shown improved outcomes and decreased mortality [10].

Heart failure caused by valvular regurgitation or obstruction is the most common indication for surgery. Outcomes for IE have historically been dire without surgery once the patient has developed refractory pulmonary edema or cardiogenic shock secondary to their IE [12]. Emergent surgery for heart failure unresponsive to medical management is crucial, and swift surgery is also recommended even if temporary stabilization of the patient with heart failure secondary to IE can be achieved.

Uncontrolled or complex infection is the second-most common indication for surgery. Abscesses and paravalvular extension of infection often cannot be cured with antibiotic therapy alone. Mortality rate is significantly reduced when early surgery is undertaken in these patients [15].

The third-most common indication for surgery is to prevent recurrent emboli from the vegetation, a devastating complication that affects 25–50% of patients [12]. Embolism is more likely when vegetations are large (>10 mm in length), highly mobile, and located on the mitral valve [12]. Emboli most often involve major arterial beds, including the brain, lungs, coronary arteries, spleen, bowel, and extremities. Up to 65% of embolic events involve the CNS, and >90% of CNS emboli lodge in the distribution of the middle cerebral artery [16]. The rate of embolic events decreases dramatically during and after the first 2–3 weeks of successful antibiotic therapy [16]. In patients with IE and evidence of CVA, regardless of the indications for anticoagulation, it is reasonable to temporarily discontinue anticoagulation [15]. This is because anticoagulation therapy may increase the risk of an embolic infarct becoming hemorrhagic. Even in most patients with prosthetic valves who experience a CNS embolic event, all anticoagulation therapy should be held for at least 2 weeks. This time should allow for thrombus organization and help to prevent acute hemorrhagic conversion of embolic lesions [16]. Most guidelines do agree on delaying valve surgery for at least 4 weeks in patients with large embolic CNS lesions or intracranial hemorrhage [14]. Other reasonable reasons to delay early surgery are very high operative risk or major neurologic impairment [17].

Indications for surgery in *right-sided* native valve endocarditis differ and include very large vegetations (>20 mm in diameter), recurrent septic pulmonary emboli, highly resistant organisms, or persistent bacteremia. HF is not a common indication for early surgery in right-sided NVE since severe TR is better tolerated than left-sided regurgitation [17].

Early surgery can also be indicated for certain pathogens (examples including *Pseudomonas aeruginosa*, Brucella, fungi, enterococci, and *S. aureus*) as these pathogens can be extremely difficult to cure with medical therapy alone and are also prone to abscess or fistula formation and other cardiac tissue destruction [15].

In patients with an implanted cardiac electronic device, the entire system, including the generator and leads, should be removed even if there is no sign of infection along the device. This is because blood stream infections can cause a biofilm of infection to coat (seed) the leads, thus making the infection impossible to irradicate with medical therapy alone. Removal can be performed at the time of infected valve surgery or at a specialized center where laser lead extractions are performed, for those not undergoing surgical valve management.

Surgical risk stratification can be quantified utilizing the Society for Thoracic Surgeon (STS) risk calculator for mitral or aortic endocarditis, but not currently for tricuspid endocarditis. Refer to Chap. 4 for surgical management of coronary artery disease and discussion on risk assessment. In all cases, decisions on intervention should be multifactorial and include discussions with the multidiscipline teams involved with the patient's care.

The risk calculator is available on the STS website:

https://riskcalc.sts.org/stswebriskcalc/calculate

Surgical risk is exceptionally high in patients with active IE; however, in many cases, the patient will not improve without surgical intervention. The average mortality risk for patients undergoing surgery for IE with associated HF is 21%, however, mortality risk for patients with medical therapy alone is 45% [10].

Table 19.8 Patient care during and after completion of antimicrobial treatment

Initiate before or at completion of therapy
• Obtain transthoracic echocardiogram to establish new baseline
• Drug rehabilitation referral for patients who use illicit injection drugs
• Educate regarding signs of endocarditis, need for antibiotic prophylaxis for certain dental/surgical/invasive procedures
• Thorough dental evaluation and treatment if not performed earlier in evaluation
• Prompt removal of intravenous catheter at completion of antimicrobial therapy
Short-term follow-up
• Obtain at least three sets of blood culture specimens from separate sites for any febrile illness and before initiation of antibiotic therapy
• Physical examination for evidence of congestive heart failure
• Evaluate for toxicity resulting from antimicrobial therapy
Long-term follow-up
• Obtain at least three sets of blood cultures from separate sites for any febrile illness and before initiation of antibiotic therapy
• Evaluation of valvular and ventricular function (echocardiography)
• Scrupulous oral hygiene and frequent dental professional office visits

Adapted from Mann et al. Braunwald's Heart Disease. A Textbook of Cardiovascular Medicine, Tenth Edition. *Elsevier*

Outpatient Management and Follow-Up Evaluation (Table 19.8)

Although novel diagnostic and therapeutic strategies have emerged, the 1-year mortality has not improved and remains at >30%, which is worse than many cancers [12]. While on antimicrobial therapy, patients should be monitored for toxicity. Weekly lab monitoring (including a complete blood count and complete metabolic panel) should be performed [18]. Historically, the entire course of antibiotics has been intravenous (typically with a peripherally inserted central catheter placed to allow home IV antibiotic administration). However, recent data have shown that transitioning certain patients to oral antibiotics, after at least 10 days of IV antibiotics, was non-inferior. This transition to an oral step-down regimen may be a possible course, with direction from an infectious disease specialist, in certain patients who are clinically stable with reassuring TEE results [15].

At the completion of antibiotic therapy, a transthoracic echocardiogram should be performed to serve as a new baseline reference for valve appearance, severity of valvular regurgitation, and quantification of left ventricular function [17].

Ongoing monitoring is recommended after hospital discharge, mainly for recurrent infection (either relapse or reinfection) and progressive valve dysfunction [12]. Patients should be informed that they remain at risk of recurrent IE, estimated to occur at a rate of 1–3% per year. At regular medical checkups, patients should be questioned about symptoms of heart failure, and a thorough physical exam should be performed [16].

Patients should be made aware that relapses can occur and that new onset of fever, chills, or other evidence of systemic infection mandates immediate evaluation, including a thorough history and physical exam and three sets of blood cultures [16]. Prescribing empirical antibiotic therapy should be avoided for undefined febrile illness until after blood cultures have been obtained (unless the patient's clinical condition warrants urgent empirical therapy) [16].

Measures to prevent IE recurrence, including good oral hygiene and consideration of antibiotic prophylaxis at the time of dental and other invasive procedures, are important [12]. Oral health and hygiene is now considered more important than antibiotic prophylaxis to reduce the risk of recurrent IE. For ongoing long-term follow up, daily dental hygiene should be stressed, with serial evaluations by a dentist who is ideally familiar with this patient population. Patients should be counseled to discuss with their team the role of antibiotic prophylaxis prior to specific types of procedures, including certain types of dental procedures [17]. The ACC and AHA do recommend ongoing use of antibiotic prophylaxis for patients undergoing certain procedures who are the highest risk of IE. Patients deemed high risk include those with a history of IE [12].

SBE prophylaxis is recommended for dental procedures only for patients with cardiac conditions at highest risk of adverse outcomes from endocarditis including prosthetic cardiac valve, previous endocarditis, congenital heart disease with unrepaired cyanotic lesions (including palliative shunts and conduits), completely repaired CHD with prosthetic material or device during the first 6 months after placement, repaired CHD with residual defects at the site or adjacent to the site of prosthetic patch or device, and/or cardiac transplant patients with cardiac valvular disease. Prophylaxis is no longer recommended for gastrointestinal or genitourinary procedures. The antibiotics used for prophylaxis are listed below (Table 19.9) and are taken 30–60 min before the procedure start. The guidelines are listed on the American Heart Association website: https://www.heart.org/en/health-topics/infective-endocarditis which also has printable cards for patients. It is critical to educate high-risk patients regarding the potential symptoms of endocarditis as the associated morbidity and mortality are high. Note: guidelines recently changed to no longer include clindamycin for prophylaxis due to potential for severe adverse drug reactions.

Table 19.9 SBE prophylaxis antibiotic regimens

Situation	Medication	Adult dosing
Oral	Amoxicillin	2 gm
Unable to take oral meds	Amoxicillin Ampicillin Cefazolin/ ceftriaxone	2 gm IM/ IV 2 gm IM/ IV 1 gm IM/ IV
Allergic to PCN or AMP-oral	Cephalexin Azithromycin/ clarithromycin Doxycycline	2 gm 500 mg 100 mg
Allergic to PCN or AMP-unable to take oral meds	Cephazolin/ ceftriaxone	1 gm IM/ IV

Clinical Pearls

- It is critically important for high-risk patients to know the signs and symptoms of IE.
- Fever and new or worsening murmur are the most common findings of IE.
- Gram positive bacteria are the most common "bug" identified in native IE.
- The diagnosis is made using the Duke Criteria.
- Annular and aortic abscesses have an increased risk of heart block and death.
- Valve repair is always preferred over replacement to avoid placement of prosthetic material.
- Right-sided endocarditis is often associated with IV drug use.
- The most common indication for surgery in left-sided lesions is heart failure.
- Embolic risk is high with large, mobile, MV vegetations.
- If a pacemaker/defibrillator is present, it is assumed to be infected with any blood stream infection and removal will need to be considered.

References

1. Mann, et al. Braunwald's Heart Disease. A textbook of cardiovascular medicine. 10th ed. Elsevier.
2. Otto CM, et al. ACC/AHA guideline for the management of valvular heart disease. Circulation. 2020;2021(143):e72–e227.
3. Nataloni M, et al. Prosthetic valve endocarditis. J Cardiovasc Med. 11:869–83.
4. Wang A, et al. Management considerations in infective endocarditis: a review. JAMA. 2018;320(1):72–83.
5. Chambers, et al. Native-valve infective endocarditis. N Engl J Med. 2020;383:567–76.
6. Baddour LM, et al. Infective endocarditis in adults: diagnosis, antimicrobial therapy, and management of complications. Circulation. 2015;132:1435–86.
7. Murdoch DR. Clinical presentation, etiology, and outcome of infective endocarditis in the 21st century. Arch Intern Med. 2009;169(5):463. https://doi.org/10.1001/archinternmed.2008.603.
8. Cahill TJ, et al. Infective endocarditis. Lancet. 2016;387:882–93.
9. UpToDate: overview of management of infective endocarditis in adults.
10. Otto CM, Nishimura RA, Bonow RO, Carabello BA, Erwin JP III, Gentile F. 2020 ACC/AHA guideline for the management of patients with valvular heart disease: a report of the American College of Cardiology/American Heart Association Joint Committee on Clinical Practice Guidelines. J Am Coll Cardiol. 2021;77(4):e25–197.
11. UpToDate: antimicrobial therapy of left-sided native valve endocarditis.
12. The Society of Thoracic Surgeons; 2022. Available from: https://www.sts.org/resources/riskcalculator.
13. Shmueli H, Thomas F, Flint N, Setia G, Janjic A, Siegel RJ. Right-sided infective endocarditis 2020: challenges and updates in diagnosis and treatment. J Am Heart Assoc. 2020;9(15).
14. Bonow RO, O'Gara PT, Adams DH, Badhwar V, Bavaria JE, Elmariah S, et al. 2019 AATS/ACC/SCAI/STS expert consensus systems of care document: operator and institutional recommendations and requirements for transcatheter mitral valve intervention. J Am Coll Cardiol. 2020;76(1):96–117.
15. Lawton JS, Tamis-Holland JE, Bangalore S, Bates ER, Beckie TM, Mischoff JM, et al. 2021 ACC/AHA/SCAI Guideline for Coronary artery Revascularization, A report of the American College of Cardiology/American Heart Association Joint Committee on Clinical Practice Guidelines. J Am Coll Cardiol. 2022;79(2):e21–e129.
16. Chung J, Shum-Tim D. The current indications and options for aortic valve surgery. J Surg. 2014;2(1):6.
17. Fedak PWM, McCarthy PM, Bonow RO. Evolving concepts and technologies in mitral valve repair. Circulation. 2008;117(7):963–74.
18. Watts TMF, Brescia AA, Murray SL, Burn DA, Wisniewski A, Romano MA. Degenerative mitral valve repair restores life expectancy. Ann Thorac Surg. 2020;109(3):494–801.
19. UpToDate: clinical Manifestations and evaluation of adults with suspected left-sided native valve endocarditis.

Part V

Cardiomyopathies/Congestive Heart Failure

Joseph Mishkin

Heart failure is a syndrome characterized by shortness of breath and fatigue and is often associated with evidence of fluid retention. This syndrome can occur due to a multitude of cardiac insults that lead to either impaired contraction or relaxation of the myocardium [1]. In some instances, the primary etiology can be due to pathology involving the pericardium as described in Chap. 23. Understanding the instigating cause of heart failure can be important in directing appropriate treatment, i.e., identifying ischemic heart disease and providing appropriate revascularization [2]. The classification of heart failure based on ejection fraction is important as most clinical trials with positive results have enrolled patients with systolic dysfunction. Fortunately, in recent years, new drug therapies have been identified to improve outcomes in those with heart failure and preserved ejection fraction [3–6]. Furthermore, advances in the treatment of cardiac amyloidosis have given optimism when targeted therapies previously did not exist [7]. In many cases, the pathophysiological cascade of neurohormonal activation and cytokine upregulation is similar regardless of the etiology of heart failure. Therefore, the pharmacological interventions to treat heart failure follow a common pathway regardless of the etiology of the heart failure syndrome [8–11].

The following chapters will define some of the most common causes of systolic and diastolic heart failure and provide the rationale for guideline directed medical therapy. Given the expected rise in incidence of heart failure in the USA and beyond, a solid foundation in identifying and treating this syndrome is important for a variety of cardiovascular and internal medicine specialties. Later sections will provide the basis for managing the more fulminant form of heart failure—cardiogenic shock.

Joseph Mishkin
Heart Failure and Transplant Services, Atrium Health/Sanger Heart and Vascular Institute, Charlotte, NC, USA
joseph.mishkin@atriumhealth.org

References

1. Braunwald E. Heart failure. JACC Heart Fail. 2013;1(1):1–20.
2. Truby L, Rogers J. Advanced heart failure: epidemiology, diagnosis, and therapeutic approaches. J Am Coll Cardiol HF. 2020;8:523–36.
3. Bhatt AS, Abraham WT, Lindenfeld J, et al. Treatment of HF in an era of multiple therapies: statement from the HF collaboratory. J Am Coll Cardiol HF. 2021;9(1):1–12.
4. Fonarow GC, Stough WG, Abraham WT, et al. Characteristics, treatments, and outcomes of patients with preserved systolic function hospitalized for heart failure: a report from the OPTIMIZE-HF Registry. J Am Coll Cardiol. 2007;50:768.
5. Anker SD, Butler J, Filippatos G, et al. Empagliflozin in heart failure with a preserved ejection fraction. N Engl J Med. 2021;385:1451–61.
6. Pitt B, Pfeffer MA, Assmann SF, et al. Spironolactone for heart failure with preserved ejection fraction. N Engl J Med. 2014;370:1383–92.
7. Ruberg FL, Grogan M, Hanna M, Kelly JW, Maurer MS. transthyretin amyloid cardiomyopathy: JACC state-of-the-art review. J Am Coll Cardiol. 2019;73:2872–91.
8. Metoprolol CR/XL Randomised Intervention Trial in Congestive Heart Failure (MERIT-HF). Effect of metoprolol CR/XL in chronic heart failure. Lancet. 1999;353:2001.
9. Packer M, Fowler MB, Roecker EB, et al. Effect of carvedilol on the morbidity of patients with severe chronic heart failure: results of the carvedilol prospective randomized cumulative survival (COPERNICUS) study. Circulation. 2002;106:2194.
10. Zannad F, McMurray JJ, Krum H, et al. Eplerenone in patients with systolic heart failure and mild symptoms. N Engl J Med. 2011;364:11.
11. Desai AS, McMurray JJ, Packer M, et al. Effect of the angiotensin-receptor-neprilysin inhibitor LCZ696 compared with enalapril on mode of death in heart failure patients. Eur Heart J. 2015;36:1990.

Heart Failure with Reduced Ejection Fraction (HFrEF)

20

Lauren Eyadiel and Bridget Rasmussen

Introduction

Heart failure is a complex systemic syndrome where inadequate blood supply due to heart dysfunction is unable to meet the metabolic demands of the tissues [1]. This clinical syndrome consists of symptoms of congestion and/or inadequate cardiac perfusion. Congestive symptoms include shortness of breath, lower extremity edema, abdominal bloating, orthopnea, and/or paroxysmal nocturnal dyspnea (PND). Symptoms of inadequate cardiac perfusion include mental status changes, cardiac cachexia, renal dysfunction, and fatigue due to decreased end organ perfusion. The clinical syndrome is combined with elevated natriuretic peptides and objective evidence of congestion and/or echocardiographic findings of structural changes to the heart including reduction in ejection fraction. Heart failure with reduced ejection fraction (HFrEF) is defined as patients with the clinical syndrome of heart failure with a left ventricular ejection fraction of less than 40% [2, 3]. This will be the focus of this chapter. Heart failure with preserved ejection fraction will be covered in Chap. 21.

L. Eyadiel · B. Rasmussen (✉)
Advanced Heart Failure, Heart Transplant, and Mechanical Circulatory Support, Cardiology, Atrium Health Wake Forest Baptist,
Winston Salem, NC, USA
e-mail: lesykes@wakehealth.edu; brasmuss@wakehealth.edu

Anatomy and Physiology

Heart failure is a complex neurohormonal process that is not completely understood. Simply put, there is an inciting event that results in damage to the homeostasis of the metabolic system resulting in activation of multiple compensatory mechanisms. These compensatory mechanisms involve the adrenergic nervous system, renin angiotensin aldosterone system (RAAS), and cytokine system. This process is initially protective, but sustained activation of these compensatory mechanisms results in adverse remodeling of the left ventricle with associated dilation and increase in left ventricular volume and mass [4, 5]. Cardiomyocyte loss leads to the inability of heart muscle to contract properly and reduces cardiac output. A reduction in cardiac output causes activation of the sympathetic nervous system and norepinephrine release, promoting peripheral vasoconstriction, increased heart failure, and increased myocardial contractility. Activation of RAAS leads to water and sodium retention, increasing circulating volume and preload. The Frank-Starling mechanism states that cardiac fiber length increases contractile strength [6] (see Chap. 2). Thus, the increased preload causes increased myocardial contractility. If this process persists, detrimental ventricular remodeling develops. Figure 20.1 summarizes this process. A basic understanding of the pathophysiology of HFrEF is required as

R. Musialowski, K. Allshouse (eds.), *Cardiovascular Manual for the Advanced Practice Provider*,
https://doi.org/10.1007/978-3-031-35819-7_20

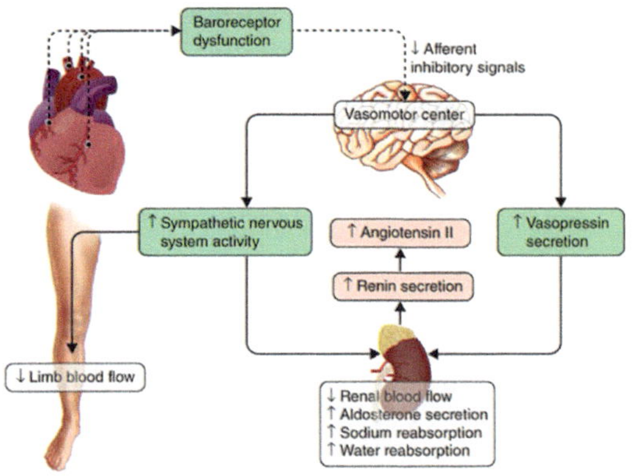

Fig. 20.1 Neurohormonal influences in HFrEF. (Adapted from Harrison's Principles of Internal Medicine)

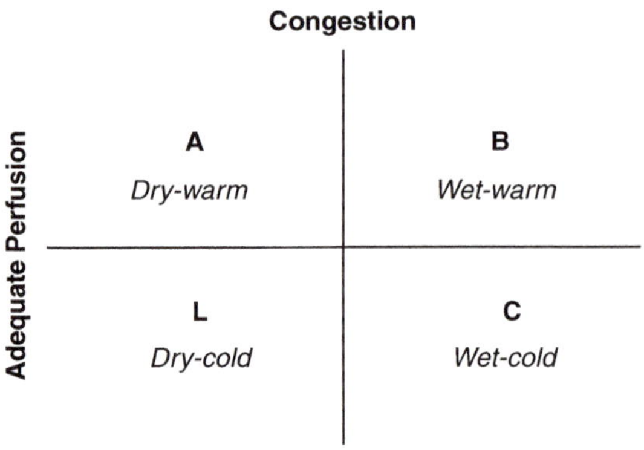

Fig. 20.2 Hemodynamic profile of heart failure patients [8]

guideline-directed medical therapies (GDMT) target these compensatory mechanisms. There are multiple etiologies of heart failure including both ischemic and nonischemic disease which are further discussed in the pathology section of this chapter.

Physical Exam

Careful clinical examination of patients with heart failure is essential. Broadly speaking, heart failure physical exam components can fall into two categories: volume status and perfusion status. Combining these assessments provides a clinical profile [7] that can drive decisions in management (Fig. 20.2).

Volume Status

Jugular vein distention, indicating an elevated jugular vein pressure (JVP), is common in patients who have increased congestion. JVP is used to estimate right atrial pressure. Waveform or pulsation is examined, typically at 45°, on both sides of the neck, which can be calculated by measuring elevation and calculating horizontal distance from the sternal angle in centimeters (cm) then estimating distance to the right atrium by adding 5 cm. Inspiratory increase in JVP is a poor prognostic indicator [9]. Pressing on the abdomen should cause transient JVP elevation that can help differentiate the waveform from carotid pulsation. This change in abdominal pressure, termed hepatojugular reflux (HJR), is pathologic if a sustained elevation is noted over 10 seconds of abdominal pressure, suggesting elevated right-sided filling pressure [9]. Likewise, the presence of orthopnea—dyspnea when lying back or supine—is indicative of elevated left ventricular filling pressures and pulmonary capillary wedge pressure (PCWP). Respiratory exam may be notable for crackles or diminished breath sounds indicative of pleural effusions, but the presence or absence of this is nonspecific. Cardiac auscultation may be notable for S3 gallop sound, a brief third heart sound in early diastole indicating increased flow rates or increased ventricular dilation. This is best heard over the apex when the patient is in a left lateral position (see Chap. 1). Pulsus alternans, alternating weak and strong pulse pressure, is an indicator of left ventricular resistance and left-sided dysfunction and may suggest decompensation. While lower extremity edema is frequently present, it is not specific for heart failure etiology. Dry oral mucosa and poor skin turgor without an obvious cause are a sign of intravascular volume depletion (Fig. 20.3).

Perfusion Status

Although a careful review of systems is vital to determining cardiac output or perfusion status,

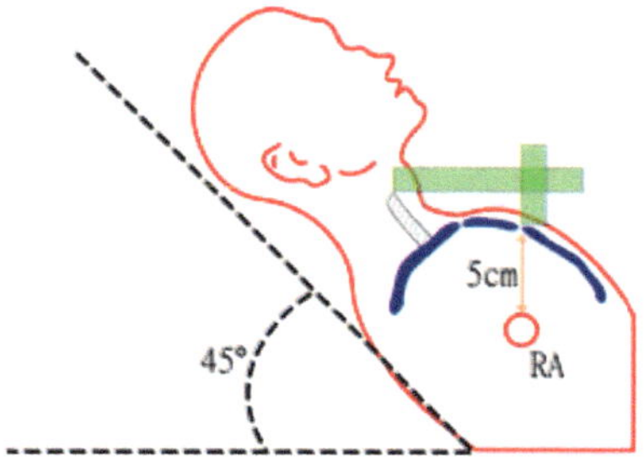

Fig. 20.3 How to measure JVP. (https://www.renalfellow.org/2011/01/02/jugular-venous-pressuredistention)

perfusion can be assessed by clinical exam as well. A narrow pulse pressure (systolic minus diastolic pressure) or low proportional pulse pressure (pulse pressure divided by systolic pressure) is a marker of low cardiac output. Cool or tepid extremities are suggestive of low cardiac output, but sensitivity is low. Prolonged or sluggish capillary refill time (greater than 2 seconds), if present, is a marker of poor perfusion.

Review of Systems

Like physical examination, a thorough review of systems can be instructive. Pertinent positive review of system findings connoting elevated volume status includes weight changes; new cough, especially when lying supine; orthopnea; paroxysmal nocturnal dyspnea (may be expressed as change in sleep habit); early satiety; abdominal bloating; and lower extremity edema. Findings that suggest poor cardiac perfusion include fatigue or malaise, decreased appetite, cold intolerance, confusion, decreased urination, and dizziness/lightheadedness. Early decompensated heart failure is often misdiagnosed as a respiratory ailment.

Clinical Classifications

There are two main tools to classify heart failure. The ACC/AHA stages of Heart Failure emphasize the development and progression of disease, and the New York Heart Association (NYHA) classes focus on exercise capacity, physical examination, and the symptomatic status of the HF disease (Table 20.1).

Table 20.1 Classification of heart failure

ACCF/AHA stages of 6F	NYHA functional classification
Stage A: At high risk for HF but without structural heart disease or symptoms of HF	I: No limitation of physical activity.
Stage B: Structural heart disease but without signs of symptoms of HF	II: Slight limitation of physical activity. Comfortable at rest, but ordinary activity results in symptoms of HF
Stage C: Structural heart disease with prior or current symptoms of HF	III: Marked limitation of physical activity. Comfortable at rest, but less than ordinary activity causes symptoms of HF
Stage D: Refractory HF requiring specialized interventions	IV: Unable to carry on any physical activity without symptoms of HF, or symptoms of HF at rest

Imaging

Imaging is utilized in heart failure to confirm the diagnosis, provide information regarding the etiology, monitor for treatment response, and to assist in prognostication. Depending on the type of imaging, information is given regarding the cardiac chamber size, architecture, global, and regional left ventricular function. Choosing the most appropriate imaging modality can be challenging and requires careful attention to patient-specific factors based on history, physical examination, and laboratory testing. Table 20.2 provides a comprehensive overview of the imaging modalities used for evaluation of patients with heart failure. The most common imaging modalities will be discussed in further detail below. Of note, routine repeat measurement of left ventricular function is not indicated in the absence of a clinical status change or treatment intervention.

Echocardiography

Two-dimensional echocardiography is considered the most useful, versatile, and cost-effective diagnostic method for patients with heart

Table 20.2 Summary of imaging modalities utilized in heart failure

Imaging modality	Most useful in defining	Conditions where most helpful	Advantages	Disadvantages
Coronary angiogram	Gold standard for evaluating coronary artery disease (CAD)	Suspected CAD	Can intervene at time of diagnosis	Invasive, radiation exposure, risk for contrast-induced nephropathy
Echocardiography	Biventricular function, wall motion, valvular lesions, structural abnormalities, pericardial effusion, estimation of right atrial and pulmonary artery pressures	Suspected CAD, valvular disease, pericardial tamponade, pulmonary hypertension	Noninvasive, no radiation exposure, ventricular function, hemodynamic information, good for initial evaluation, and monitoring of treatment response in HF	Difficult in patient with poor acoustic windows
Computed tomography (coronary CT)	Coronary disease, biventricular function and volumes, congenital heart disease anatomy	Suspected CAD, adult congenital disease	High negative predictive value for CAD with reliable ejection fraction (EF) measurement	Radiation exposure, risk for contrast-induced nephropathy, difficult with rapid heart rate
Magnetic resonance (CMR)	**Gold standard for EF and volume assessment.** Etiology (ischemic versus nonischemic CMP) and characterization of nonischemic CMP, myocardial viability, biventricular volumes, congenital heart disease anatomy	Ischemic CMP: Viability Nonischemic CMP: Diagnosis Myocarditis, sarcoidosis, amyloidosis, arrhythmogenic RV cardiomyopathy, LV non-compaction, constrictive pericarditis	No radiation exposure, best noninvasive evaluation of myocardial tissue	Limited to magnet compatible metals, poor visualization in the presence of pacemakers or implantable cardiac defibrillators, difficult to evaluate in arrhythmias
Cardiopulmonary exercise testing (CPET)	Objective measurement of functional limitation in advanced HF	Advanced HFrEF, consideration for advanced HF therapies, determining pulmonary versus cardiac etiology of dyspnea	Noninvasive, objective measurement of functional status, monitoring of functional decline over time	Orthopedic issues that limit patient ability to ride bike or walk on treadmill, can be affected by beta blocker use and obesity
Nuclear imaging				
Multigated acquisition scan (MUGA)	LV function and volumes	Determining LVEF in patients with poor acoustic windows	Highly reproducible measurement of LVEF	Radiation exposure
Positive emission tomography (PET)	Myocardial perfusion and viability, LV function and volumes, sarcoidosis	Suspected CAD, "hibernating" myocardium, sarcoidosis	Allows for noninvasive diagnosis of sarcoidosis	Exposure to radiation, variable accuracy given specific diet prior to testing, may miss three vessel CAD
Single-photon emission computed tomography (SPECT)	Myocardial perfusion, amyloidosis	Suspected CAD, amyloidosis	Noninvasive diagnosis of amyloidosis	Exposure to radiation, may miss three vessel CAD, poor assessment of ejection fraction

Adapted from Heart Failure: A Companion to Braunwald's Heart Disease [10]. *CMP* cardiomyopathy

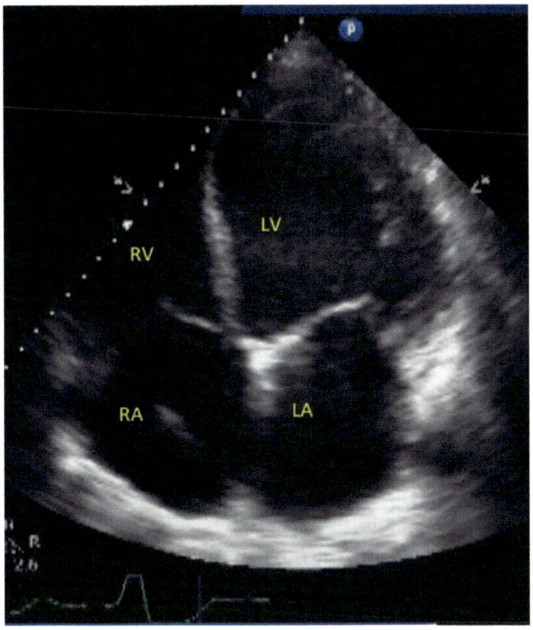

Fig. 20.4 Cardiac chamber enlargement on echo due to HFrEF

failure [11]. Transthoracic echocardiography (TTE) is readily available, noninvasive, and provides information regarding the type of ventricular dysfunction (systolic versus diastolic), left ventricular ejection fraction (LVEF), assessment of right ventricular function, dimensions of the cardiac chambers, valvular function, structural abnormalities, as well as the presence or absence of a pericardial effusion. This information is useful at the time of diagnosis as well as for monitoring treatment response and prognosis over time. Below are images that demonstrate HFrEF based on echocardiography (Fig. 20.4).

Cardiac Magnetic Resonance Imaging

Cardiac MRI (CMR) is considered to provide a higher-quality image than TTE and has become the noninvasive gold standard for determining LV volume, LVEF, and LV mass [10, 12, 13]. Compared with TTE, it is felt that there is less interrater variability. This imaging modality typically utilizes gadolinium contrast which assists in differentiating tissue characteristics to guide management [13]. The presence of late gadolinium enhancement is representative of scar in the myocardium, which is important for treatment considerations, including placement of implantable cardiac defibrillators. The pattern of enhancement gives information regarding HF etiology and can differentiate between dilated cardiomyopathy, ischemia, hypertrophic cardiomyopathy, myocarditis, as well as more rare cardiomyopathies [10, 12]. This method is superior in identification and characterization of left ventricular thrombi when compared with TTE [10]. In ischemic cardiomyopathy, CMR images can assist in evaluating viability with and without stress images [10].

Unfortunately, the presence of cardiac devices, including cardiac resynchronization therapy devices, can cause artifact, making the images difficult or impossible to interpret. This may render the test inadequate; therefore, alternative imaging methods are preferred in these patients. In addition, CMR is contraindicated in patients with metallic elements that are not MRI compatible. MRI can cause these metals to heat up during the test, can cause forces on magnetic metals, or cause severe image degradation.

Pathology/Description

Ischemic Heart Failure

Despite advances in revascularization and treatment of coronary artery disease, myocardial infarction (MI) is the most common cause of heart failure. Heart failure development at the time of MI, during index hospitalization, or following MI may manifest with different clinical attributes and outcomes. Myocardial compromise secondary to necrosis, stunning, or structural rupture causes rapid structural changes, myocyte edema, and progressive myocyte death within three hours of ischemic time. Even revascularization causes insult through an oxidative stress reaction and embolization of thrombotic debris [14]. The incidence of heart failure at the time of presentation has increased, possibly because of improvement in prehospital care. Conversely, heart failure development during hospitalization has fallen in the setting of improvements in revascularization. However, the incidence of heart failure with preserved ejection fraction after myocardial infarction has increased.

Heart failure with reduced ejection fraction (HFrEF) following hospitalization for MI is secondary to scar formation and cardiomyocyte death triggering activation of neurohormonal and sympathetic nervous system processes that initiate and perpetuate left ventricular remodeling. Infarction size and location impact the risk for development of HFrEF. Multivessel disease and anterior MI pose the highest risk [14]. Comorbidities including hypertension, atrial fibrillation, diabetes, and chronic kidney disease further compound the risk for HFrEF development post MI. Female gender and older age also increase the risk of heart failure.

Natriuretic peptide elevation, biphasic pattern of BNP elevation, and glomerular filtration rate are associated with HFrEF development post MI. Troponin elevation can correspond to infarct size on CMR, but association with HFrEF development is unclear [14].

Wall motion abnormalities on TTE predict mortality in HFrEF more accurately than LV ejection fraction alone. Right ventricular dysfunction seen on TTE also contributes to HFrEF development. Left ventricular enlargement post MI is more commonly seen in relation to transmural MI, larger infarct size, intramyocardial hemorrhage, microvascular obstruction, and advanced age and confers an increased risk of HFrEF hospitalization [14]. CMR is the gold standard imaging modality to define infarct size and scar formation.

Guideline-directed medical therapy including beta blockers, ACEIs/ARBs, and mineralocorticoid receptor antagonists has shown mortality benefit following MI. Early administration of statins within 24 h of MI is associated with a reduction in heart failure hospitalization and in-hospital mortality [15]. Patients should be risk stratified for wearable defibrillator prior to hospital discharge (see Chap. 13).

Nonischemic Cardiomyopathy (NICM)

Cardiomyopathy is a myocardial disorder in which heart muscle structure and/or function is abnormal in the absence of coronary artery disease, hypertension, valvular disease, or congenital heart defect [16]. Non Ischemic Cardiomyopathy categorization has evolved through advances in imaging and knowledge. The American Heart Association (AHA) defined cardiomyopathies as primary, or confined to the heart, or secondary, as part of generalized systemic disorders.

Three primary categories exist:

1. Genetic: channel disorders, arrhythmogenic right ventricular cardiomyopathy (ARVC), hypertrophic cardiomyopathy (HCM), left ventricular non-compaction (LVNC), and glycogen storage disorders
2. Acquired: inflammatory/myocarditis, stress induced (Takotsubo), peripartum, tachycardia-induced
3. Mixed acquired and genetic (dilated (DCM) and restrictive (RCM) cardiomyopathy) [17]

The European Society of Cardiology 2008 position paper on cardiomyopathy classification sought to group cardiomyopathies according to functional and morphological phenotypes which could be used to guide clinical practice [18]. Cardiomyopathies were divided into five categories which could have either familial or nonfamilial subclassifications: HCM, DCM, ARVC, RCM, and unclassified cardiomyopathies (Fig. 20.5).

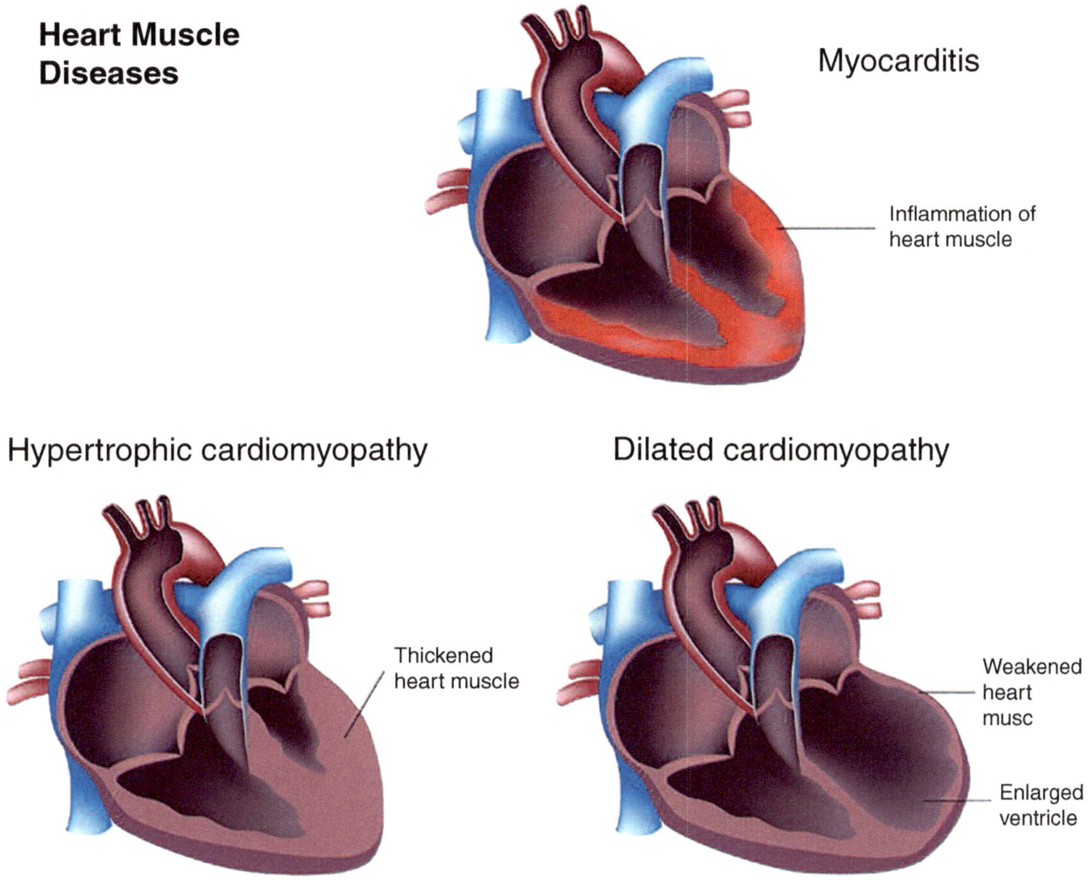

Fig. 20.5 ESC classification of myocarditis, dilated cardiomyopathy, and hypertrophic cardiomyopathy. (Used with permission, Shutterstock)

Hypertrophic Cardiomyopathy (HCM)

HCM is an autosomal dominant sarcomere protein mutation cardiomyopathy in which non-dilated left ventricular hypertrophy (LVH) is present in the absence of a systemic or valvular disease [16, 17]. There are greater than 30 genes known that can be evaluated for by genetic testing for prognostic education of family members. It is the most common cause of sudden cardiac death (SCD) in athletes younger than 35 years of age [19]. It can be associated with congenital syndromes and glycogen storage disease disorders or metabolic disorders such as Anderson-Fabry disease. Presenting symptoms characteristic of HCM include atypical chest pain (particularly associated with exertion or dehydration) and SCD. Evaluation of family history for unexplained SCD is imperative. A systolic murmur that increases with intensity during Valsalva maneuver may be present [20]. Electrocardiographic T wave inversions, generally in the lateral leads, are the most common electrocardiogram abnormality; ST segment depression, pathological Q waves, and ventricular arrhythmias have also been observed, particularly after exercise [19, 20]. On TTE, small ventricular chamber size with LVH is noted with an irregular localization of septal or apical hypertrophy (Fig. 20.6), which can result in left ventricular outflow tract obstruction (LVOTO) or mitral valve dysfunction (Fig. 20.7) (systolic anterior motion of the mitral valve against the intraventricular septum causing dynamic LVOTO) (Fig. 20.8). In cases of mild LVH in athletes, CMR can help differentiate pathologic and physiologic LVH [19]. Contrasted CMR studies differentiate the extent of myocardial fibrosis which is associated with increased risk of ventricular arrhythmias [21].

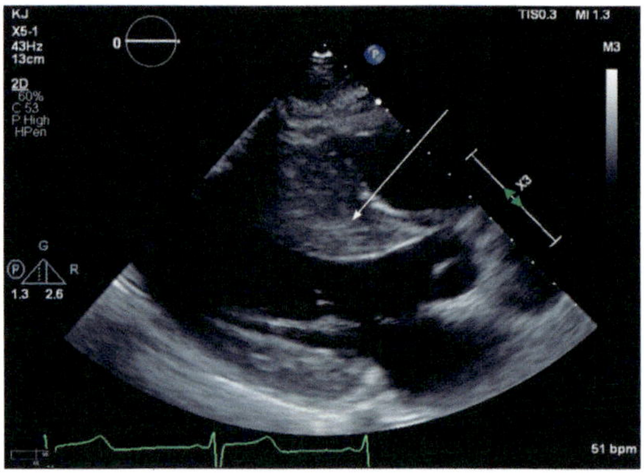

Fig. 20.6 Echocardiography of HCM. Arrow points to asymmetric septal hypertrophy of HCM

Beta blockers are the initial therapy for symptomatic HCM, with non-dihydropyridine calcium channel blockers used if beta blockers are not well tolerated. These medications decrease myocardial oxygen demand of the hypertrophied muscle, decrease the rate of fibrosis formation, and reduce the severity of the obstruction. They also can help prevent and treat potential arrhythmias. Reduction of symptoms and improvement of the murmur is the goal of therapy. If LVOTO is refractory to maximally tolerated medical therapy or hemodynamics are compromised, septal reduction procedures such as surgical myomectomy or alcohol ablation should be considered. Cardiac transplantation is reserved for end-stage systolic dysfunction [21]. Regardless of medical course, moderate or high intensity competitive sports are prohibited. Shared decision-making between the patient and physician is critical

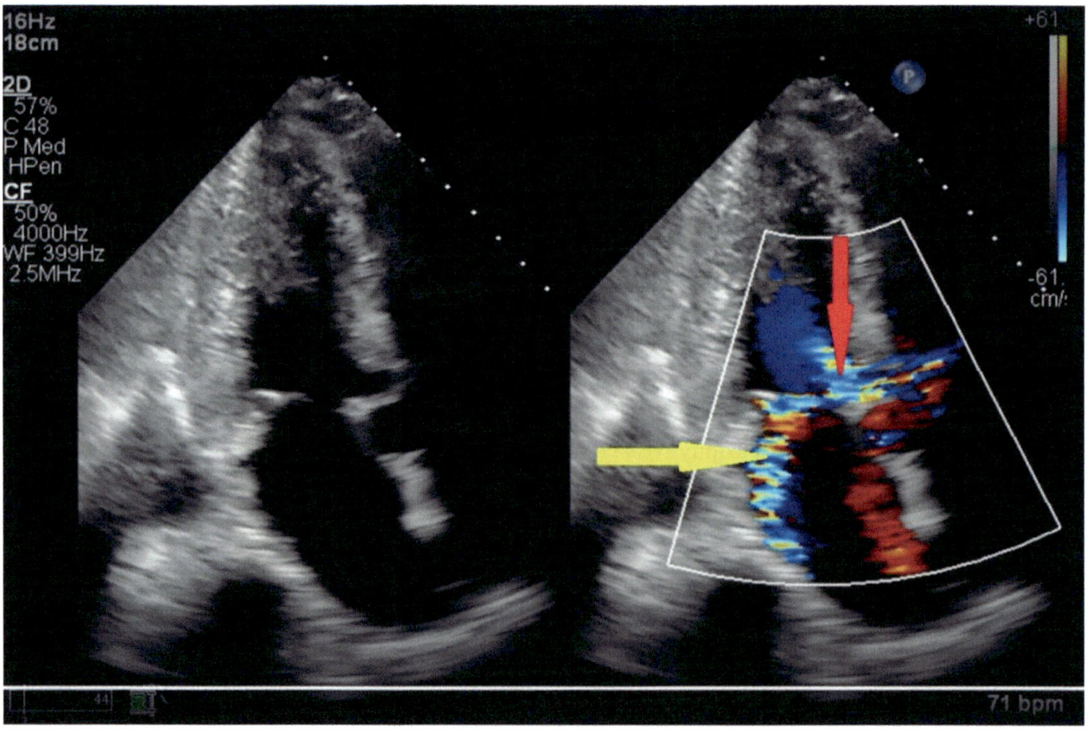

Fig. 20.7 Dynamic outflow tract gradient-induced MR. Red arrow shows turbulent flow below the aortic valve from a dynamic LVOT obstruction. The yellow arrow demonstrates eccentric MR caused by abnormal anterior leaflet function

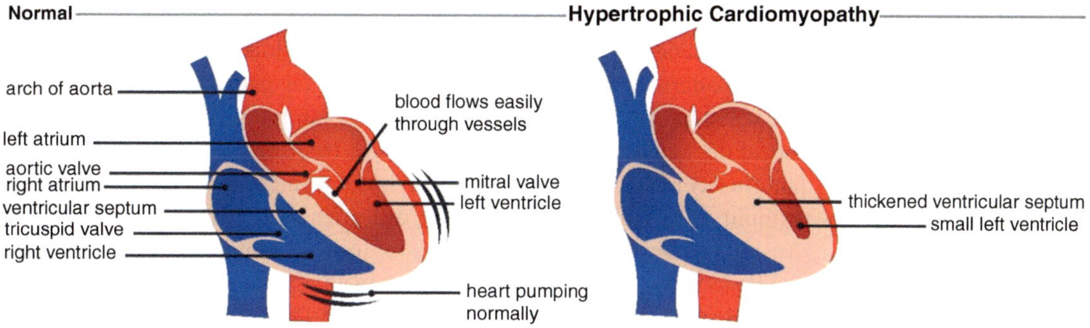

Fig. 20.8 Structural differences in normal and hypertrophic heart. (Used with permission, *Journal of Imaging*, *8*(4), 102. https://doi.org/10.3390/jimaging8040102)

regarding activity restriction. Patients should be risk stratified for SCD and evaluated for implantable cardioverter-defibrillator (ICD) placement. This evaluation considers percentage of scar burden seen on MRI (>12–15%), frequency of non-sustained ventricular tachycardia on ambulatory monitoring, the specific genetic defect, and family history of SCD.

Restrictive Cardiomyopathy (RCM)

Unlike the anatomic basis for HCM, restrictive cardiomyopathies are characterized by a functional pattern in which impaired myocardial compliance results in reduced ventricular filling and increased ventricular pressure, diastolic dysfunction, and preserved ejection fraction [16]. Heterogeneity of culprit pathologies makes defining RCM difficult. RCM can be idiopathic, familial, or secondary to systemic disorders. It can involve infiltration of the myocardium with abnormal proteins, glycogen, minerals, or other substances or demonstrate restrictive physiology without infiltration. Common causes of RCM in adults are amyloidosis, sarcoidosis, hemochromatosis, and sequelae of radiation therapy [22].

Diagnosis of RCM is based on clinical, laboratory, and imaging findings. The primary clinical presentation is heart failure, particularly right heart failure, with dyspnea on exertion and fatigue being most common. Signs of right heart failure, such as elevated jugular vein distention, peripheral edema, and ascites are commonly observed. A right-sided S3 or left ventricular S4 sound may be present, indicating rapid filling within a stiffened ventricle [23] (see Chap. 1). Diffuse reduced QRS voltage or prolonged PR interval can be seen on electrocardiogram, although their presence is unnecessary for diagnosis. Bi-atrial enlargement is often present with restrictive physiology and is reflected in widened more prominent P waves on EKG. Atrial or ventricular dysrhythmia may also be present [23]. Common TTE findings are bi-atrial enlargement and diastolic dysfunction. Further imaging is guided by disease suspicion. Laboratory finding of elevated B-type natriuretic peptide (BNP) marker is common.

Amyloidosis

Amyloidosis is an infiltrative RCM in which amyloid, an abnormal fibrillar protein made up of unstable precursor proteins, deposits in the heart (or other organs) leading to functional organ loss [24]. The most common types are immunoglobulin light chain amyloidosis (AL) or transthyretin amyloidosis, further divided into "wild type" (ATTR-wt) and mutant (ATTR-m) subtypes. Patients present with differing organ involvement patterns with disease course dependent on the involved organs. In general, cardiac involvement increases mortality [22]. History of bilateral carpal tunnel syndrome, peripheral neuropathy, or syncope raises suspicion of disease presence. Physical exam may be notable for macroglossia and periorbital purpura. Orthostatic hypotension or baseline hypotension is often present.

In addition to the restrictive pattern findings above, TTE imaging is also significant for LV, right ventricular, and intra-atrial thickening, possibly with a "speckled" pattern seen on ultrasound imaging due to amyloid fibrils in the myocardium. Pericardial effusion can be present. Longitudinal strain imaging shows more significant impairment in the left ventricular basal versus apical segments, producing a "cherry on top" pattern [23] (Fig. 20.9). On CMR, amyloid deposits produce a unique subendocardial late gadolinium enhancement in the ventricles and atria [22]. Nuclear imaging tracers (pyrophosphate scan) can detect ATTR with high sensitivity and specificity differentiate between AL and ATTR types.

High sensitivity cardiac troponin and BNP are useful markers of disease progression but not specific. After TTE, electrocardiogram, and clinical evaluation, laboratory markers of AL amyloidosis should be considered. These include serum free light chains, serum, and urine immunofixation electrophoresis. While endomyocardial biopsy (EMB) is the gold standard for cardiac amyloidosis, it is invasive and not without complication risk. A negative biopsy cannot rule out disease process because of patchy amyloid deposition pattern. If EMB is pursued, Congo red staining identifies amyloid presence. A less invasive biopsy test is fat pad biopsy, which has a higher yield in AL amyloid [22].

Heart failure treatment involves addressing conduction blocks and managing volume overload with diuretics or aldosterone antagonists [20]. AL amyloid is treated systemically with chemotherapeutic agents and potentially stem cell transplant. ATTR amyloid (both wild type and mutant) can be treated with early initiation of tafamidis, which binds to transthyretin and slows amyloid formation. Beta blockers should be used cautiously since the cardiac output in amyloid patients is often heart rate dependent.

Cardiac Sarcoidosis

Sarcoidosis is a multi-organ granulomatous disease in which noncaseating granulomatous inflammation can lead to fibrosis in affected organs. Cardiac sarcoidosis (CS) most commonly presents as conduction abnormalities (including ventricular abnormalities and atrioventricular (AV) node blocks) and heart failure symptoms. Patients may complain of palpitations, syncope, presyncope, or even have SCD [25]. In clinically

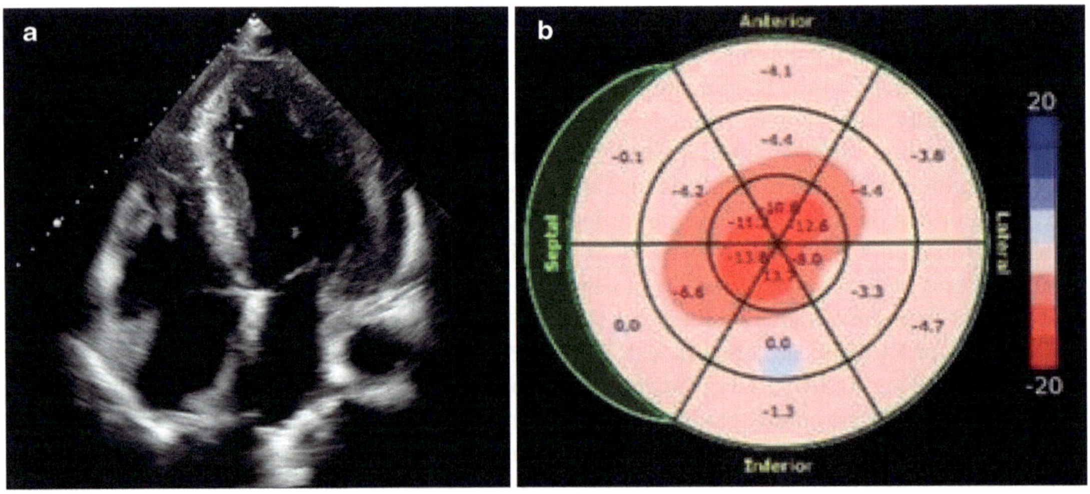

Fig. 20.9 (**a**) Typical echogenic findings of cardiac amyloidosis with LV and septal thickening and (**b**) strain imaging. (Used with permission, *Biomedicines*, *10* (4), 903. https://doi.org/10.3390/biomedicines10040903)

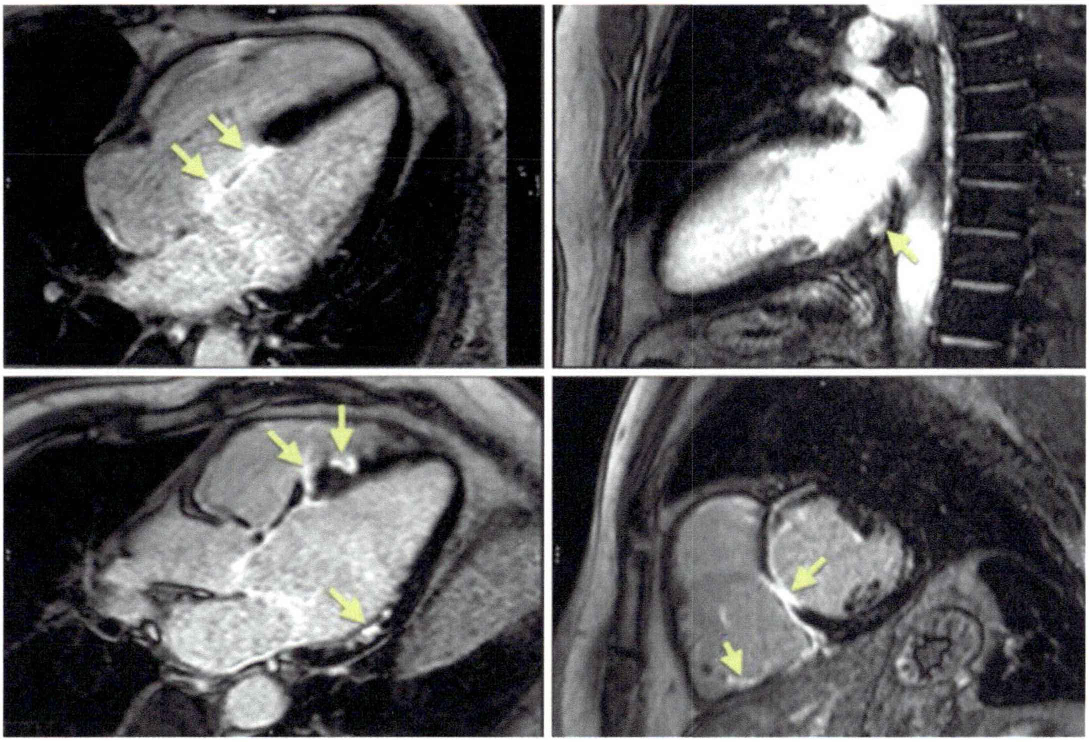

Fig. 20.10 Late gadolinium enhancement in a patient with pulmonary sarcoidosis and extensive cardiac involvement. There are several focal non-subendocardial based LGE areas with infiltration (arrows) in a variable pattern of transmural distribution

evident disease, electrocardiogram abnormalities in addition to conduction blocks can include QRS complex fragmentation, pathological Q waves, and ST changes. TTE findings are not pathognomonic but may show basal interventricular thinning [26] (Fig. 20.10). Endomyocardial biopsy is felt to be low yield secondary to the patchy nature of the CS.

CMR is the optimal study to determine the presence of cardiac sarcoidosis. Late gadolinium enhancement, seen in basal segments of the septal and lateral wall in a non-infarct pattern, commonly represents fibrosis although can also indicate inflammation. In active disease, inflammation can be seen with fluorodeoxyglucose positron emission tomography (FDG-PET), with FDG uptake patterns indicating active CS inflammation [25], guiding treatment. These two imaging modalities are complementary in the diagnosis and management of CS.

Corticosteroids are the treatment of choice in active disease, with methotrexate as a second-line agent. Antiarrhythmic medication and possible transcatheter ablation may be necessary in cases of ventricular arrhythmia. Patients should be risk-stratified for SCD and implantable cardiac defibrillator discussed. Cardiac resynchronization defibrillator therapy is indicated for high-grade heart blocks.

Dilated Cardiomyopathy (DCM)

Dilated cardiomyopathy is defined as an enlargement of the left ventricle with contractile dysfunction. It is a common form of heart muscle disease and the most frequent cause of heart transplantation [17]. Familial cases account for up to 35% of DCM [27]. Presentation can be accompanied by thromboembolic events and arrhythmias. Pathophysiologic changes of ventricular remodeling and ventricular dilation are discussed in detail above.

While heterogeneous in etiology (*see* Table 20.3), initial heart failure symptoms (lower extremity swelling, orthopnea, fatigue after mild exertion) are typically present and may be accompanied by nausea, abdominal fullness, early satiety, and anorexia. Physical exam can reveal peripheral and generalized edema, elevated jugular vein pulsation, tachycardia, inferolateral displacement of apical pulse, S3 gallop, delayed capillary refill, and crackles in lung field auscultation.

Electrocardiography is nonspecific but can include tachyarrhythmias and bundle branch blocks. Chest X-ray imaging will show cardiomegaly, often with pulmonary venous congestion. Diagnosis is confirmed with echocardiography which may include wall motion abnormalities, right ventricular involvement, and functional mitral regurgitation [27].

Table 20.3 Common causes of dilated cardiomyopathy

Genetic/familial	Syndromic disease/inborn errors of metabolism
Neuromuscular disorders	Drugs
Duchenne muscular dystrophy Becker muscular dystrophy	Antineoplastic agents Psychiatric drugs
Infection (myocarditis)	Endocrine disorders
Viral Bacterial Fungal Parasitic Protozoal Rickettsia	Hypothyroidism Hyperthyroidism Cushing's disease Addison's disease Diabetes mellitus Acromegaly
Autoimmune disorders	Nutritional deficiency
Giant cell myocarditis Dermatomyositis Systemic lupus erythematosus	Selenium Thiamine Zinc Copper
Peripartum	
Toxicity and overload	
Ethanol Cocaine Amphetamines Anabolic steroids	

Table adapted from Weintraub, R. et al. (2017). Dilated Cardiomyopathy. *The Lancet*, *390*(10092), 401–402 [27]

Myocarditis

Myocarditis is an inflammatory disease of the heart which can be a consequence of infection, toxic substance exposure, or immune system activation. It can exist along a continuum from acute to chronic and is characterized by those stages as well as etiology and severity. The initial presentation can range from prodromal symptoms to fulminant myocarditis with circulatory collapse [28, 29]. Myocarditis progresses from acute inflammation to interstitial edema to myocyte necrosis to fibrosis. Ventricular size may be preserved in the early phase, but damage to the myocardium over time leads to LV dilation [17]. Patients with acute myocarditis present with a variety of signs and symptoms as seen in Table 20.4 [17, 28].

Over a quarter of presentations represent fulminant myocarditis presenting with ventricular arrhythmias and cardiogenic shock (Table 20.5). More commonly, symptoms are accompanied by abnormal electrocardiogram with ST elevation, frequently in the inferior and lateral leads [28].

Endomyocardial biopsy is necessary in arrhythmogenic or fulminant presentation with cardiogenic shock [29]. EMB is recommended in the following settings:

- Other causes of HF have been excluded or when it may influence treatment (Table 20.5).
- For patients with unexplained fulminant HF (new-onset HF of less than 2 weeks duration associated with hemodynamic compromise).
- Unexplained new-onset HF of 2 weeks to 3 months duration associated with a dilated LV and new ventricular arrhythmias, Mobitz type II second-degree AV block, third-degree AV block, or failure to respond to usual care within 1–2 weeks.

CMR is recommended in clinically suspected acute myocarditis within 2–3 weeks from onset of symptoms to evaluate for myocardial inflammation. Hyperemia is suggested with early gadolinium enhancement, tissue edema seen with increased T2-weighted imaging, and necrosis/fibrosis seen with late gadolinium enhancement. These are the

Table 20.4 Presentation of myocarditis

Signs and symptoms	Clinical features	Differential cause
New or worsening heart failure/ cardiomegaly	Excessive fatigue or exercise intolerance Pulmonary edema, S3 gallop	All causes
Chest pain/ACS-like presentation	Ischemic features on EKG such ST depression or elevation/T-wave inversion	All causes
Acute pericarditis	Pleuritic chest pain. PR depression/diffuse ST elevation	
Cardiac arrhythmias or EKG changes	Sinus tachycardia. Atrial or ventricular arrhythmia; new bundle branch block, heart block	Giant cell myocarditis Cardiac sarcoidosis
Cardiogenic shock	May see rapid decompensation with or without associated multisystem organ failure	Giant cell myocarditis Cardiac sarcoidosis
Nonspecific myalgias or recent viral illness/URI		Viral myocarditis Eosinophilic myocarditis
Sudden cardiac death		All causes

Table 20.5 Clinical criteria for myocarditis

Clinical presentation: at least one or more of the following	Diagnostic criteria: at least one or more of the following	Ancillary supportive findings
Acute chest pain (pericarditis)	New EKG findings of any of the following: First-third degree AV block or BBB; ST/T wave changes; sinus arrest; VT; VF; asystole; Afib; IVCD; low voltage; SVT	Fever ≥38.0 °C at presentation or within prior 30 days +/− associated symptoms such as chills, myalgias, HA, N/V/D
New onset or worsening dyspnea at rest or exercise, and/or fatigue, with or without left and/or right HF signs	Elevated troponin	Prior clinical suspected or definite myocarditis
Palpitations or unexplained arrhythmia symptoms and/or syncope and/or sudden cardiac death	LV or RV dysfunction	Exposure to toxic agents
Unexplained cardiogenic shock	Tissue characterization by CMR	Extra-cardiac autoimmune disease

Adapted from Cooper, Leslie. Up to date. Clinical manifestations and diagnosis of myocarditis in adults. Jul 13, 2021

established cardinal findings to support myocarditis. PET imaging can be considered as alternative imaging if CMR is not possible or if other organs or a systemic process is suspected [28].

One specific consideration is giant cell myocarditis. This disease presents as a rapidly progressive necrotizing myocarditis with generally fulminant presentation and involving refractory ventricular arrhythmias. It should be diagnosed promptly with endomyocardial biopsy, and immunosuppressive therapy should be initiated as soon as possible. Even with early and aggressive therapy, mortality and need for cardiac transplantation are very high in this cohort of critically ill patients. There should be early consideration of extracorporeal membrane oxygenation and mechanical support.

Immune checkpoint inhibitor inflammation is another specific disease. Patients on this class of chemotherapeutic agents can have a rapidly progressive decompensation resulting in death. This type of myocarditis needs an early diagnosis, and high-dose corticosteroids are necessary to avoid cardiogenic shock and death. Fortunately, early intervention results in normalization of the ventricular function.

Treatment is directed at underlying cause and therapies aimed at clinical presentation. Inotropic and advanced mechanical support may be needed in severe disease. The immune modulation therapies are reserved for a small subset of acute myocarditis (Table 20.6).

Table 20.6 Myocarditis etiologies to consider early biopsy and immune modulating agents

Giant cell myocarditis-related shock and arrhythmias
Immune checkpoint inhibitor inflammation
Acute sarcoidosis shock and related arrhythmias

Peripartum Cardiomyopathy

Peripartum cardiomyopathy is left ventricular systolic dysfunction associated with pregnancy, most commonly presenting in the peripartum or postpartum period. Risk factors include increased age, African American race, hypertension and preeclampsia, multiple gestations, prior cardiomyopathy during pregnancy, and obesity [17, 20]. In addition to the hemodynamic stress of pregnancy, genetics, nutritional deficiencies, and autoimmune processes have been implicated [30]. Because symptoms of heart failure such as fatigue, dyspnea, or lower extremity edema can be mistaken for common pregnancy symptoms, diagnosis may be delayed. TTE imaging is nonspecific and notable for LV systolic dysfunction and dilation [20]. Peripartum cardiomyopathy is treated with guideline-directed medical therapy (GDMT) aimed at preventing further LV remodeling, with the caveat that angiotensin receptor blockers and angiotensin-converting enzyme inhibitors are contraindicated during pregnancy and diuretics should be used carefully to avoid hypotension and poor uterine perfusion. Planned delivery with a cardio-obstetrics team is important, as is risk stratification for SCD and careful contraceptive measures postdelivery [30] (see Part XI).

Arrhythmogenic Right Ventricular Cardiomyopathy (ARVC)

ARVC is a familial disease process of the heart muscle, predominantly impacting the right ventricle in which myocardial tissue is replaced with adipose and fibrous tissue. Subepicardial RV free wall segments impacted by mechanical stress during cardiac contraction are most frequently impacted [16, 31]. It is defined by right ventricular regional or global dysfunction, with or without LV dysfunction, with histological and/or electrocardiographic abnormalities present [16]. The disease process may have immunologic mediation since inflammatory infiltrate is frequently present. Presentation with arrhythmias (ventricular ectopy or ventricular tachycardia with left bundle branch morphology), exercise-induced syncope, or sudden cardiac death is common [17, 31]. The electrocardiogram commonly exhibits T-wave inversions in V1-V3, and progression beyond V3 is associated with advanced disease [31]. Additionally, a right bundle branch block can be seen in severe structural disease. Likewise, the presence of an epsilon wave, a deflection at the end of the QRS complex and before the T wave, connotes significant disease [31] (Fig. 20.11). Other conduction criteria and family history are important considerations in diagnosis and therapy options. TTE findings include right ventricular hypertrophy, dilation of right ventricular outflow tract and ventricle, and most frequently right ventricular global or segmental abnormalities [31]. CMR is the image modality of choice to show functional and morphological abnormalities associated with ARVC

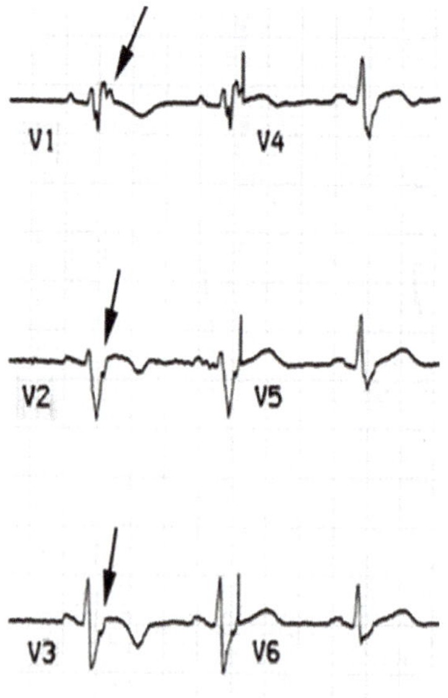

Fig. 20.11 Post excitation epsilon waves in right precordial leads. (Used with permission, *Orphanet Journal of Rare Diseases*, 2 (1), 45. https://doi.org/10.1186/1750-1172-2-45)

including intramyocardial fat infiltration and RV dilation.

Treatment involves risk stratification for ICD consideration, as well as treatment with antiarrhythmic medications, beta blockers, and standard heart failure therapies. Anticoagulation may be warranted. Finally, ARVC diagnosis precludes patients from participating in competitive or resistance sports [31].

Unclassified

Takotsubo Cardiomyopathy

Stress cardiomyopathy or "broken heart syndrome" is defined by acute decline in LVEF in response to profound stress, primarily affecting older/postmenopausal women. Presentation of acute chest pain is common. Diffuse T-wave inversions, possibly with ST elevations, are seen on electrocardiogram, and cardiac biomarkers may be mildly elevated. The echocardiography findings of regional wall motion abnormalities impacting the LV apex ("apical ballooning") in the absence of obstructive coronary disease are pathognomonic for Takotsubo cardiomyopathy [16]. This apical ballooning is the most common form (85%), but isolated mid-wall and basal wall motion abnormalities may occur (15%). With supportive medical management, LV function is rapidly reversible in days to weeks [17]. A previous stress-induced cardiomyopathy increases the risk of subsequent stress-induced recurrence.

Management

Guideline-Directed Medical Therapy (GDMT)

Based on the guidelines, patients with HFrEF should be maintained on beta blockers, RAAS inhibition (angiotensin-converting enzyme inhibitors (ACEi)), angiotensin receptor blockers (ARB), or angiotensin-neprilysin inhibitors (ARNi), and a mineralocorticoid receptor antagonist (MRA) [32] (Fig. 20.11). However, since publication of the 2017 American Heart Association and American College of Cardiology comprehensive heart failure guidelines, ongoing clinical trial data has indicated reduction of mortality and benefit with four specific groups of medications which are now known as the "four pillars of heart failure therapy" [33] (Fig. 20.12). The four pillars of heart failure therapy include a beta blocker, ARNI, MRA, and sodium-glucose cotransporter 2 inhibition (SGLT2i). Isosorbide dinitrate and hydralazine have mortality benefit but are often second-line agents. There are additional medical therapies that improve morbidity but not mortality, including loop and thiazide diuretics, ivabradine, digoxin, and vericiguat. The focus of this section will be on the four pillars of heart failure therapies and diuretics for

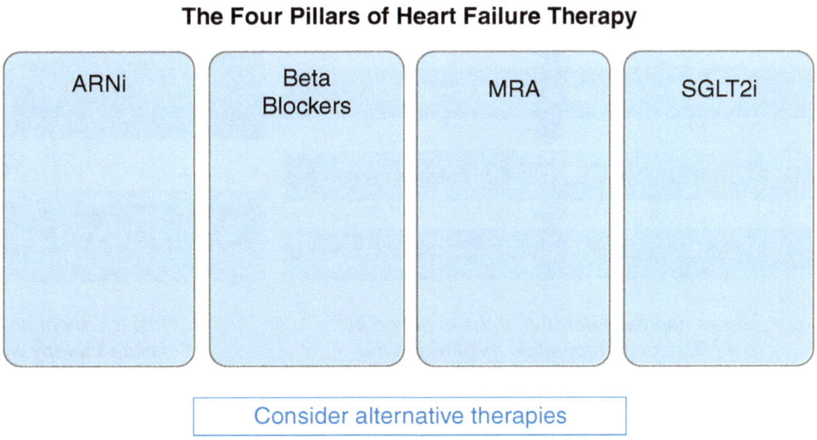

Fig. 20.12 Adapted from Sam Straw et al. Open Heart 2021;8:e001585

relief of congestion. Target doses of these medications and data-driven agents within each category are summarized in Table 20.7. The mortality benefit of these agents has been shown to be dose dependent. There is a newer concept in management of HFrEF of the "need for speed" with regard to rapid initiation and up-titration of the four pillars of heart failure therapy to further reduce morbidity and mortality for patients with HFrEF [34] (Fig. 20.13). A recommended rapid sequencing for initiation of GDMT is shown in the figure below [35].

Table 20.7 Target doses of the four pillars of heart failure guideline-directed medical therapies

	Starting dose	Target dose
Beta blockers		
Bisoprolol	1.25 mg once daily	10 mg once daily
Carvedilol	3.125 mg twice daily	25 mg twice daily for weight <85 kg and 50 mg twice daily for weight ≥85 kg
Metoprolol succinate	12.5–25 mg daily	200 mg daily
ARNI		
Sacubitril/valsartan	24/26 mg twice daily	97/103 mg twice daily
ACEis		
Captopril	6.25 mg three times daily	50 mg three times daily
Enalapril	2.5 mg twice daily	10–20 mg twice daily
Lisinopril	2.5 mg daily	40 mg daily
Ramipril	1.25 mg daily	10 mg daily
ARBs		
Candesartan	4 mg daily	32 mg daily
Losartan	25 mg daily	150 mg daily
Valsartan	40 mg twice daily	160 mg twice daily
Mineralocorticoid receptor antagonists		
Eplerenone	25 mg daily	50 mg daily
Spironolactone	25 mg daily	50 mg daily
SGLT2i		
Dapagliflozin	10 mg daily	10 mg daily
Empagliflozin	10 mg daily	10 mg daily

Adapted from: https://www.jacc.org/doi/pdf/10.1016/j.jacc.2020.11.022

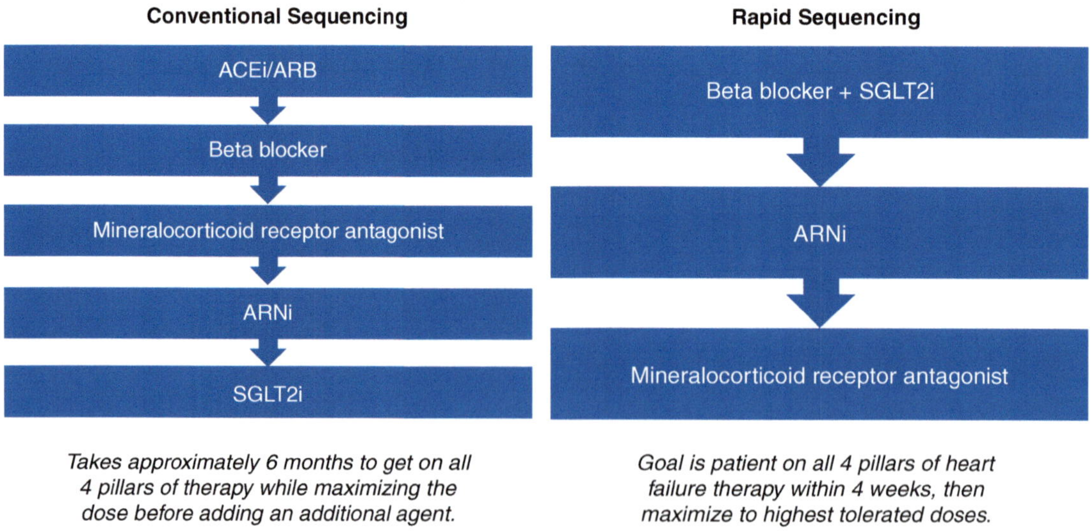

Fig. 20.13 Adapted from Packer and McMurray (2021), European Journal of Heart Failure [35]

Beta Blockers

Beta blockers are utilized to decrease sympathetic stimulation resulting in improved prognosis in patients with HF. These medications are considered the cornerstone of HFrEF therapy. While many beta blockers exist, only bisoprolol, metoprolol succinate, and carvedilol have shown a mortality benefit in patients with HFrEF. Initiation of beta blockade should be done with caution as they may worsen volume overload and precipitate cardiogenic shock if initiated or up-titrated during acute decompensation. Withdrawal or dose reduction of beta blockade in patients who are acutely decompensated and in those at baseline has been shown to increase mortality. Therefore, these should be continued, if possible, on admission. In a stable, compensated patient, the goal is to increase to the target dose as noted in Table 20.7. A good rule of thumb with beta blockers in heart failure is to "start low and titrate slow." Common side effects of beta blockers include fatigue, exercise intolerance, erectile dysfunction, and bradycardia.

RAAS Inhibition

ACE Inhibitors (ACEIs)

Angiotensin-converting enzyme inhibitors (ACEIs) were the initial drug utilized in early trials showing a reduction in mortality for patients with heart failure. These medications inhibit RAAS by inhibiting angiotensin-converting enzymes. While on these medications, renal function and potassium levels should be monitored as these can cause acute kidney injury and hyperkalemia. Because of this, ACEIs should not be started in patients with rapidly changing renal function. Patients on these medications can have a side effect of cough which can be mitigated by changing to an ARB or ARNI. Rare, more serious side effects include severe allergic reactions including anaphylaxis and angioedema. ACEIs and ARBs should not be administered as part of the same HfrEF regimen.

Angiotension Receptor Blockers: ARBs

ARBs are an alternative agent to ACEIs with similar mortality benefits in patients with heart failure with fewer adverse effects. These medications block the angiotensin receptor as the name indicates. These medications do not cause cough and are generally better tolerated than ACEIs. Patients who have had angioedema with ACEIs can be carefully challenged with an ARB as cross reactivity is rare. Monitoring for ARBs is the same as with ACEIs.

Angiotensin Receptor-Neprilysin Inhibitor: ARNIs

ARNIs are superior regarding reduction in mortality and HF hospitalizations when compared with ACEIs or ARBs making these medications one of the four pillars of heart failure therapy and the drug of choice for RAAS inhibition. RAAS inhibition is achieved by blocking both angiotensin and neprilysin. Neprilysin is an enzyme that breaks down endogenous brain natriuretic peptide (BNP). BNP causes a natriuresis and diuresis via the kidney. ARNIs inhibit the breakdown of BNP and improve sodium and fluid excretion. These medications are indicated for patients with chronic symptomatic HFrEF with any ejection fraction and NYHA Class II-IV symptoms. These medications are more blood pressure lowering than ACEIs or ARBs thus should be used with caution in patients with hypotension. The use of ARNIs causes a transient elevation in BNP levels due to neprilysin inhibition but not in NT-pro BNP levels. ARNIs are contraindicated in patients who have had angioedema to ACEIs. In addition, due to cross-reactivity, a 36-h washout period is required when transitioning from ACEI to ARNI but not when transitioning from ARB to ARNI.

Mineralocorticoid Receptor Antagonists

These medications work by blocking the RAAS through inhibition of aldosterone production. MRAs are indicated in patients with symptomatic heart failure with NYHA Class II-IV symptoms. The two agents include spironolactone and eplerenone, both of which have a proven mortality benefit in patients with HFrEF. Due to RAAS inhibition, renal function must be monitored. These agents are potassium-sparing diuretics, and while their diuretic effect is weak, caution should be used in patients with hyperkalemia or baseline potassium levels of >5.0 mmol/L. Gynecomastia is a common side effect of spironolactone, and patients can be changed to eplerenone. Newer literature indicates this agent reduces blood pressure in patients who are hypertensive but does not have a significant effect on blood pressure in patients who are normotensive at baseline.

Sodium-Glucose Cotransporter 2 Inhibition (SGLT2i)

SGLT2i works by blocking the sodium-glucose cotransporter in the kidney, but the exact mechanism of benefit in patients with HFrEF is unknown [33]. However, SGLT2 inhibition leads to osmotic diuresis and natriuresis resulting in decreased arterial pressure and stiffness [36]. This, in turn, reduces preload and afterload which results in reduction of adverse cardiac remodeling. These medications have been shown to reduce all-cause mortality in patients with HFrEF which is likely driven by the statistically significant reduction in heart failure hospitalizations in patients with and without diabetes. The medications which have been studied for use in HFrEF include dapagliflozin and empagliflozin. Common adverse effects include dehydration, renal dysfunction, and yeast infections. When used in conjunction with loop diuretics, the dose of loop diuretics should be decreased in anticipation of natriuresis with initiation of SGLT2i. However, the exact dose adjustment of loop diuretics has not yet been investigated. Like ACEIs, ARBs, and ARNIs, SGLT2is have been shown to be renal protective in patients with chronic kidney disease.

Diuretics

Loop diuretics are the cornerstone of management of congestion in patients with HF. That said, these medications have never shown a mortality benefit for patients with heart failure and thus are not considered one of the pillars of heart failure therapy. The ideal dose is the lowest dose the patient needs to achieve and maintain euvolemia. If this is not possible with loop diuretics alone, the use of thiazide diuretics for augmentation can be considered. Diuretics are best given in the morning due to frequent urination. Twice daily dosing can be considered with a second dose midday to prevent nocturia if once daily dosing is insufficient. Table 20.8 shows loop and thiazide diuretic agents and dosing options.

Furosemide is the initial loop diuretic of choice due to cost but overall has variable oral bioavailability. In the setting of diuretic resistance, or lack of diuresis with optimal dosing, transitioning to an alternative loop diuretic with better oral bioavailability such as torsemide or bumetanide should be considered.

When considering equivalent diuretic dosages, 40 mg of oral furosemide = 20 mg of oral torsemide = 1 mg of oral bumetanide = 20 mg of IV furosemide.

Device Therapy

Implantable Cardiac Defibrillators (ICDs)

About 50% of patients with HFrEF have ventricular arrhythmias resulting in sudden cardiac

Table 20.8 Diuretic dose ranges

Diuretics	Dose range
Loop diuretics	
Furosemide	20–240 mg
Bumetanide	0.5–5 mg
Torsemide	20–200 mg
Thiazide diuretics	
Metolazone	2.5–10 mg
Hydrochlorothiazide	25–100 mg

death [37]. Therefore, ICDs are indicated in NYHA II/III patients with an LV ejection fraction of ≤35% on optimal GDMT for 3 months for prevention of sudden cardiac death [36]. Interestingly, patients who have a higher New York Heart Association (NYHA) functional class have a higher risk for sudden cardiac death. While GDMT reduces the risk of sudden cardiac death, this is not eliminated. Antiarrhythmic drug therapies increase the sudden death risk. ICDs are not indicated in patients who have a life expectancy of less than 12 months. It is important to note that ICDs do not provide any direct therapeutic benefit for HFrEF but instead act solely to prevent sudden cardiac death from ventricular arrhythmias.

Cardiac Resynchronization Therapy (CRT)

CRT is indicated in patients who have a left bundle branch block with a QRS of ≥150 ms (Fig. 20.14), NYHA class II-IV symptoms, with an LV ejection fraction of ≤35% on maximally tolerated GDMT for 3–6 months. There are two forms of CRT—one where this device acts solely as a biventricular pacemaker (CRT-P) and the other where a defibrillator lead is added to the right ventricle (CRT-D). Unlike ICDs, CRT has been shown to reduce mortality in patients with HFrEF by reducing heart failure events and improving LVEF [38]. CRT-D is a three-lead device with a lead in the right atrium, defibrillator coil in the right ventricle, and a left ventricular lead which is placed in the coronary sinus. An alternative indication for CRT-D is high right ventricular pacing burden in patients with dual-chamber ICDs. The EKG of a standard RV apical pacemaker is a LBBB morphology in lead V1. CRT will have a more RBBB morphology in lead V1. The higher the biventricular pacing percentage, the more likely the patient is to have effective CRT. Higher dose of beta blockers may be used to optimize pacing as well.

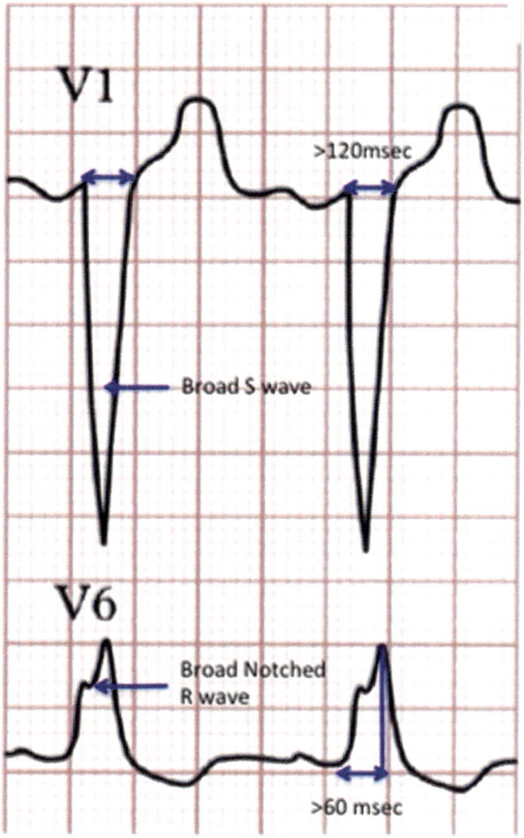

Fig. 20.14 Findings of left bundle branch block morphology on EKG. (Used with permission, *The American Journal of Cardiology*, *111* (2), 291–300 https://doi.org/10.1016/j.amjcard.2012.09.029)

Advanced Heart Failure Therapies

If patients do not have improvement in LVEF and functional status with GDMT or addition of CRT when indicated, one should consider referral to an advanced heart failure specialist for consideration of advanced heart failure therapies. The high-risk features which indicate appropriateness of referral are summarized in the acronym I-NEED-HELP [33].

I: IV inotropes
N: NYHA IIIB/IV or persistently elevated natriuretic peptides
E: End-organ dysfunction
E: Ejection fraction ≤35
D: Defibrillator shocks
H: Hospitalizations >1
E: Edema despite escalating diuretics
L: Low blood pressure, high heart rate
P: Prognostic medication: progressive intolerance or down-titration of GDMT

Advanced heart failure therapies include left ventricular assist devices and cardiac transplantation. Cardiac transplantation is considered for patients with advanced heart failure who have an acceptable BMI, are compliant with medications and follow-up, do not have substance abuse including current tobacco use, and are 70 years of age or younger.

Management of Comorbidities

The 2017 American College of Cardiology (ACC) consensus statement identified cardiovascular and non-cardiovascular heart failure comorbidities: coronary artery disease, atrial dysrhythmias, mitral regurgitation, aortic stenosis, hypertension, dyslipidemia, peripheral vascular disease, cerebrovascular disease, obesity, chronic lung disease, chronic renal disease, anemia, iron deficiency, thyroid disorders, and sleep-disordered breathing [32].

Mitral Regurgitation

Recent trials (Coapt) in patients after optimization of GDMT and at least moderate residual secondary mitral regurgitation have shown mortality benefit with intervention on the mitral valve. Transcatheter edge-to-edge mitral repair (TEER) has been shown to confer additional mortality benefit. Consideration of intervention upon the valve should be considered (see Chap. 17).

Hypertension

While no clinical trials evaluating optimal blood pressure lowering agents and blood pressure reduction in the setting of HFrEF and hypertension are available, ACC guidelines recommend management of HFrEF with concurrent hypertension with GDMT to a goal threshold associated with improved clinical outcomes in other high-risk populations: less than 130/80 mmHg. In clinical practice, the goal is to reduce patients' blood pressure in HFrEF to as low as a patient will tolerate without symptoms of orthostasis. In addition to GDMT, diuretics can be used in patients with volume overload to control blood pressure. Avoidance of non-dihydropyridine calcium channel blockers and alpha-adrenergic blockers are recommended [39].

Sleep-Disordered Breathing (SDB)

There is a strong association of both central sleep apnea and obstructive sleep apnea with worse heart failure outcomes. Sleep-disordered breathing leads to increased inflammation, oxidative stress-induced endothelial dysfunction, increased sympathetic nervous system activation, and increased intrathoracic pressure fluctuations. This in turn causes an increase in LV afterload and possibly contributes to atrial fibrillation which is strongly associated with SDB [40]. Addressing and treating SDB through oxygen therapy or positive airway pressure therapy are imperative in heart failure management.

Iron Deficiency

Iron deficiency, even in the absence of anemia, is prevalent among heart failure patients and associated with decreased functional capacity and survival [41]. The ACC guidelines recommend that patients with iron deficiency defined as ferritin <100 ng/L or ferritin 100–300 ng/L if transferrin saturation is less than 20% be considered for intravenous iron therapy to improve functional status [41].

Clinical Pearls

- Never forget, *there is no substitute for a good history and physical exam*. Heart failure is a *clinical diagnosis* which is confirmed with imaging and laboratory testing.
- Physical exam: Jugular venous pressure assessment is an important skill learned over time.
- Ischemic evaluation: All patients with a new diagnosis of heart failure or a new decline in LV ejection fraction need an ischemic evaluation to rule out a reversible cause or a contributing factor to the reduction in ejection fraction.
- GDMT: Do not repeat imaging until your patient is on maximally tolerated GDMT to determine ICD candidacy or advanced therapy. Maximal GDMT means the highest doses

of medications (the four pillars plus adjunct medical therapies) with a goal heart rate of 60–70 beats per minute and a blood pressure as low as they can tolerate without symptoms of orthostasis.
- Tachycardia: Make sure sinus tachycardia is not a compensatory mechanism in a patient with impending cardiogenic shock. **Slowing the heart rate may precipitate shock and may be fatal.**
- Diuretics: If your patient on oral furosemide is no longer responding, consider a transition to torsemide, especially in cases where abdominal edema is present.
- Remember diuretic conversion: 40 mg of oral furosemide = 20 mg of oral torsemide = 1 mg of oral bumetanide = 20 mg of IV furosemide.
- If inadequate diuresis or significant worsening of end-organ function occurs, patients may have low cardiac output and require inotropic or advanced mechanical support.
- Iron deficiency: Remember, even if a patient with heart failure is not anemic but iron deficient, they benefit from iron supplementation.

References

1. Ponikowski P, et al. 2016 ESC guidelines for the diagnosis and treatment of acute and chronic heart failure: the task force for the diagnosis and treatment of acute and chronic heart failure of the European Society of Cardiology (ESC) developed with the special contribution of the Heart Failure Association (HFA) of the ESC. Eur Heart J. 2016;37:2129–200. https://doi.org/10.1093/eurheartj/ehw128.
2. Gibson G, Blumer V, Mentz RJ, Lala A. Universal definition and classification of heart failure: a step in the right direction from failure to function. 2020. https://www.acc.org/latest-in-cardiology/articles/2021/07/12/12/31/universal-definition-and-classification-of-heart-failure.
3. Bozkurt B, et al. Universal definition and classification of heart failure: a report of the Heart Failure Society of America, Heart Failure Association of the European Society of Cardiology, Japanese Heart Failure Society and Writing Committee of the Universal Definition of Heart Failure. J Card Fail. 2021;S1071-9164(21):00050-6. https://doi.org/10.1016/j.cardfail.2021.01.022.
4. Schwinger RHG. Pathophysiology of heart failure. Cardiovasc Diagn Ther. 2021;11(1):263–76. https://doi.org/10.21037/cdt-20-302.
5. Briasoulis A, Androulakis E, Christophides T, et al. The role of inflammation and cell death in the pathogenesis, progression and treatment of heart failure. Heart Fail Rev. 2016;21:169–76. https://doi.org/10.1007/s10741-016-9533-z.
6. Moss RL, Fitzsimons DP. Frank-Starling relationship. Circ Res. 2002;90(1):11–3. https://doi.org/10.1161/res.90.1.11.
7. Nohria A, Tsang SW, Fang JC, Lewis EF, Jarcho JA, Mudge GH, Stevenson LW. Clinical assessment identifies hemodynamic profiles that predict outcomes in patients admitted with heart failure. J Am Coll Cardiol. 2003;41(10):1797–804. https://doi.org/10.1016/s0735-1097(03)00309-7.
8. Albakri A. Low-output heart failure: a review of clinical status and meta-analysis of diagnosis and clinical management methods. Clin Med Invest. 2019;4 https://doi.org/10.15761/CMI.1000179.
9. Thibodeau JT, Drazner MH. The role of the clinical examination in patients with heart failure. JACC Heart Fail. 2018;6(7):543–51. https://doi.org/10.1016/j.jchf.2018.04.005.
10. Mann DL, Zipes DP, Libby P, Bonow RO, Braunwald E. Braunwald's heart disease: a textbook of cardiovascular medicine. 10th ed. Philadelphia, PA: Elsevier/Saunders; 2015.
11. Mieres JH, et al. Noninvasive imaging. Am Fam Physician. 2007;75(8):1219–28.
12. Peterzan MA, Rider OJ, Anderson LJ. The role of cardiovascular magnetic resonance imaging in heart failure. Card Fail Rev. 2016;2(2):115–22. https://doi.org/10.15420/cfr.2016.2.2.115.
13. Leiner T, et al. SCMR position paper (2020) on clinical indications for cardiovascular magnetic resonance. J Cardiovasc Magn Reson. 2020;22(1):76. https://doi.org/10.1186/s12968-020-00682-4.
14. Jenča D, et al. Heart failure after myocardial infarction: incidence and predictors. ESC Heart Fail. 2021;8(1):222–37. https://doi.org/10.1002/ehf2.13144.
15. Elgendy IY, Mahtta D, Pepine CJ. Medical therapy for heart failure caused by ischemic heart disease. Circ Res. 2019;124(11):1520–35. https://doi.org/10.1161/circresaha.118.313568.
16. Elliott P, et al. Classification of the cardiomyopathies: a position statement from the European Society of Cardiology working group on myocardial and pericardial diseases. Eur Heart J. 2007;29(2):270–6. https://doi.org/10.1093/eurheartj/ehm342.
17. Maron BJ, et al. Contemporary definitions and classification of the cardiomyopathies. Circulation. 2006;113(14):1807–16. https://doi.org/10.1161/circulationaha.106.174287.
18. McKenna WJ, Maron BJ, Thiene G. Classification, epidemiology, and global burden of cardiomyopathies. Circ Res. 2017;121(7):722–30. https://doi.org/10.1161/CIRCRESAHA.117.309711.

19. Malhotra A, Sharma S. Hypertrophic cardiomyopathy in athletes. Eur Cardiol Rev. 2017;12(2):80. https://doi.org/10.15420/ecr.2017:12:1.
20. Brieler J, Breeden MA, Tucker J. Cardiomyopathy: an overview. Am Fam Physician. 2017;96(10):640–6.
21. Ommen SR, et al. 2020 AHA/ACC guideline for the diagnosis and treatment of patients with hypertrophic cardiomyopathy. Circulation. 2020;142(25):e558. https://doi.org/10.1161/cir.0000000000000937.
22. Madan N, Kalra D. Clinical evaluation of infiltrative cardiomyopathies resulting in heart failure with preserved ejection fraction. Rev Cardiovasc Med. 2020;21(2):181–90. https://doi.org/10.31083/j.rcm.2020.02.65.
23. Geske JB, Anavekar NS, Nishimura RA, Oh JK, Gersh BJ. Differentiation of constriction and restriction. J Am Coll Cardiol. 2016;68(21):2329–47. https://doi.org/10.1016/j.jacc.2016.08.050.
24. Muchtar E, Blauwet LA, Gertz MA. Restrictive cardiomyopathy. Circ Res. 2017;121(7):819–37. https://doi.org/10.1161/circresaha.117.310982.
25. Markatis E, Afthinos A, Antonakis E, Papanikolaou IC. Cardiac sarcoidosis: diagnosis and management. Rev Cardiovasc Med. 2020;21(3):321–38. https://doi.org/10.31083/j.rcm.2020.03.102.
26. Sun BJ, et al. Prevalence of echocardiographic features suggesting cardiac sarcoidosis in patients with pacemaker or implantable cardiac defibrillator. Korean Circ J. 2011;41(6):313. https://doi.org/10.4070/kcj.2011.41.6.313.
27. Weintraub RG, Semsarian C, Macdonald P. Dilated cardiomyopathy. Lancet. 2017;390(10092):400–14. https://doi.org/10.1016/s0140-6736(16)31713-5.
28. Ammirati E, et al. Management of acute myocarditis and chronic inflammatory cardiomyopathy. Circ Heart Fail. 2020;13(11):e007405. https://doi.org/10.1161/circheartfailure.120.007405.
29. Kociol RD, et al. Recognition and initial management of fulminant myocarditis. Circulation. 2020;141(6):e69. https://doi.org/10.1161/cir.0000000000000745.
30. Davis MB, Arany Z, McNamara DM, Goland S, Elkayam U. Peripartum cardiomyopathy: JACC state-of-the-art review. J Am Coll Cardiol. 2020;75(2):207–21. https://doi.org/10.1016/j.jacc.2019.11.014.
31. Elias Neto J, Tonet J, Frank R, Fontaine G. Arrhythmogenic right ventricular cardiomyopathy/dysplasia (ARVC/D)—what we have learned after 40 years of the diagnosis of this clinical entity. Arq Bras Cardiol. 2018;112:91. https://doi.org/10.5935/abc.20180266.
32. Yancy CW, et al. 2017 ACC/AHA/HFSA focused update of the 2013 ACCF/AHA guideline for the management of heart failure. J Am Coll Cardiol. 2017;70(6):776–803. https://doi.org/10.1016/j.jacc.2017.04.025.
33. Maddox TM, et al. 2021 Update to the 2017 ACC expert consensus decision pathway for optimization of heart failure treatment: answers to 10 pivotal issues about heart failure with reduced ejection fraction. J Am Coll Cardiol. 2021;77(6):772–810. https://doi.org/10.1016/j.jacc.2020.11.022.
34. Greene SJ, Butler J, Fonarow GC. Simultaneous or rapid sequence initiation of quadruple medical therapy for heart failure—optimizing therapy with the need for speed. JAMA Cardiol. 2021;6(7):743–4. https://doi.org/10.1001/jamacardio.2021.0496.
35. Packer M, Mcmurray JJV. Rapid evidence-based sequencing of foundational drugs for heart failure and a reduced ejection fraction. Eur J Heart Fail. 2021;23(6):882–94. https://doi.org/10.1002/ejhf.2149.
36. Zelniker TA, Braunwald E. Mechanisms of cardiorenal effects of sodium-glucose cotransporter 2 inhibitors: JACC state-of-the-art review. J Am Coll Cardiol. 2020;75:422–34.
37. Al-Khatib SM, et al. 2017 AHA/ACC/HRS guideline for management of patients with ventricular arrhythmias and the prevention of sudden cardiac death: executive summary: a report of the American College of Cardiology/American Heart Association task force on clinical practice guidelines and the Heart Rhythm Society. Circulation. 2018;138(13):e210–71. https://doi.org/10.1161/CIR.0000000000000548.
38. Moss AJ, et al. Cardiac-resynchronization therapy for the prevention of heart-failure events. N Engl J Med. 2009;361(14):1329–38. https://doi.org/10.1056/nejmoa0906431.
39. Whelton PK, et al. 2017 ACC/AHA/AAPA/ABC/ACPM/AGS/APhA/ASH/ASPC/NMA/PCNA guideline for the prevention, detection, evaluation, and management of high blood pressure in adults. J Am Coll Cardiol. 2018;71(19):e127–248. https://doi.org/10.1016/j.jacc.2017.11.006.
40. Cowie MR, Gallagher AM. Sleep disordered breathing and heart failure. JACC Heart Fail. 2017;5(10):715–23. https://doi.org/10.1016/j.jchf.2017.06.016.
41. Von Haehling S, Ebner N, Evertz R, Ponikowski P, Anker SD. Iron deficiency in heart failure. JACC Heart Fail. 2019;7(1):36–46. https://doi.org/10.1016/j.jchf.2018.07.015.

Additional References

Gudigar A, Raghavendra U, Samanth J, Dharmik C, Gangavarapu MR, Nayak K, Ciaccio EJ, Tan R-S, Molinari F, Acharya UR. Novel hypertrophic cardiomyopathy diagnosis index using deep features and local directional pattern techniques. J Imaging. 2022;8(4):102. https://doi.org/10.3390/jimaging8040102.

Kumar V, Venkataraman R, Aljaroudi W, Osorio J, Heo J, Iskandrian AE, Hage FG. Implications of left bundle branch block in patient treatment. Am J Cardiol. 2013;111(2):291–300. https://doi.org/10.1016/j.amjcard.2012.09.029.

Thiene G, Corrado D, Basso C. Arrhythmogenic right ventricular cardiomyopathy/dysplasia. Orphanet J Rare Dis. 2007;2(1):45. https://doi.org/10.1186/1750-1172-2-45.

Waldmeier D, Herzberg J, Stephan F-P, Seemann M, Arenja N. Advanced imaging in cardiac amyloidosis. Biomedicines. 2022;10(4):903. https://doi.org/10.3390/biomedicines10040903.

21 Heart Failure with Preserved Ejection Fraction (HFpEF)

Carolina D. Tennyson

Anatomy and Physiology

Heart failure (HF) is a complex clinical syndrome that results from any structural or functional impairment of cardiac output. Heart failure with preserved ejection fraction (HFpEF) is a chronic HF syndrome in the setting of an EF > 50%. It is estimated that HFpEF accounts for at least one-half of all HF cases. The initial diagnosis of HFpEF frequently progresses to a chronic clinical course of HFrEF (*see* Tables 21.1 and 21.2).

Patients with HFpEF typically have one or more of the following underlying pathophysiologic processes acting together: (1) diastolic dysfunction due to impaired left ventricular (LV) relaxation, or LV diastolic stiffness; (2) LV remodeling; (3) increased ventricular and arterial stiffness; (4) right HF due to pulmonary venous hypertension; (5) chronotropic incompetence; and (6) endothelial dysfunction. Underlying comorbidities like chronic kidney disease, hypertension, and diabetes mellitus contribute to a systemic proinflammatory state. This activates the renin-angiotensin-aldosterone system (RAAS), which is a critical regulator of blood volume and systemic vascular resistance. The activation of the RAAS system and altered perfusion affects end-organ function, and clinicians should monitor for cardiorenal and cardio-hepatic syndromes in all forms of clinical heart failure.

Table 21.1 Risk factors for HFpEF

Risk factors for heart failure [1]
Sedentary lifestyle
Cigarette smoking
Obesity
Excessive alcohol intake
Influenza
Cardiotoxic drugs
Chest radiation
Hypertension
Dyslipidemia
Diabetes mellitus
Coronary artery disease

Acute HF can result in rapid decompensation and can be attributed to neurohormonal activation, venous congestion, endothelial dysfunction, myocardial injury, and renal dysfunction [3]. This constellation of physiological changes causes the patient symptoms of dyspnea, fatigue, peripheral pitting edema, and jugular vein distention. Exercise intolerance, weight gain, early satiety, and dyspnea are common presentations of HFpEF exacerbation.

C. D. Tennyson (✉)
Duke University School of Nursing, Durham, NC, USA
e-mail: carolina.tennyson@duke.edu

R. Musialowski, K. Allshouse (eds.), *Cardiovascular Manual for the Advanced Practice Provider*,
https://doi.org/10.1007/978-3-031-35819-7_21

Table 21.2 Some etiologies of HFpEF

Hypertensive heart disease [2]
Coronary artery disease
Ischemic cardiomyopathy
Severe, chronic, stable coronary disease
Restrictive cardiomyopathy
Infiltrative diseases (amyloidosis, sarcoidosis, hemochromatosis)
Primary diabetic cardiomyopathy
Idiopathic
Hypertrophic cardiomyopathy
Obstructive or nonobstructive
Primary valvular heart disease
Aortic stenosis
Aortic regurgitation
Mitral stenosis
Mitral regurgitation
Pericardial disease
Constrictive pericarditis
Cardiac tamponade
Primary right ventricular dysfunction
Pulmonary arterial hypertension
Arrhythmogenic right ventricular dysplasia
Congenital heart disease
High-output cardiac failure (uncommon)
Severe anemia
Thyrotoxicosis
Cirrhosis
Shunt due to large arteriovenous fistulae

Physical Exam (See Chap. 20)

A full physical exam should be completed. Special attention should be paid to:

- Lung fields should be assessed for crackles/rales that may indicate pulmonary edema
- Jugular venous distension +/ hepatojugular reflex
- Edema in the legs, hips, and abdomen
- Heart sounds: rate, rhythm, S3 and/or S4 sound may indicate volume overload
- Signs of low cardiac output (cool and/or diaphoretic skin, weak pulses)

Volume status and vital signs should be assessed at each patient encounter. This includes serial assessment of body weight, as volume overload will result in weight gain.

Classification (See Chap. 20)

Imaging (See Chap. 20)

Diagnosis

The diagnosis of HFpEF can be challenging because it requires exclusion of other potential noncardiac causes of symptoms suggestive of HF. There is no single diagnostic test for HF because it is largely a clinical diagnosis based on a careful history and physical exam. The European Society of Cardiology recommends a simple diagnostic approach that includes all of the following:

1. Symptoms and signs of HF
2. Evidence of an LVEF ≥50%
3. Objective evidence of cardiac structural and/or functional abnormalities consistent with the presence of LV diastolic dysfunction/raised LV filling pressures, including raised natriuretic peptides [2]

In patients presenting with dyspnea, measurement of natriuretic peptide biomarkers is useful to support a diagnosis or exclusion of HF but is not diagnostic itself [1].

Management

Medical Therapy

There are fewer medications with demonstrated benefit for HFpEF as compared to HFrEF. For patients with HFpEF, the diagnosis and treatment of contributing factors such as atrial fibrillation, hypertension, coronary artery disease, diabetes, and chronic kidney disease are essential to prevent the progression of HF. Beta blockers should be used cautiously in patients with amyloidosis as the cardiac output is very heart rate dependent.

Patients with HFpEF and persistent hypertension should be treated to attain a systolic blood pressure less than 130 mmHg. There are limited data to guide the choice of antihypertensive therapy in HFpEF, but medications that inhibit the renin-angiotensin-aldosterone system are preferred (i.e., mineralocorticoid receptor antagonist, angiotensin receptor neprilysin inhibitor) [1].

Patients with HFpEF are more likely than the general population to have atrial fibrillation. Heart rhythm and rate control are important mainstays of HFpEF treatment. It is very important to consider occult unrecognized paroxysmal atrial fibrillation as a cause of decompensation and recurrent hospitalization, even if the patient presents through ED in normal sinus rhythm. Management of atrial fibrillation is reasonable to improve symptomatic HF. Beta blockers are the preferred agent for achieving rate control, and digoxin may be an effective adjunct therapy. Diltiazem has a mild negative inotropic effect and should be used with caution. When rate or rhythm control is not achievable, AV nodal ablation and resynchronization therapy device placement can be useful [4].

The SGLT2 inhibitor empagliflozin is the agent approved for reducing the risk of cardiovascular death and hospitalization for HF in patients with HFpEF. Multiple mechanisms of action are thought to contribute to this cardiovascular benefit including the lowering of glucose, blood pressure, and body weight. SGLT2 inhibits also induce a mild diuretic effect, reduction of uric acid, and higher red cell mass [5]. Empagliflozin does not need to be titrated for HF benefit. Reduction of a patient's insulin regimen should be considered when initiating an SGLT2 inhibitor. Additionally, evidence is mounting that the prescription of SGLT2 inhibitors even during hospitalization for acute heart failure can also provide clinical benefit within 90 days [6].

HFpEF is a preload driven diagnosis. The diastolic filling curve is very steep. Thus, the ventricle progresses rapidly from volume depletion to pulmonary edema. This pathology leads to the frequent and recurrent emergency department evaluations for either of these two volume states. Loop diuretics like torsemide, furosemide, and bumetanide have not been found to improve survival but are the main agent for symptom management and decongestion. Intravenous delivery should be used for patients needing immediate relief or who are decompensated.

Periodically, all HF patients should be screened for iron deficiency anemia. Symptomatic, ambulatory HF patients with iron deficiency anemia and EF ≤45% or hospitalized HF patients with EF ≤50% should be supplemented with ferric carboxymaltose.

Nonmedical Management

Patients who are admitted to the hospital for the primary problem of heart failure exacerbation should have a follow-up appointment within 1 week to evaluate fluid volume status, review any changes made in medication regimen, and provide patient education. Fluid restriction is beneficial to minimize readmissions, and dietary salt restriction is recommended, but this recommendation is currently being reevaluated in clinical trials.

Clinical Pearls

- The evidence-based medication to treat HFpEF is an SGLT2 inhibitor.
- Treating comorbidities like hypertension, obesity, and atrial fibrillation can help mitigate the progression and exacerbation of HF.
- Volume status can sometimes be tenuous in the HFpEF population. Use the lowest dose of effective loop diuretic in conjunction with SGLT2 inhibitors to maintain euvolemia. Educate the patient regarding daily weights and PRN dosing to avoid hospitalization.
- Preferred treatment of HTN for patients with HFpEF is medications that work to modify the RAS system (ACE-I/ARB/ARNI, MRA).
- When patients with HFpEF have persistent symptoms and/or HF hospitalizations despite optimal medical therapy, refer to an advanced HF program.

References

1. Yancy CW, Jessup M, Bozkurt B, Butler J, Casey DE, Colvin MM, et al. 2017 ACC/AHA/HFSA focused update of the 2013 ACCF/AHA guideline for the management of heart failure. J Am Coll Cardiol. 2017;70(6):776–803.
2. McDonagh TA, Metra M, Adamo M, Gardner RS, Baumbach A, Böhm M, et al. 2021 ESC guidelines for the diagnosis and treatment of acute and chronic heart failure: developed by the task force for the diagnosis and treatment of acute and chronic heart failure of the European Society of Cardiology (ESC) with the special contribution of the Heart Failure Association (HFA) of the ESC. Eur Heart J. 2021;42(36):3599–726.
3. Mentz RJ, O'Connor CM. Pathophysiology and clinical evaluation of acute heart failure. Nat Rev Cardiol. 2016;13(1):28–35.
4. Yancy CW, Jessup M, Bozkurt B, Butler J, Casey DE, Drazner MH, et al. 2013 ACCF/AHA guideline for the management of heart failure. J Am Coll Cardiol. 2013;62(16):e147–239.
5. Rangaswami J, Bhalla V, de Boer IH, Staruschenko A, Sharp JA, Singh RR, et al. Cardiorenal protection with the newer antidiabetic agents in patients with diabetes and chronic kidney disease: a scientific statement from the American Heart Association. Circulation. 2020;142(17):e265–86.
6. Voors AA, Angermann CE, Teerlink JR, Collins SP, Kosiborod M, Biegus J, et al. The SGLT2 inhibitor empagliflozin in patients hospitalized for acute heart failure: a multinational randomized trial. Nat Med. 2022;28:1–7.

Pulmonary Vascular Disease

22

Lyn Shelton and Joe Mishkin

Introduction

Pulmonary hypertension, in its basic definition, is the elevation of pulmonary artery pressures. The elevated pulmonary artery pressures result from pulmonary vasculature remodeling due to an underlying disease process. Over time the resultant progressive workload imposed via the pulmonary vasculature overworks the right ventricle. PAH without intervention may be progressive, leading to right heart failure and death.

Regarding formal diagnostic criteria, however, pulmonary hypertension consists of a mean pulmonary artery pressure greater than 20 mmHg. Previously, the cutoff was a mean PA pressure greater than or equal to 25 mmHg based upon an arbitrary number. Evidence suggested that patients in the borderline range of a mean PA pressure 21–24 mmHg had suffered worse outcomes which prompted the guideline update. The Sixth World Symposium on Pulmonary Hypertension further defines PH in updated terms of Pre- and Post-capillary pulmonary hypertension. Patients may also have a combination of both forms of pulmonary hypertension. These designations require hemodynamic assessment via right heart catheterization for pulmonary artery pressures and pulmonary capillary wedge pressure measurements, respectively.

Precapillary pulmonary hypertension is defined as a mean pulmonary artery pressure (mPAP) greater than 20 mmHg at rest in addition to pulmonary capillary wedge pressure (mPCWP) less than or equal to 15 mmHg and a pulmonary vascular resistance (PVR) greater than or equal to 3 Wood units. PVR is a function of mean pulmonary artery pressure minus mean wedge giving us transpulmonary gradient. (TPG). The TPG divided by cardiac output equals PVR.

$$\text{TPG} = \text{Mean PA pressure} - \text{Mean pulmonary capillary wedge pressure}$$

$$\text{PVR} = \text{TPG} / \text{cardiac output}\left(\text{COL} / \text{min}\right)$$

L. Shelton (✉)
Atrium Health/SHVI Heart Failure/Transplant Clinic, Pulmonary Hypertension Clinic, Charlotte, NC, USA

Asheville Cardiology, Asheville, NC, USA
e-mail: doyle.shelton@atriumhealth.org

J. Mishkin
Atrium Health/SHVI Heart Failure/Transplant Clinic, Pulmonary Hypertension Clinic, Charlotte, NC, USA

Atrium Health/Sanger Heart and Vascular Institute, Charlotte, NC, USA
e-mail: Joseph.mishkin@atriumhealth.org

R. Musialowski, K. Allshouse (eds.), *Cardiovascular Manual for the Advanced Practice Provider*,
https://doi.org/10.1007/978-3-031-35819-7_22

As you can see from the above equations, specific factors can drive pulmonary vascular resistance. The higher the PA pressure versus the mean wedge pressure, the higher the PVR. PVR is augmented when there is lower cardiac output. Try to think of PVR as a factor of the difficulty of moving blood from the right heart through the lungs to reach our left heart circulation.

Precapillary PH entails elevated pulmonary pressures in the absence of left-sided heart disease/volume overload (i.e., therefore excludes WHO Group II PH). Isolated post-capillary pulmonary hypertension is defined as mPAP greater than 20 mmHg with mPCWP greater than 15 mmHg and a PVR <3 Wood units. This is consistent with higher filling pressures secondary to left-sided heart disease (WHO Group II or also can include WHO Group V). There is also combined pre- and post-capillary pulmonary hypertension where mPCWP is greater than 15 mmHg and, PVR is greater than 3 Wood units. Typically, the pulmonary vascular bed can vasodilate in response to enhanced flow. However, if we examine PAH histologically, we find remodeling of the distal pulmonary vasculature with the growth of endothelial and smooth muscle cells as well as infiltration of inflammatory cells [1–3]. This is manifested by constriction via vascular remodeling with fibrosis and stiffness. In addition, there is in situ thrombosis [4]. Factors in PH patients that lead to these changes include decreased nitric oxide (NO) levels and increased endothelial levels. NO is an antiproliferative and a vasodilator, while endothelin is a vasoconstrictor. Prostacyclin levels are also decreased. Prostacyclin is antiproliferative, inhibits platelet function, and is a vasodilator. The pathophysiology of PAH has led to the development of medications that affect these pathways and are targets for treatments [5].

Classifications

We need to further categorize pulmonary hypertension based upon the underlying disease process. The World Health Organization (WHO) designates five classification groups of pulmonary hypertension (Table 22.1). It should be noted that although patients may have a diagnosis of PH, often these patients possess a combination of underlying etiologies, placing them in more than one WHO group. Pharmacological treatment strategies will be outlined in further detail later but focus on WHO group I PAH as well as a pharmacological indication for WHO group IV.

Table 22.1 WHO group classifications of pulmonary hypertension

I. PAH	Idiopathic Drug and toxin-induced Heritable Associated with PAH: Examples include connective tissue disorders, portal hypertension, congenital heart disease, HIV infection, Pulmonary venous occlusive disease (PVOD)
II. Pulmonary hypertension due to left-sided heart disease	LV systolic or diastolic dysfunction, valvular heart disease
III. Pulmonary hypertension due to lung disease and/or hypoxia	Examples include COPD, ILD, OSA
IV. Chronic thromboembolic pulmonary hypertension (CETPH).	Pulmonary embolism
V. Pulmonary hypertension with unclear or multifactorial mechanisms	Examples include end-stage renal disease on dialysis, myeloproliferative disorders, sarcoidosis

The Global prevalence of PAH is often difficult to assess. European registries have reported rates of 5–52 per million people. Regarding WHO Group I, statistics note an annual incidence of 2–5 cases per million people and affects 25 persons per one million population in Western countries. Contrasting this with WHO group 2, valvular left-sided heart disease accounts for more than 100 million persons [6, 7].

Presentation/Physical Exam Findings

As an APP, you will be required to evaluate and treat patients with primary cardiac issues, but often they possess concomitant comorbidities. Patients frequently present with complaints of

Table 22.2 Physical exam findings that may be suggestive of pulmonary hypertension

An increased pulmonic component of the second heart sound [11].	High-pitched early diastolic murmur of pulmonic regurgitation	Abnormal pulmonary exam may be associated with underlying pulmonary diseases such as interstitial lung disease (ILD), COPD/emphysema. These include velcro-like dry crackles, wheezing, or severely diminished airflow
Holosystolic murmur of tricuspid regurgitation	Elevated jugular venous distention corresponding to right ventricular fluid overload as well as tricuspid regurgitation	The examination may also include a large A wave in the jugular venous pulse or may also have prominent V waves in the jugular venous pulse secondary to tricuspid regurgitation
Liver tenderness or enlargement on exam	Right heart failure signs may include peripheral edema or ascites	Patients may have a palpable RV heave given right ventricular hypertrophy/dilation
Cyanosis and evidence of clubbing may be present in patients with underlying shunts or congenital heart disease	Scleroderma patients may have associated skin changes, telangiectasias, digital ulcerations.	

dyspnea, fatigue and progressive functional limitations. This presentation may be consistent with pulmonary HTN, but the differential diagnosis is lengthy. Given that presenting symptoms can often be attributed to other comorbidities, PH patients may have a delay in diagnosis and subsequent treatment.

REVEAL (Registry to Evaluate Early and Long-Term PAH Disease Management) data review in 2011 noted 21.1% of patients experienced symptoms greater than 2 years before PAH was recognized. Patients less than 36 years of age showed the highest likelihood of delayed disease recognition as well as those patients with a documented history of common respiratory diseases with obstructive sleep apnea/obstructive airways disease [8]. Therefore, a detailed history and proper examination combined with appropriate diagnostic testing are paramount. Higher risk comorbidities, such as a history of connective tissue disorder, liver disease, HIV disease, thromboembolic history, or methamphetamine abuse, should imply a higher suspicion for pulmonary arterial hypertension [1]. This should also include those with a history of congenital heart disease.

More advanced PAH may present with chest pain, syncope, and evidence of right heart failure/strain. Chest pain can be seen due to reduced cardiac output as a factor of RV strain and overload in combination with higher pulmonary vascular resistance. Chest pain may also be caused by left main coronary artery compression secondary to an enlarged pulmonary artery [9]. Syncope in patients with underlying pulmonary arterial hypertension is highly concerning for poor cardiac output with RV dysfunction, reduced forward flow, and high pulmonary vascular resistance. Patients with right heart failure and strain may present with prominent abdominal distention/ascites as well as lower extremity edema and JVD (see discussion on cor pulmonale). Rare findings may include hoarseness via Ortner's syndrome, in which the left laryngeal nerve becomes paralyzed secondary to compression by dilated pulmonary artery [10]. Work-up and subsequent treatment options will be based on the type of diagnosed pulmonary hypertension and associated comorbidities. A detailed physical exam is an essential component of assessing the pulmonary hypertension patient (Table 22.2).

Diagnostic Modalities/Imaging

Diagnostic testing is necessary to assist in elucidating the form of pulmonary hypertension to guide your treatment strategy. Testing should aid in confirming or excluding forms of pulmonary hypertension, for which the management strategy should be focused on the underlying disease process versus PAH. Examples include PH secondary to obstructive sleep apnea, chronic pulmonary disease, systolic and diastolic heart failure.

Echocardiography

Transthoracic echo (TTE) is one of the hallmarks of pulmonary hypertension screening tests. One benefit is that's it's noninvasive and widely available. It can be a useful initial screening study in the setting of presenting subjective symptoms. TTE is effective at identifying structural changes that may be associated with pulmonary hypertension. These include right ventricular size and systolic function, presence of pericardial effusion, and presence and severity of tricuspid regurgitation. It can assess for flattening of the interventricular septum (D-shaped LV) associated with right ventricular pressure and/or volume overload (Fig. 22.1). In addition, an echocardiogram can identify other potential contributing factors to pulmonary hypertension including diastolic dysfunction, valvular heart disease, and left ventricular systolic dysfunction.

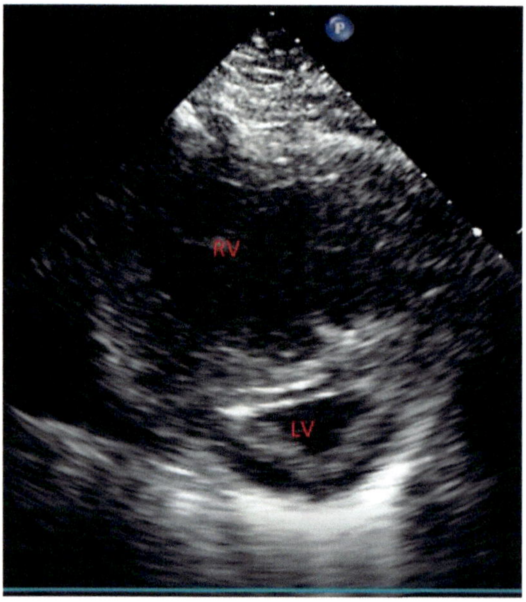

Fig. 22.1 D-shaped interventricular septum of PH and RV enlargement. The RV is severely dilated and larger than the LV. High RV pressures flatten the septum into a D-shape

TTE has been used to estimate pulmonary artery systolic pressure (PASP) or right ventricular systolic pressure (RVSP) at times. It is not recommended to use estimated pulmonary artery pressure, however, via echo for diagnosis. This given potential inaccuracies of estimated right atrial pressure as well as suboptimal tricuspid regurgitation signal or interpretation, which are used to estimate PA pressures [12]. Furthermore, TTE findings should never be utilized in the place of right heart catheterization for documenting definitive pulmonary artery systolic pressure for initiation or alteration of therapies for PAH.

However, tricuspid regurgitation velocity (TRV) has been utilized for assigning the echocardiographic probability of pulmonary hypertension in patients suspected of having pulmonary hypertension. TRV greater than 3.4 m/sec confers a high risk of pulmonary hypertension, whereas below 2.8 m/sec without other signs of pulmonary hypertension changes on echo confers a low probability if no other parameters of PH findings on echo are met [13]. A TRV of less than 2.8 m/sec without other presence of pulmonary hypertension signs on echo confers a low probability.

Computerized Tomographic Angiography (CTA) of the Chest

CTA is used to assess for acute pulmonary embolism given concern for thromboembolic phenomenon as acute potential cause for pulmonary hypertension and right ventricular systolic dysfunction. It should be noted that CTA is an appropriate modality for the evaluation of underlying acute pulmonary emboli. However, its sensitivity may be suboptimal for defining chronic thromboembolic phenomenon in WHO IV. (Please see V/Q scan discussion below).

CT of the Chest

Obtained for parenchymal lung disease, assess for RV dilation, assess enlarged main pulmonary artery.

Ventilation Perfusion Scan

This scan can identify potential chronic thromboembolic phenomenon as CTA chest has diminished sensitivity in identifying chronic thromboembolic pulmonary disease. Even if a patient has a negative CTA chest for pulmonary embolism, this does not exclude the potential for chronic thromboembolic disease.

V-Q scan utilizes an inhaled radiolabeled aerosol and injectable radioactive tracer to assess lung ventilation/perfusion. A nuclear camera is utilized to register distribution of the radioactive material on the alveoli and pulmonary arteries, looking for mismatches. Results are noted as high, intermediate, or low probability and non-diagnostic [14].

PFTs: Pulmonary Function Studies

This functional test helps identify pulmonary hypertension attributed to WHO group III with the suggestion of underlying restrictive or obstructive lung disease. PFTs also utilize DLCO (diffusion capacity), which can be noted to be decreased in pulmonary arterial hypertension and concern for PVOD (pulmonary venous occlusive disease.)

Cardiac MRI

CMRI is the gold standard for right ventricular assessment as it can give accurate measurements of anatomy, ejection fraction, flow, and even assess for myocardial perfusion.

Right Heart Catheterization

This invasive study is required for the diagnosis of pulmonary arterial hypertension as it provides direct hemodynamic assessment. It is mandatory to confirm the presence of and help delineate the type of pulmonary hypertension (pre/post/combined), and assist with risk stratification. It also provides the hemodynamic data to initiate PAH therapy and subsequent titrations based on follow-up hemodynamics after therapy is initiated. (See Chap. 2).

Chest X-ray

May show enlargement of the pulmonary arteries/RV enlargement.

12 Lead ECG

EKG Findings in pulmonary hypertension may include right axis deviation, p pulmonale c/w right atrial enlargement, signs of RV hypertrophy, RV strain, RBBB, and in some cases QTc prolongation [15].

OSA Evaluation

Sleep apnea may be a contributing factor to WHO Group III pulmonary hypertension which, can be readily diagnosed and treated. We will discuss sleep apnea in further detail later.

Vasoreactivity Study

This study is done at the time of the initial right heart cath. This involves assessing pulmonary pressure changes with a Vaso-reactive agent: typically, this is inhaled nitric oxide. Vaso-reactive patients demonstrate a reduction in mean pulmonary artery pressure of $\geq$10 mmHg to an absolute value of $\leq$40 mmHg with either an increase or no change in cardiac output (CO). Treatment of Vaso reactive patients will be discussed under treatment options.

6-min Walk

This easy evaluation is the measurement of distance walked in 6 min but is a vital data point linked to survival rates. This must be measured in a consistently.

Pulmonary Artery (PA) Angiogram

A PA angiogram is a catheterization-based procedure to assess for pulmonary emboli. It is typically indicated if abnormal VQ Scan or high suspicion for chronic thromboembolic disease (WHO Group IV PH).

Initial Routine Lab Work

1. Complete blood count. Rule out anemia or potential for possible blood dyscrasias.
2. Complete metabolic panel for assessment of renal function, liver function studies (portopulmonary HTN).
3. Hepatitis panel.
4. Thyroid panel.
5. HIV serologic testing.
6. Genetic testing: BMPR2. BMPR2 mutation accounts for 80% of heritable and 20% of idiopathic pulmonary hypertension [16].
7. Assessment for connective tissue disorders. For example: ANA.
8. Cardiac BNP or NTProBNP.

Treatment

In terms of pulmonary hypertension management, it is important to verify the type/types of pulmonary hypertension and risk stratify patients. Tools are readily available to clinicians to risk stratify pulmonary hypertension patients into low, intermediate, and high-risk groups. These classifications are based on functional, clinical, and hemodynamic measurements. There are many comprehensive risk stratification tools available. The following parameters appear to have the greatest predictive accuracy: 6-min walk distance, BNP/NTproBNP, right atrial pressure, cardiac index, and mixed venous oxygen saturation [17].

The REVEAL registry uses variables to calculate 1-year mortality and is predictive of survival at baseline, 1-year follow-up, and 5-year follow-up. In the absence of or in conjunction with PAH pharmacologic therapy when indicated, supportive treatments for PAH are an essential component of the treatment paradigm. Basic supportive treatments should be indicated in the treatment of an underlying disease process (Table 22.3).

Patients with confirmed WHO Group 4 PH secondary to thromboembolic disease should be referred early to a specialty center for pulmonary endarterectomy. If they are not candidates for surgery, balloon pulmonary angioplasty (BPA) and medical therapy should be considered.

Table 22.3 Supportive treatment options

Treatment	Recommendations
Supervised exercise	Avoid over-strenuous exertion/ symptomatic exercise
Supplemental oxygen	When required to maintain appropriate oxygen sats with rest, exercise, or sleep
Anticoagulation	As indicated in WHO Group IV (CTEPH)
	In idiopathic PAH-must be determined on an individual basis
Diuretics	Cautious use for right heart failure as it can cause reduced right heart preload
	Diuretics for patients with high left-sided filling pressures (WHO Group II)
Arrhythmias	Aggressive treatment of SVTs. Often poorly tolerated in severe PAH
	Typically try to avoid negative inotropic medications with right heart failure
Avoidance of pregnancy	High mortality risk in PAH and pregnancy. Necessity for appropriate contraception
Underlying pulmonary disease	Needs appropriate treatment of underlying pulmonary disease
Smoking cessation	
Immunizations	Including PNA/pneumococcal vaccinations
Psychosocial support	
Hematology	Correction of iron deficiencies given increased metabolic demand with anemia/iron deficiency
WHO Group IV (CTEPH)	Early referral to a special center for potential pulmonary thromboendarterectomy or balloon pulmonary angioplasty (BPA) if a candidate

Pharmacological therapy has been shown via clinical trial results to be indicated in pulmonary arterial hypertension (WHO Group I) and WHO Group 4. Patients with WHO Group 2 and 3 PH should not be treated with PAH- specific therapy due to the high risk of complications. The exception is pulmonary hypertension associated with interstitial lung disease (WHO Group III), with recent data demonstrating the benefits of inhaled prostacyclin, Treprostinil [18]. Goals of therapy and factors associated with better prognosis include functional class I–2, 6-min walk distance greater than 400 m, and normal right ventricular function per echocardiogram and hemodynamic parameters (Table 22.4).

Current treatment recommendations call for upfront oral combination therapy for low to intermediate-risk patients with PAH and upper combination therapy that should include prostacyclin therapy for patients with high-risk features. Patients should be reevaluated 3–6 months from the start of combination therapy, and if goals are not met, sequential triple therapy or escalation of therapy from oral to parenteral prostacyclin is most likely to be considered [19].

Vasoreactivity testing is recommended to evaluate the response to calcium channel blocker only for patients with idiopathic PAH, heritable PAH, and PAH associated with drugs and toxins. If positive, then high-dose calcium channel blocker is used, If goals of therapy are not achieved after 3–6 months, it is recommended to start specific PAH therapy.

Regarding pharmacologic therapy for PAH, there are three main pathways typically targeted. These include the prostacyclin pathway, endothelium pathway, and nitric oxide.

Table 22.4 Goals of therapy/factors associated with better prognosis

Functional class	NYHA class 1–2
6-minute walk distance	Greater than 400 meters
Right ventricular function	Normal
Treatment regimen	Combination therapy

Prostacyclin Pathway

Prostacyclin induces potent vasodilatation of all vascular beds. This decreases pulmonary vascular resistance and reduces pressure. It inhibits platelet aggregation and appears to have both cytoprotective and antiproliferative activities [20]. It can be delivered orally, via IV or subcutaneously, or inhaled.

Common side effects include local site pain (SQ route), vasodilatory side effects such as headache, flushing, and GI upset. The side effects can be dose-dependent. IV or SQ is initiated at a low dose (usually 1–2 ng/kg/min) and titrated upward slowly over time to achieve clinical improvement or occasionally limited due to side effects. IV requires an indwelling catheter which can increase the risk of line-associated infections. Therefore, appropriate hygiene measures are necessary. In addition, we always recommend IV prostacyclin infuse via a single-lumen catheter. You must avoid flushing the line containing the prostacyclin, which, if given as a bolus, can induce profound hypotension, GI side effects, or even reports of deaths associated with boluses. See Table 22.5.

Table 22.5 Prostacyclins

Prostacyclin	Utilization/description
IV	Prostacyclin analog
Epoprostenol	Demonstrated survival benefit in randomized clinical trials
	Half-life few minutes: Potential for rebound effects if interruptions in therapy
	Common side effects: Diarrhea, jaw pain, muscle pain, flushing, headache
Iloprost	Inhaled prostacyclin therapy
	Short half-life, therefore, must be given 6x a day
	Common side effects: Cough, headache, flushing
Treprostinil	Longer half-life than Epoprostentol
	Available via IV, subcutaneous route
	Subcutaneous route may experience infusion site pain, swelling, redness
Selexipag	Selective prostacyclin receptor agonist. Orally dosed
	Starts 200 mcg bid and titrate up to 1600 mcg bid if tolerating
	Similar side effects to others with headache, flushing, arthralgias, jaw pain, and GI side effects with nausea/diarrhea. SEs may be dose-dependent

Table 22.6 Endothelin Receptor Antagonists

ERA generic	Brand	Dosing	Monitoring
Ambrisentan	Letairis®	5, 10 mg	Selective ETA receptor antagonist, low risk of liver injury Risk of edema (class effect)
Macitentan	Opsumit®	10 mg	Risk of edema. Potential for anemia
Bosentan	Tracleer®	62.5 mg,125 mg	Liver toxicity potential so close monitoring required Pre/post-initiation/ongoing treatment <40 kg: start with 62.5 mg bid >40 kg: Start 62.5 mg bid and then increase to 125 mg bid in 4 weeks

Endothelin Receptor Antagonists

Endothelial -1 is a vasoconstrictor and has Type A and B receptors. Binding to these receptors is utilized to reduce pulmonary vascular resistance. Dependent upon the ERA used, it may bind to type A only (Ambrisentan) or to type A and B (Bosentan and Macitentan). See Table 22.6.

ERA Clinical Points

- PAH patients may often require low-dose diuretics with mild symptoms of edema.
- ERA should not be utilized in patients with diastolic dysfunction or PAH patients with elevated capillary wedge pressure on right heart cath.
- ERA's are potentially teratogenic. Therefore, it is imperative that women patients of childbearing age use appropriate contraception and obtain monthly pregnancy tests while on therapy.
- Common side effects other than edema include nasal congestion, and headache.

Nitric Oxide Pathway

PDE-5 Inhibitors (Phosphodiesterase-5 Inhibitors)

PDE-5 inhibiton results in vasoldilation of the pulmonary arteries via the nitric oxide pathway. This class is utilized in the treatment of PAH as our pulmonary vasculature contains phosphodiesterase 5. It should be noted that these drugs are used to treat erectile dysfunction but have different indications and dosing with regard to pulmonary hypertension. See Table 22.7.

Table 22.7 PDE-5 Inhibitors

PDE-5i generic	Brand	Dosing
Sildenafil	Revatio®	20 mg three times a day
Tadalafil	Adcirca®	20 mg, 40 mg once daily

PDE-5 Inhibitors (Phosphodiesterase-5 Inhibitors) Clinical Pearls

- They are *contraindicated in the setting of baseline nitrates,* given the potential for prominent hypotension.
- Common side effects include the following: Headache, nasal congestion, epistaxis, flushing, joint pain, GI side effects.
- May lower blood pressure.
- *Contraindicated with Riociguat.*

Soluble Guanylate Cyclase Stimulator

Riociguat (Adempas®): Works by enhancing cGMP production, which is a vasodilator.

Indications:

- It is indicated for PAH and PAH secondary to chronic thromboembolic etiology.

Potential Side effects:

- Hypotension.
- Syncope potential.
- Bleeding.
- It has demonstrated antiproliferative/antiremodeling properties in animals [18].

Dosing

- Dosing is typically 0.5–1.0 mg TID and monitor for hypotension.

- It can be titrated up to a max dose of 2.5 mg tid.

Major Contraindication

- *Concurrent use with PDE 5 inhibitors is contraindicated,* given potential for hypotension.

Most patients with PAH are treated initially with combination therapy consisting of two agents. Select patients may be candidates for monotherapy as per the outline. PAH requires ideally early disease detection and proactive treatment with multiple classes of drugs targeting multiple pathogenic pathways [2]. Treatment combinations have been shown to demonstrate improved 6-min walk distance and delay in time to clinical worsening. In patients whom medical therapy fails to reduce their risk to low or intermediate level, referral for lung transplation is recommended. [21]. Atrial septostomy may be considered in end-stage PAH or those awaiting lung transplant. It unloads the right atrium and right ventricle and delays right ventricular failure. This in turn improves left ventricular preload but at the price of reduced oxygenation given right to left shunting [21].

Clinical Pearls

- Patients on IV prostacyclin therapy: DO NOT flush the line infusing the prostacyclin agent. This can accidentally bolus the patient and lead to significant consequences not limited to hypotension, prominent flushing, and even death.
- Always make sure patients are not on active nitrate medications if you are prescribing a PDE-5 inhibitor. The combination can cause prominent hypotension.
- Care with aggressive diuresis in true PAH patients as they can be right heart preload dependent and you can cause hypotension, worsening of cardiac output if they become volume depleted.
- Always verify names and dosages of PAH medications—this may be through the patient or may have to be verified via their specialty pharmacy.
- If they are on IV or SQ prostacyclin therapy, always verify their current weight and dosing weight. Often their prescribing pharmacy or info may be detailed on their infusion pump. Occasionally adjustments need to be made for prominent weight changes to make sure they are on the appropriate dosing.
- A combination of Riociguat (Adempas) and a PDE-5 inhibitor is contraindicated due to ®hypotension.
- Not all pulmonary hypertension is pulmonary arterial hypertension.

Pulmonary Embolism

Introduction

Acute pulmonary embolism remains one of the most challenging cardiovascular disorders to manage. The heterogeneity in presentation, complex nomenclature for risk stratification and multiple treatment modalities now available create a need for a multidisciplinary approach to the management of this disease process. Despite advances in technology, mortality for acute PE remains high [22]. The following section reviews the contemporary approach to diagnosis, risk stratification, and treatment of acute pulmonary thromboembolic disease. The evaluation and management of chronic thromboembolic will be addressed in pulmonary hypertension section of this chapter.

Physiology

Acute PE results in sudden increase in pulmonary vascular resistance (PVR) which can cause right ventricular (RV) dilation, tricuspid regurgitation, and subsequent RV failure. This can rapidly escalate to systemic hypotension and cardiogenic shock. The mechanism of this deterioration is multifactorial including shifting of the interventricular septum toward the left ventricle (LV) causing decreased LV filling as well as increased RV wall stress and causing myocardial ischemia (Fig. 22.1). Acute PE can lead to severe ventilation-perfusion mismatching and subsequent hypoxemia. Patients may also develop a respiratory alkalosis due to hyperventilation.

Classification and Risk Stratification

Classification and risk stratification in acute PE incorporates clinical indicators, imaging findings, and biomarkers to help determine severity of disease and best interventions [23]. The classification has differing risk and therapeutic options (Table 22.8). Most patients who present with PE are normotensive without imaging or biomarker evidence of RV strain or dysfunction. PE with signs of RV dysfunction but normotension is termed intermediate-risk PE, while the presence of hemodynamic instability is indicative of high-risk PE [24]. High-risk PE is also termed massive PE. These patients may present with syncope, systemic arterial hypotension, cardiogenic shock, or cardiac arrest. The term "supermassive" or catastrophic PE is used to describe patients with fulminant cardiopulmonary collapse that require cardiopulmonary resuscitation.

Intermediate-risk PE patients represent a considerable challenge as they can experience a sudden decline in clinical status despite early identification and institution of anticoagulation therapy. The significant heterogeneity of this patient population can lead to confusion regarding appropriate treatment strategies. Intermediate-risk PE patients are sometimes further subclassified into intermediate-low and intermediate-high risk depending on presence or absence of both RV dysfunction in conjunction with a positive troponin or elevated brain natriuretic peptide (BNP) level.

Table 22.8 Classification of Pulmonary embolus

Risk	Hemodynamics
Intermediate low	RV dysfunction with normotension with negative troponin and BNP
Intermediate high	RV dysfunction with normotension with elevated troponin and BNP
High risk/massive	Hemodynamic instability
Catastrophic/ super massive	Cardiovascular collapse

Adapted from Piazza G. Submassive pulmonary embolism. JAMA 2013;309:171–80

Scoring systems exist to help characterize the severity of acute PE to help guide therapeutic decision-making. The PESI (Pulmonary Embolism Severity Index) and simplified PESI (sPESI) scores are common tools used to identify patients with increased 30-day mortality risk [25, 26]. In addition to these risk scores, an increased RV-to-LV ratio on computed tomography (CT) imaging is associated with high 30-day mortality risk as well.

History and Presentation

The presentation of pulmonary embolus is diverse. Patients may be asymptomatic with an embolus seen as an incidental finding on imaging. This diagnosis should be considered in patients with the common findings in Table 22.9. Most often patients will present with chest pain that is pleuritic in nature accompanied by shortness of breath. In some cases, presenting symptoms can be vague and nonspecific and attributed to anxiety. In severe cases, acute PE may present as sudden cardiac death. Risk factors for PE include recent surgery, trauma, immobilization or active malignancy. In some instances, patients may harbor a genetic predisposition to thrombus formation.

Physical Findings

Physical exam findings for acute PE can range from normal vital signs to tachycardia and hypotension. In cases of massive PE, patients may

Table 22.9 Common presenting signs and symptoms of PE

Unexplained tachycardia
Dyspnea on exertion
Pleuritic and localized chest pain
Syncope
Cardiac arrest

present with syncope or fulminant cardiogenic shock.

There can be evidence of right heart strain including elevated jugular venous pressure and a third heart sound. Evidence of malperfusion may include altered mental status and cool extremities in conjunction with cyanosis.

Imaging

An EKG most commonly shows sinus tachycardia, but atrial arrhythmias may occur. The classic EKG is described as S1Q3T3. This describes a new S wave in lead I with a new Q wave and inverted T wave in lead III. These findings are consistent with acute RV dilatation and strain.

CTA of the chest is the best diagnostic modality to image acute PE (Fig. 22.2). The rapid avail ability of CT is essential in these patients as hemodynamic collapse may occur suddenly.

Treatment and Management

Multidisciplinary PE response teams (PERT) have emerged to help standardize the approach to treatment of PE, particularly cases where the quality of evidence is limited or in the presence of conflicting recommendations. The utilization of the PERT is like what has been done in response to other common cardiovascular conditions, such as myocardial infarction, stroke, and acute aortic syndromes. As previously stated, acute PE can lead to cardiogenic shock, an area where a team-based approach to care has been successful in improving outcomes. The goal of the PERT is to improve access to care, reduce variability in treatment strategies and identify best practices [27, 28].

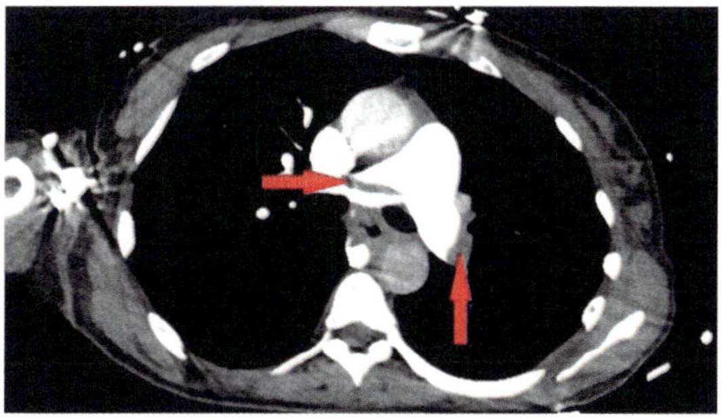

Fig. 22.2 CTA chest showing PE. Red arrows point to bilateral thrombus in the right and left pulmonary arteries

Pharmacologic Therapies

Anticoagulation remains the cornerstone for treatment of PE. Regimens include intravenous unfractionated heparin, subcutaneous low molecular weight heparin, fondaparinux, or direct oral anticoagulants.

Systemic fibrinolysis is utilized to attempt immediate reversal of RV dysfunction and prevent deterioration into hemodynamic collapse and improve mortality [29, 30]. In a large, randomized-control trial full-dose systemic fibrinolysis consisting of 100 mg tissue plasminogen activator (t-PA), reduced the risk of hemodynamic collapse in intermediate-risk PE, though with an associated increased risk of bleeding in the form of intracranial hemorrhage [31]. Subsequent clinical trials investigating half-dose t-PA did not demonstrate improvement in mortality or reduction in adverse bleeding events. There was also an increased need for escalation of therapy with this strategy [32, 33].

Pharmacologic hemodynamic support is important for the initial stabilization of patients and to maintain end organ perfusion while instituting more definitive therapy for PE. Epinephrine and norepinephrine are drugs of choice due to their ability to enhance RV contractility without promoting systemic vasodilation. Avoidance of excessive volume loading is critical in the setting of RV dysfunction and should be avoided when central venous pressure exceeds 15 mmHg. Although pulmonary vasodilator therapy can reduce pulmonary vascular resistance and RV afterload, the use of inhaled nitric oxide has not been shown to improve outcomes in intermediate-risk PE [34].

Advanced Therapies

Advanced therapies for PE include catheter-based Intervention, surgical pulmonary embolectomy, and mechanical circulatory support [35]. Catheter-based therapy includes catheter-directed fibrinolysis and mechanical embolectomy. These modalities can also be employed in combination. While the frequency of catheter-based therapy utilization has increased, the overall efficacy of this approach with respect to mortality has not been studied in large, randomized-control trials. Ultrasound-facilitated, catheter-directed fibrinolysis (EkoSonic Endovascular System™) has been FDA approved in the USA for the treatment of intermediate and high-risk PE. The main endpoint noted in trials utilizing ultrasound-facilitated, catheter-directed fibrinolysis has been improvement in RV-LV ratio [36, 37]. Ultrasound waves are pulsed into the thrombus to break up the clot and facilitate the effect of thrombolytics.

Percutaneous mechanical thrombectomy is another catheter-based technique that does not utilize thrombolysis therapy. The FlowTriever™ system (Inari Medical, Irvine, California) and the Indigo Thrombectomy System™ (Penumbra, Inc., Alameda, California) are two such devices that have been undergone single-arm studies, both demonstrating improvement in imaging outcomes. Further research is needed to determine the best utilization of these catheter-based technologies along with timing of their deployment. These devices mechanically remove the thrombus from the pulmonary artery. They work best on proximal thrombus.

Surgical pulmonary embolectomy should be considered in patients with intermediate–high- or high-risk PE when fibrinolysis has failed or is contraindicated [38, 39]. Surgical intervention should also be considered when "clot-in-transit" is present (Fig. 22.3), patients experience hemodynamic collapse or respiratory failure requiring cardiopulmonary resuscitation. It is most effective in patients with large centrally located PE and when performed before onset of multisystem organ failure and high vasoactive medication requirement. In this scenario, a Cardiothoracic surgeon will mechanically remove thrombus from inside the pulmonary arteries via a median sternotomy approach. Most often these patients require temporary mechanical circulatory support after the procedure.

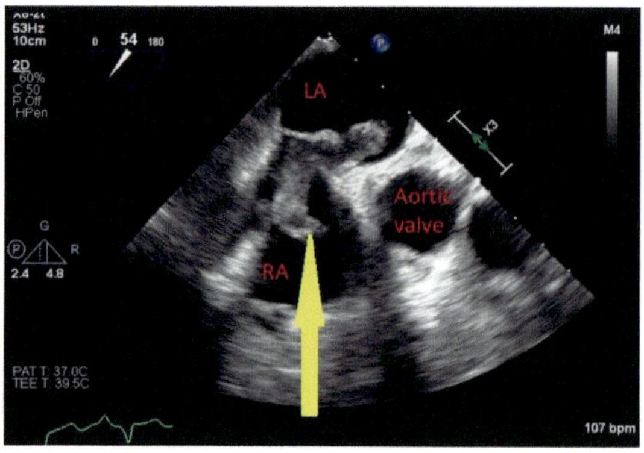

Fig. 22.3 TEE image showing Clot (yellow arrow) in transit across a PFO

Extracorporeal membrane oxygen (ECMO) has been increasingly utilized for management of high-risk PE. Patient selection and timing of deployment are critical aspects that have yet to be well-defined. Like other forms of cardiogenic shock, utilization of temporary mechanical circulatory support demonstrates improved outcomes when employed prior to onset of severe multisystem organ failure. While ECMO has been utilized as an adjunctive measure in PE, recently it has been shown that some patients may recover on ECMO without the addition of fibrinolysis or mechanical thrombectomy (Chap. 25) [40].

Conclusion and Future Considerations

The management of acute PE depends not only on timely diagnosis, but also appropriate and accurate risk stratification to guide the utilization of pharmacologic therapies. Furthermore, accurate risk assessment can help identify those patients that may benefit from a broadening availability of catheter-based interventions.

Intermediate-risk PE patients remain a significant challenge as many data points need to be assimilated in a timely fashion to balance the risk-benefit ratio of various treatment modalities. High-risk and catastrophic PE patients who previously experienced dismal outcomes, may have better opportunity for survival with mechanical circulatory support and deployment of catheter-based technology or surgical thrombectomy in selected patients. There is optimism that utilization of multidisciplinary PERT will help improve outcomes moving forward.

Clinical Pearls

- The management of acute PE depends not only on timely diagnosis, but also appropriate and accurate risk stratification to guide the utilization of pharmacologic therapies.
- Anticoagulation remains the cornerstone for treatment of PE.
- Intermediate-risk PE patients remain a significant challenge as many data points need to be assimilated in a timely fashion to balance the risk-benefit ratio of various treatment modalities.
- High-risk and catastrophic PE patients who previously experienced dismal outcomes, may have better opportunity for survival with mechanical circulatory support and deployment of catheter-based technology or surgical thrombectomy in selected patients.
- There is optimism that utilization of multidisciplinary PERT will help improve outcomes moving forward.

Cor Pulmonale

We will briefly outline Cor Pulmonale in conjunction with our pulmonary hypertension section. Cor Pulmonale is defined by alteration in the structure and function of the right ventricle caused by a primary respiratory system disease [41]. It refers to the combination of hypertrophy, pressure overload, and dilation of the right ventricle in the face of pulmonary hypertension [42]. It is the result of pulmonary hypertension developed from any underlying process. In the presence of an underlying pulmonary disease, there can be alveolar hypoxia which can be a main cause of pulmonary vasoconstriction, as discussed in the PH section prior. Hypoxemia also leads to smooth muscle cell proliferation of small pulmonary arteries with vascular mediated changes in nitric oxide, endothelin 1 as outlined for PH prior [41]. This leads to hyper viscosity from pulmonary vasoconstriction and polycythemia. Subsequently, the pulmonary vasculature does not allow increases in cardiac output without significant increases in pulmonary artery pressure [42]. The cascade ultimately results in RV systolic dysfunction with limitations in cardiac output in response to exercise.

Cor pulmonale can be further defined as acute or chronic. Chronic cor pulmonale can be seen in the setting of pulmonary hypertension etiologies outlined prior for WHO Groups from PH discussion earlier. These include diseases such as COPD and interstitial lung disease. It may also occur in upper airway obstruction/sleep apnea, and chest wall changes with kyphoscoliosis or pulmonary vasculature with pulmonary arterial hypertension [41]. Other findings include autoimmune diseases such as scleroderma, cystic fibrosis, and obesity hypoventilation syndrome [41].

Acute cor pulmonale, on the other hand, is most commonly due to acute pulmonary embolism. The right heart is better equipped to handle volume load as opposed to a pressure load. Therefore, even small increases in pulmonary artery pressure may result in large increases in right ventricular work and right ventricular hypertrophy [43].

Presenting symptoms are like those of pulmonary hypertension and are often related to the underlying disorder. Common symptoms include dyspnea on exertion as well as exertional fatigue. Also, RV failure signs with abdominal distention and lower extremity edema may be seen.

Physical Exam

See the Pulmonary hypertension exam above given similarities.

Evaluation

Evaluation for cor pulmonale is consistent with pulmonary hypertension evaluation. Assessment for acute or chronic PE, underlying pulmonary disease with cxr/pulmonary function test/parenchymal lung disease should be considered. Echo can assess for structural changes of the right heart and estimated pulmonary pressures. Cardiac MRI can further assess right heart morphology and include right heart ejection fraction/volumetric indices. Assess EKG for signs of right ventricular hypertrophy, P pulmonale, and right bundle branch block.

Treatment

Cor pulmonale treatment should be aimed at treating the underlying condition. This includes the correction of hypoxia to improve pulmonary vasoconstriction. In patients with evidence of right ventricular failure, diuretics may also be utilized for decongestion. Treatment of the underlying pulmonary process is indicated. Examples include treatment of pulmonary arterial hypertension, OSA, and pulmonary emboli if indicated. Smoking cessation is imperative.

If COPD is diagnosed, advise appropriate treatment of the disease, which may include bronchodilators and avoidance of pulmonary irritations.

Clinical Pearls

- Smoking cessation!
- Assess and treat the underlying etiology.
- Diuretics for symptomatic relief of right-sided congestion.
- Hypotension and renal failure are poor prognostic indicators.

Sleep Apnea and Cardiovascular Disorders

Obstructive sleep apnea (OSA) is a disorder characterized by obstructive apnea, hypopnea, and/or respiratory effort-related arousals caused by repetitive collapse of the upper airway [44]. It is the most common sleep-related breathing disorder. It can be characterized by hypoxia and hypercapnia with full or partial airway constriction while sleeping [45]. Central sleep apnea results from the removal of wakefulness stimulus to breathe in patients with compromised neuromuscular ventilatory control [46]. These include patients with neuromuscular disease or chest wall disease. They may have central nervous system disease, neuromuscular disease or severe abnormalities in pulmonary mechanics such as kyphoscoliosis. Central sleep apnea is felt to be secondary to mechanisms that trigger central respiratory events, including post hyperventilation central apnea or central apnea secondary to hypoventilation, as can be seen with opioid use [46].

Presentation

Presenting symptoms of OSA often include patient complaints of waking up gasping for air or choking. Partners or family members may also reiterate the patient frequently snores or may have witnessed apneic periods. Patient may have daytime somnolence, dyspnea on exertion, and easy fatigability. Complaints of restless sleep, nocturia, headache on awakening, and sore throat can be common. Sleep apnea often goes undiagnosed and untreated as the symptoms may not be readily noticeable or not attributed to sleep apnea.

Physical Exam

Physical exam typically focuses on the assessment of risk factors and limited exam with oral assessment, BMI, and neck measurements (*see* Table 22.10).

Approximately 30% of patients with BMI > 30 and 50% of those with BMI > 40 have OSA [47].

Mallampati score provides a score of 1–4 based upon anatomic features of the airway when patients have their mouth open, and their tongue

Table 22.10 Risk Factors for OSA

Obesity with BMI greater than 30
Large neck circumference: Greater than 17 in. in men (43 cm), 15 inches in women (37 cm)
Increased Mallampati score

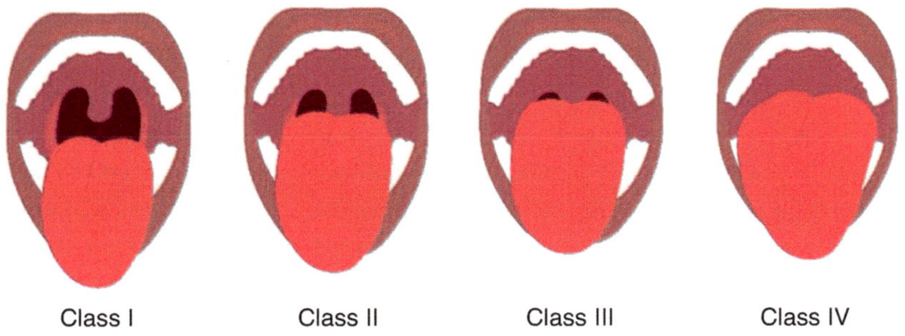

Fig. 22.4 Anatomy of the Mallampati score

Table 22.11 STOP-bang questionnaire

S: "Do you snore loudly, loud enough to be heard through a close door?"			
T: "Do you feel tired or fatigued during the daytime almost every day?"			
O: "Has anyone observed that you stop breathing during sleep?"			
P: "Do you have a history of high blood pressure with or without treatment?"			
B: BMI greater than 35			
A: Age older than 50 years			
N: Neck circumference greater than 17 in (43 cm)			
G: Gender, male			
SCORE	0–2	3–4	5–8
OSA risk for moderate to severe OSA	Low	Assess risk factors	High

protruded. The score is calculated based on the physical exam of the soft palate in relationship to the tongue. Less visualization of the uvula is scored higher and has a higher likelihood of OSA (Fig. 22.4). For every one-point increase in the Mallampati score, the odds of having obstructive sleep apnea increased more than twofold, independent of more than 30 variables that reflected body habitus, airway anatomy, symptoms, and medical history [48].

Screening tools at the time of assessment may also be used to further stratify potential risk for OSA and the necessity for a referral.

The STOP-BANG screening tool is outlined below and widely utilized, given its ease of use/limited time required. Chung et al. developed initially as pre-surgery screening tool for OSA and is easily completed for risk stratification. The score is from 0 to 8. Sensitivity to detect OSA based upon score of ≥3 to detect moderate to severe OSA (AHI > 15) and severe OSA (AHI > 30) was 93% and 100%, respectively (Table 22.11). (AHI defined as an average number of episodes of apnea and hypopnea per hour.)

Patients with scores of 0–2 on STOP-BANG are at low risk for moderate to severe OSA and with scores 5–8 are considered high risk for OSA. Patients with scores of 3–4 require further criteria for classification as having a higher risk for moderate to severe OSA [49]. Typically, they are considered higher risk if they have one additional risk factor to include BMI >35, male gender, neck circumference >16 in (40 cm), or a serum bicarbonate level > or equal to 28 mmol/L [49].

Physiology

Sleep apnea can lead to a cascade of changes from the pathophysiology standpoint. Parasympathetic activity increases during our sleep cycle. However, during periods of apnea with airway obstruction, hypoxia, and increased CO_2 leads to an increase in sympathetic output. Other potential changes include the activation of the renin angiotensin-aldosterone system (RAAS) in the setting of sympathetic activation. Sleep apnea patients often have elevated angiotensin II and aldosterone levels. These cause water retention of the kidneys and vasoconstriction of the peripheral vasculature, which can lead to hypertension [50]. OSA may also lead to endothelial dysfunction. Nitric oxide, a vasodilator, can be impaired with obstructive sleep apnea but can improve with treatment [51].

Obstructive sleep apnea may also increase inflammatory markers and reactive oxygen species, which is postulated as a possible mechanism by which OSA increases the risk of cardiovascular disease and overall mortality [52]. Patients with untreated sleep apnea are at higher risk of hypertension or difficult to control hypertension. Other potential complications include an increased risk of arrhythmia given hypoxic induced events. Patient may have atrial arrhythmias/bradycardia arrhythmias, Increased risk of heart failure, myocardial infarction, stroke, and pulmonary hypertension. Sleep apnea occurs in obese population which have other concomitant comorbidities associated with obesity, including diabetes, dyslipidemia, and underlying CAD.

Typical risk factors for sleep apnea include obesity. Obesity leads to mechanical obstruction from adipose tissue causing airway collapse.

Diagnosis

In patients with risk factors or symptoms concerning for obstructive sleep apnea, prompt referral should be entertained to sleep medicine physicians. These specialized physicians can then determine the appropriateness for further testing, including polysomnography.

Sleep Study

Polysomnography (PSG) is performed in the laboratory with technicians. This study is beneficial as it provides an opportunity to directly assess potential for obstructive sleep apnea and directly observed rapid eye movements, sleep-associated disturbances such as periodic leg movements, apneas, and seizures [47]. Nocturnal seizuresare are an ominous sign which may lead to sudden death during sleep if treatment is not rapidly initiated. AASM guidelines require EEG or EMG, heart rhythm monitoring, monitoring of leg movements, breathing with monitoring airflow at the nose and mouth.

The Centers for Med"care and Medicaid Services criteria recognize a positive polysomnography study for OSA as:

AHI or RDI greater than or equal to 15 events per hour

AHI or RDI greater than or equal to 5 and less than or equal to 14 events per hour with documented symptoms of excessive daytime sleepiness, impaired cognition, mood disorders, insomnia, or documented hypertension, ischemic heart disease, or history of stroke [47].

Patients with a higher risk PSG during the first 2 h of diagnostic PSG may undergo a split-night PSG study. The second portion of the testing involves titrating a CPAP device [47]. Alternatively, home sleep study evaluations are becoming popular and more cost-effective.

Management

Non-surgical treatment options include CPAP (continuous positive airway pressure) or BiPAP (bilevel positive airway pressure in which the inhaled/exhaled pressures are adjusted independently.)

These devices provide airflow into the airway via a facemask/nasal covering. It is considered a first-line intervention for sleep apnea and decreases symptoms. Benefits of therapy include improvement in blood pressure, improvement in right heart function, pulmonary hypertension, daytime sleepiness, and cognition.

The treatment process for sleep apnea also includes general and behavioral measures, including:

- Weight loss which has been shown to improve obstructive sleep apnea symptoms and severity.
- Avoidance of sleeping in the supine position to reduce airway collapse.
- Sleep hygiene: consistent sleep/wake cycle and avoidance of device/light stimulation at bedtime.
- Avoidance of sedating pharmacologic agents, including alcohol, 4–6 h before bedtime.
- Compliance with CPAP or BiPAP, including nocturnal oxygen if utilized.

Potential surgical treatments for OSA also exist. Options include Uvulopalatopharyngoplasty (UPPP) and maxillomandibular advancement (MAD). These should be done via centers specializing in surgical intervention. Maxillomandibular advancement (MAD) changes the position of the maxilla and the mandible, which enlarges the airway. It moves to the lower jaw forward to prevent closing in the upper airway [53]. Uvulopalatopharyngoplasty (UPPP) removes a section of the uvula, soft palate, and tonsil to enlarge the airway. These treatments are reserved for those who do not respond to CPAP or mandibular advancement device [53].

Oral appliance therapy may also be utilized to assist the movement of the mandible. This is recommended for the treatment of primary snoring without obstructive sleep apnea and for adult patients with obstructive sleep apnea who are intolerant to CPAP as opposed to no treatment. It is recommended that a qualified dentist provide oversight and use a custom titratable appliance over non-custom oral devices [54].

Tracheostomy may even be considered in select patients who have failed standard medical therapies.

If the patient still has daytime somnolence despite adherence to CPAP, CNS stimulants may be prescribed. Currently, armodafinil, modafinil, or solriamfetol (DNRI-dopamine/norepinephrine reuptake inhibitors) are FDA approved for residual sleepiness despite optimal treatment of OSA using PAP [47].

Clinical Pearls

- STOP-BANG questionnaire to make the clinical diagnosis of OSA.
- First line of management is to advocate lifestyle modification/sleep hygiene habits, including weight loss if BMI is elevated.
- OSA is an underrecognized cardiovascular risk factor that requires management and therapy.
- OSA can cause sudden death, atrial fibrillation, and poorly controlled hypertension.
- CPAP compliance should always be discussed.
- Long-term evaluation with sleep medicine is important as CPAP settings may need to be adjusted over time to optimally treat OSA.

References

1. Paul H. Pulmonary arterial hypertension. N Engl J Med. 2021;385:2361–76.
2. Wagenvoort CA. The pathology of primary pulmonary hypertension. J Pathol. 1970;101:Pi.
3. Price LC, Wort SJ, Perros F, et al. Inflammation in pulmonary arterial hypertension. Chest. 2012;141:210–21.
4. Marc H, Lau Edmund MT, David M, Xavier J, Oliver S, Gerald S. Pulmonary vascular remodeling in PAH from a pathological perspective involves vasoconstriction, arterial remodeling, and in situ thrombosis. Advances in Therapeutic Interventions for Patient with Pulmonary Arterial Hypertension. Circulation. 2014;130:2189–208.
5. Thenappan T, Ormiston M, Ryan J, Archer S. Pulmonary arterial hypertension: pathogenesis and clinical management. BMJ. 2018;360:j5492.
6. Humbert M, Sitbon O, Chaouat A. PAH in France: results from a national registry. Am J Respir Crit Care Med. 2006;173(9):1023.
7. Stephen A, Kenneth WE, Wilkins MR. Basic science of pulmonary arterial hypertension for clinicians: new concepts and experimental therapies. Circulation. 2010;121:2045–66.
8. Brown LM, Chen H, Halpern S, Taichman D, McGood MD, Farber HW, Frost AE, Liou TG, Turner M, Feldkircher K, Miller DP, Elliott CG. Delay in recognition of pulmonary arterial hypertension: factors identified from the REVEAL Registry. Chest. 2011;140(1):19.
9. Rich S, McLaughlin VV, O'Neill W. Stenting to reverse left ventricular ischemia due to left main coronary artery compression in primary pulmonary hypertension. Chest. 2001;120(4):1412.
10. Braunwald E, Zipes D, Libby P. Heart disease. A textbook of cardiovascular medicine, vol. 2, 6th ed. 2001.
11. Sutton G, Harris A, Leatham A. Second heart sound in pulmonary hypertension. Br Heart J. 1968;30(6):743.
12. Amsallem M, Sternbach JM, Adigopula S, Kobayashi Y, Vu TA, Zamanian R, Liang DD, Dhillon G, Schnittger I, McConnell MV, Haddad F. Addressing the controversy of estimating pulmonary arterial pressure by echocardiography. J Am Soc Echocardiog. 2016;29(2):93–102.
13. Galie N, Humbert M, Vachiery JL, Gibbs S, Lang I, Torbicki A, Simonneau G, Peacock A, Vonk Noordegraaf A, Beghetti M, et al. ESC/ERS guidelines for the diagnosis and treatment of pulmonary hypertension: the joint task force for the diagnosis and treatment of pulmonary hypertension of the European Society of Cardiology (ESC) and the European Respiratory Society (ERS): endorsed by: Association for European Paediatric and Congenital Cardiology (AEPC), International Society for Heart and Lung Transplantation (ISHLT). Eur Heart J. 2015;2016(37):67–119. https://doi.org/10.1093/eurheartj/ehv317.

14. Mirza H, Hashmi M. Lung ventilation perfusion scan. StatPearls Publishing; 2022.
15. Bossone E, Paciocco G, Iarussi D, et al. The prognostic role of the ECG in primary pulmonary hypertension. Chest. 2002;121:513–8. https://doi.org/10.1378/chest.121.513.
16. Evans JDW, Girerd B, Montani D, Wang X-J, Galie N, Austin ED, et al. BMPR2 mutations and survival in pulmonary arterial hypertension:an individual participant data meta-analysis. Lancet Respir Med. 2016;4(2):129–37.
17. Boucly A, Weatherald J, Humbert M, et al. Risk assessment in pulmonary arterial hypertension. Eur Respir J. 2018;51(3):pii: 1800279. https://doi.org/10.1183/13993003.00279-2018.
18. Waxman A, Restrepo-Jaramillo R, Thenappan T, et al. Inhaled Treprostinil in pulmonary hypertension due to interstitial lung disease. NEJM. 2021;384:325–34.
19. The 6th world symposium of PH: risk stratification and medical treatment in PH, 6 part series. ACC. Franco Veronica. 2019.
20. Salim Y, Anastasia N, Theo T. Clinical update on pulmonary hypertension. J Investiagt Med. 2020;68(4):821–7.
21. Hassoun Paul M. Pulmonary arterial hypertension: review article. NEJM. 2021;385:2361–76.
22. Casazza F, Becattini C, Bongarzoni A, et al. Clinical features and short term outcomes of patients with acute pulmonary embolism. The Italian pulmonary embolism registry (IPER). Thromb Res. 2012;130:847–52.
23. Konstantinides SV, Meyer G, Becattini C, et al. 2019 ESC guidelines for the diagnosis and management of acute pulmonary embolism developed in collaboration with the European Respiratory Society (ERS). Eur Heart J. 2019;41:543–603.
24. Piazza G. Submassive pulmonary embolism. JAMA. 2013;309:171–80.
25. Aujesky D, Obrosky DS, Stone RA, et al. Derivation and validation of a prognostic model for pulmonary embolism. Am J Respir Crit Care Med. 2005;172:1041–6.
26. Jiménez D, Aujesky D, Moores L, et al. Simplification of the pulmonary embolism severity index for prognostication in patients with acute symptomatic pulmonary embolism. Arch Intern Med. 2010;170:1383–9.
27. Dudzinski DM, Piazza G. Multidisciplinary pulmonary embolism response teams. Circulation. 2016;133:98–103.
28. Giri JS, Piazza G. A midterm report card for pulmonary embolism response teams. Vasc Med. 2018;23:72–4.
29. Chatterjee S, Chakraborty A, Weinberg I, et al. Thrombolysis for pulmonary embolism and risk of all-cause mortality, major bleeding, and intracranial hemorrhage: a meta-analysis. JAMA. 2014;311:2414–21.
30. Marti C, John G, Konstantinides S, et al. Systemic thrombolytic therapy for acute pulmonary embolism: a systematic review and meta-analysis. Eur Heart J. 2015;36(10):605–14.
31. Meyer G, Vicaut E, Danays T, et al. Fibrinolysis for patients with intermediate-risk pulmonary embolism. N Engl J Med. 2014;370:1402–11.
32. Wang C, Zhai Z, Yang Y, et al. Efficacy and safety of low dose recombinant tissue-type plasminogen activator for the treatment of acute pulmonary thromboembolism: a randomized, multicenter, controlled trial. Chest. 2010;137:254–62.
33. Kiser TH, Burnham EL, Clark B, et al. Half-dose versus full-dose alteplase for treatment of pulmonary embolism. Crit Care Med. 2018;46:1617–25.
34. Kline JA, Puskarich MA, Jones AE, et al. Inhaled nitric oxide to treat intermediate risk pulmonary embolism: a multicenter randomized controlled trial. Nitric Oxide. 2019;84:60–8.
35. Piazza G. Advanced management of intermediate- and high-risk pulmonary embolism: JACC focus seminar. J Am Coll Cardiol. 2020;76:2117–27.
36. Kucher N, Boekstegers P, Muller O, et al. Randomized controlled trial of ultrasoundassisted catheter-directed thrombolysis for acute intermediate-risk pulmonary embolism. Circulation. 2014;129(479–86):23.
37. Piazza G, Hohlfelder B, Jaff MR, et al. A prospective, single-arm, multicenter trial of ultrasound-facilitated, catheter-directed, lowdose fibrinolysis for acute massive and submassive pulmonary embolism: the SEATTLE II study. J Am Coll Cardiol Intv. 2015;8:1382–92.
38. Poterucha TJ, Bergmark B, Aranki S, Kaneko T, Piazza G. Surgical pulmonary embolectomy. Circulation. 2015;132:1146–51.
39. Goldberg JB, Spevack DM, Ahsan S, et al. Survival and right ventricular function after surgical management of acute pulmonary embolism. J Am Coll Cardiol. 2020;76:903–11.
40. Ghoreishi M, DiChiacchio L, Pasrija C, et al. Predictors of recovery in patients supported with VA-ECMO for acute massive pulmonary embolism. Ann Thorac Surg. 2020;110(70–5):37.
41. Garrison DM, Pendela VS, Memon J. Cor pulmonale. [Updated 2021 Aug 11]. In: StatPearls [Internet]. Treasure Island, FL: StatPearls Publishing; 2022. Available from: https://www.ncbi.nlm.nih.gov/books/NBK430739/.
42. Hosenpud JD, Greenbert BH. CHF pathophysiology, diagnosis, and comprehensive approach to management. 2nd ed. 2000. p. 368–69.
43. Valentin F, Wayne AR, O'Rourke RA, et al. Hurst's the heart. 10th ed. 2001.
44. Kline LR. Clinical presentation and diagnosis of obstructive sleep apnea in adults. Up to Date. 2021.
45. Jordan AS, McSharry DG, Malhotra A. Adult obstructive sleep apnoea. Lancet. 2014;383:736–47.
46. Aurora RN, Bista SR, Casey KR, Chowdhuri S, Kristo DA, Mallea JM, Ramar K, Rowley JA, Zak RS, Heald JL. Updated adaptive servo-ventilation recommendations for the 2012 AASM guideline: "the treatment of central sleep apnea syndromes in adults: practice parameters with an evidence-based litera-

ture review and meta-analyses". J Clin Sleep Med. 2016;12(5):757–61.
47. Wickramasinghe H, et al. Obstructive sleep apnea clinical presentation. Medscape; 2020.
48. Nuckton TJ, Glidden DV, Browner WS, Claman DM. Physical examination: Mallampati score as an independent predictor of obstructive sleep apnea. Sleep. 2006;29(7):903–8. https://doi.org/10.1093/sleep/29.7.903. PMID: 16895257.
49. Chung F, Yegneswaran B, Liao P, et al. STOP questionnaire: a tool to screen patients for obstructive sleep apnea. Anesthesiology. 2008;108:812–21.
50. Jin Z-N, Wei Y-X. Meta-analysis of effects of obstructive sleep apnea on the renin-angiotensin-aldosterone system. J Geriatr Cardiol. 2016;13:333.
51. Ip MS, Lam B, Chan LY, Zheng L, Tsang KW, Fung PC, et al. Circulating nitric oxide is suppressed in obstructive sleep apnea and is reversed by nasal continuous positive airway pressure. Am J Respir Crit Care Med. 2000;162(6):2166–71.
52. Ladan P, George U, Steven H, Brett K, Jason M. Review of the management of OSA and pharmacological symptom management. Medicina. 2021.
53. Basyuni S, Barabas M, Quinnell T. An Update on mandibular advancement devices for treatment of obstructive sleep apnoea hyponoea syndrom. J Thoracic Dis. 2018;10(Suppl 1):S48–56.
54. Ramar K, Dort LC, Katz SG, Lettieri CJ, Harrod CG, Thomas SM, Chervin RD. Clinical practice guideline for the treatment of obstructive sleep apnea and snoring with Oral appliance therapy: an update for 2015. J Clin Sleep Med. 2015;11(7):773–827. https://doi.org/10.5664/jcsm.4858. PMID: 26094920; PMCID: PMC4481062.

Pericardial Disease

23

Ashley McDaniel and Richard Musialowski

Pericardial Disease

The heart is protected by tissue layers that make up the pericardial sac. The parietal pericardium is a thick fibrous structure that can be congenitally absent without clinical significance. The visceral pericardium is adherent to the epicardial layer of the heart. The potential space between the two layers contains a small amount of serous pericardial fluid to cushion and protect the heart, allowing it to move freely within the pericardial sac. It is important to recognize that the parietal pericardium extends up to and includes the ascending root of the aorta (Fig. 23.1). This becomes clinically relevant with aortic dissection. Blood tracking outside the aorta will collect in the pericardial space with resultant hemodynamically significant effusion and clinical tamponade (Chap. 28).

Pericarditis

Pericarditis is inflammation of the pericardial sac surrounding the heart. Acute pericarditis is the most common disorder involving the pericardium and is often secondary to a viral process [1]. Other common causes are systemic autoimmune diseases and neoplastic disease with pericardial involvement (Table 23.1) [2]. The clinical diagnosis is made when two of the four criteria listed in Table 23.2 are present. Commonly, a patient will present with inability to lay flat due to sharp and stabbing chest pain. The pain is usually sudden in onset and often described as centrally located, worse with deep inspiration, and pleuritic in nature. Pain frequently improves when sitting forward. Patients may describe radiation to the trapezius ridge, the area from the neck to the shoulder region. Recurrence of inflammation will have very similar symptoms to initial presentation. Many also complain of associated fatigue, shortness of breath, orthopnea, or PND.

The classification of pericarditis is related to the duration and recurrence of symptoms (Table 23.3).

A. McDaniel (✉) · R. Musialowski
Sanger Heart and Vascular Institute, Atrium Health, Charlotte, NC, USA
e-mail: ashley.mcdaniel@atriumhealth.org; Richard.musialowski@atriumhealth.org

Physical Exam

Commonly, the physical exam is unremarkable. Occasionally, a pericardial rub may be heard with the patient leaning forward, during expiration at the left lower sternal edge. It may have one, two, or three components. Usually, a single sound during ventricular systole can be heard intermittently. It has been described sounding like the separation of Velcro™ and can be mistaken for a systolic murmur. The presence of a pericardial effusion often negates the presence of the rub as

R. Musialowski, K. Allshouse (eds.), *Cardiovascular Manual for the Advanced Practice Provider*, https://doi.org/10.1007/978-3-031-35819-7_23

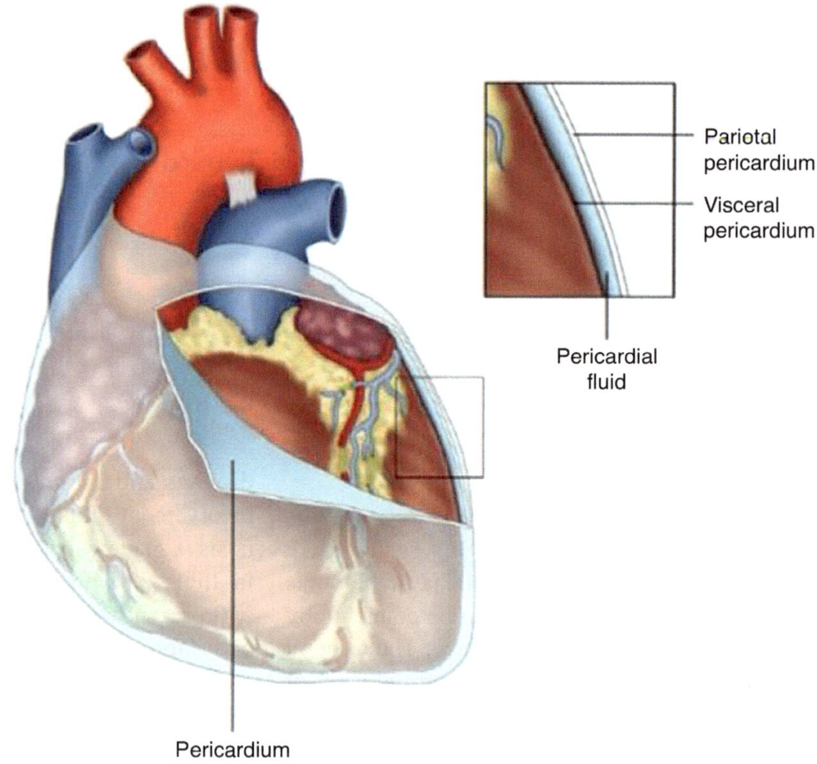

Fig. 23.1 Anatomy of pericardium. (Adapted from Poorsattar, S.P., Maus, T.M. (2022). Pericardium. In: Maus, T.M., Tainter, C.R. (eds) Essential Echocardiography. Springer, Cham. https://doi.org/10.1007/978-3-030-84349-6_14)

Table 23.1 Causes of pericarditis

Etiologies	Examples
Infectious	Viral: Idiopathic. COVID-19-common Bacterial: TB—more common in underdeveloped countries Fungal-rare
Uremic pericarditis	ESRD patients
Post-myocardial infarction (Dressler's syndrome)	Less commonly seen due to early MI intervention
Autoimmune disease	RA, SLE serositis—common
Malignancies	Metastatic cancer-lung, melanoma, and breast—common

Table 23.2 Diagnostic criteria by the American College of Cardiology requires two of four criteria

Chest pain that is positional and pleuritic
Physical exam finding of friction rub
EKG changes characteristic of pericarditis
New or worsening pericardial effusion

Table 23.3 Classification of pericarditis

Acute	Criteria present in Table 23.2, CRP and sedimentation rate elevation, CT or MR imaging showing pericardial inflammation
Incessant	Symptoms lasting >4–6 weeks and less than 3 months
Recurrent	Symptom recurrence after 4–6 weeks or longer of a symptom-free interval
Chronic	Symptoms greater than 3 months

Adapted from Yehuda Adler, Philippe Charron, Massimo Imazio, Luigi Badano, Gonzalo Barón-Esquivias, Jan Bogaert, Antonio Brucato, Pascal Gueret, Karin Klingel, Christos Lionis, Bernhard Maisch, Bongani Mayosi, Alain Pavie, Arsen D Ristić, Manel Sabaté Tenas, Petar Seferovic, Karl Swedberg, Witold Tomkowski, ESC Scientific Document Group, 2015 ESC Guidelines for the diagnosis and management of pericardial diseases: The Task Force for the Diagnosis and Management of Pericardial Diseases of the European Society of Cardiology (ESC) Endorsed by: The European Association for Cardio-Thoracic Surgery (EACTS), European Heart Journal, Volume 36, Issue 42, 7 November 2015, Pages 2921–2964, https://doi.org/10.1093/eurheartj/ehv318

the fluid lubricates the inflamed pericardial layers. A current or recent fever may be associated if infectious process is present.

Diagnostic Testing

EKG may show diffuse concave or saddle-shaped ST elevation in multiple vascular distributions. If these changes were all true STEMI, hemodynamic collapse and cardiogenic shock would be clinically present. Diffuse PR segment depression with isolated PR segment elevation in aVR is usually present simultaneous with the ST segment changes (Fig. 23.2).

Transthoracic Echocardiogram: Since pericarditis is a clinical diagnosis, there are no specific echocardiographic findings in acute pericarditis. The imaging modality may be a helpful diagnostic tool to assess for pericardial effusion and tamponade physiology. Assessment for a focal wall motion abnormality should be undertaken potentially indicating post-infarct pericarditis or myocarditis.

Labs: Inflammatory markers may be elevated including white blood cell count, C-reactive protein, and sedimentation rate. High sensitivity troponin is used to assess for myocardial damage and associated myocarditis or ischemic etiology. If there is a classic presentation of positional chest pain with other clinical signs of pericarditis, an elevation of troponins suggests myopericarditis (Table 23.6).

Cardiac MRI (cMRI) may be useful to assess for pericardial inflammation and to evaluate associated myocarditis (Fig. 23.3).

Management of Acute Pericarditis

Uncomplicated pericarditis should be managed in the ambulatory setting (Table 23.4). High-risk features including an effusion with hemodynamic compromise necessitating admission for inpatient management (Fig. 23.4). Acute inpatient management includes Ketorolac 15–30 mg IV for 1–2 doses for initial pain management and immediate initiation of colchicine.

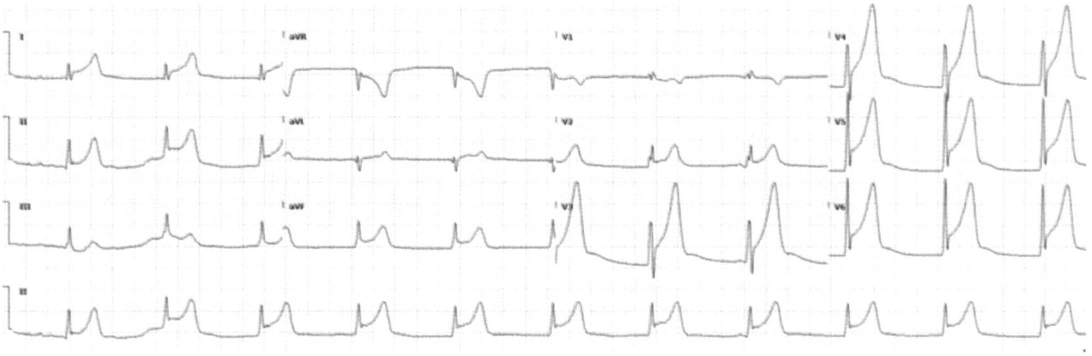

Fig. 23.2 EKG suggestive of acute pericarditis

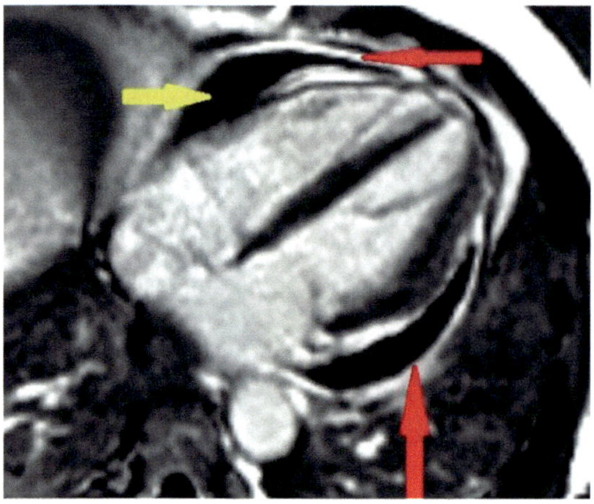

Fig. 23.3 MRI of pericarditis and effusion. Yellow arrows indicate pericardial effusion. Red arrows are gadolinium enhancement of inflamed pericardium

Table 23.4 Treatment options for acute pericarditis

Drug	Usual dosing	Duration of therapy	Tapering
High-dose aspirin	750–1000 mg every 8 h	1–2 weeks	Decrease by 250–500 mg every 1–2 weeks
Ibuprofen	600 mg every 8 h	1–2 weeks	Decrease by 200–400 every 1–2 weeks
Colchicine	0.5 mg daily (<70 kg) or 0.5 mg twice daily (≥70 kg)	3 months	Continue for duration

Adapted from Yehuda Adler, Philippe Charron, Massimo Imazio, Luigi Badano, Gonzalo Barón-Esquivias, Jan Bogaert, Antonio Brucato, Pascal Gueret, Karin Klingel, Christos Lionis, Bernhard Maisch, Bongani Mayosi, Alain Pavie, Arsen D Ristić, Manel Sabaté Tenas, Petar Seferovic, Karl Swedberg, Witold Tomkowski, ESC Scientific Document Group, 2015 ESC Guidelines for the diagnosis and management of pericardial diseases: The Task Force for the Diagnosis and Management of Pericardial Diseases of the European Society of Cardiology (ESC)

Corticosteroids should be avoided as initial treatment since corticosteroids could suppress the patient's immune response to a virus and therefore maintain the trigger for inflammation [3]. This may lead to increased risk of chronic pericarditis and constrictive pericardial physiology. If recurrent pericarditis does occur, colchicine for 6 months along with NSAIDs or

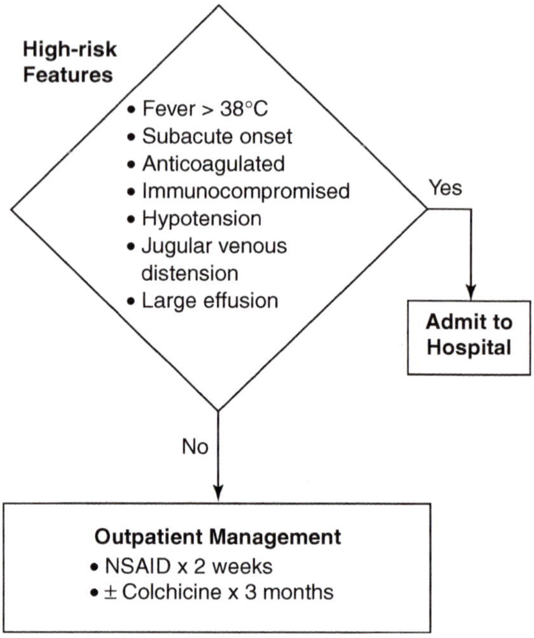

Fig. 23.4 Pathway for treatment of acute pericarditis. (Adapted from Lilly, L., 2013. Treatment of Acute and Recurrent Idiopathic Pericarditis. *Circulation*, 127(16), pp.1723–1726)

high-dose ASA should be continued until the relief of symptoms occurs [4]. Cardiac MRI is now recommended in cases of recurrent pericarditis. Corticosteroids are considered to treat recurrence if the serum CRP is low and the patient is without cardiac MRI abnormalities. Recently, a new agent, rilonacept, was approved to treat recurrent pericarditis, especially if abnormal MRI findings of late gadolinium enhancement are seen within the pericardium. This injectable agent inhibits IL-1 alpha and IL-1 beta and thus alters the autoinflammatory pathway associated with recurrent pericarditis.

Clinical Pearls

- Pericarditis is a clinical diagnosis. A good history of present illness is all that is needed.
- Inquire about recent cold symptoms or fever as recent viral illness is a very common cause of pericarditis.
- Always obtain an EKG to rule out ischemia as an etiology.
- If hemodynamically unstable, echocardiography and clinical bedside assessment to evaluate for tamponade.

- Avoid corticosteroids as they can often lead to recurrent pericarditis.
- Exercise restriction for 3 months or until resolution of symptoms and normalization of CRP, ECG, MRI, and echocardiogram.

Myocarditis

Myocarditis is inflammation of the heart muscle tissue. Clinically, myocarditis and pericarditis can present at the same time. Similar to pericarditis, viral infection and replication in myocarditis can cause myocardial injury and cell death. The injury occurs through direct invasion, production of cardiotoxic substances, or chronic inflammation [5]. Clinical pericarditis with significant troponin elevation and LV dysfunction suggests myocarditis (see Chap. 20). This diagnosis should be suspected in patients who present with or without new cardiac symptoms with a rise in cardiac biomarkers, abnormal LV function, or change in EKG [6].

Constrictive Pericarditis

Constrictive pericarditis is typically a chronic condition that results when granulation tissue forms scar/fibrosis that encases the heart. This causes a loss of elasticity of the pericardial sac. Scarring can become calcified and lead to a compressive syndrome where the ventricles are unable to adequately fill [7]. The disease is often progressive in nature, and nonspecific early signs of cor pulmonale often delay the diagnosis. Traditional treatment often is not successful, and this diagnosis must be considered if there are risk factors for constriction (Table 23.5).

Table 23.5 Common causes of constrictive pericardial disease

Acute or relapsing viral or idiopathic pericarditis
Any type of cardiac surgery
Trauma with organized blood within pericardial space
Mediastinal irradiation
Neoplastic disease
Rheumatoid arthritis
Systemic lupus erythematosus
ESRD/chronic dialysis patients

Adapted from Hoit, B., 2022. *UpToDate*. [online] Uptodate.com

Physiological Characteristics

Constriction causes hemodynamic compromise due to the fixed obstruction to rapid early diastolic filling. An effusion does not need to be present for constrictive pericardial disease. If it is present, it is referred to as constrictive-effusive disease. Pericardiocentesis can alleviate the additional obstruction if an effusion is present, but the underlying constriction will still cause clinical cor pulmonale.

Normally, LV filling is independent of respiratory variation. In constrictive pericarditis, elevated pericardial pressures impede diastolic filling of the RV and eventually the LV. As respiration occurs, there is increased blood return to the fixed RV. The pressures equilibrate due to constriction or an effusion, and the septum pushes into the LV. The abnormal septal motion will impede LV filling and results in lower stroke volume and cardiac output. When this occurs, the ventricles become interdependent. This interdependence causes variation of LV filling associated with respiration. Echocardiography can image this interdependence, and the abnormal septal motion with inspiration is easily seen. Constriction is a clinical diagnosis supported by cardiac imaging. Occasionally, cardiac catheterization is necessary to confirm equalization of diastolic pressures.

Constriction and restrictive cardiomyopathy can be a clinical dilemma. The main difference is the presence of pericardial abnormalities with ventricular interdependence on imaging in constrictive disease. Restriction has abnormalities of the myocardium with evidence of pulmonary hypertension due to chronic HFpEF [8].

Physical Exam

The examination is very similar to pericardial tamponade. The chronicity of the constriction results in more extensive signs of cor pulmonale as seen in Table 23.6.

Table 23.6 Clinical examination findings of constrictive pericarditis

Elevated JVP with a deep, steep Y descent
Kussmaul sign—lack of an inspiratory decline in JVP
Peripheral edema
Ascites and hepatomegaly
Pleural effusion
Pericardial knock—slightly earlier than a third heart sound
Pulsus paradoxus—uncommon without effusion

Adapted from Hoit, B., 2022. *UpToDate*. [online] Uptodate.com

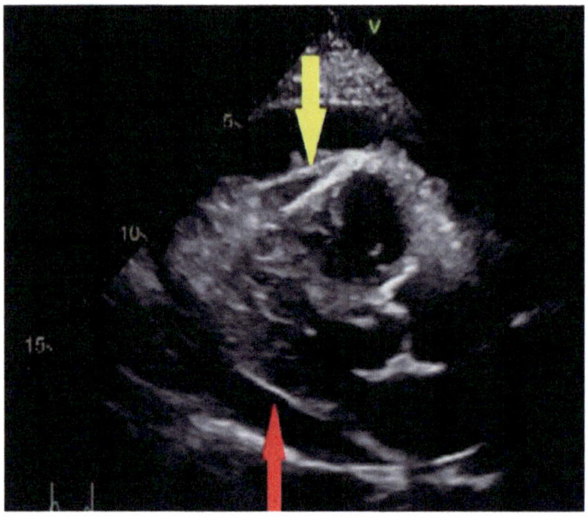

Fig. 23.5 Constrictive effusive pericarditis. The yellow arrows show the thickened parietal pericardium with fibrinous exudate attached suggestive of a chronic disease. The red arrow shows the pericardial effusion

Noninvasive Testing

Echocardiography is the initial test of choice. Signs of chronic effusion with thickening of the visceral and parietal pericardium are often noted. Abnormal septal bounce (ventricular interdependence) is seen with ventricular contraction and varies with respiration (Fig. 23.5).

Cardiac CT is a very good test to evaluate for pericardial thickening as is MRI. CT imaging is more readily available and has excellent diagnostic accuracy. An effusion does not have to be present for constriction physiology (Fig. 23.6).

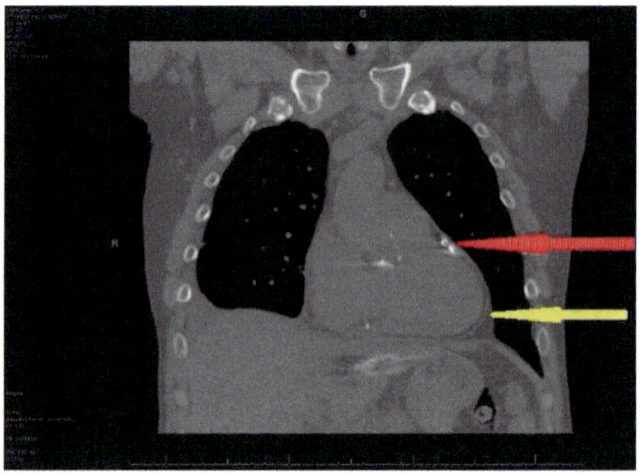

Fig. 23.6 CT of pericardium. Red arrow shows calcification of the pericardium. Yellow arrow shows marked thickening of the pericardium. Both finding suggest constrictive pericardial disease. Note the absence of a significant effusion

Treatment

Constrictive pericardial disease is difficult to diagnose and treat. Diuretic therapy to manage symptoms of cor pulmonale is the cornerstone of treatment. Often, this becomes inadequate and signs of intravascular volume depletion and end-organ hypoperfusion become problematic. Surgical pericardial stripping can be performed but only after the failure of conservative management. This is a high-risk procedure that has high surgical mortality but can significantly improve this disease. During this procedure, parietal pericardium is removed allowing passive filling of the ventricles. If the disease has progressed significantly, the visceral pericardium may be involved, and the patient may have minimal improvement postoperatively. Appropriate patient selection is essential prior to this procedure.

Clinical Pearls

- Consider constriction in patients with risk factors and treatment-resistant cor pulmonale
- Diuretics are used aggressively before high-risk surgery is considered

Pericardial Effusion

The normal pericardial sac contains 10–50 ml of serous fluid. This fluid is designed to lubricate the heart during contraction. Certain disease states result in an increased production of this physiologic fluid. A pericardial effusion may be present and asymptomatic. The effusion is often an incidental finding on other imaging studies and only significant if its size causes hemodynamic instability. A pericardiocentesis may be performed to rapidly treat hemodynamic instability or may be performed for diagnostic evaluation to determine the etiology (Table 23.7).

Physical Examination

Heart sounds may be faint due to increased distance between the chest and the heart. Clinically, the measurement of pulsus paradoxus is the bedside examination finding of ventricular interdependence. Pulses paradoxus is a clinical clue to tamponade and consists of a greater than 10 mmHg inspiratory decline in systolic arterial pressure. This evaluation is performed by increasing the pressure of sphygmomanometer cuff until there are no Korotkoff sounds. Air is slowly released from the cuff until sounds are intermittently heard. The cuff is deflated until the sounds are present continuously. The difference in numbers from beginning of intermittent and continuous is calculated. You should also palpate the radial pulse, and if you note the pulse weakens or disappears during inspiration, this is also a positive sign [5]. Normal is less than 10 mmHg. Hemodynamic significance is seen at 30 mmHg.

Table 23.7 Common causes of pericardial effusion

Common causes of cardiac tamponade	Uncommon causes of cardiac tamponade
Pericarditis	Collagen vascular disease (SLE, RA, scleroderma)
Tuberculosis	Radiation induced
Iatrogenic/procedure	Post myocardial infarction
Trauma	Uremia
Neoplasm/malignancy	Aortic dissection
	Bacterial infection
	Pneumopericardium

Adapted from Yehuda Adler, Philippe Charron, Massimo Imazio, Luigi Badano, Gonzalo Barón-Esquivias, Jan Bogaert, Antonio Brucato, Pascal Gueret, Karin Klingel, Christos Lionis, Bernhard Maisch, Bongani Mayosi, Alain Pavie, Arsen D Ristić, Manel Sabaté Tenas, Petar Seferovic, Karl Swedberg, Witold Tomkowski, ESC Scientific Document Group, 2015 ESC Guidelines for the diagnosis and management of pericardial diseases: The Task Force for the Diagnosis and Management of Pericardial Diseases of the European Society of Cardiology (ESC)

Diagnosis

The gold standard for diagnosis of a pericardial effusion is with echocardiography (Fig. 23.7). It is rapidly available and simple test to evaluate hemodynamic stability. Stable pericardial effusion can be appreciated on a CT scan or MRI. Hemodynamic abnormalities can be seen on these imaging modalities, but echocardiography is more readily available. CT can sometimes overestimate the size of effusion, and the size should be confirmed with echocardiography.

EKG findings are nonspecific. When a pericardial effusion is present and large, you may see electrical alternans on the EKG. This is caused by the heart "floating" in the fluid and moving with respiration and contraction toward and away from the EKG leads.

The cardiac silhouette may be enlarged on chest X-ray due to the presence of fluid.

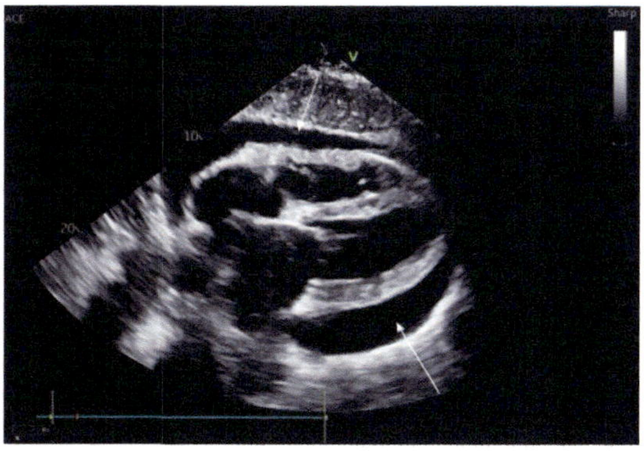

Fig. 23.7 Pericardial effusion on echocardiography. White arrows point to large circumferential pericardial effusion

Treatment

Asymptomatic effusions are usually observed without treatment. If the etiology is unclear and enough fluid is present, pericardiocentesis may be used as a diagnostic test. Treatment of an underlying disease is often indicated. Rarely, empiric anti-inflammatory agents are given if the sed rate and CRP are elevated (Table 23.4).

Cardiac Tamponade

Cardiac tamponade is a life-threatening condition that occurs when the accumulation of fluid in the pericardial space compresses the ventricle resulting in obstruction to ventricular filling. The quantity of fluid is of less concern but more so how rapidly it accumulates. The amount of fluid needed to cause tamponade could be as small as 200 ml if it develops rapidly. When pericardial effusions are chronic or develop more slowly, the pericardium has time to adapt, and there is less chance of hemodynamic compromise.

Clinical Signs

Three principal clinical features of tamponade are hypotension, soft or absent heart sounds, and jugular venous distention with a prominent descent during systole. These three clinical features are known as Beck's triad. Since the main issue is reduced preload to the ventricles from external compression, the heart rate increases to maintain a cardiac output. The SVR increases to maintain blood pressure. The patient in tamponade presents cool, diaphoretic, tachycardic, and hypotensive. *Never* give beta blockers to reduce the heart rate as this will result in cardiovascular collapse.

Diagnosis

Echocardiography will show collapse of the RA and RV walls during diastole. The collapse confirms impaired filling of the ventricle. Blood flow across the mitral valve is also assessed to determine if there is variation with respiration. These signs together confirm tamponade.

Treatment

Pericardiocentesis is indicated if there is hemodynamic compromise with tamponade physiology. If immediate removal of fluid is not possible, aggressive fluid resuscitation should be administered to optimize preload. Occasionally, recurrent significant effusions may require surgical removal of a section of pericardium (pericardial window) to avoid recurrent tamponade, often seen with malignant effusions and is usually palliative in nature [9].

Clinical Pearls

- CT scan can sometimes overestimate the size of effusion. Always confirm size and hemodynamic significance with echocardiography
- Tamponade is an emergency and requires immediate action
- Never give beta blockers to a patient in tamponade

References

1. Imazio M. Acute pericarditis: clinical presentation and diagnosis. UpToDate. [online] Uptodate.com. 2022. Available at: https://www.uptodate.com/contents/acute-pericarditis-clinical-presentation-and-diagnosis?search=pericarditis%20adult&source=search_result&selectedTitle=1~150&usage_type=default&display_rank=1.
2. Bach DS. American College of Cardiology: 2015 ESC guidelines for pericardial disease. 2015.
3. Ismail TF. Acute pericarditis: update on diagnosis and management. Clin Med (Lond). 2020;20(1):48–51. https://doi.org/10.7861/clinmed.cme.20.1.4.
4. Lilly L. Treatment of acute and recurrent idiopathic pericarditis. Circulation. 2013;127(16):1723–6.
5. Jameson JL, Fauci A, Kasper D, Hauser S, Longo D, Loscalzo J. Harrison's principles of internal medicine, 20th ed.
6. Cooper, L. Up to date. Treatment and prognosis of myocarditis in adults.
7. Hoit B. UpToDate. [online] Uptodate.com. 2022. Available at: https://www.uptodate.com/contents/constrictive-pericarditis?search=constrictive%20pericarditis&source=search_result&selectedTitle=1~110&usage_type=default&display_rank=1. Accessed 16 Aug 2022.
8. Sorajja P, Hoit B. UpToDate. [online] Uptodate.com. 2022. Available at: https://www.uptodate.com/contents/differentiating-constrictive-pericarditis-and-

restrictive-cardiomyopathy?source=history_widget. Accessed 12 Aug 2022.

9. Adler Y, Charron P, Imazio M, Badano L, Barón-Esquivias G, Bogaert J, Brucato A, Gueret P, Klingel K, Lionis C, Maisch B, Mayosi B, Pavie A, Ristić AD, Tenas MS, Seferovic P, Swedberg K, Tomkowski W, ESC Scientific Document Group. 2015 ESC Guidelines for the diagnosis and management of pericardial diseases: the Task Force for the Diagnosis and Management of Pericardial Diseases of the European Society of Cardiology (ESC) Endorsed by: the European Association for Cardio-Thoracic Surgery (EACTS). Eur Heart J. 2015;36(42):2921–64. https://doi.org/10.1093/eurheartj/ehv318.

Part VI

Shock

24 Cardiogenic Shock

Courtney Bennett and Amanda Solberg

Introduction

Cardiogenic shock (CS) is a life-threatening state of end-organ hypoperfusion secondary to low cardiac output (CO). CS is associated with significant in-hospital mortality and significant healthcare cost. Mortality rates have been documented in excess of 80% despite modern therapies [1, 2].

Over the last several years, there has been a subtle shift in etiology of CS as early identification and treatment of acute coronary syndrome (ACS) have become the standard of care. Myocardial infarction (MI) remains the most prevalent etiology with mortality reported as greater than 35% [1], but CS secondary to advanced heart failure is now commonly seen in the cardiac intensive care unit (CICU) setting around the country [1, 3].

Differentiating Shock

Shock is a state of circulatory failure, which leads to cellular and tissue hypoxia. There are multiple underlying etiologies of shock based on the mechanism of hypoperfusion. The classifications include cardiogenic, distributive, obstructive, hypovolemic, and neurogenic (Table 24.1). In this chapter, we will focus on cardiogenic shock, but it is important to recognize the other causes and that patients may have a combination of more than one type of shock.

C. Bennett · A. Solberg (✉)
Mayo Clinic, Rochester, MN, USA
e-mail: Bennett.Courtney@mayo.edu; Solberg.Amanda@mayo.edu

R. Musialowski, K. Allshouse (eds.), *Cardiovascular Manual for the Advanced Practice Provider*,
https://doi.org/10.1007/978-3-031-35819-7_24

Table 24.1 Classification of shock and expected hemodynamic responses

Classification of Shock					
	Heart Rate	**Cardiac Output**	**CVP**	**PCWP**	**SVR**
Cardiogenic	↑	↓	↔↑	↑	↑
Distributive -Septic -Anaphylactic	↑	↑	↔↓	↓	↓
Obstructive -Tamponade -PE -Pneumothorax	↑	↓	↑	↓	↑
Hypovolemia	↑	↓	↔↓	↓	↑
Neurogenic	↑	↓	↔↓	↓	↓

Pathophysiology

Cardiogenic shock is a condition of decreased myocardial contractility secondary to underlying cardiac dysfunction and hypotension causing hypoperfusion of the myocardium and other end organs. This hypoperfusion causes even more ischemia to cardiac tissue, which further reduces low stroke volume and worsens diastolic filling. This cycle can progress rapidly leading to patient death if not treated.

As cardiac output decreases, intrinsic compensatory mechanisms designed to raise blood pressure cause vasoconstriction and fluid retention. This is reflected as increased systemic vascular resistance (SVR) and elevated pulmonary capillary wedge pressure (PCWP). In CS, these mechanisms become maladaptive and cause an increase in myocardial oxygen requirements, further worsening myocardial dysfunction.

Catecholamines are released by the sympathetic nervous system in an attempt to increase stroke volume by raising the heart rate and constricting blood vessels. Simultaneously, the renin-angiotensin-aldosterone system is activated when the renal system is poorly perfused and attempts to increase blood volume. Fluid is then retained in an attempt to raise blood pressure, which increases both preload and afterload. As the myocardium is stretched, brain natriuretic peptide (BNP) is released and further contributes to the physiologic cycle.

The goal of these intrinsic mechanisms is to increase cardiac output by raising preload, stroke volume, and heart rate. However, if left unchecked, they increase the myocardial workload leading to worsening cardiac output, decreased tissue perfusion, hypotension, ischemia, and ultimately myocardial dysfunction with remodeling [4].

End-organ dysfunction occurs secondary to tissue hypoperfusion. When systemic tissue is hypoperfused, an inflammatory process is triggered. This inflammatory process leads to the release of cytokines and nitric oxide, which cause vasodilation in the microcirculation, further affecting blood pressure and worsening hypoperfusion. As vasodilation occurs, oxygen delivery decreases and ischemia develops [5, 6]. Poor tissue perfusion and hypoxia lead to the development of lactic acidosis.

Clinical Presentation

History and Physical

Past medical history is key to the workup of CS. Myocardial infarction, particularly ST-elevation MI, is the most common cause of CS, and anterior MI is the most likely to develop CS. Any primary cardiac diagnosis that causes myocardial dysfunction can deteriorate to CS. Chronic heart failure (HF) can deteriorate into an acute decompensated state and now accounts for as much as 30% of CS presentations [2]. Other causes of CS include cardiac arrest, valvular heart disease, tamponade, myocarditis, congenital heart disease, hypertrophic cardiomyopathy, refractory ventricular tachycardia, apical ballooning, pulmonary hypertension, and PE [3, 5, 6].

Patients may present with a variety of symptoms and/or feelings that include chest pain, dyspnea, PND/orthopnea, syncope, presyncope, progressive fatigue, and palpitations. Physical exam findings may include pallor, cyanosis, or mottling of the skin. Assessment of the extremities for strength of pulses and temperature can provide an understanding of the patient's perfusion status. Cardiac auscultation may reveal extra heart sounds, particularly an S3 being indicative of HF, or murmurs. Evaluation of elevated jugular venous pressure, pulsatile liver, significant hepatojugular reflex, ascites, and lower extremity edema may be helpful in determining the patient's volume status, as well as assessment of the lungs for rales suggestive of pulmonary edema.

Patients with CS may present with symptoms consistent with their underlying pathology, and the physical exam will be dictated by the CS phenotype [2]. Three phenotypes of CS exist. These phenotypes are categorized according to volume status and cardiac output or peripheral exam. Clinically, phenotypes can be broken down into warm or cold and wet or dry (Table 24.2). The first phenotype is described as classic CS. Patients will have evidence of decreased CO, increased SVR, and evidence of increased preload. Euvolemic CS also has evidence of decreased cardiac output and increased SVR, but preload is normal. Mixed or vasodilatory CS is a decrease in CO and increase in preload, but the SVR is normal to low. Lastly, vasodilatory shock which is non-cardiogenic is described as an increase in CO, with decreased preload and afterload.

When there is clinical evidence for CS, assessment of the severity is crucial to understanding the patient's risk for deterioration and overall prognosis. Clinical evidence of CS may include ashen or mottled appearance, cold and clammy to the touch, elevated lactate (>2.0), rales on physical exam, evidence of organ involvement including transaminitis or rise in creatinine (double in creatine or 50% decrease of GFR), hypotension (systolic BP <90, MAP <60), and altered mental status [7].

The Killip classification assessment can be of value when attempting to determine the patient's overall clinical picture and mortality risk [8]. This system relies on the physical exam for appropriate classification. Killip Class I was defined as no evidence of heart failure. Class II was defined as heart failure with the presence of an S3 and rales on physical exam. Class III was defined as severe heart failure which included the presence of significant pulmonary edema. Class IV was defined as frank cardiogenic shock.

Table 24.2 Clinical presentation of CS

		Volume status	
		Wet	Dry
Peripheral exam	Cold	Cardiogenic shock	Euvolemic cardiogenic shock
	Warm	Mixed shock	Vasodilatory shock (not CS)

Identification and management of early stages of CS can prevent further deterioration. The Society for Cardiovascular Angiography and Intervention (SCAI) has developed a classification for CS (Fig. 24.1) [7]. The SCAI classification includes five stages of increased CS severity. Stage A identifies patients at risk. Stage B identifies patients beginning to show signs of deterioration. These patients develop hypotension and/or tachycardia without evidence of hypoperfusion but require intervention to prevent the development of end-organ damage. Stage C is classic CS. The patient has frank evidence of hypoperfusion and requires hemodynamic intervention. Stage D is CS that continues to worsen despite intervention and escalation of therapy. Stage E is refractory CS [7].

Diagnostic Studies

An electrocardiogram (ECG) should be performed within 10 min of patient arrival [4, 5]. As MI is the most common cause of CS, assessment of ST-segments and T-wave abnormalities is crucial. In addition, ECG can determine rhythm and underlying conduction.

Laboratory workup is a crucial part of evaluating end-organ involvement. Troponins should be drawn at baseline. Troponin I or T is acceptable, although recently institutions have transitioned to high sensitivity troponins. Isolated troponin elevation in the absence of ACS is not specific but is a strong predictor of mortality when significantly elevated. A complete blood count to include hemoglobin and white blood cell count will be important to assess for underlying signs of anemia and infection. Electrolytes, creatinine, and cystatin C for kidney function assessment, liver function tests with INR, LDH, and lactate. Elevated lactate levels are associated with increased mortality in patients with CS [4].

NT proBNP can be helpful for differentiating the etiology of shortness of breath and for prognosis. ACS patients with increased BNP levels are at increased risk of mortality [4].

A point-of-care ultrasound (POCUS) exam of the heart, lungs, and IVC can add valuable infor-

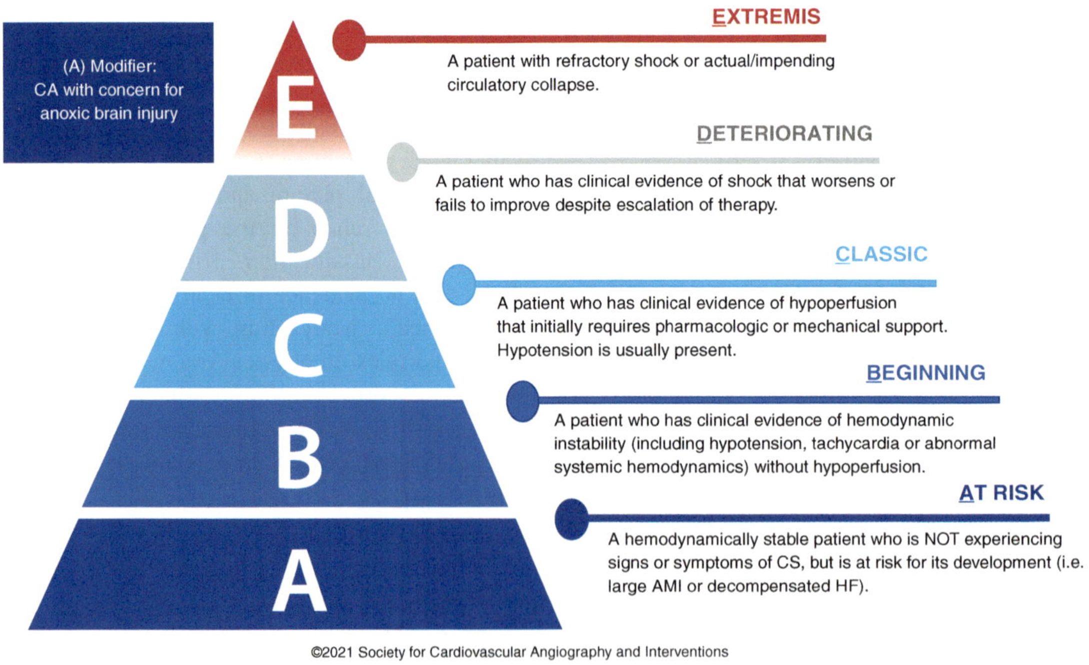

Fig. 24.1 SCAI cardiogenic shock stages classifies patients in or at risk for CS according to clinical status. (Permission granted by Naidu et al. [9])

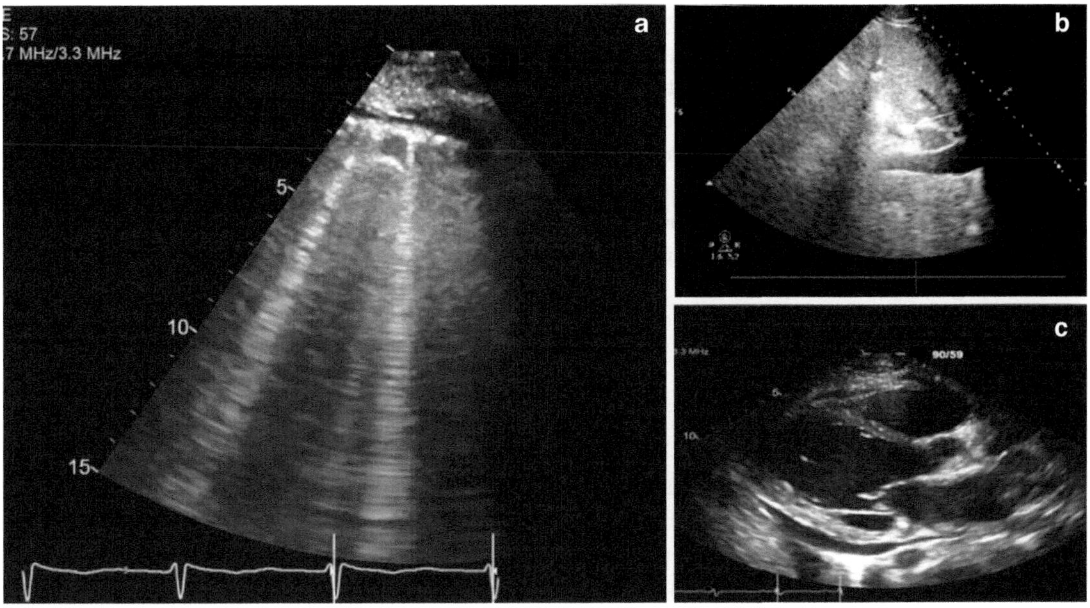

Fig. 24.2 (**a**) B-lines consistent with pulmonary edema present on lung imaging, (**b**) dilated IVC consistent with increased preload, and (**c**) dilated left ventricle with a small circumferential pericardial effusion

mation to your physical exam. POCUS is a goal-directed ultrasound and does not take the place of a formal transthoracic echocardiogram (TTE). Figure 24.2 demonstrates an example of the constellation of finding on POCUS in a patient with CS. Formal TTE should be a standard of care and be performed as part of the CS repertoire. A TTE adds valuable information about cardiac structure and function and will further define the direction of care.

Chest X-ray should also be performed and can help differentiate infection from pulmonary edema or other etiology during evaluation for CS.

Management

Once CS has been identified, the goal of therapy is to maintain adequate tissue perfusion. Management should be geared toward circulatory support, ventricular unloading, and myocardial perfusion. The underlying cause of CS must be identified and managed while simultaneously providing supportive care. As the most common cause of CS remains ACS, early consideration for reperfusion therapy will be of utmost importance [5].

The cornerstone of treating patients with confirmed or suspected CS is getting the patient to the correct level of care. Patients with CS should be triaged to a setting that offers percutaneous coronary intervention (PCI), mechanical circulatory support (MCS), a Cardiac Intensive Care Unit (CICU), and cardiac transplant capabilities [10].

As patients with CS are commonly volume overloaded and develop pulmonary edema, ensuring an adequate airway and oxygenation is crucial. In the setting of acute decompensated heart failure and CS, noninvasive positive pressure ventilation (NIPPV) is required to optimize ventilation and oxygenation. NIPPV recruits lung tissue resulting in an increase in oxygenation and a decrease in work of breathing. If noninvasive positive pressure ventilation is felt to be inadequate, then consider mechanical ventilation with the goal of lung protection ventilation and oxygenation [10, 11].

Continuous hemodynamic monitoring is an important aspect of managing CS. Using arterial lines for continuous blood pressure management and pulmonary artery catheters (PAC) to titrate medications and guide additional therapy can be helpful. If a PAC is unavailable or there is a contraindication, then a central line or a PICC line can also provide the ability to monitor hemodynamics and give central access for vasoactive medications. There are also minimally invasive hemodynamic monitors available, and noninvasive measures of hemodynamic parameters can be obtained with echocardiography.

Historically, PAC were used regularly in post MI patients. Subsequent literature demonstrated a correlation between PA catheter use and increase in mortality, and routine PAC use is no longer recommended for MI. Despite decline in use, PAC remain the standard for hemodynamic monitoring in the setting of moderate to severe CS. Careful patient assessment and risk evaluation should continue when deciding on monitoring. Complications include bleeding, embolism, infection, pulmonary infarct or hemorrhage, and inaccurate data collection.

Continuous hemodynamic monitoring with PAC can provide real-time feedback for care teams to react and adjust treatments. PAC consist of ports enabled to transduce right atrial pressure, pulmonary arterial pressure with the ability to measure a PCWP tracing, and mixed venous oxygen saturation. From these measurements, CO, SVR, PVR, cardio power output (CPO), and pulmonary artery pulsatility index (PAPi) can be calculated.

CO and cardiac index (CI) can be obtained via thermodilution, which is considered the most accurate, or by Fick calculation. Thermodilution is a procedure performed at the bedside ideally using a dedicated rapid injector. Normal saline is rapidly injected into the RA port of the PAC, and a thermistor monitors the temperature from the RA to the PA. Limitations to the thermodilution method include less reliable readings associated with tricuspid valve regurgitation and ventricular septal defects [12].

A CO and CI calculated by Fick can be done as an alternative. The Fick calculation takes into account oxygen consumption (VO_2), height, weight, SaO_2 from an ABG, SvO_2 from a PAC, hemoglobin, heart rate, and age.

$$CO = \frac{VO_2}{\left[\left(SaO_2 - SvO_2\right) \times hgb \times 13.4\right]}$$

$$CI = \frac{CO}{BSA}$$

To maintain tissue perfusion, CS management should be focused on increasing CO. CO is improved by increasing the heart rate and the stroke volume. Inotrope support is the first line for increasing stroke volume, improving contractility, and off-loading pressures working against failing ventricles. In the CICU, there are common IV inotropes used regularly for the treatment of CS (Tables 24.3 and 24.4). Each has pros and cons for use, and each should be chosen carefully based on the patient's clinical picture. Monitoring should be based on signs of end-organ function including lactate, creatinine, urine output, skin temperature, and mottling.

Dobutamine is a fast-acting beta receptor agonist with strong beta-1 stimulation and some beta-2 stimulation. It is a typical first-line IV agent for inotropic support in the treatment of CS [13]. In addition to inotropy, dobutamine causes vasodilation and therefore has some afterload reduction effect. The combination of increased cardiac contractility and decreased afterload improves stroke volume and therefore increases CO. Dobutamine has side effects including increased heart rate and is known to be proarrhythmic. The onset of action of dobutamine can be seen within minutes of initiation. Dosing should be started low and increased as needed. Typical dose initiation is 2.5 μg/kg/min.

Milrinone is a phosphodiesterase inhibitor, which helps to activate beta receptors. This results in an inotropic effect in the heart with beta-1 receptor activation and pulmonary and

Table 24.3 Differentiating SVO_2 and $ScVO_2$ when trending in CS

SVO_2 vs $ScVO_2$
• **SVO_2** is a true mixed venous sample from the distal port of PAC
• **$ScVO_2$** can be used as a substitute and is obtained from a central line, or proximal port of PAC. Central venous saturation is higher because the low oxygen content from the coronary sinus is not included

Table 24.4 Common inotropes and vasopressors used for management of CS

Inotropes and vasopressors				
	Mechanism	Half-life	Dose range	Considerations
Milrinone	Phosphodiesterase inhibitor	2.3 h	0.1–0.5 µg/kg/min	– Can accumulate in renal failure
Dobutamine	Strong beta receptor agonist	<2 min	2–10 µg/kg/min	– Proarrhythmic
Dopamine	Dopaminergic receptor agonist, alpha and beta agonist at higher doses	<2 min	2–10 µg/kg/min	– Known to be proarrhythmic – Associated with higher mortality – First choice when heart rate is low
Epinephrine	Strong alpha and beta agonist	<5 min	0.01–0.3 µg/kg/min	– Proarrhythmic – Associated with high lactate levels
Norepinephrine	Strong alpha agonist, weaker beta agonist	1–2 min	0.01–0.3 µg/kg/min	– Offers some mild inotrope effect – Associated with less arrhythmia side effects
Vasopressin	Vasopressin receptor agonist in vascular smooth muscle	10–20 min	0.03–0.06 µg	– Pure vasoconstrictor

systemic vasodilation with beta-2 receptor activation. Milrinone has a slower onset of action than dobutamine. In addition, because milrinone is renally cleared, accumulation of the drug can occur and cause worsening side effects including arrhythmias and hypotension.

Studies suggest increased mortality with the use of dopamine in patients with CS [2]. It has both inotropic and vasopressor activity. At low doses (0.5–2 µg/kg/min), the effects are primarily dopaminergic with peripheral vasodilation. Intermediate doses (2–10 µg/kg/min) have primarily beta-1-adrenergic effect with increased cardiac contractility, heart rate, and blood pressure. Doses >10 µg/kg/min have alpha-adrenergic effect with primary vasoconstriction and increased blood pressure.

Epinephrine is considered a second-line medication that acts as both inotrope and vasopressor. At lower doses, epinephrine acts more as an inotrope given strong beta receptor agonist properties. Epinephrine is proarrhythmic and can therefore be problematic in the setting of underlying cardiac dysfunction. In addition, epinephrine is associated with high lactate levels. Dose range is similar to norepinephrine ranging from 0.01 to 0.3 µg/kg/min.

Vasopressor support in the setting of hypotension should be used to support tissue perfusion with the goal to maintain MAP greater than 65 mmHg in conjunction with other therapies. Norepinephrine has been a standard first-line vasopressor agent commonly used to treat hypotensive states like septic shock. Norepinephrine offers vasoconstriction and mild inotrope effect.

Afterload reduction should be considered if tolerated by blood pressure. Afterload reduction can assist with improving CO by decreasing cardiac oxygen demands. If IV afterload reduction is necessary, consider nitroglycerin, clevidipine, or nitroprusside for short-term therapy with plans to transition to an oral agent based on clinical picture including kidney function.

Long-Term Care

Although mortality is high, patients can recover. The patient should be supported while decompensated with plans to intervene and treat their underlying cardiac dysfunction.

Guideline-directed medical therapy (GDMT) for the treatment of heart failure should be considered in patients who have recovered from CS. Beta blockers, ACE inhibitors, and other evidence-based therapies can be initiated when the patient is close to a euvolemic state and weaning off IV inotrope and vasopressor agents. Afterload reduction can be transitioned to an oral regimen based on kidney function and diagnosis. Inotrope support may continue. Some patients remain on long-term inotropes in the outpatient setting as a bridge to transplant or as palliative support for quality of life.

Clinical Pearls

- Patients with confirmed or suspected CS should be triaged to a setting that offers PCI capabilities and a CICU.
- Evaluation and treatment of underlying cardiac dysfunction should continue while supporting patients in CS. ACS is the most common etiology of CS and should be ruled out immediately upon presentation.
- To maintain tissue perfusion, CS management should be focused on increasing CO. Inotrope support is the first line for increasing stroke volume, improving contractility, and offloading pressures working against failing ventricles.
- Ongoing risk assessment in the setting of CS is crucial. Risk assessment tools including the SCAI shock stages and Killip classification should be considered for mortality prediction.
- MCS consideration and cardiac transplant evaluation are warranted in patients with refractory CS.
- Early involvement of palliative care can assist with goals of care discussions and symptom management and can be particularly useful in the setting of chronic end-stage heart failure.
- GDMT for the treatment for heart failure should be considered in patients who have recovered from CS.

References

1. O'Brien C, Beaubien-Souligny W, Amsallem M, Denault A, Haddad F. Cardiogenic shock: reflections at the crossroad between perfusion, tissue hypoxia, and mitochondrial function. Can J Cardiol. 2020;36(2):184–96.
2. van Diepen S, Katz JN, Albert NM, Henry TD, Jacobs AK, Kapur NK, et al. Contemporary management of cardiogenic shock: a scientific statement from the American Heart Association. Circulation. 2017;136(16):e232–e68.
3. Brener MI, Rosenblum HR, Burkhoff D. Pathophysiology and advanced hemodynamic assessment of cardiogenic shock. Methodist Debakey Cardiovasc J. 2020;16(1):7–15.
4. Vahdatpour C, Collins D, Goldberg S. Cardiogenic shock. J Am Heart Assoc. 2019;8(8):e011991.
5. Bertini P, Guarracino F. Pathophysiology of cardiogenic shock. Curr Opin Crit Care. 2021;27(4):409–15.
6. Lim HS. Cardiogenic shock: failure of oxygen delivery and oxygen utilization. Clin Cardiol. 2016;39(8):477–83.
7. Baran DA, Grines CL, Bailey S, Burkhoff D, Hall SA, Henry TD, et al. SCAI clinical expert consensus statement on the classification of cardiogenic shock: this document was endorsed by the American College of Cardiology (ACC), the American Heart Association (AHA), the Society of Critical Care Medicine (SCCM), and the Society of Thoracic Surgeons (STS) in April 2019. Catheter Cardiovasc Interv. 2019;94(1):29–37.
8. Killip T III, Kimball JT. Treatment of myocardial infarction in a coronary care unit. A two year experience with 250 patients. Am J Cardiol. 1967;20(4):457–64.
9. Naidu SS, Baran DA, Jentzer JC, Hollenberg SM, van Diepen S, Basir MB, et al. SCAI SHOCK stage classification expert consensus update: a review and incorporation of validation studies: this statement was endorsed by the American College of Cardiology (ACC), American College of Emergency Physicians (ACEP), American Heart Association (AHA), European Society of Cardiology (ESC) Association for Acute Cardiovascular Care (ACVC), International Society for Heart and Lung Transplantation (ISHLT), Society of Critical Care Medicine (SCCM), and Society of Thoracic Surgeons (STS) in December 2021. J Am Coll Cardiol. 2022;79(9):933–46.
10. Jentzer JC, Tabi M, Burstein B. Managing the first 120 min of cardiogenic shock: from resuscitation to diagnosis. Curr Opin Crit Care. 2021;27(4):416–25.
11. Alviar CL, Miller PE, McAreavey D, Katz JN, Lee B, Moriyama B, et al. Positive pressure ventilation in the cardiac intensive care unit. J Am Coll Cardiol. 2018;72(13):1532–53.
12. Argueta EE, Paniagua D. Thermodilution cardiac output: a concept over 250 years in the making. Cardiol Rev. 2019;27(3):138–44.
13. Jentzer JC, Coons JC, Link CB, Schmidhofer M. Pharmacotherapy update on the use of vasopressors and inotropes in the intensive care unit. J Cardiovasc Pharmacol Ther. 2015;20(3):249–60.

25 Introduction to Mechanical Support

Courtney Bennett and Amanda Solberg

Intro to Support Devices

Mechanical circulatory support (MCS) devices are designed to support patients, while they are acutely decompensated, or to support them through high-risk procedures to prevent decompensation. MCS devices are designed to augment vasopressor and inotrope therapy as a way to decrease preload, afterload, and oxygen consumption by the heart. Long-term mechanical support devices are also available and are used as a bridge to transplantation, bridge to decision, destination therapy, or bridge to recovery.

There are several MCS options, each with varying evidence supporting their use (Table 25.1). MCS devices can be placed surgically or percutaneously. The main MCS devices used today include intra-aortic balloon pump (IABP), percutaneous ventricular assist device (pVAD), extracorporeal membrane oxygenation (ECMO), and implanted ventricular assist devices (VAD).

Complications include death, infection, limb ischemia, embolic events, bleeding, hemolysis, and malposition [1]. These complications may be worsened depending on patient comorbidities. Careful patient selection for MCS is warranted. Each patient should undergo a robust multidisciplinary evaluation to determine candidacy if able. It is also recommended that prompt evaluation by the MCS team should be made in patients with CS to facilitate recovery [1].

C. Bennett · A. Solberg (✉)
Mayo Clinic, Rochester, MN, USA
e-mail: Bennett.Courtney@mayo.edu; Solberg.Amanda@mayo.edu

R. Musialowski, K. Allshouse (eds.), *Cardiovascular Manual for the Advanced Practice Provider*,
https://doi.org/10.1007/978-3-031-35819-7_25

Table 25.1 MCS devices, their level of support, mechanism of action, and helpful information for each

Device	Description	Level of support (CO)	Placement	Mechanism of action	Indication/ contraindication Pros/cons
IABP (temporary)	– Increase SV – Decrease afterload – Perfuse coronary arteries	0.5–1 L/min	– Femoral access – Sits in descending aorta	– Timed balloon inflation during diastole increases coronary artery perfusion, and rapid deflation during systole reduces afterload	– Risk for limb and organ ischemia, atherosclerotic embolization, and hemolysis – Monitor distal pulses, device placement with CXR, CBC, and renal function – Used as first-line MCS despite mixed evidence – Patient is limited to best rest with maximum HOB elevation to 30° – Recent ability to place axillary to allow patient ambulation at some institutions
pVAD (temporary)	– Reduce oxygen consumption of LV – Decrease diastolic volume of LV	2.5–5.5 L/min depending on the device	– Femoral access – Sits in the ventricle, flows into aorta	– An axillary flow catheter pulls blood from the ventricle and pushes blood to aorta	– High risk for hemolysis and leg ischemia – Monitor distal pulses, CBC, LDH, plasma-free hemoglobin
V-A ECMO (temporary)	– Provides both respiratory and circulatory support	Up to 6 L/min	– Peripheral or central cannulation – Venous cannula at the level of the right atrium, and arterial cannula in the aorta or femoral artery	– Blood is pumped to an extracorporal machine, blood is oxygenated, and carbon dioxide is removed	– High risk for limb ischemia with peripheral cannulation – The left ventricular may requiring venting
LVAD (long term)	– Reduce oxygen consumption of LV – Decrease diastolic volume of LV	Up to 8 L/min	– Placed via sternotomy	– Blood is removed from left ventricle and returned to the aorta	– Destination therapy bridge to decision, bridge to transplant, or bridge to recovery – No pulses will be auscultated in continuous flow devices – High risk of thrombotic events, GI bleed, and infection

Reference

1. van Diepen S, Katz JN, Albert NM, Henry TD, Jacobs AK, Kapur NK, et al. Contemporary management of cardiogenic shock: a scientific statement from the American Heart Association. Circulation. 2017;136(16):e232–68.

Part VII

Peripheral Vascular Disease

Frank R. Arko III

Introduction

Vascular disease encompasses a wide span of disease processes involving the arterial and venous systems. Much of the pathology in vascular surgery is chronic in nature but each disease process can present in the acute setting and when this occurs, we see high incidences of morbidity and mortality. In this chapter, we will define the common diagnoses seen in the vascular surgery scope to include aortic dissection and aneurysms, peripheral arterial disease (PAD), carotid artery disease, and deep vein thrombosis (DVT).

Aortic pathology can be life threatening if not appropriately managed and regularly followed in the outpatient setting. Therefore, it is imperative that we discuss in detail the acute management of aortic disease as well as the long-term goals of therapy for our patients. Complicated acute type B aortic dissection (TBAD) can present with life threatening end organ ischemia, aortic rupture, spinal cord ischemia, or limb ischemia. Chronic aortic dissections can present with aneurysmal degeneration, arterial stenosis, compressive symptoms, and risk of aortic rupture. A mainstay of treatment in aortic disease centers around adequate blood pressure control and regular vascular surgery follow-up with imaging to survey aortic size.

PAD is a chronic process that develops over time due to atherosclerosis of the arteries related to common risk factors including age, cholesterol, smoking history, diabetes, and hypertension. Atherosclerotic disease is important to discuss and understand as patients present with a wide scope of symptoms from asymptomatic, to lifestyle limiting claudication and in severe cases of PAD, rest pain and even limb loss. PAD can affect the great vessels of the aortic arch, the aorta, iliac arteries, arteries of the lower extremities and is commonly seen in areas of arterial bifurcations. The mainstay of treatment is

F. R. ArkoIII
Vascular and Endovascular Surgery, Atrium Health/Sanger Heart and Vascular Institute, Charlotte, NC, USA
e-mail: Frank.Arko@atriumhealth.org

medical therapy and modification of risk factors and interventional therapy is usually guided based on the patient's quality of life with the goal of reducing symptoms.

Initially a DVT is an acute thrombotic event that over time will develop into chronic thrombus and scarring within the venous system. Many patients presenting with DVT can be treated with anticoagulation alone but in the select group of patients with proximal DVT, interventional therapy can be recommended to reduce the long-term effects of thrombus burden. A major goal in the treatment of DVT is to reduce post-thrombotic syndrome and venous hypertension which can lead to chronic swelling, heaviness, leg fatigue, hemosiderin deposition, and lastly venous ulceration.

Carotid Artery Stenosis (CAS)

26

Trent Gabriel and Frank R. Arko III

Anatomy and Physiology

The carotid arteries are the predominate vessels that supply blood to the head and neck. The right common carotid artery (RCCA) originates from the brachiocephalic artery, whereas the left common carotid artery (LCCA) originates directly from the aortic arch. Both CCAs bifurcate in the neck at the level of the carotid sinus into two branches. The external carotid arteries (ECAs) supply the neck and face with arterial blood, whereas the internal carotid arteries (ICAs) supply the brain. To further specify location, the carotid arteries are located posterior to the sternoclavicular joints and are protected as they lie within the carotid sheath, which is a fibrinous connective tissue that also contains the internal jugular veins and the vagus nerve. For most patients, the bifurcation of the CCAs into the ECAs and ICAs occurs at the level of the upper border of the thyroid cartilage and roughly the level of the fourth or fifth cervical vertebrae. At the bifurcation, there is the carotid body as well as the carotid sinus. The carotid body is a chemoreceptor that works to detect the levels of PO_2, PCO_2, and pH of the blood that passes through the bifurcation into the brain and face. This mainly works to alert the brain of the need to increase respiratory rate. The carotid sinus is a baroreceptor that responds to changes in the stretch of the blood vessel and helps to maintain blood pressure (Fig. 26.1).

T. Gabriel (✉)
Atrium Health/Sanger Heart and Vascular Institute, Charlotte, NC, USA
e-mail: benjamin.gabriel@atriumhealth.org

F. R. Arko III
Vascular and Endovascular Surgery, Atrium Health/Sanger Heart and Vascular Institute, Charlotte, NC, USA
e-mail: Frank.Arko@atriumhealth.org

R. Musialowski, K. Allshouse (eds.), *Cardiovascular Manual for the Advanced Practice Provider*,
https://doi.org/10.1007/978-3-031-35819-7_26

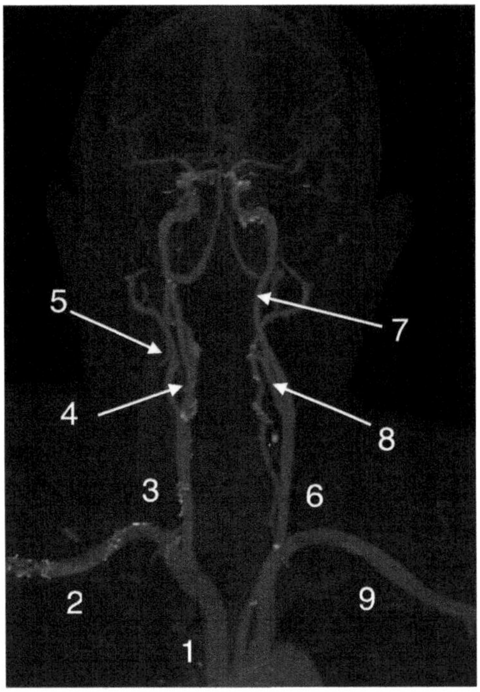

1. Brachiocephalic artery
2. Right subclavian
3. Right common carotid artery
4. Right internal carotid artery
5. Right external carotid artery
6. Left common carotid artery
7. Left internal carotid artery
8. Left external carotid artery
9. Left subclavian artery

Fig. 26.1 Carotid anatomy

Pathology/Pathophysiology of Carotid Artery Stenosis

There are several potential causes of CAS with the most common being the development of atherosclerosis, fibromuscular dysplasia, anatomical variances, carotid artery aneurysms, Takayasu's arteritis, radiation therapy injuries, and carotid body tumors.

Far and away the most common cause of CAS is the development of atherosclerosis. One of the prominent reasons the development of atherosclerosis can specifically affect the CCAs is the anatomy of the arterial bifurcation. The hemodynamics of the blood flow through this channel with associated fluctuations of shear stress can predispose regions with lower flow velocity (i.e., the carotid bifurcation) to development of atherosclerotic plaques. The hemodynamics of arterial flow at the carotid bifurcation can significantly increase the likelihood of atherosclerotic plaque, reducing vessel lumen diameter, and increasing risk of thrombotic or embolic event (Fig. 26.2).

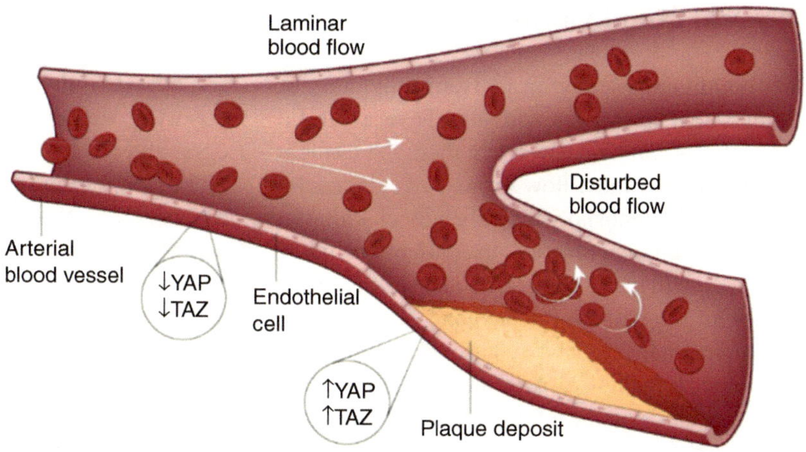

Fig. 26.2 Turbulent flow in CAS development ([1], Figure 1)

Plaques form in part due to the inflammatory response (platelet deposition, smooth muscle cell proliferation, and slow accumulation of lipoproteins) involved in the repair process. The atherosclerotic plaques form due to several reasons, including elevated blood cholesterol, long-term damage from smoking on the intima of the vessel wall, chronically elevated blood glucose, and genetic predisposition (Chap. 27).

Presentation of CAS

Patients with carotid artery disease can present with or without neurological symptoms. Symptomatology and degree of stenosis are both considered when evaluating for surgical revascularization. Patients with symptomatic carotid artery disease may present with a myriad of neurological symptoms (Table 26.1) and may be revascularized at a lower degree of stenosis, whereas patients with asymptomatic carotid artery disease may be revascularized at a higher degree of stenosis.

Table 26.1 Common historical features to consider with CAS

Suggestive of symptomatic CAS	Commonly not associated with CAS
Amaurosis fugax—loss of vision in one eye	Dizziness/vertigo without loss of balance
Difficulty speaking or understanding	Syncope or near syncope
Loss of strength on contralateral side	Muscle tension headache
Numbness and sensory loss on contralateral side	Tinnitus
Facial droop	
Slurred speech	
Sudden severe headache	

Physical Examination

It is common to see referrals from providers for patients that have been found to have a carotid bruit. Bruits can be heard when there is turbulent blood flow that must flow around an atherosclerotic plaque (stenosis) within the vessel wall.

For best clinical practice, the patient should be evaluated with their head secure and slightly tilted back with the chin elevated. Stand or sit next to the patient on the right when auscultating the right ICA and ask them to look to their left. Repeat the same technique on the left (sit or stand to their left and have them look right). Stethoscope should be placed approximately 2–3 cm above the clavicle, and patient asked to briefly hold their breath as they are expiring. Reposition the stethoscope two to three times moving caudally toward the level of the bifurcation on both sides [2].

The presence or absence of a carotid bruit is not diagnostic for whether the patient has significant carotid artery stenosis. Additionally, carotid artery bruits are most often found to be benign. Multiple studies have shown varying degrees of specificity and sensitivity, with a consistent trend showing a positive bruit to be more specific than sensitive.

Imaging/Diagnostic Testing

There are four main diagnostic tests that are used to evaluate the degree of stenosis within carotid arteries: cerebral angiography, carotid duplex ultrasound (DUS), magnetic resonance angiography, and computed tomographic angiography. Also, there are three main methods of measuring the degree of stenosis: NASCET, ECST, and CC.

The first method of measuring carotid artery stenosis, the North American Symptomatic Carotid Endarterectomy Trial (NASCET), measures the residual lumen diameter at the most stenotic portion of the vessel and compares this with the lumen diameter in the normal ICA distal to the stenosis. This differs from the European Carotid Surgery Trial (ECST) which measures the lumen diameter at the most stenotic portion and compares this with the estimated probable original diameter at the site of maximum stenosis (Fig. 26.3). Lastly, the third most common method to measure carotid artery stenosis is the common carotid (CC) method which measures the residual lumen diameter at the most stenotic portion of the vessel and compares it to the lumen diameter in the proximal CCA.

Conventional Cerebral Angiography Pros of this diagnostic modality includes being able to evaluate the entire carotid artery system while also showing information about atherosclerotic disease, plaque morphology, and collateral circulation as well. However, the downside to this diagnostic imaging and the main reasons that it is rarely used are that it is invasive, quite expensive, and places patients at a slightly increased risk of morbidity (due to CVA) and mortality.

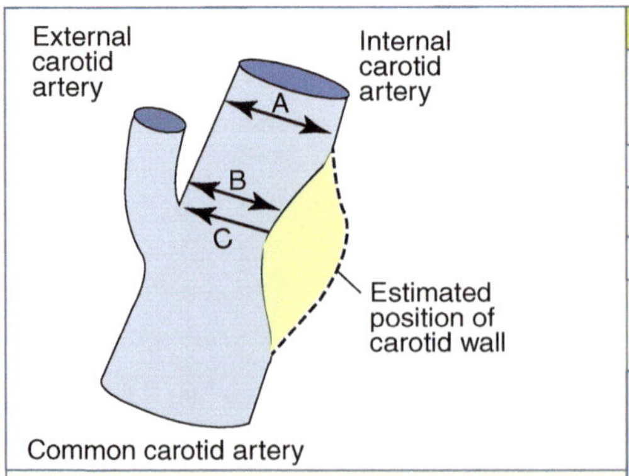

NASCET $\frac{A-B}{A}$ ECST $\frac{C-B}{C}$

NASCET	ECST
30	65
40	70
50	75
60	80
70	85
80	91
90	97

Approximate equivalent degrees of internal carotid artery stenosis used in NASCET and ESCT according to recent direct comparisons

Fig. 26.3 Assessing carotid stenosis severity ([3], Fig 4)

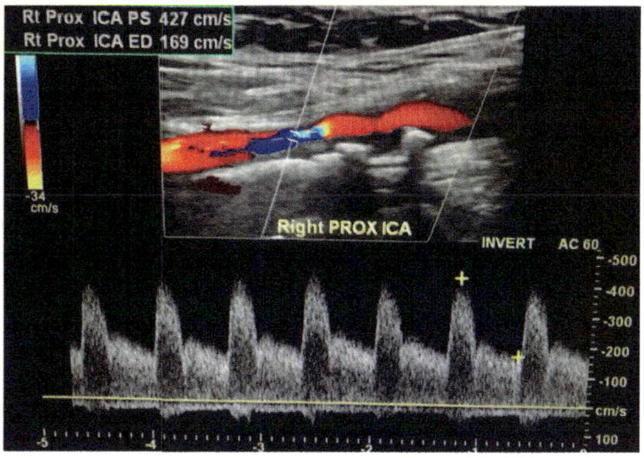

Fig. 26.4 Carotid duplex ultrasound with high-grade stenosis of the proximal ICA. *PS* peak systolic, *ED* end diastolic

Table 26.2 Duplex ultrasound evaluation for carotid severity: Atrium health vascular laboratory standardization values

Stenosis	ICA PSV (cm/s)	Plaque	ICA EDV (cm/s)	ICA/CCA PSV ratio
Normal	<125	None	<40	<2.0
<50%	<125	<50% diameter reduction	<40	<2.0
50–69%	≥125–230	>50% diameter reduction	≥40– ≤100	2.0–4.0
> 70%	>230	>50% diameter reduction	>100	>4.0
Near occlusion	High, low, or undetectable	Visible	Variable	Variable
Occlusion	Undetectable	Visible, no detection	Not applicable	Not applicable

CCA common carotid, *ICA* internal carotid, *EDV* end-diastolic velocity, *PSV* peak systolic velocity, *PSV ratio* carotid index

Carotid Artery Duplex Ultrasound (US) This imaging modality (Fig. 26.4) utilizes B-mode and Doppler US techniques to find focal increases in blood flow velocity which can be indicative of carotid artery stenosis. It combines data from the peak systolic velocity (PSV), end-diastolic velocity (EDV), spectral configuration, and the carotid index (ICA PSV to CCA PSV ratio). This imaging modality has been shown to be highly specific or highly sensitive for detecting a residual lumen diameter of <1.5 mm (Table 26.2). The benefits of this imaging modality include that it is noninvasive, safe, and relatively inexpensive. The downside to this specific imaging modality includes that near occlusions can be missed, the degree of stenosis can be overestimated, and the cervical portion of the ICA is best seen. The natural anatomic variances of patients make it difficult to obtain accurate results as well.

Magnetic Resonance Angiography This diagnostic image shows a 3D image of the carotid bifurcation with good sensitivity for detecting high-grade stenosis but less accurate for detecting moderate stenosis. Contraindications to potentially utilizing this modality are that MRA is more expensive, time-consuming, and less readily available. In addition, MRA is not a safe option for patients with significantly reduced kidney function.

Computed Tomography Angiography This imaging modality shows an in-depth anatomic depiction of the lumen, adjacent soft tissues, and bony structures (Fig. 26.5). It can be particularly useful when carotid duplex is not reliable. CTA is more readily available than MRA but still expensive. Lastly, impaired renal function is a relative contraindication.

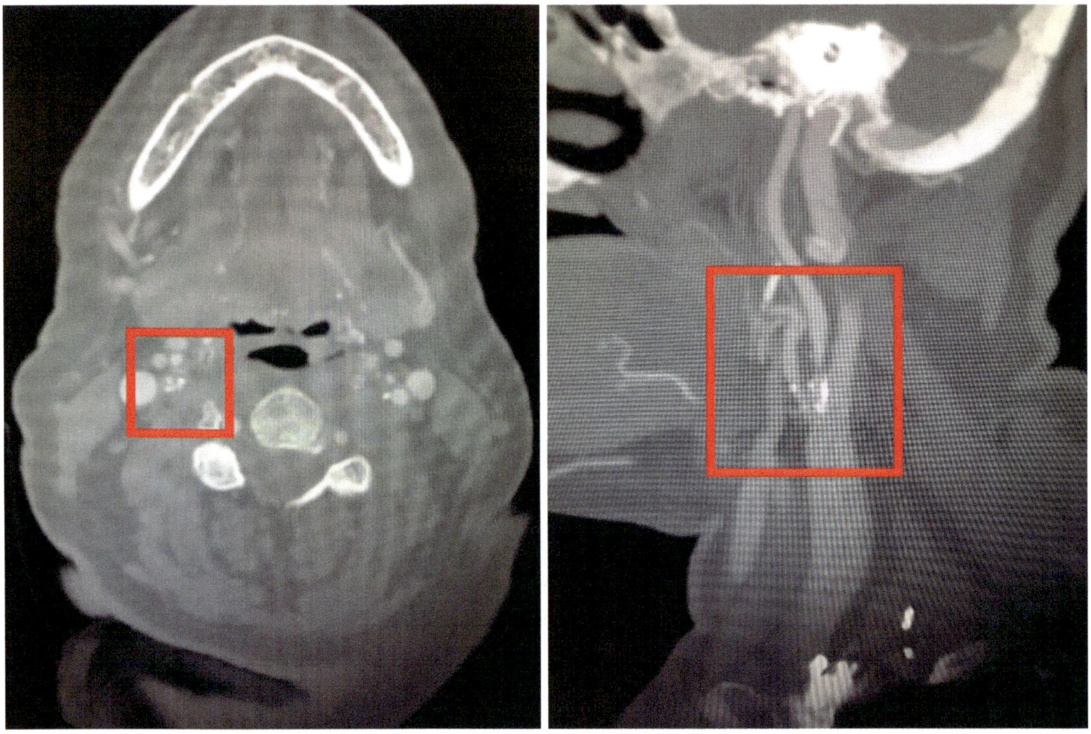

Fig. 26.5 CT angiography of the neck with 90% ICA stenosis (coronal and orbital views)

Management of Carotid Artery Stenosis

If the patient is asymptomatic, and there is less than <70% ICA stenosis, conservative management is the best option. Optimal medical therapy includes aspirin 81 mg and statin therapy. Statin medications have been proven through many studies to be very beneficial at reducing atherosclerotic plaque buildup as well as stabilizing existing plaque. Atorvastatin and rosuvastatin are most common as they have been shown to be the most efficacious as high potency statins. Dual antiplatelet therapy may be recommended. Modifiable risk factors that are encouraged include smoking cessation, routine exercise, adequate blood pressure control, blood glucose control, and adherence to medical regimen.

Surgical options for carotid revascularization include TCAR (transcarotid artery revascularization), transfemoral carotid artery stenting, CEA (carotid endarterectomy), and carotid artery bypass. These modalities are usually considered in symptomatic patients with stenotic disease.

Table 26.3 Qualifying characteristics for TCAR

>75 years of age
HFrEF <35%
CAD with >75% stenosis
Abnormal stress testing
Severe pulmonary disease
Prior head and neck radiation
Prior CEA with restenosis
Surgically inaccessible lesion
Contralateral occlusion
Able to use clopidogrel for 60 days

CEA This surgery is an open surgical procedure where the carotid artery is opened and the plaque within the vessel is removed, and the artery is repaired.

TCAR This surgery can be ideal for many high-risk surgical patients. Direct visualization of the diseased carotid and a reversal of flow away from the brain are established with a small pump removing debris and reducing embolic potential. A filter is utilized, and the blood is removed from the carotid artery and returned to the femoral vein. Once this reversed flow is safely established, stenting of the carotid lesion is undertaken with a reduction in the risk of neurologic injury. There are several qualifying factors for patients (Table 26.3).

Surveillance

Doppler ultrasound imaging is traditionally used for postoperative surveillance after carotid revascularization to evaluate patency or recurrent disease. Restenosis can occur after revascularizations due to in-stent restenosis or thrombosis in TCAR, intimal hyperplasia, thrombosis, or recurrent atherosclerotic disease after CEA.

Clinical Pearls

- The presence or absence of a carotid bruit does not correlate with the severity of extracranial carotid disease.
- Patients with risk factors, or known coronary, neurovascular, or peripheral arterial disease, should be screened for carotid artery disease.
- Symptomatology in conjunction with degree of stenosis will determine the need for carotid revascularization.
- TCAR may be a good surgical option for high-risk surgical patient meeting TCAR criteria.
- Ultrasound surveillance is needed after carotid intervention to assess for restenosis.

References

1. Mehta V, Tzima E. A turbulent path to plaque formation. Nature. 2016;540:531–2. https://doi.org/10.1038/nature20489.
2. Kass J, Krishnamohan P. Clinical overview: carotid artery stenosis. Elsevier. 1 Jan 2022. ClinicalKey. Accessed 14 Mar 2022.
3. Saxena A, Ng EYK, Lim ST. Imaging modalities to diagnose carotid artery stenosis: progress and prospect. Biomed Eng OnLine. 2019;18:66. https://doi.org/10.1186/s12938-019-0685-7.

Peripheral Arterial Disease (PAD) 27

Trent Gabriel, Amber Amick, and Frank R. Arko III

Anatomy

The body's circulatory system is made of an amazing network of vessels. Systemic arteries bring oxygenated blood flow from the heart to all the tissues and organs throughout the body, through tiny capillaries, and back to the heart via the venous system. The arterial system is continuous from the heart and structured to accommodate the high pressures of blood being ejected from the heart with each heartbeat. Arteries have three layers, the innermost being the intima, which is lined with endothelium. This single-celled layer is a continuous layer present throughout the arteries, capillaries, veins, heart valves, and endocardial surfaces. The intima secretes multiple factors that adjust vessel tone (vasodilation) and affect platelet aggregation and formation of thrombus. The middle layer, or media, of arteries is made of smooth muscles, elastin, and collagen and responds to signals along the intima. The outermost wall of arteries is the adventitia, made up of long fibrinous collagen chains, autonomic nerves, and vasa vasorum (perfuse external walls of larger vessels) [1] (*see* Fig. 28.1).

When evaluating the total arterial anatomy (Fig. 27.1), it may be easiest to start from the heart and follow the aortic arch into the brachiocephalic, common carotids, and subclavian arteries and continue into the head/neck/chest. These arteries are also called the great vessels. From the subclavian arteries, the arm will further perfuse via the axillary, brachial, radial, and ulnar arteries into the palmar arch and smaller arteries of the hands. Blood flow also continues from the arch to the descending aorta just left of the left subclavian artery and follows the thoracic aorta through the chest and past the diaphragm where the abdominal aorta will lead you to the visceral segment. Here you will find the celiac, superior mesenteric, bilateral renal, and inferior mesenteric arteries that supply blood flow to structures and organs of the abdomen. Proceed distally, and you will reach the common iliac arteries, where the aorta bifurcates into smaller arteries of the pelvis and provides inflow to the bilateral lower extremities. The iliac arteries will bifurcate into internal and external iliac arteries and then continue to the femoral arteries. The common femoral arteries will bifurcate into the profunda and superficial femoral arteries. The superficial femoral arteries will travel along the medial thighs posteriorly behind the knee where the popliteal artery will lead to the tibioperoneal trunk, peroneal artery,

T. Gabriel · A. Amick (✉)
Atrium Health/Sanger Heart and Vascular Institute, Charlotte, NC, USA
e-mail: benjamin.gabriel@atriumhealth.org; Amber.amick@atriumhealth.org

F. R. Arko III
Vascular and Endovascular Surgery, Atrium Health/Sanger Heart and Vascular Institute, Charlotte, NC, USA
e-mail: Frank.Arko@atriumhealth.org

R. Musialowski, K. Allshouse (eds.), *Cardiovascular Manual for the Advanced Practice Provider*,
https://doi.org/10.1007/978-3-031-35819-7_27

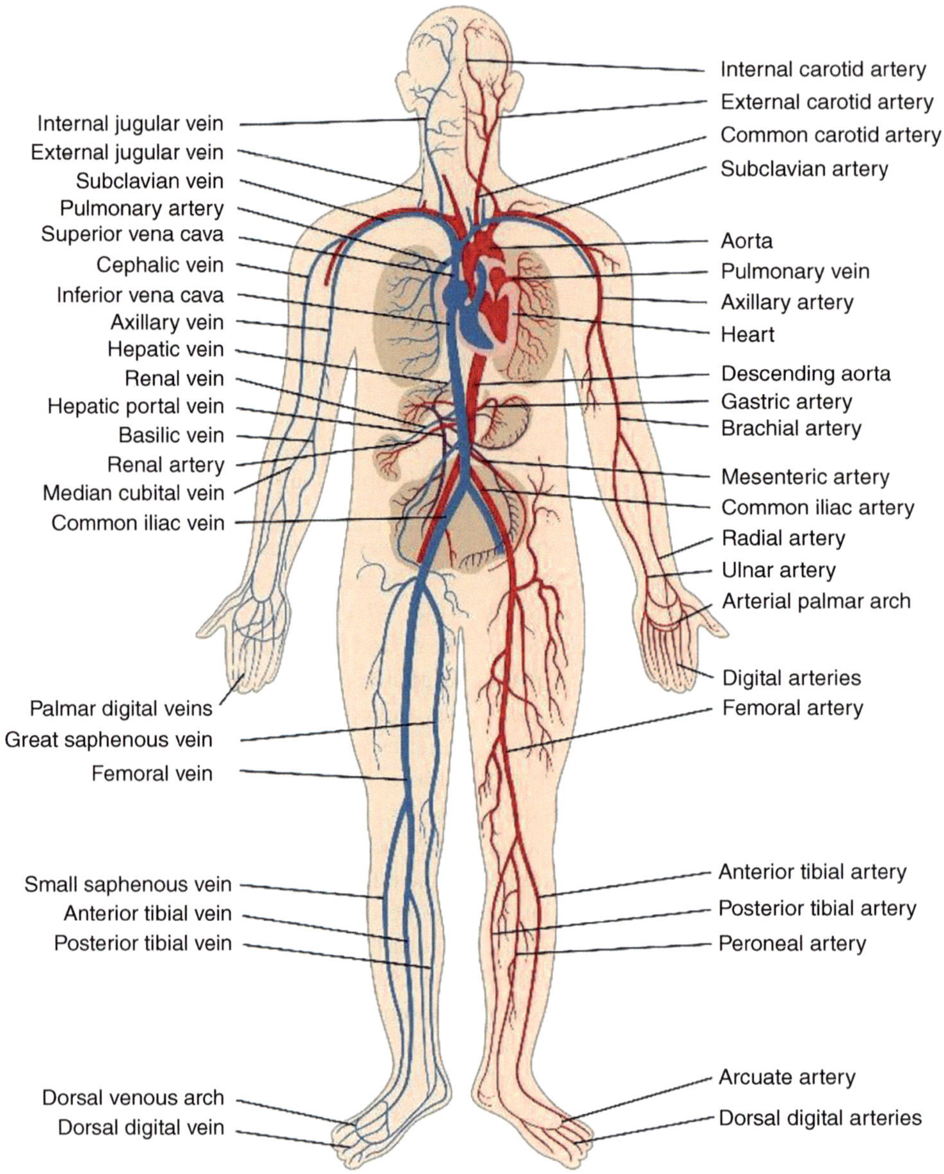

Fig. 27.1 Human circulatory system

posterior tibial artery, and the anterior tibial artery. These distal arteries will then perfuse the arteries of the foot.

Physical Examination

A clinician's physical exam should be thorough to best evaluate for PAD as well as to determine potential need for intervention. Upon inspection, a clinician may appreciate muscle atrophy, hair loss, color changes (cyanosis or pallor), ischemic tissue changes, wounds, or decreased motor function of an area affected by arterial insufficiency. When palpating, the clinician may note cooler temperatures along the skin which may correspond with the level of disease. The clinician should evaluate motion and sensation along the extremities, including hands, fingers, feet, and toes where the most distal arteries may be compromised. A clinician should evaluate their patient for palpable pulses (brachial, radial, ulnar, femoral, popliteal, posterior tibial, and dorsalis pedis), their quality, as well as if there is variation in laterality.

Pulse may be qualified as 0, absent; 1, diminished; 2, normal; and 3, bounding.

If pulses are nonpalpable, a clinician can further evaluate with a handheld Doppler while listening to the quality of arterial signals in the same anatomical locations – these may be described as triphasic, biphasic, monophasic, or absent arterial signals. In addition to auscultation via Doppler, a clinician may apply the bell of a stethoscope to evaluate for turbulent blood flow (i.e., bruit), which could indicate stenosis, fistula, and other vascular pathologies.

Pathology/Pathophysiology

Peripheral arterial disease (PAD) is a condition which is caused by atherosclerosis which reduces tissue perfusion over time. Atherosclerosis is the pathophysiologic process of accumulation of lipids and fibrous materials between the layers of the arterial wall, reducing the diameter of the arterial lumen, thereby limiting arterial blood flow to tissue [2]. This development of atherosclerosis over time leads to the formation of plaque which can eventually thrombose or rupture, causing occlusion of distal vessels (Fig. 27.2). PAD effects the lower extremities more often than the upper; however, PAD may occur anywhere in the body and manifests through varying degrees of symptoms based on the severity of disease, as well as collateralized blood flow. PAD is a chronic and progressive disease in which the severity of symptoms will worsen with time if not appropriately managed. In its mildest form, patients may present with abnormal test results but without symptoms. In mild to moderate disease, patients may experience symptoms such as nonlimiting or limiting claudication. The Rutherford Classification System is the gold standard among most vascular practices within the United States to aid in classifying severity of claudication (Fig. 27.3).

Patients who suffer from severe disease may develop tissue injury, nonhealing wounds, or ischemic pain. Patients who suffer from ruptured atherosclerotic plaque may present with acute limb ischemia and need to be revascularized quickly to minimize irreversible ischemic injury—please refer to The Rutherford

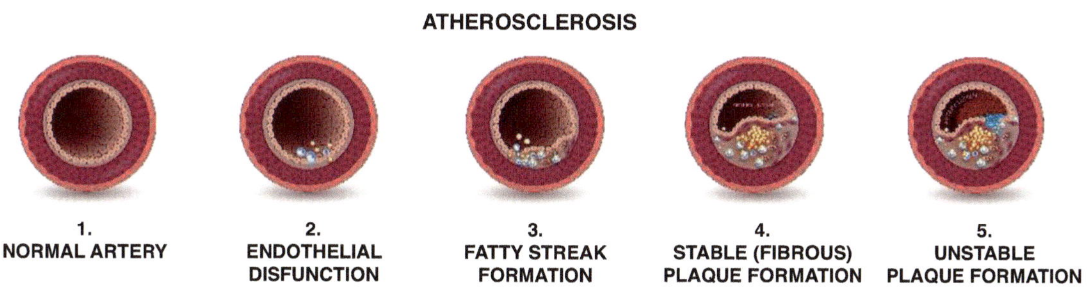

Fig. 27.2 PAD progression of arterial disease

Fig. 27.3 The Rutherford classification system of claudication

Grade	Category	Clinical description
I	0	Asymptomatic; not hemodynamically correct
	1	Mild claudication
	2	Moderate claudication
	3	Severe claudication
II	4	Ischemic rest pain
	5	Minor tissue loss; non-healing ulcer, focal gangrene with diffuse pedal ischemia
III	6	Mojor tissue loss extending above transmetatarsal level; foot no longer salvageable

Grade	Category	Sensory loss	Motor deficit	Prognosis	Doppler signals	
					Arterial	Venous
I	Viable	None	None	No immediate threat	Audible	Audible
IIA	Marginally threatened	None or minimal (toes)	None	Salvageable if promptly treated	Inaudible*	Audible
IIB	Immediately threatened	More than toes	Mild/moderate	Salvageable if promptly revascularised	Inaudible	Audible
III	Irreversible	Profound, anaesthetic	Profound, paralysis (rigor*)	Major tissue loss amputation. Permanent nerve damage inevitable	Inaudible	Inaudible

This is an identical replica of the table in the 1997 publication by Rutherford *et al.*,[2] with the exception of the asterisks (*).
*In the original 1997 classification it was stated that arterial Doppler sounds are never present in Stage IIA, and that rigor (mortis) is always present in Stage III. However, it is the opinion of the Writing Committee that exceptions to these rules do exist, and a slight modification of the Rutherford classification from 1997 may be appropriate in the future.

Fig. 27.4 Rutherford classification of acute limb ischemia

Classification of Acute Limb Ischemia (Fig. 27.4).

Imaging/Diagnostic Testing

Ankle Brachial Index

Physiologic testing is used to establish the diagnosis of PAD. Depending on the specific type of testing, this can assist in defining the severity and extent of disease in patients with risk factors or suspicion for PAD. A cost-effective, easily available, and appropriate diagnostic tool to first evaluate a patient for PAD is by obtaining an ankle-brachial index (ABI). This simple and noninvasive test can determine the presence and extent of PAD. An ABI can be calculated on each leg by using the systolic blood pressure at the ankle, divided by the *highest* brachial systolic blood pressure.

A normal ABI is ≥1 as the systolic blood pressure in the ankle is typically higher than in the arm. An ABI of ≤0.9 is diagnostic of the presence of PAD. An ABI of 0.4–0.9 is suggestive of a degree of arterial obstruction often associated with claudication. An ABI of less than 0.4 represents severe, multilevel, disease that risks non-healing ulcerations, ischemic rest pain, and pedal gangrene (Fig. 27.4). ABI results of >1.3 are falsely/artificially elevated which signifies that the lower extremity ankle arteries are calcified and/or noncompressible. In this case, the values recorded are considered nondiagnostic. If the values are nondiagnostic, then the use of toe-brachial indices (TBI) and toe pressures (TP) becomes even more valuable in predicting the ability to heal a current wound. TBIs are obtained by plac-

Table 27.1 Toe pressure utilization for nondiagnostic ABI >1.3

Toe-brachial index 0.7–0.8 normal
Toe pressure >30 mmHg in diabetic favorable wound healing
Toe pressure >50 mmHg nondiabetic favorable wound healing

ing a pneumatic cuff on one of the toes (usually the great toe) (Table 27.1).

Arterial Duplex Ultrasound

Arterial duplex ultrasound is considered the mainstay and often the initial noninvasive vascular imaging obtained when PAD is suspected. Duplex evaluation visualizes perfusion through the arteries in real time and measures peak systolic velocities (PSV) of arterial blood flow. Ratios are then determined from the change in PSV, which indicate a particular degree of stenosis.

Computed Tomography Angiography (CTA)

CT imaging uses contrast to obtain large series of still images to better visualize and evaluate arterial blood flow. CTA can be used when considering open operative approach or concern for inability to cannulate for endovascular intervention. CT evaluation requires intravenous contrast for adequate visualization of vessels, thus consider risk of contrast exposure in renal patients.

Management

Medical management and risk factor modification are crucial in maintaining vascular wellness, reducing complication and recurrent ischemic events, minimizing atherosclerotic progression, and achieving limb salvage. Medical therapies may include antiplatelet therapy, lipid-lowering agents (statins), and full anticoagulation when deemed appropriate. High-dose/high-potency statin therapy is recommended for all patients with atherosclerotic disease regardless of baseline LDL level [2]. Hypertension impacts plaque formation; thus, adequate blood pressure management according to guidelines is important. Glucose management in diabetics is important for long-term vascular health, as well as minimizing risk of lower extremity wounds. Tobacco cessation is important for overall cardiovascular health, as well as maintaining patency of prior vascular interventions. Lifestyle modification should also include regular exercise or implementing a regular walking program. Many patients can avoid (or at least delay) the need for endovascular or surgical intervention by adhering to a walking program and successfully modifying risk factors.

Currently, there is no definitive evidence for the efficacy of aspirin in patients with asymptomatic PAD. The guidelines vary in their treatment recommendations for patients with asymptomatic PAD. The American Heart Association/American College of Cardiology PAD guideline recommends antiplatelet therapy as reasonable if the ankle-brachial index is ≤0.90; the European Society of Cardiology guideline recommends against routine antiplatelet therapy in asymptomatic patients; and the Society for Vascular Surgery guideline provides no specific recommendations for this. Patients with symptomatic PAD should be treated with antithrombotic therapy to reduce cardiovascular risk. Single antiplatelet therapy with either aspirin or clopidogrel is recommended. Patients who undergo revascularization for PAD should be prescribed lifelong antithrombotic therapy. With respect to surgical revascularization, aspirin, clopidogrel, and rivaroxaban are all reasonable strategies [3].

Revascularization management and procedures of the lower extremities include a variety of endovascular and open surgical techniques. Age, risk factors, acute vs. chronic disease, and a multitude of variables are considered in a patient's plan of care. Generally, endovascular approach is preferred to an open surgery procedure. An endovascular approach consists of a surgeon evaluating and treating arterial blockages from within the lumen of an artery. After accessing the artery, an angiogram will be performed to visualize disease along the vessel, and then interventions such as angioplasty, atherectomy, thrombectomy, drug-coated balloon angioplasty, stenting, and administration of medications (i.e., nitroglycerin, thrombolytics) may be performed.

There are multiple open revascularization options depending on a patient's extent of disease. Some examples of open surgical revascularization are provided below:

- Aortobifemoral bypass—performed to treat aortoiliac occlusive disease or aneurysmal disease. A bypass is placed from the aorta to both femoral arteries.
- Iliofemoral bypass—used to treat iliofemoral occlusive disease. A bypass is placed from the iliac to femoral artery.
- Axillofemoral bypass—extra-anatomic bypass performed axillary artery to the femoral artery. Lower patency rates long term.

Revascularization may be performed using autologous vein harvest, synthetic material, or donor vessel.

Autogenous vein conduit bypass generally is preferred over synthetic grafts.

Prosthetic conduit bypass has an increased risk of needing graft explantation in the setting of infection.

Surveillance

Patients having undergone vascular intervention will need lifelong management and surveillance. This is often done with duplex ultrasound follow-up at least annually. CTA may be more appropriate for certain patients. Ankle- and toe-brachial index pressures are typically followed long term for reassessment of trending patient's baseline arterial flow. At every follow-up, symptoms are evaluated in conjunction with testing results to determine potential need for reintervention. It is important to maintain close follow-up as the patient will require lifelong medical therapy and potentially require repeat intervention.

Clinical Pearls

- Critical limb ischemia (CLI) is a classification of severe peripheral arterial disease. These patients suffer ischemic rest pain and/or tissue loss. If revascularization is unsuccessful, amputation may be needed.
- Patients with severe PAD as evidenced by testing may not require surgical intervention if asymptomatic but warrant medical management and a regular walking program.
- Patients with severe peripheral arterial disease should be considered for screening of disease in other vascular beds (neurovascular, coronary, carotid).
- After revascularization in patient with acute limb ischemia, evaluate for compartment syndrome, an acute process that leads to repeat occlusion of arterial perfusion and potential nerve damage.

Deep Vein Thrombosis

Anatomy and Physiology

Deep vein thrombosis (DVT) is when thrombus forms within a deep vein of the leg. Deep veins are identified as they have corresponding arterial vessels, whereas superficial veins do not (Fig. 27.5).

Superficial veins can be found in the subcutaneous tissues, while deep veins travel among muscles and bones below the fascia [1]. Perforator veins drain superficial venous blood flow into the deep vein system. Veins differ from arteries in that they are a low flow system and have a thin muscular wall, and blood is traveling against gravity. Veins have one-way valves which prevent regurgitation of blood flow back down the leg, while it travels back to the heart for recirculation [12]. Skeletal muscle contraction of the lower extremities also aids in propulsion of blood flow up through the low flow venous system. DVTs are more common in the lower extremities due to this flow against gravity.

DVTs should be classified as either provoked or unprovoked, which guides management.

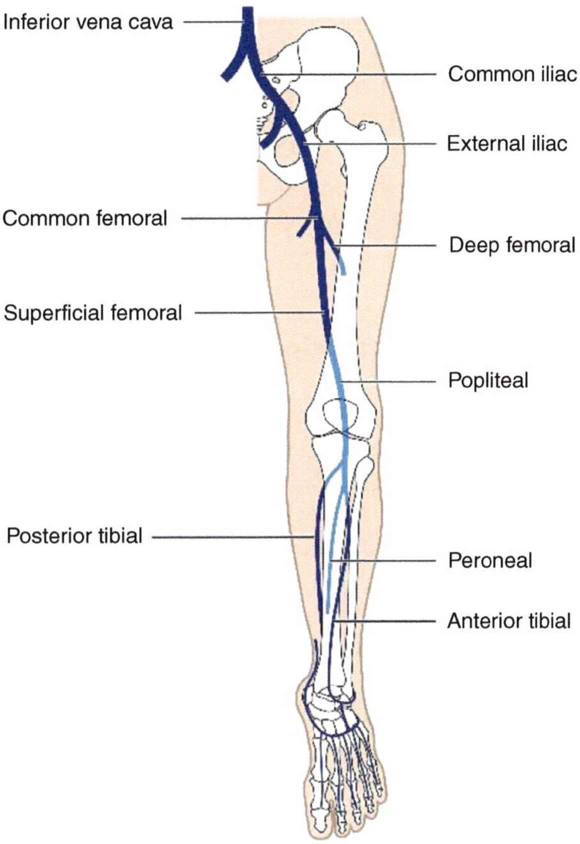

Fig. 27.5 Deep veins of lower extremity

Anatomical location of DVT also helps guide management, taking into consideration proximal or distal involvement in the extremities [5] (Table 27.2).

A myriad of other complications may arise from DVT, including post-thrombotic syndrome (PTS), venous insufficiency, venous wound development (venous stasis ulceration), and potential limb loss.

Post-thrombotic syndrome (PTS) occurs in 20–50% of patients with DVT, with 5% developing severe PTS. [7] Patients can develop chronic leg pain, itching, neuropathy, erythema, edema, ulcers, and limited activity tolerance (Table 27.3). PTS is managed with compression garments (usually 30–40 mmHg), wound care, and medical therapy (i.e., moisturizer, topical steroids, anti-inflammatories) [8].

Table 27.2 DVT location and risk [13]

Proximal—higher risk of PE and mortality	Distal—lower risk
Iliac	Peroneal
Femoral	Posterior Tibial
Popliteal	Anterior Tibial

Table 27.3 Risk factors for post-thrombotic syndrome (PTS)

DVT above the knee
Recurrent DVT in the ipsilateral limb
Persistent symptoms beyond 1 month of therapy
Therapy noncompliance/subtherapeutic AC levels
Obesity
Residual thrombus

Physical Exam

Patients with DVT may exhibit swelling, tenderness, erythema, firmness along the leg, as well as a positive Homan's sign. Patients with Homan's sign experience increased calf pain with dorsiflexion of the foot; however, this is a poor predictor of DVT.

Pathology/Description

DVTs can develop due to stasis of blood flow within the deep vein system, endothelial injury, or because of a hypercoagulable state, known as Virchow's Triad [9]. DVTs occur in 300,000–600,000 people in the United States per year [7]. For common risk factors, see Table 27.4.

Symptoms will develop in the affected limb. Most patients will experience pain, swelling, warmth, erythema, hyperpigmentation, aching, throbbing, and limb heaviness. If patients experience chest pain, shortness of breath, tachypnea, tachycardia, or unexplained cough with DVT, they should be screened for pulmonary embolus [10] (Chap. 22).

Table 27.4 Risk factors for DVT

Family history/genetics	History of prior thrombotic event
Malignancy	Spinal cord injury/paralysis
African American race	Tobacco use
Oral contraceptives	Pregnancy (6 weeks postpartum)
Surgery within 3 months	Venous catheters
Prolonged immobility-travel, cast	Hospitalization
Age >40 years and risk doubles with every 10 years	Hypertension
Congestive heart failure	Sickle cell disease
Autoimmune disorders	Hypercoagulable states

Imaging and Diagnosis

D-dimer can be tested, but it is not recommended given low specificity. Diagnosis of DVT is obtained via visualization of thrombus in the vein. Venous duplex for evaluation of DVT is the gold standard (Fig. 27.6); however, computed tomography venography (CTV) can also be obtained (Fig. 27.7). Interventional venogram can be diagnostic as well therapeutic. Patients

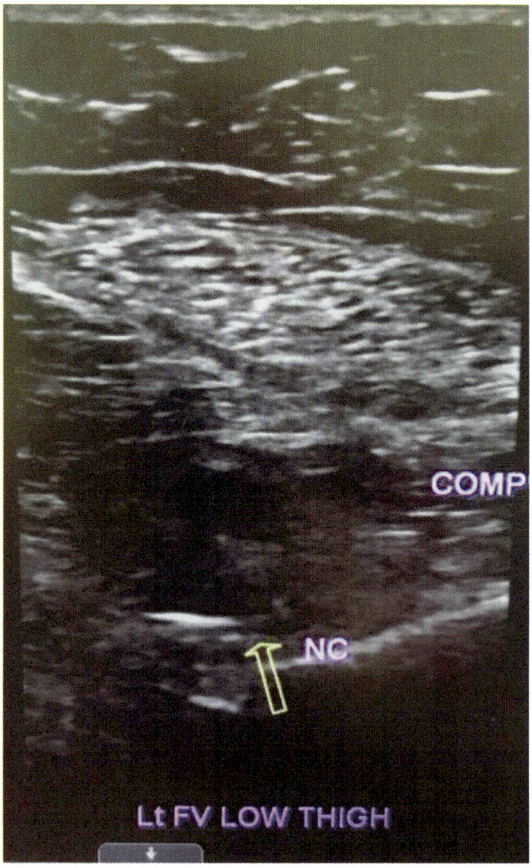

Fig. 27.6 Femoral vein that does not collapse with pressure. The lack of compression is suggestive of thrombus and DVT at the yellow arrow

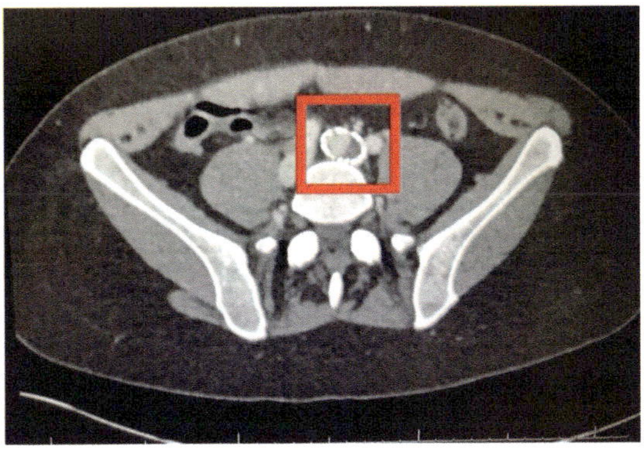

Fig. 27.7 CTV to evaluate IVC stented segment. Dark thrombus formation is seen on the right side of the stented IVC segment

who have unprovoked DVT should undergo hypercoagulable workup. EKG, echocardiogram (to evaluate for right heart strain), CT angiography of the chest, or ventilation-perfusion (VQ) scan may be used to evaluate for pulmonary embolism.

Management

The aim of DVT management is to reduce risk of thrombus propagation and embolization, relieve acute symptoms, and reduce risk of lasting complications [11]. DVTs are managed with anticoagulation (AC). Intravenous options for this include systemic regular dose unfractionated heparin in the acute setting. Therapeutic low-molecular-weight heparin (enoxaparin) or oral anticoagulation can be used in the acute, subacute, or chronic phase. Oral anticoagulants include direct-acting oral anticoagulants (DOACs) (apixaban, dabigatran, edoxaban, rivaroxaban) or warfarin (vitamin k antagonists-VKA).

The CHEST Guidelines can help aid clinician decision-making based on DVT classification. CHEST recommends serial imaging (weekly venous ultrasound) for 2 weeks instead of anticoagulation in patients with isolated ***distal DVT*** of the leg without severe symptoms or risk factors for extension. Upon repeat imaging, AC is not recommended if no extension is seen and is recommend if thrombus has propagated (even if remaining in the distal veins).

CHEST recommends AC for patients with isolated DVTs who are experiencing severe symptoms. Apixaban, dabigatran, edoxaban, or rivaroxaban over VKA is recommended in the first 3 months (treatment phase), and AC alone over interventional therapies (thrombolytic, mechanical, or pharmacochemical) for acute DVTs. Oral Xa inhibitor (apixaban, edoxaban, rivaroxaban) over LMWH is recommended for initiation and treatment phases for patients with cancer. VKA (with INR target 2.5) is recommended for patients diagnosed with triple antiphospholipid syndrome.

The CHEST guidelines also provide recommendations on duration of treatment. Patients with acute DVT without contraindication for AC should begin a treatment phase of 3 months of AC. At the completion of 3 months, patients should be assessed for extended therapy. Therapy should be extended for patients if the VTE was unprovoked or provoked by a persistent risk factor (prefer DOAC over VKA).

Surgical interventions for management of DVT include thrombolysis, catheter-directed therapy, and thrombectomy. Thrombolysis, catheter-directed thrombolysis, and surgical thrombectomy are reserved for extensive proximal lower extremity DVT (iliofemoral) for those with severe symptoms, threatened limb (phlegmasia), and with thrombus burden for <14 days [11] (*see* Table 27.5). For these patients, the benefit of more aggressive intervention may outweigh the associated risks [13]. The 2016 AC Forum and 2020 NICE recommend individual risk-to-benefit analysis for catheter-directed therapy (CDT) and that patients with iliofemoral DVT who have symptoms for <14 days, good functional status, life expectancy of 1+ years, and low risk for bleeding be considered for CDT [13].

Patients should undergo repeat venous ultrasound to evaluate DVT if symptoms worsen—this will evaluate for thrombus propagation. Swelling and leg heaviness may persist for those with extensive DVTs, despite surgical intervention and post intervention therapies. This can be alleviated by consistent use of com-

Table 27.5 Contraindication to thrombolysis and DVT [12]

Absolute	Relative
Recent intracranial hemorrhage (ICH)	History of uncontrolled HTN
Severely uncontrolled HTN	Severe hypertension at presentation (SBP >180, DBP >110)
Cerebral vascular lesion-neoplasm	CPR >10 min within last 3 weeks
Ischemic stroke within 3 months	Remote ischemic stroke
Possible aortic dissection	Dementia
Head trauma or facial trauma within 3 months	Pregnancy
Recent intracranial or spinal surgery	Major surgery within 3 weeks
Active bleeding (except menses)	Internal bleeding within 2–4 weeks
Streptokinase within 6 months	Active peptic ulcer disease
	Noncompressible vascular puncture

pression garments, leg elevation, and regular exercise. Patients can begin wearing compression garments once a DVT is deemed stable, and not propagating. Compression garments help support venous structure and reduce venous stasis. There is no evidence that the use of graduated compression garment reduces the risk of DVT. Bed rest is not recommended after DVT diagnosis while starting anticoagulation therapy [11].

Clinical Pearls

- Aside from patient with asymptomatic distal DVT, patients without contraindication to AC should be treated for a minimum of 3–6 months with the option of extending duration of therapy.
- When selecting AC, DOACs are preferred over VKA EXCEPT in patients with moderate-severe liver disease or antiphospholipid syndrome [7].
- Oral Xa inhibitor (apixaban, edoxaban, rivaroxaban) over LMWH is recommended for initiation and treatment phases for patients with cancer.
- Clinicians should weigh risk of bleeding when considering anticoagulation. Risk factors for major bleeding while taking AC include age >65, alcohol use, liver failure, renal failure, anemia, antiplatelet therapy, cancer, reduced functional capacity, frequent falls, prior bleeding issues, prior stroke, and recent surgery [11].
- An inferior vena cava (IVC) filter may be placed in patients with acute proximal DVT of the leg who have contraindication to AC.
- It is important to educate patients on modifiable risk factors to prevent new or recurrent thrombotic events. These risk factors include medication compliance, smoking cessation, heart healthy diet, regular exercise, weight management, and surgical prophylaxis.
- Phlegmasia dolens is a rare and life-threatening complication of extensive, acute DVT [14]. Surgical intervention due to arterial perfusion compromise and risk of limb loss may be needed.

References

1. Britannica, The Editors of Encyclopaedia. “artery”. Encyclopedia Britannica, 6 Jun. 2023, https://www.britannica.com/science/artery. Accessed 29 July 2023.
2. Berger J, Davies M. Overview of lower extremity peripheral arterial disease. UpToDate. 2021. www.uptodate.com/contents/overview-of-lower-extremity-peripheral-artery-disease?source=history_widget#H16453723. Accessed 14 Mar 2022.
3. Hussain MA, Al-Omran M, Creager MA, Anand SS, Verma S, Bhatt DL. Antithrombotic therapy for peripheral artery disease: recent advances. J Am Coll Cardiol. 2018;71:2450–67.
4. Douketis J. Overview of the venous system. 2021. https://www.merckmanuals.com/home/heart-and-blood-vessel-disorders/venous-disorders/overview-of-the-venous-system.
5. Moore KJ, Tabas I. Macrophages in the pathogenesis of atherosclerosis. Cell. 2011;145(3):341–55, www.cell.com/abstract/S0092-8674(11)00422-3. https://doi.org/10.1016/j.cell.2011.04.005.
6. Lip, et al. Overview of the treatment of lower extremity deep vein thrombosis. 2022. https://www.uptodate.

com/contents/overview-of-the-treatment-of-lower-extremity-deep-vein-thrombosis-dvt.
7. Ortel, et al. American Society of Hematology 2020 guidelines for management of thromboembolism: treatment of deep vein thrombosis and pulmonary embolism. 2020. https://ashpublications.org/bloodadvances/article/4/19/4693/463998/American-Society-of-Hematology-2020-guidelines-for.
8. Kushner A, West P, Pillarisetty L. Virchow triad. 2021. https://www.ncbi.nlm.nih.gov/books/NBK539697/.
9. Themes, UFO. Peripheral vascular disease. Thoracic Key. Southern California Vascular Institute. 2017. https://thoracickey.com/peripheral-vascular-disease-2/, https://calvascular.net/peripheral-vascular-disease/. Accessed 14 Mar 2022.
10. Venous thromboembolism. n.d.. https://www.nhlbi.nih.gov/health-topics/venous-thromboembolism.
11. Wilburn & Shian. Deep venous thrombosis and pulmonary embolism: current therapy. 2017. https://www.aafp.org/afp/2017/0301/p295.html.
12. Baig & Bodle. Thrombolytic therapy. 2021. https://www.ncbi.nlm.nih.gov/books/NBK557411/.
13. Stevens, et al. Antithrombotic therapy for VTE disease: second update of the chest guidelines and expert panel report. 2021. https://journal.chestnet.org/article/S0012-3692(21)01507-5/fulltext?_ga=2.38742947.1844619104.1647184408-751823456.1647184408.
14. Chaochankit & Akaraborworn. Phlegmasia cerulea dolens with compartment syndrome. 2018. https://www.ncbi.nlm.nih.gov/pmc/articles/PMC6200621/.

Diseases of the Aorta

28

Tracy Totten and Frank R. Arko III

Aneurysm

Anatomy and Physiology

The term aneurysm describes dilatation of any blood vessel greater than 1.5× increase in diameter compared with expected normal diameter. Excluding intracranial vessels, arterial aneurysms are most prevalent in the infrarenal aorta [1]. Aortic aneurysms are commonly associated with concomitant aneurysm of the ascending aorta, thoracic aorta, iliac, femoral, or popliteal arteries.

Arterial walls are made up of three layers: tunica intima, media, and adventitia. A true aneurysm involves dilation of all intact layers of the arterial wall due to remodeling of the extracellular matrix (ECM) (Fig. 28.1).

Pathology/Description

Aneurysmal degeneration of the aorta is a multifactorial, systemic process generally felt to be due to alterations in vascular wall biology leading to a loss of vascular structural proteins (viz., collagen) and wall strength. Biomechanical forces, including stress across the arterial wall, are also felt to play a role [3]. As the aorta enlarges, turbulent flow develops within the aneurysm due to the flow dynamics and can lead to thrombus formation along the aortic wall [4]. This can lead to distal embolization.

Classification

The shape of aneurysms is defined as fusiform or saccular. A fusiform aneurysm is a ballooning on all sides of the aorta, whereas a saccular aneurysm is a focal enlargement which is one sided. A false aneurysm (pseudoaneurysm) develops from arterial injury with subsequent hematoma formation and does not involve all three layers of the arterial wall (Fig. 28.2).

Aneurysms can occur throughout the entirety of the aorta. Location of aneurysms includes the aortic root, ascending aorta, aortic arch, thoracoabdominal aorta (Type I, II, III, IV), suprarenal aorta, juxtarenal, and infrarenal aorta. Abdominal aortic aneurysms (AAAs) are a leading cause of death in the United States [1]. AAAs are classi-

T. Totten (✉)
Atrium Health/Sanger Hearth and Vascular Institute, Charlotte, NC, USA
e-mail: tracy.totten@atriumhealth.org

F. R. Arko III
Vascular and Endovascular Surgery, Atrium Health/Sanger Heart and Vascular Institute, Charlotte, NC, USA
e-mail: Frank.Arko@atriumhealth.org

R. Musialowski, K. Allshouse (eds.), *Cardiovascular Manual for the Advanced Practice Provider*,
https://doi.org/10.1007/978-3-031-35819-7_28

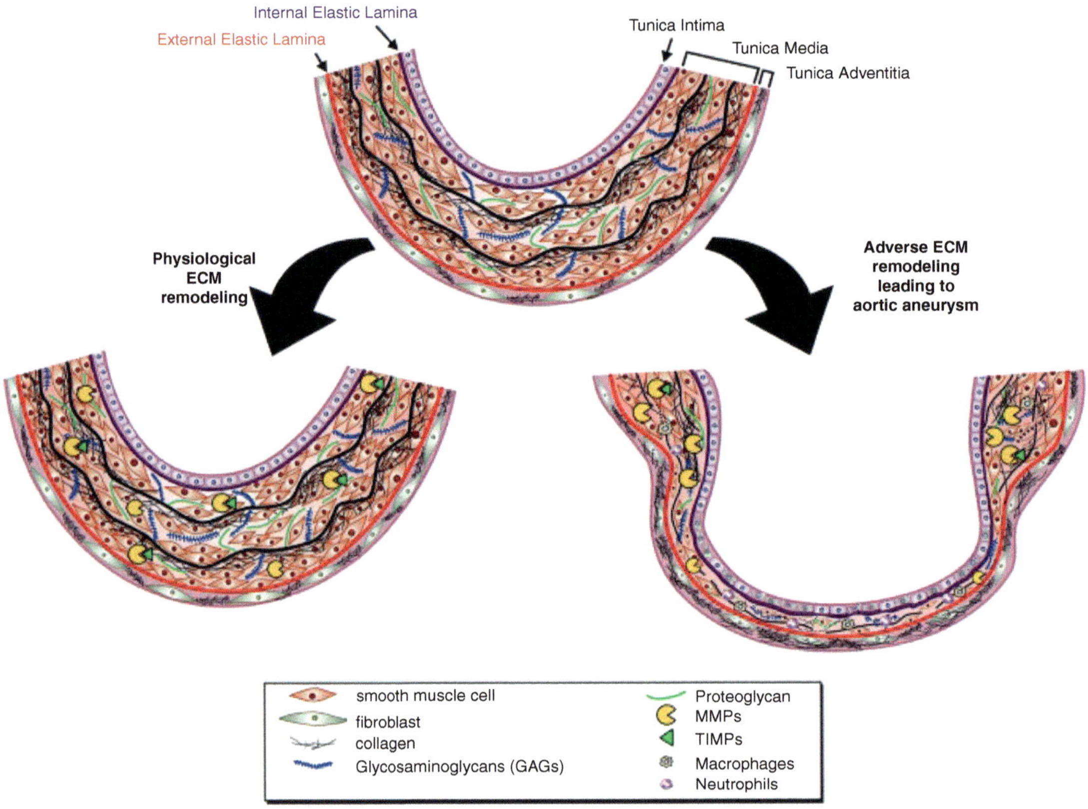

Fig. 28.1 Extracellular matrix, regional heterogeneity of the aorta, and aortic aneurysm [2]

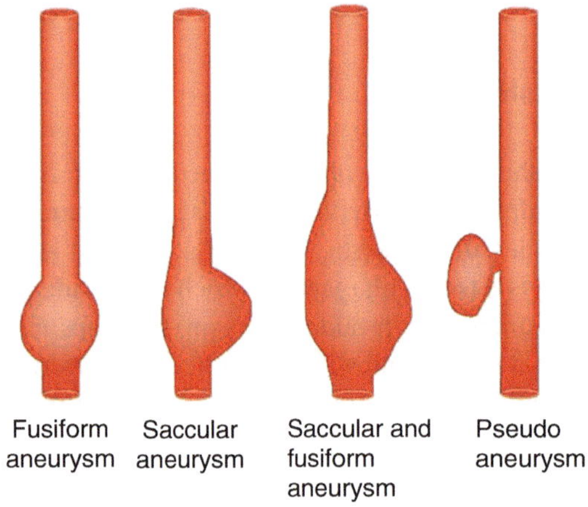

Fig. 28.2 Types of aneurysm

fied based on anatomical location, shape, and size (Fig. 28.3).

Depending on the location and size of the aneurysmal segment, the management and classification can vary. Aneurysm size is described by diameter and length, with diameter being the important risk factor for rupture (Table 28.1).

Risk Factors

Aortic aneurysms often occur in the setting of other concomitant diseases. Most AAAs are related to atherosclerotic *disease* (Table 28.2).

Incidence of AAA increases in males age greater than 60 years and females greater than 70 years of age. Males are more likely to develop AAA than females. However, females are more likely to rupture at a smaller size than males [5]. Genetic conditions that are known to be associated with developing aortic aneurysms include Ehlers-Danlos syndrome (EDS) and Marfan's syndrome. These conditions are more concerning in patients who present with aneurysms at a younger age. There is high association between smoking and development of aneurysm.

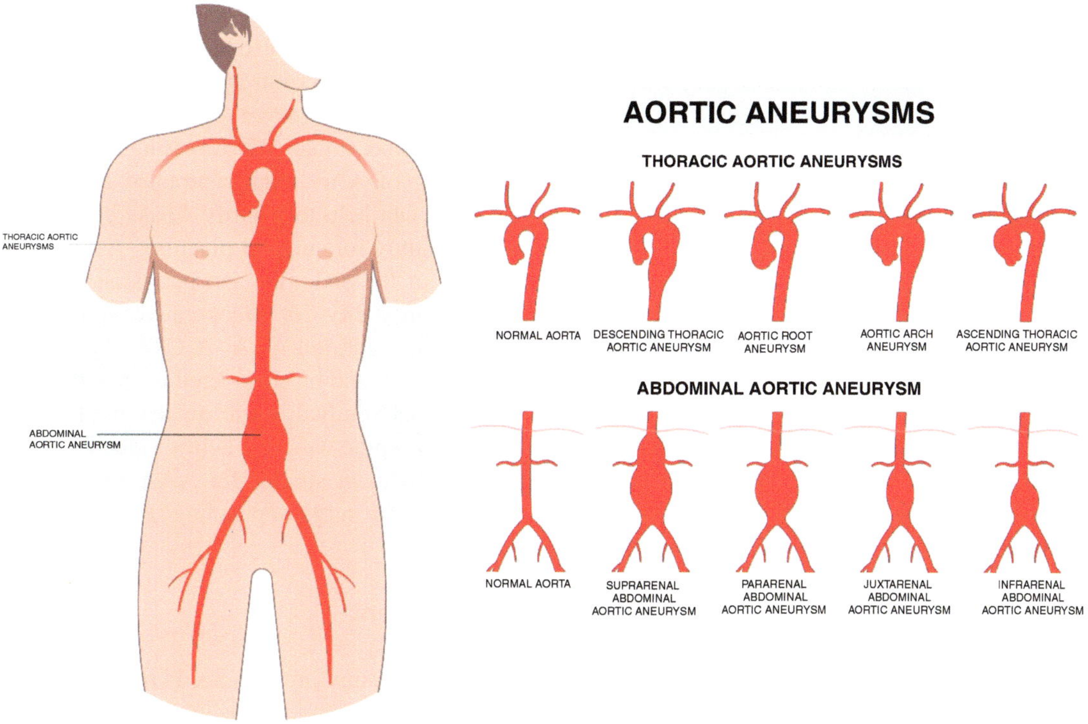

Fig. 28.3 Aortic aneurysm morphology and location

Table 28.1 Size and rupture risk [5]

Size of aneurysm	Annual risk of rupture
Small (3–3.9 cm)	No increased risk
Medium (4–4.9 cm)	1%
Large (5–5.9 cm)	5–10%
Very large (6–6.9 cm)	10–20%
Giant (7–7.9 cm)	20–40%
>8 cm	30–50%

Table 28.2 Risk factors for aneurysm development

Atherosclerotic *disease*	Any tobacco use
Family history	Male sex
Genetic predisposition	PAD/PVD
Autoimmune/inflammatory process	Remote aortic surgery
Infection	Hypertension
Age >60 years	Caucasian race
Obesity	Trauma

Asymptomatic screening is recommended in patients with tobacco use.

Signs and Symptoms

AAAs are commonly asymptomatic and found incidentally during workup for other disease processes or on an age-related screening exam. Symptomatic patients can present with a wide array of symptoms. This may include abdominal, back, or flank pain. If there is evidence of a large AAA, the patient can present with obstructive symptoms such as gastric outlet obstruction (GOO), nausea/vomiting, urinary symptoms due to obstruction of ureters, and inferior vena cava compression and deep vein thrombosis (DVT). If an AAA has evidence of thrombus along the aortic wall, a patient may present with embolic changes (i.e., claudication, discoloration of toes, and feet).

Physical Exam

When examining the vascular patient for a concern of aortic aneurysm, it is important to complete a full vascular exam. This includes a full abdominal examination, lower extremity, and peripheral pulse examination including palpation of the popliteal fossa for pulsatile masses, auscultation of carotid bruits, and cardiac auscultation. The provider must keep in mind the following list of physical exam findings as the patient may present with any of the following (Table 28.3). Do not rely on a physical exam to diagnose a AAA since it is a difficult clinical diagnosis. Always check distal pulses due to risk of embolic disease and concomitant PAD.

Imaging

When working up an AAA, there are many different imaging modalities. Duplex ultrasound (DUS) is the modality of choice for screening and surveillance of AAA and lower extremity aneurysms [5]. This is also the cheapest and least invasive. It is not uncommon that an abdominal CT scan will be ordered for a patient during workup of abdominal pain revealing an incidental finding of AAA. Non-contrasted abdominal CT scans can help to identify AAAs but are not an ideal study for surgical planning. A CT angiography of the abdomen and pelvis is the most accurate modality for preoperative workup or concern for ruptured AAA. A CTA chest/abdomen/pelvis should be considered for any thoracic or thoracoabdominal aortic aneurysm. MRI of the lumbar spine can also help to identify AAA but are not ideal studies for AAA and are not appropriate for surgical planning (Fig. 28.4).

Management

Aortic aneurysms are managed medically with regular imaging surveillance until they reach size criteria for surgical intervention. A goal of aneu-

Table 28.3 Physical findings consistent with AAA

Abdominal pulsatile mass	Enlarged popliteal pulse
Aortic bruit	Painful aortic palpation
Abdominal, inguinal, or flank pain	Embolic changes in lower extremity

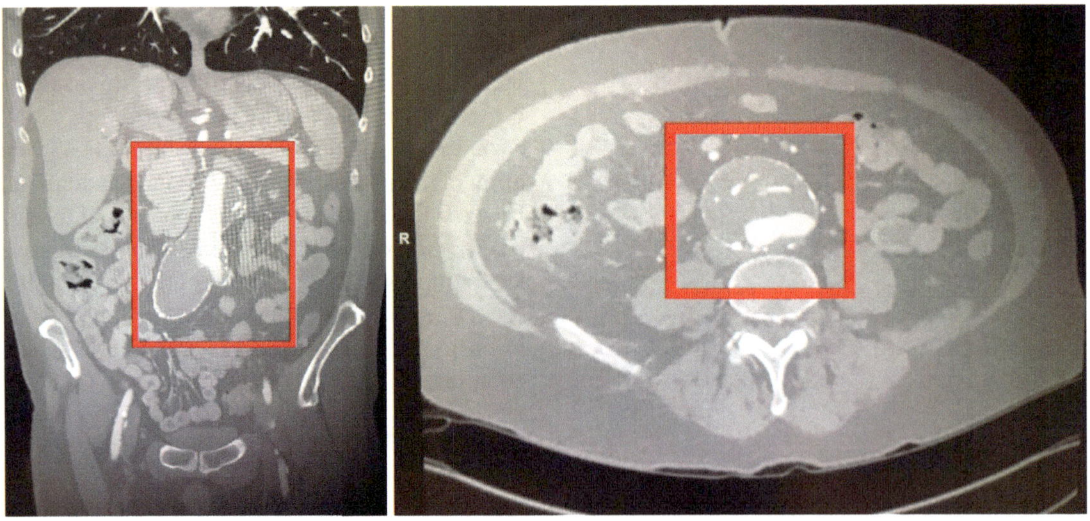

Fig. 28.4 Infrarenal AAA pre-EVAR with heavy thrombus (DARK) and atherosclerotic burden (calcification in wall of aorta) on CT imaging

rysmal disease is early detection, surveillance, and elective repair to prevent complications of rupture, thrombosis, or embolism. The diagnosis and treatment will depend on stability of the aneurysm [5]. Vascular surgery referral can be placed for any aortic aneurysm. Any incidence of ruptured aortic aneurysms requires emergent operative repair.

Medical management is indicated for stable aortic aneurysms of less than 5.5 cm in males and less than 5.0 cm in women. Modifiable risk factors in the medical management of aortic aneurysms include smoking cessation, management of hypertension, cholesterol, obesity, and atherosclerotic disease. Medical therapy includes antiplatelet therapy, statin drugs, and blood pressure management with a goal of normotension. Beta-blocker therapy is preferred as first-line agent. Full anticoagulation is needed if thromboembolic disease distal to an aneurysm is identified with mural thrombus within the aneurysm. Avoid the use of fluoroquinolones as they have been shown to increase size of AAA and complications associated with rupture or dissection.

Once an aneurysm is diagnosed, DUS surveillance is obtained and is based on size and location (Table 28.4).

The timing of surgical intervention is often guided by size of the aneurysm (Table 28.5).

Table 28.4 Aneurysm surveillance AAA

Aneurysm size	Duplex imaging frequency
<4.0 cm	Annually
4.0–5.0 cm	Every 6 months
>5.0	CTA

Table 28.5 Aneurysm size and indication for surgical intervention

Rapid growth 0.5 cm over 6 months
Ascending and abdominal >5.5 cm males, >5.0 cm females
Ascending and abdominal Marfan's >5.0 cm male, 4.5 cm female
>4.5 cm ascending root if aortic valve disease involvement
Isolated aortic arch >5.5 cm
Popliteal >2.5 cm asymptomatic
Common iliac >3.5 cm asymptomatic

Surgical intervention is then further defined based on endovascular repair versus open repair. EVAR is the most common repair, but there are still cases in which open repair is preferred. Endovascular repair is defined as EVAR (endovascular aortic repair), TEVAR (thoracic endovascular repair), and FEVAR (fenestrated endovascular aortic repair).

Open aortic repair is completed with aortic bypass grafting with either aortoiliac, aortobifemoral bypass graft, or straight aortic tube graft for patients without iliac artery involvement. Open repair may be indicated in younger patients who are otherwise healthy; patients with anatomy not conducive to EVAR, including short or angulated infrarenal aortic neck; and multiple branch vessels increasing risk for endoleak. Patients with connective tissue disorders may be favored for open repair.

Endovascular aortic repair is completed via percutaneous or open arterial access. Straightforward EVAR can be completed with procedural sedation versus general sedation. Open access may be indicated in patients with concomitant peripheral arterial disease, small access vessels, or prior surgical interventions. Depending on the complexity of the repair, alternative access sites may also be indicated including brachial artery or open axillary artery conduit. Repair is completed by placing a bifurcated endograft within the aorta thereby excluding the aneurysm sac (Fig. 28.5). Prior to completion, a final angiogram is imaged to ensure no evidence of endoleak at the remainder of the case. Occasionally, assistive devices are used to aid with the seal zone including fixation devices, coiling, or onyx glue in patients with a short neck.

Open aortic repair is completed via midline or retroperitoneal incision (Fig. 28.6). The extent of repair is based on anatomical involvement of iliac and femoral arteries or concomitant PAD. The incision is carried down to the abdominal cavity exposing the aorta. A retroperitoneal approach is performed with the patient in right lateral decubitus position through a left flank incision. The proximal and distal arteries are then clamped, repair is completed

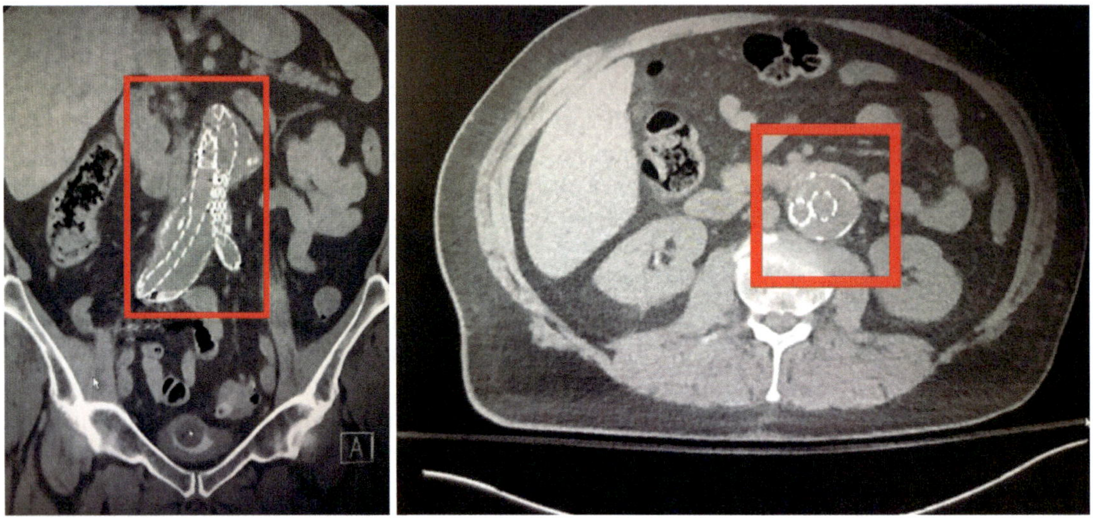

Fig. 28.5 EVAR treatment of AAA with exclusion of residual thrombus

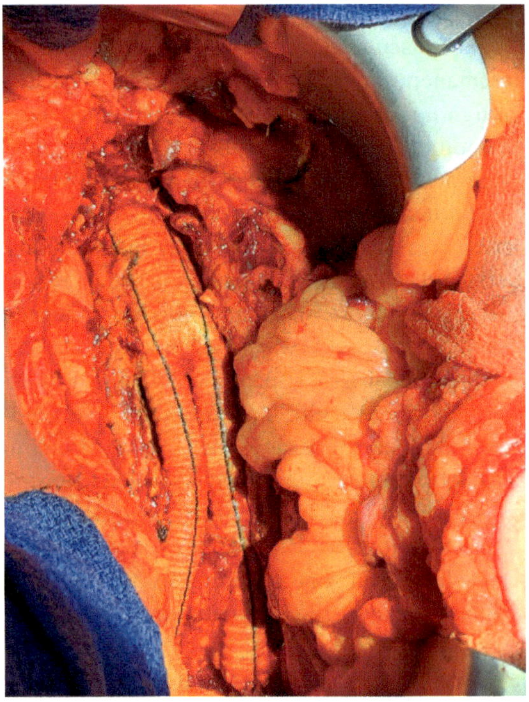

Fig. 28.6 Open aorto-bi-iliac bypass with Dacron graft

by replacing the aneurysmal segment with synthetic graft, the aneurysm is then oversewn, and the abdomen is closed.

Postoperative surveillance of EVAR of the infrarenal segment can be completed with aortic duplex in the vascular surgery clinic. An endoleak is defined as flow outside of the endograft and within the remaining AAA sac, risking continued aneurysm growth (Table 28.6).

Table 28.6 Types of endoleaks (EL)

1 ab	Proximal (a) distal (b) graft attachment site leaks
2	Retrograde flow into the sac via aortic side branches (i.e., lumbar, mesenteric)
3	Defect in the graft either d/t fabric tear or disconnection of modular overlap
4	Graft wall porosity
5	Increase in maximum aneurysm diameter with no identifiable endoleak; endotension

[a] Intervention is indicated for Types 1, 3, and 2 when EL sac with increasing aortic size [6]

Clinical Pearls

- Consider screening patients with risk factors for AAA given they are commonly asymptomatic.
- Fluoroquinolones are contraindicated in patients with history of aortic aneurysm or dissection as there is an increased risk of aneurysm and dissection with this drug class.
- Consider TTE screening for ascending aortic aneurysm with new diagnosis of AAA and vice versa.
- Endocarditis prophylaxis should be recommended with any patient s/p aortic graft.
- There is risk for genetic inheritance of aneurysms, thus recommend family screening.

Aortic Dissection

Anatomy and Physiology

An aortic dissection is a tear within the layers of the aorta. The tear occurs within the intima which causes a separation of the media, creating a new channel which is defined as the false lumen. The native channel is defined as the true lumen. Throughout the aortic dissection, there are many communications between the true and false lumen defined as fenestrations. The presence of an "intimal flap," representing the intimomedial septum between the true and false lumen, is the most characteristic pathology in acute aortic dissection [7] (Fig. 28.7). Aortic dissections are classified as acute versus chronic based onset timing and on the location of the entry tear. An acute aortic dissection is defined as onset of symptoms within 2 weeks, subacute >14 days to 90 days, and chronic >90 days.

Historically, there were two classification systems: Debakey (1965) and Stanford (1970). The Debakey classification defines the intimal tear and the extent of aortic dissection. The standard Stanford classification describes only the tear and defines a type A as involving the proximal aorta or type B (TBAD) which is distal to the left subclavian artery [7] (Fig. 28.8).

DeBakey

Type 1. Dissection originates in the ascending aorta, extending to descending and abdominal aorta

Type 2. Dissection originates and is confined to the ascending alone

Type 3. Dissection originates in the descending aorta

3a = Supra-diaphragm

3b = Below diaphragm

The newest classification system as defined by the Society for Vascular Surgery (SVS) in 2020 helps to overcome previous limitations and further develop more accurate communication when describing the complex aortic dissection patient. Within the new SVS classification scheme for aortic dissection, the distinction between Type A and Type B is predicated on entry tear location alone and defined in zones [8].

When discussing aortic syndromes, intramural hematoma (IMH) as well as the penetrating aortic ulcer (PAU) should also be included. IMH does not have a clear tear or communication as an aortic dissection but rather appears as hemorrhage within the aortic wall [8]. A PAU is defined as atherosclerotic plaque that penetrates the aortic wall. PAU rupture risk is directly associated with the ulcer depth [8].

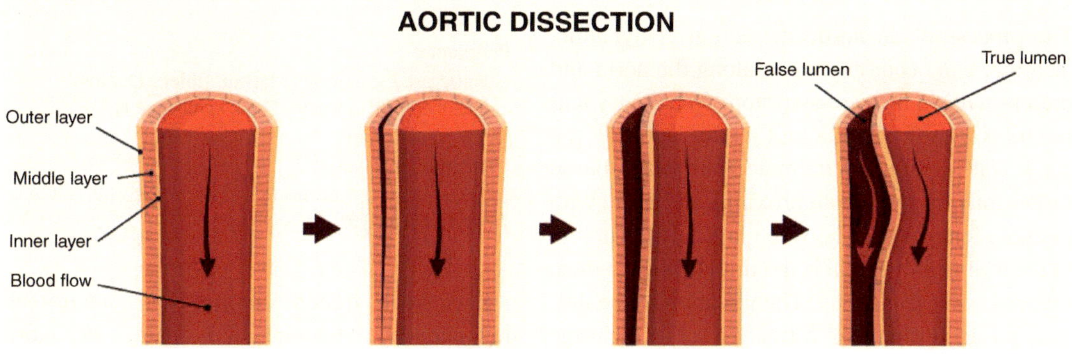

Fig. 28.7 Development and progression of aortic dissection

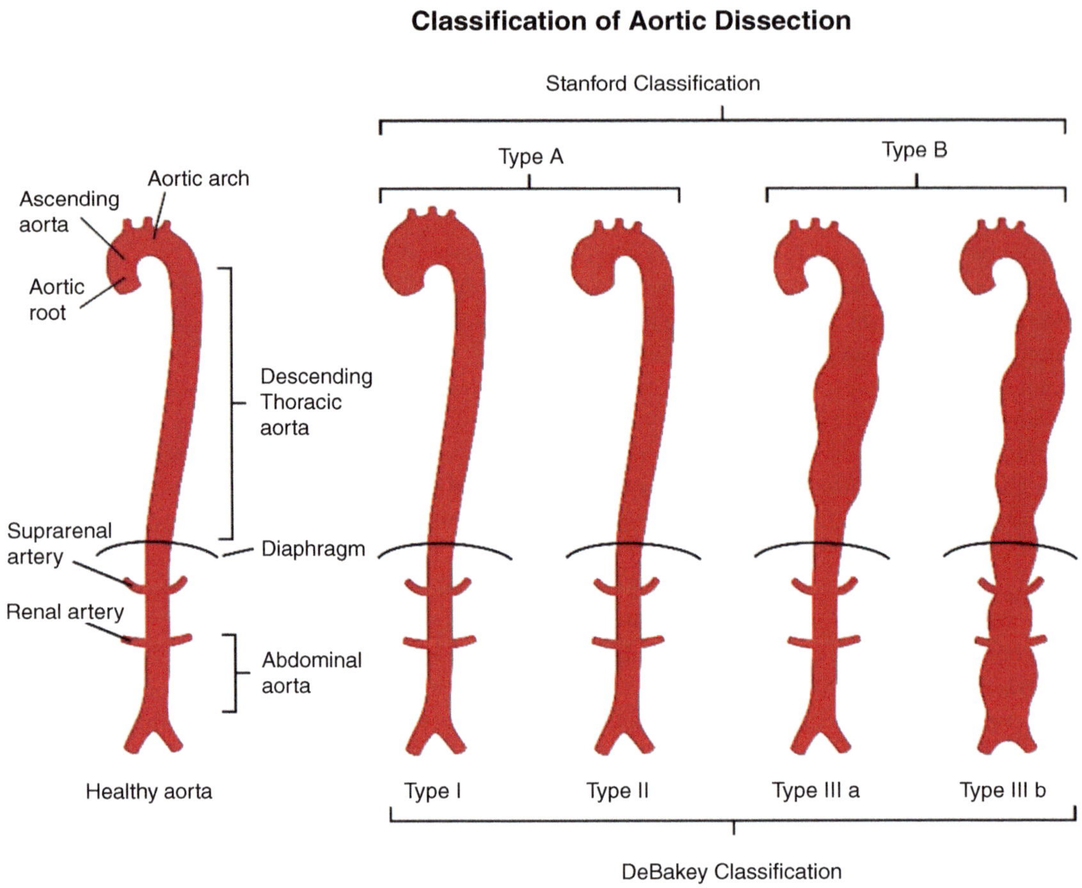

Fig. 28.8 Dissection classification: Stanford and Debakey

Pathology/Description

The process of an aortic dissection is dynamic, therefore can occur anywhere along the aorta and present with an array of symptoms. The entry tear occurs within the intima and media layers of the aortic wall, creating an intimal flap in which blood rushes into the space both proximal and distal with multiple fenestrations between layers [7]. Rupture of the intima and media is the initial event in most cases of aortic dissection. The violation of the intimal surface results in formation of a cleavage plane into the outer media and subsequent propagation for a varying distance in this plane, either antegrade or retrograde [7] (Fig. 28.7).

Aortic dissections are classified as complicated versus uncomplicated. Complicated dissections are defined by malperfusion of end organs, true lumen compression, aneurysmal degeneration, uncontrolled pain, or aortic rupture.

Table 28.7 Risk factors for dissection

Uncontrolled and sudden variation in blood pressure
Cocaine
Pregnancy
Genetic predisposition (Marfan, Ehlers-Danlos syndrome (EDS), Loeys-Dietz syndrome (LD)
Blunt force trauma
Bicuspid aortic valve
Inflammatory conditions of Giant cell arteritis (GCA), Takayasu arteritis

Risk Factors for Dissection

See Table 28.7.

Physical Exam

The patient may present with a wide array of symptoms. The classic description is described as a ripping, tearing, sharp, "worst ever" anterior chest or back pain. There may be evidence of an anxious appearing patient with tachycardia and tachypnea. If there is a flow-limiting dissection, the patient can present with hypoperfusion symptoms and commonly abdominal pain. The medical provider should always obtain blood pressure readings in both upper extremities as the patient may present with loss of pulses to extremities which could represent ischemia. Always complete a thorough cardiac exam and auscultate for cardiac murmur. If the dissection involves the intracranial vessel, there could be evidence of neurologic changes presenting with stroke, Horner's syndrome, voice hoarseness, and spinal cord ischemia.

Imaging

When working up, aortic dissections consider the following imaging modalities. The gold standard imaging is a CT angiogram of the chest, abdomen, and pelvis. An acute dissection flap (Fig. 28.9) is thin in appearance compared with a chronic dissection which will appear as a clearly defined dissection flap that usually is thicker and more dense [8]. IMH will appear as a hyperdensity within the aortic wall. PAU will appear as an atherosclerotic lesion with ulcer-like projection within the aortic wall. A chest X-ray can reveal widening of the cardiac or aortic silhouette with widened mediastinum. A TTE or TEE can be used to evaluate for any evidence of cardiac tamponade or aortic insufficiency in the setting of a type A aortic dissection. A TTE should be ordered with diagnosis of acute aortic dissection. MR angiograms are not recommended. An EKG should always be obtained in the setting of acute type A aortic dissection. Proximal dissection into a coronary artery (RCA) can create STEMI in addition to aortic dissection.

Management

Prompt diagnosis and management are key, and aortic dissections are associated with high morbidity and mortality. Type B aortic dissections are either managed medically or occasionally surgically. The cornerstone of medical therapy is reduction of arterial blood pressure [7]. Acute aortic dissection patients will be admitted to ICU for anti-impulse therapy and vasodilator therapy.

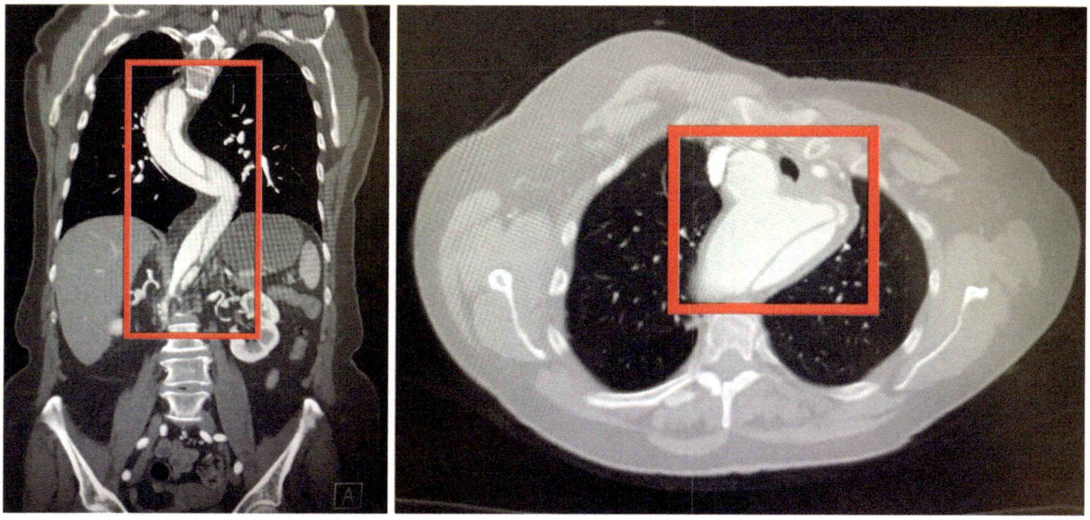

Fig. 28.9 CTA with acute thoracic aortic dissection

Beta blockade (labetalol or esmolol) is always initiated first as vasodilators can cause a reflex tachycardia, which can worsen the dissection. Intravenous nicardipine is commonly used as a vasodilator. The goal is prompt control of heart rate and systolic blood pressure goal <120 mmHg or HR <70 bpm.

Urgent surgical repair is indicated of acute type A aortic dissections because medical treatment is associated with 60% in-hospital death rate [7]. The anatomic goal is resection of the aortic intimal tear to eliminate the threat of rupture and to reconstruct the aortic wall layers. Type A dissection may require aortic valve repair/replacement, aortic root/aortic arch/hemiarch repair/replacement. Acute tamponade may develop with dissection into the pericardium. This is a surgical emergency, and pericardial tap should be avoided as this may worsen hemodynamic collapse and delay emergent surgical intervention.

In patients with uncomplicated type B dissection (TBAD), surgical therapy has not shown superiority over medical therapy [7]. Therefore, most TBAD are managed medically if uncomplicated. The goal of medical therapy is anti-impulse control, pain control, and evaluating for malperfusion or disease progression. TEVAR or surgical intervention may be warranted in TBAD with persistent/recurring pain, uncontrolled hypertension despite medical therapies, advancing aortic expansion, or any evidence of malperfusion. A TEVAR may be performed to prevent late complications and promote aortic remodeling as well. During this procedure, a stent graft is deployed in the true lumen to cover the entry tear with the goal of improved aortic perfusion and encouraging thrombosis of the false lumen (Fig. 28.10).

Surveillance

The principal late complication of aortic dissection is aneurysmal dilatation of the outer wall of the false lumen [7]. Regular follow-up with serial imaging for routine surveillance is recommended lifelong with a vascular surgery clinic. False lumen patency or thrombosis is an important predictor of regional luminal growth and reintervention rate [8]. In follow-up, maximal aortic diameter is documented and followed over time. Patients with aortic dissection undergo at least annual surveillance with CT angiogram.

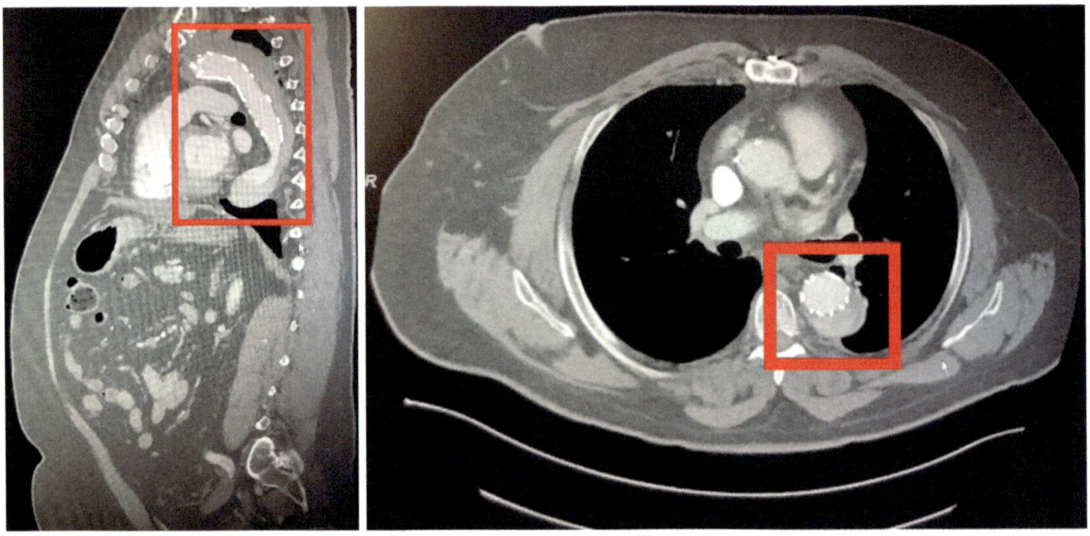

Fig. 28.10 TEVAR within true lumen excluding thrombus in false lumen

Clinical Pearls

- Patients diagnosed with aortic dissection should be referred to an aortic center when possible.
- Anti-impulse therapy is the mainstay of treatment for heart rate and blood pressure in patients with aortic dissection.
- A bicuspid aortic valve is associated with increased risk of aortic dissection and thoracic aortic aneurysm.
- Genetic referral for screening should be considered in patients with acute aortic dissections, especially in the younger population.

References

1. Lawrence PF, Rigberg DA. Arterial aneurysms, epidemiology, and natural history. Rutherford's vascular surgery and endovascular therapy. 2019. p. 875–83. https://www-clinicalkey-com.ahecproxy.ncahec.net/#!/content/book/3-s2.0-B9780323427913000694?scrollTo=hl0000575.
2. Jana S, Hu M, Shen M, Kassiri Z. Extracellular matrix, regional heterogeneity of the aorta, and aortic aneurysm. Exp Mol Med. 2019;51:1–15.
3. Dalman R, Mell M. Overview of abdominal aortic aneurysm. 2022. https://www.uptodate.com/contents/overview-of-abdominal-aortic-aneurysm#!.
4. Schermerhorn M, Cronenwett JL. Arterial aneurysms: abdominal and iliac aneurysms. Rutherford vascular surgery. 6th ed. Elsevier; 2005.
5. Abdominal aortic aneurysm. Elsevier BV; 2021. https://www-clinicalkey-com.ahecproxy.ncahec.net/#!/content/67-s2.0-7c5e261c-ea6f-4cab-aae7-cb8155587799.
6. White SB, Stavropoulos SW. Management of Endoleaks following Endovascular Aneurysm Repair. Semin Intervent Radiol. 2009 Mar;26(1):33-8. https://doi.org/10.1055/s-0029-1208381. PMID: 21326529; PMCID: PMC3036461.
7. Black J, Cambria RP. Aortic dissection: perspectives for the vascular/endovascular surgeon. Rutherford's vascular surgery. 2005. p. 1512–31.
8. Lombardi JV, Hughes GC, Appoo JJ, et al. Society for Vascular Surgery (SVS) and Society of Thoracic Surgeons (STS) reporting standards for type B aortic dissections. 2020. https://www.jvascsurg.org/article/S0741-5214(19)32649-7/fulltext.

Part VIII

Adult Congenital Heart Disease (ACHD)

Jana Reid Arwa Saidi

1.1 Introduction

Congenital heart disease is a rapidly growing subspecialty of cardiology. Nearly 1% of infants born in the USA have congenital heart disease [1–4]. Initially considered a disease of the pediatric population, many advances in the field have led to more adults now living with congenital heart disease than children. Prior to 1940, in the absence of any meaningful treatment options, 90% of infants born with complex congenital heart disease died before adulthood [2]. Following major advancements in diagnosis and treatment, a majority of infants now live into adulthood. As such, there are currently well over one million adults living with congenital heart disease [4, 5].

The evolution of treatment of congenital heart disease has been dramatic over the last 60 years. The development and advances in surgical, interventional, and diagnostic tools have changed the landscape of management and have profoundly affected outcomes. The first PDA ligation was performed in 1938. In 1944, Dr. Blalock, Dr. Taussig and Mr. Thomas devised the first shunt to improve pulmonary blood flow in a patient with Tetralogy of Fallot. The invention of the heart-lung bypass machine in 1955 led to the first repair of an ASD, which was the start of decades of advancement in congenital heart surgery. Catheter based procedures were developed in the 1960s and initially treated lesions such as PDAs and ASDs and are now used in complex disease. The first Fontan procedure was performed in 1968, allowing children born with a single functional ventricle to live past one year of age. The advent of 2D echocardiography in the 1970s permitted a major step forward in the diag-

J. Reid · A. Saidi
UF Health Congenital Heart Center, University of FL, Gainesville, FL, USA
e-mail: reidja@shands.ufl.edu; asaidi@pedcard.ufl.edu

nosis and management of congenital heart disease. Transposition of the Great Arteries was treated with the first arterial switch procedure in 1975, eventually replacing the previously performed atrial switch procedure and dramatically altering the long-term course for patients with TGA. The first minimally invasive heart valve replacement was performed in 2000, leading the way for non-surgical options for a variety of congenital heart defects. 3D imaging is now being used to help map out complex anatomy in advance of intricate surgical interventions and stem cell therapy is an emerging field that is the source of many exciting research studies [6].

Hundreds of thousands of infants and children have benefitted from these advances in diagnosis, intervention, and clinical care, such that they are living well into adulthood. While initially thought to be curative, it has been recognized over time that many of these interventions allowed children to grow up without severe limitations, but with increased long-term morbidity and mortality, often becoming evident in the adult years. The need for uninterrupted specialized care in an ACHD center cannot be overstated, as outcomes for adults who have been lost to follow-up are notably worse than those who have consistent access to care. As childhood palliative interventions reach the end of their lifespan, adults with congenital heart disease are prone to atrial and ventricular arrhythmias, infective endocarditis, heart failure, pulmonary hypertension, and the need for pacemakers and/or defibrillators [3, 4, 7]. They may require additional interventions for their congenital heart disease, either via surgical or transcatheter intervention. For those with advanced disease processes that cannot be otherwise salvaged, advanced therapies including mechanical circulatory support and transplantation, sometimes multi-organ, may be considered. Additional factors for adults with congenital heart disease include contraception, pregnancy risk and delivery considerations, perioperative care for non-cardiac surgery and the management of acquired cardiac and non-cardiac co-morbidities [4–7]. A multidisciplinary model of care for adult congenital heart disease is critical to long-term health and wellness.

Adults with congenital heart disease make up an ever growing and intriguing subset of general cardiology. Whether a simple or complex lesion, these patients have special considerations for management. There have been many advances in care over the last 60 years and certainly the future is full of more revolutionary innovations for those living with congenital heart defects.

References

1. Allen HD, Penny DJ, Feltes TF, Cetta F. Moss and Adams' heart disease in infants, children, and adolescents including the fetus and young adult. 9th ed. Wolters Kluwer; 2016.
2. Tennant PW, Pearce MS, Bythell M, Rankin J. 20-year survival of children born with congenital anomalies: a population-based study. Lancet. 2010;375(9715):649–56. https://doi.org/10.1016/S0140-6736(09)61922-X.

3. Gurvitz M, Dunn JE, Bhatt A, et al. Characteristics of adults with congenital heart defects in the United States. J Am Coll Cardiol. 2020;76(2):175–82.
4. Stout KK, Daniels CJ, Aboulhosn JA, et al. 2018 AHA/ACC Guideline for the Management of Adults With Congenital Heart Disease: a report of the American College of Cardiology/American Heart Association Task Force on Clinical Practice Guidelines [published correction appears in J Am Coll Cardiol. 2019 May 14;73(18):2361–2362]. J Am Coll Cardiol. 2019;73(12):e81–e192.
5. Baumgartner H, De Backer J, Babu-Narayan SV, et al. 2020 ESC guidelines for the management of adult congenital heart disease. Eur Heart J. 2021;42:563–645.
6. Kiess M. History and evolution of the treatment of adult congenital heart disease. BCMJ. 2016;58(7):368–72.
7. Warnes CA. Adult congenital heart disease: the challenges of a lifetime. Eur Heart J. 2017;38(26):2041–7. https://doi.org/10.1093/eurheartj/ehw529.

ACHD

29

Amanda Green and Jorge Alegria

Simple Defects

Atrial Septal Defect (ASD) A communication between the atria, allowing blood flow between the systemic and pulmonary circulations [1]. These can occur in isolation or as a part of a more complex diagnosis/constellation of defects.

Anatomy and Physiology

Defect in the atrial septum. These can be in the septum primum, secundum, or associated with anomalous pulmonary veins in the case of a sinus venosus defect (superior or inferior location).

The degree of shunting across the ASD is determined by the size of the defect as well as the degree of ventricular compliance. In older adults who have decreased ventricular compliance and a stiffer ventricle, there is a greater risk of transient heart failure after closure of the atrial defect, given that the stiff ventricle now must accept a greater volume load and no longer has the "pop off" of the atrial septum [1, 2]. The development of left ventricular diastolic dysfunction with subsequent increase in left atrial pressure may result in an increase left to right shunt in adults, especially in the presence of hypertension or coronary artery disease.

A. Green
Atrium Health/Sanger Heart and Vascular Institute, Greenville, SC, USA
e-mail: amanda.green1@atriumhealth.org

J. Alegria (✉)
Atrium Health/Sanger Heart and Vascular, Congenital Heart Center, Charlotte, NC, USA
e-mail: Jorge.Alegria@atriumhealth.org

Types of ASD

Secundum ASD: Located in septum primum, in the region of the fossa ovalis. This is more common in females who make up 65–75% of the patient population with secundum ASD [3]. Depending on the defect size and pulmonary vascular resistance, it can often be closed by transcatheter techniques.

Primum ASD: Also known as endocardial cushion or AV septal defects and are associated with abnormalities of the atrioventricular valves [3]. Anatomically located in the septum secundum, these ASDs usually require surgical repair. In the electrocardiogram a first-degree atrioventricular block and left axis deviation can be found. Left ventricular outflow tract obstruction can be present. Long-term complications in adults may result in need of permanent pacemaker, left sided atrio-ventricular valve replacement.

Sinus Venosus ASD: These are located along the superior or inferior portion of the atrial septum near the junction of the SVC or IVC. They are often associated with partial

R. Musialowski, K. Allshouse (eds.), *Cardiovascular Manual for the Advanced Practice Provider*,
https://doi.org/10.1007/978-3-031-35819-7_29

anomalous pulmonary venous return. Superior sinus venosus is the most common form of the two, and accounts for 5–10% of all ASDs [3]. These commonly requires surgical repair of defect and baffling of the pulmonary veins to the left atrium.

Coronary Sinus Septal Defect: This is a defect in the wall of the coronary sinus also known as an "unroofed coronary sinus," which can result in left to right shunting (LA CS defect RA) [3]. This is also commonly associated with a persistent left superior vena cava.

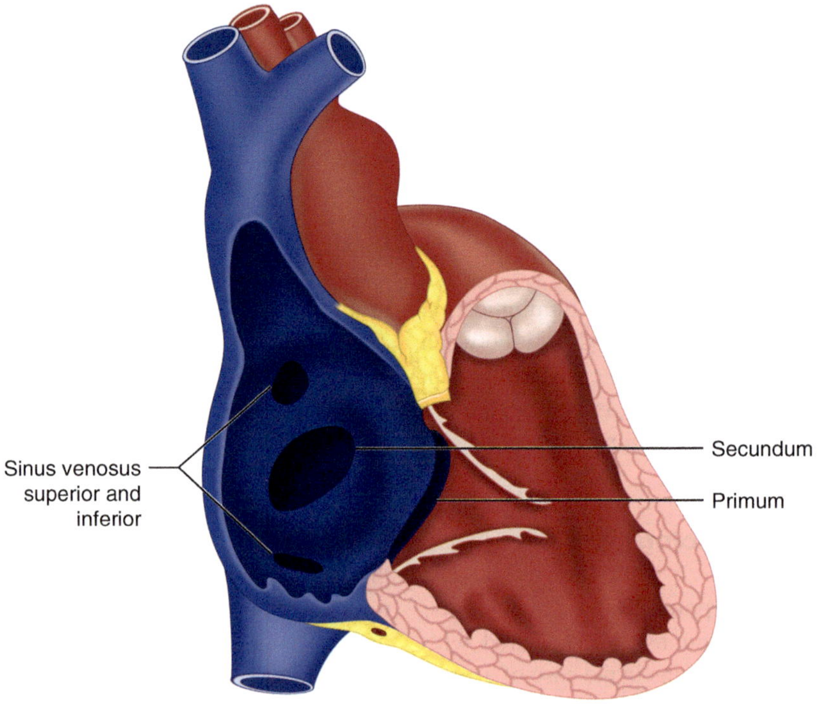

Physical Exam Correlations

On physical exam, there may or may not be a murmur if the ASD is small with a low degree of shunting. If a higher degree of left to right shunt is present, there may be a soft systolic ejection murmur given the increased blood flow across the pulmonary valve annulus. S2 may have fixed splitting but this finding is not always present [3]. In patients with pulmonary hypertension, P2 may be loud or "snappy" [3].

Adults with undiagnosed ASDs may present with a chief complaint of fatigue, exercise intolerance, and/or palpitations [1]. Paradoxical embolism may also occur.

EKG may demonstrate a right bundle branch block or rSr' pattern in secundum atrial septal defect [1, 3].

Pathology/Description

This defect may be associated with Down Syndrome, Holt Oram syndrome, DiGeorge syndrome, and Ellis Van Creveld syndrome [2]. There is an approximate 10% inheritance risk from a parent with an ASD to their child [2].

Imaging: CMR, Cardiac CT, and/or TEE are useful to evaluate ASD size, shape, rim tissue, and pulmonary venous connections in adults with

ASD. These imaging modalities are helpful in the decision-making regarding ASD closure type and timing [3].

Management

Management of the ASD depends on the type and location of the defect. Secundum ASDs can often be closed with transcatheter techniques and devices, while primum ASDs, coronary sinus septal defects, and sinus venosus ASDs require surgical repair.

The ACC/AHA guidelines recommend that adults with an unrepaired ASD or a repaired ASD with residual shunt have pulse oximetry at rest and during exercise performed. This will help assess for systemic desaturation, which would indicate the presence of right to left shunting across the defect.

Indications for Repair [4]:

- Qp:Qs (pulmonary: systemic blood flow) of >/= 1.5:1 and/or right heart enlargement.
- ASDs should not be closed in adults where the pulmonary arterial systolic pressure is >2/3 of systemic, PVR greater than 2.3 systemic, and/ or there is a net right to left shunt.

Long-term surveillance for ASD depends on the type of ASD and repair needed and are specified in the AHA/ACC Guidelines for the Management of Adults with Congenital Heart Disease.

Simple (I): a small, isolated ASD. This includes a native isolated small ASD, or repaired secundum ASD or sinus venosus defect without significant residual shunt or chamber enlargement.

Moderate Complexity (II): Primum ASD, moderate to large unrepaired secundum ASD.

ACHD expertise may improve outcomes in procedures such as diagnostic and interventional cardiology procedures including EP procedures [4].

Pearls

- Approximately 34% of adults with unrepaired ASD have complaints of palpitations, which typically is sinus tachycardia [1]. In patients aged 40–60 years, 15% may have atrial flutter [1].
- ASD may have fixed splitting of S2, more common in defects with greater shunting (higher Qp:Qs) [3].
- If pulmonary hypertension is present, may have loud P2 [3].
- RV lift may be felt in the subxiphoid area on deep inspiration [3].
- EKG may show a rSr' pattern in the right precordial leads, and right bundle branch block may also be seen [1, 3].

Ventricular Septal Defect (VSD)

Anatomy and Physiology

A VSD is a hole/communication between the ventricular septum (wall that separates right and left ventricles) that allows for blood communication from the left sided systemic circulation to the right sided circulation or pulmonary circulation. Ventricular septal defects can occur in various parts of the ventricular septum and are classified based on their location [5]. In both children and adults (excluding bicuspid aortic valve in the adult population), VSDs are the most common congenital heart defect [5]. In many cases the VSD may close spontaneously from either muscle occlusion in muscular defects, or closure from aneurysmal tricuspid valve tissue in perimembranous defects. With reduction in size, the burden of shunt is also decreased [5].

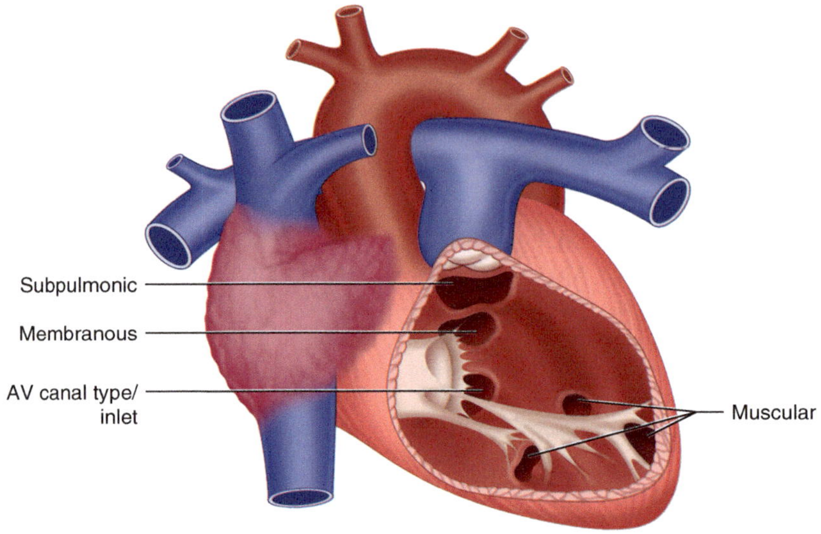

Physical Exam Correlations

- Systolic Murmur typically present.
  - Very small Muscular VSD - Murmur can be a short "squeaky" type murmur as the defect may close part way through systole.
  - Muscular VSD: This will be a pansystolic murmur, usually harsh in quality, along the second to third left intercostal spaces. Patient may have an associated thrill, so the provider should always palpate precordium to determine if this is present [6].

    The louder the murmur, typically the more restrictive the defect (greater drop in pressure across the defect = louder murmur).
  - Large VSD: Systolic murmur may not be as loud if there is not a dramatic pressure gradient change across the ventricular septum. If the VSD is large, patient will have a soft murmur, may have fixed splitting of S2 or "snappy" P2 component of S2 given the elevated pulmonary arterial pressures [7].

    If there is significant volume overload from left to right shunting, patient may also have a diastolic rumble.
  - Nonrestrictive VSD: Typically, this is a large VSD with equalization of pressures in both ventricles and associated pulmonary hypertension. If this is long- standing, patients can develop Eisenmenger syndrome which is classified as irreversible pulmonary hypertension with cyanosis. These patients may have a left to right shunting at rest with reversal to right to left shunting with ambulation. Consider ambulatory saturation testing to evaluate for desaturation with activity [7].

Pathology/Description

VSD is a defect located in the ventricular septum which initially creates a volume load on the left heart. Long-standing VSDs can ultimately lead to elevation in pulmonary artery pressures and pulmonary hypertension.

Imaging

VSD can be evaluated by echocardiogram. Modalities such as Cardiac MRI may also be helpful as this will give you detailed anatomic information as well as information regarding the degree of shunting. Cardiac CT can be used to obtain information regarding anatomy (size and location) of the defect [5, 7].

If there is a concern for cyanosis, ambulatory saturation monitoring with a hall walk test is helpful.

Right heart catheterization is helpful to gather information regarding the degree of pulmonary hypertension, PH reversibility testing, as well as degree of shunting (Qp:Qs) [5, 7].

Management

- Most isolated muscular and Perimembranous VSDs close spontaneously.
- If repair is indicated:
- Membranous, Inlet, Subpulmonary, all require surgical repair if hemodynamically significant.
  - Clinically symptomatic
  - Qp:Qs $\geq$ 1.5:1
  - Chamber enlargement (left heart)
- Muscular VSD can be repaired in the cath lab or surgically depending on anatomy/size.
- Closure of a large VSD with associated pulmonary hypertension may not be recommended if pulmonary vascular bed not responsive or if there is a concern that the pulmonary vascular resistance is too high, although in some cases a "fenestrated" patch or device can decompress the right heart [4].

Pearls
- In patients with unrepaired VSD, there is an increased risk of infective endocarditis. This will typically affect the tricuspid and pulmonary valves [4, 8].
- Survival in Unoperated VSD:
  - Small restrictive defects have a high 25-year survival of 87% [4, 8]. In patients with a small VSD, low Qp:Qs <1.5:1 and low pulmonary vascular resistance had survival rate of 96% [9].
  - Moderate and large defects have a lower 25-year survival of 86 and 61%, respectively [4].
  - Patients with large shunt and Eisenmenger syndrome had even lower 25-year survival at 42% [4].
- Survival in repaired VSD: Significantly improved but remains abnormal [4].
- The majority of small restrictive VSDs located in the membranous or muscular septum can be observed and do not need intervention [4]. For the small number of patients who develop progressive aortic insufficiency related to their perimembranous VSD, surgical repair may be indicated [4, 8].
- Patients with unrepaired VSDs, that are moderately restrictive, may have mild-moderate pulmonary hypertension. Some patients with large nonrestrictive defects may develop Eisenmenger syndrome, and have shunt reversal and systemic desaturation [4, 8].
- Patients with previous closure of their VSD may have patch leak or residual VSD [4].

Bicuspid Aortic Valve (BAV)

Bicuspid AV is the most common congenital heart defect with incidence of 4.6 per 1000 live births. It is 1.5 times more prevalent in males than females. It has a high degree of disease progression leading to aortic stenosis and/or regurgitation, as well as association with aortic root dilation, aortic dissection, and thoracic aortic aneurysm [4, 10].

Anatomy and Physiology

Bicuspid AV is caused by fusion of the aortic valve leaflet commissure creating a two-leaflet valve instead of a three-leaflet valve. This results in a "fish mouth"- appearing opening of the aortic valve rather than a round unobstructed opening. The most common anatomic forms of bicuspid aortic valve include fusion of the right and left coronary commissures or right and non-coronary commissures. Fusion of the right and non-coronary commissure is associated with a more rapid deterioration of the valve leading to stenosis or insufficiency, whereas fusion of the right and left coronary commissure has a greater incidence of association with coarctation of the aorta [10, 11].

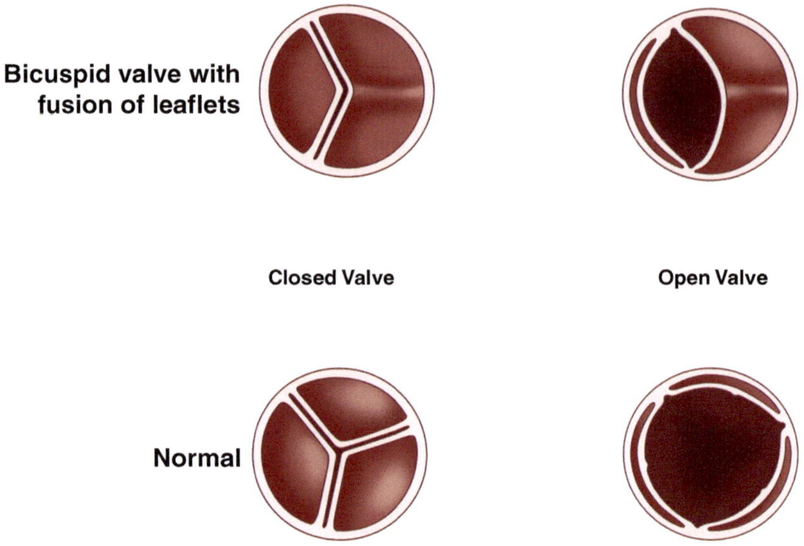

Physical Exam Correlations

Patients may have an audible click (systolic ejection noise) [12]. Murmur may only be present if there are other associated diagnoses such as coarctation of the aorta, or valvular disease with obstruction or insufficiency [12]. Providers need to assess for coarctation of the aorta. Coarctation of the aorta and bicuspid valve are commonly associated [10, 11].

Pathology/Description

BAV has aortic valve morphology but with two functional leaflets of unequal size, instead of three, due to incomplete commissural separation during fetal development [3, 5]. There is a familial heritability in an autosomal dominant pattern. In one study, the incidence of asymptomatic bicuspid aortic valve in first-degree relatives is 9% with a 32% incidence of those first-degree relatives having an abnormal aorta [4, 12].

Given the abnormal flow pattern of blood across the aortic valve leaflets in bicuspid aortic valve, there may be calcification or obstruction of the leaflets, which can happen at a higher rate than for those with a tricuspid aortic valve [10]. There may also be incomplete coaptation of the valve leaflets resulting in aortic insufficiency.

Imaging

Evaluation of bicuspid aortic valve is with transthoracic echocardiogram. The valve can be evaluated in more detail with TEE, Cardiac MRI and Cardiac CT to look at valve morphology and evaluate degree of aortic stenosis and regurgitation.

If AS or AI is present, stress testing can also be used to evaluate and risk stratify the patient's need for intervention, either transcatheter or surgical [4, 12].

Management

Surgical and/or transcatheter management of bicuspid valves can be considered in patients with severe obstruction or regurgitation. In the younger population, balloon aortic valvuloplasty in the cath lab is more common; however, in adults, transcatheter valve therapies or surgical valve repair/replacement is more common [12, 13].

Clinical Pearls

- Bicuspid aortic valves can often be asymptomatic but can also present with aortic stenosis or insufficiency earlier in life. One study found that patients with bicuspid aortic valve presented at age 40 ± 20 years vs. 67 ± 16 years for patients with tricuspid valve [12].

- If a Bicuspid valve found, assessment for coarctation of the aorta (supine 4 extremity BPs and imaging) and other aortopathies (ascending aorta/aortic root, thoracic aorta) should be undertaken [10–12].
- First-degree relatives of patients with bicuspid valve should have routine screening echocardiograms [4].

Valvar Pulmonary Stenosis (PS)

PS is typically associated with a conical or dome-shaped pulmonary valve or can be a result of thickening of the pulmonary valve leaflets. The narrowing of the opening of the valve between the right ventricle and pulmonary arteries with obstruction at the level of the valve, results in hypertension of the right ventricle [14].

Anatomy and Physiology

Valvar PS occurs in approximately 7% of children born with CHD. PS can be isolated or can occur in combination with other defects, such as in Tetralogy of Fallot [14]. Pulmonary stenosis is associated with Noonan syndrome, Alagille syndrome, Williams syndrome, and congenital rubella [14]. Isolated valvar PS can be associated with a dilated main PA and dysplastic valve leaflets [4]. Valvar PS results in RV hypertrophy and hypertension, which varies based on the degree of obstruction [14].

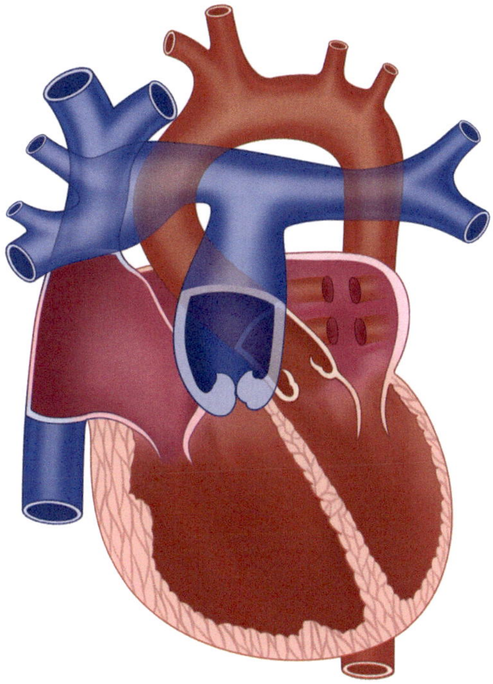

Valvar pulmonary stenosis with dysplastic /thickened leaflets of the pulmonary valve, and right ventricular hypertrophy, as well as dilation of the main and branch pulmonary arteries which can be secondary to the high velocity jet across the pulmonary valve leaflets.

Physical Exam Correlations

Physical exam findings may include a crescendo-decrescendo systolic murmur which radiates out into the axillae or to the back. The murmur varies in intensity and can have associated thrill [14]. If the patient has pulmonary insufficiency, you may also hear a diastolic murmur or a “to-fro” murmur.

Pathology/Description

Pulmonary valve stenosis is primarily a congenital diagnosis and includes pulmonary valve abnormalities such as uni-commissural, dome-shaped, dysplastic, and bicuspid [4, 14] valves. Pulmonary stenosis can be seen in Noonan, Alagille, and Williams syndromes, and with congenital rubella [4, 14].

Imaging

Echocardiograms are done for routine surveillance of the degree of obstruction and/or insufficiency. Cardiac MRI can be helpful to evaluate RV size and volumes as well as the dimensions of the pulmonary valve and main pulmonary artery if interventions are being considered [4]. EKG is also recommended [4].

Management

Intervention for valvar pulmonary stenosis can often be done by transcatheter techniques, balloon pulmonary valvuloplasty. If failure of balloon pulmonary valvuloplasty occurs or there is progressive insufficiency, surgical intervention may be considered [4].

Clinical Pearls

- Adults with the history of pulmonary stenosis require ongoing cardiac follow-up and monitoring for evidence of progressive valve stenosis or regurgitation, RV hypertrophy, heart failure, and arrhythmias [4, 14].
- Patients with PS (mild, moderate, and severe)—usually have a good long-term outcome. Some will require intervention in adulthood either for progressive PS or significant pulmonary insufficiency due to prior intervention (Transcatheter or surgical) [4, 14].

Tetralogy of Fallot (TOF)

The most common cyanotic congenital heart defect is Tetralogy of Fallot (TOF), and it accounts for 7% to 10% of congenital heart defects [15].

Anatomy and Physiology

Tetralogy of Fallot (TOF) is comprised of four defects including a large VSD, overriding aorta, pulmonary stenosis, and RV hypertrophy. Unrepaired TOF can either be "pink" (acyanotic) or "blue" (cyanotic) depending on the degree of pulmonary stenosis and amount of pulmonary blood flow/right to left shunting across the VSD. Repair of TOF is typically done when the patient is an infant, and consists of VSD closure, transannular patch, and resection of RV muscle bundles [4]. This repair typically leaves the patient with little to no PS and free pulmonary insufficiency. In the present day, TOF is repaired in infancy. However, there may be adult patients that have not had complete repair given when/where they were born.

Unrepaired Tetralogy of Fallot

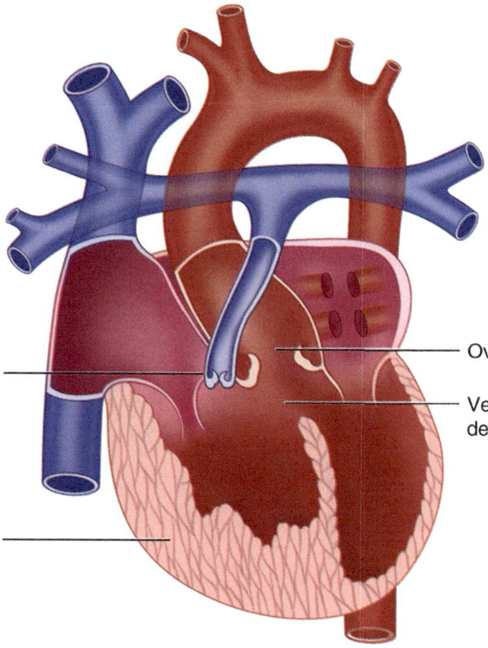

Physical Exam Correlations

In repaired TOF, the physical exam may consist of a to-fro systolic murmur. This is secondary to the movement of blood back and forth across the RVOT (systolic murmur secondary to pulmonary stenosis) and diastolic murmur from the pulmonary insufficiency.

Pathology/Description

In tetralogy of Fallot, the aorta overrides the ventricular septum, which "crowds out" the pulmonary artery and subpulmonic area, resulting in a small MPA, potentially small branch PA's, valvar, and subvalvar pulmonary stenosis [15]. Adults with tetralogy of Fallot who have undergone complete repair may require pulmonary valve replacement in adulthood given ongoing PS/PI and RV dilation and dysfunction [4].

Imaging

EKG, Echo, Cardiac MRI, and stress testing are recommended at certain intervals. Cardiac MRI is helpful for quantification of RV size and function, especially when considering the timing of pulmonary valve replacement [4].

Management

Repair of tetralogy of Fallot usually consists of resection of RV muscle bundles, and use of a patch to enlarge the main pulmonary artery and branch pulmonary arteries. The VSD is closed with a patch and any residual ASD is closed [4]. Adults with repaired tetralogy of Fallot may often require pulmonary valve replacement. This can either be done via surgical techniques or in the cath lab via transcatheter techniques. There are now FDA approved transcatheter valve therapies for replacement of pulmonary valve in the native RVOT [4].

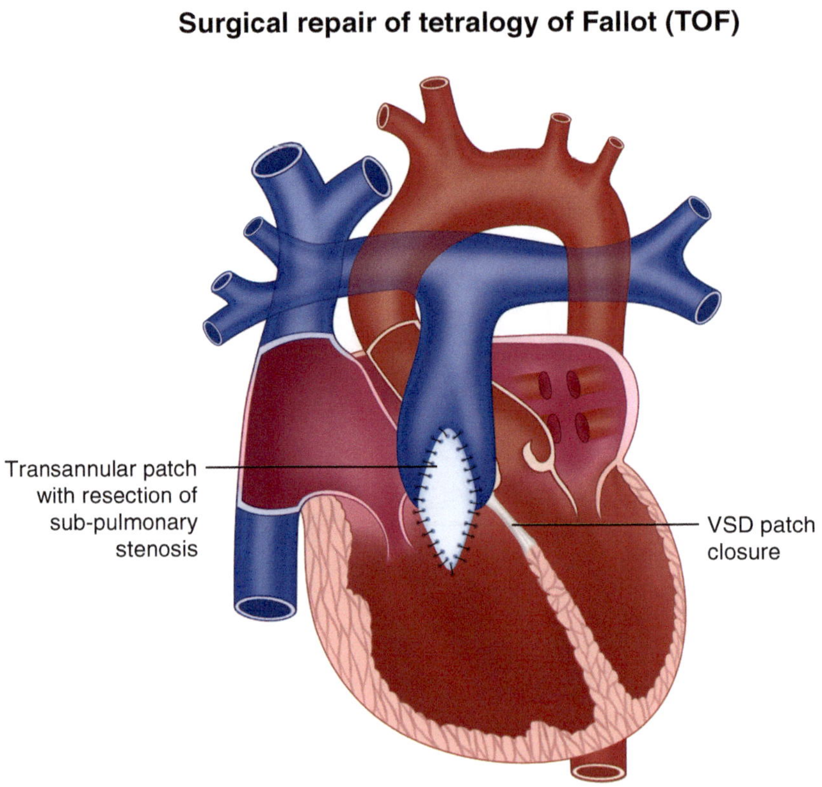

Clinical Pearls

- Cardiac MRI is the gold standard for evaluation of RV size, function, and valve regurgitation in patients with repaired TOF [4].
- Prior to any intervention, the proximal coronaries and their origins need to be outlined [4].
- Leading causes of mortality in adults with repaired TOF are arrhythmia, heart failure, and complications from reoperations [15].
- In adults with TOF, inducible VT is associated with increased risk of clinical VT or SCD. Programmed ventricular stimulation is useful in risk-stratifying patients who are at moderate risk of SCD, rather than as a routine surveillance tool in low-risk patients [4].
- Bundle Branch Block >180 ms is associated with higher risk of sudden death.
- Syncope in a repaired TOF must be considered VT until proven otherwise.
- Pulmonary hypertension can occur in repaired TOF.

Coarctation of the Aorta

Anatomy and Physiology

Coarctation is a narrowing or stricture in the aorta. This most commonly occurs near the ductal remnant and takeoff of the left subclavian artery (proximal descending aorta) [4, 16]. It is frequently associated with a bicuspid aortic valve and may be seen in Turner's Syndrome. First-degree relatives of patients diagnosed with obstructive left heart disease are at a significantly higher risk (as high as 10%) for coarctation and other left heart lesions [16].

Physical Exam Correlations

Hypertension is common in both repaired and unrepaired patients with coarctation of the aorta [4, 16]. If a patient has recurrent obstruction, four extremity blood pressures, done with the patient laying supine, may reveal decreased BP in the lower extremities. A systolic murmur may be heard at the left mid-clavicular line and/or posteriorly along the spine. Brachial femoral pulse delay may be present if there is obstruction [4].

Pathology/Description

There are several theories of why coarctation occurs:

1. Ductal tissue extends into the aortic arch and as the ductus closes and becomes a ligament the aorta is also constricted.
2. Flow: poor flow through the aortic arch during fetal development secondary to other left heart lesions resulting in poor growth of the aorta this is often associated with hypoplasia of the aortic arch, not just coarctation.

Post-repair of coarctation, aneurysm formation in the proximal descending aorta at the site of repair can occur. Dissection can also occur, primarily in the setting of uncontrolled hypertension [4]. Ascending aortic aneurysm can occur in those patients with bicuspid aortic valve.

Imaging

Transthoracic echocardiogram, Cardiac CT and MRI can all be helpful for evaluating the structure of the aortic arch and gradient across the coarctation. Upper and lower extremity BPs are also helpful in evaluating gradient (using the right arm for upper extremity measurement). EKG and stress testing are used in evaluation with the EKG evaluating for LVH and stress testing is used to evaluate BP measurements with exercise as well as look for any evidence of ischemia [4].

Management

Surgical repair or stent angioplasty in the cath lab is recommended for adults with hypertension and significant native or recurrent coarctation of the aorta [4, 17]. Hypertension management is critical. Complications of coarctation repair include re-coarctation, pseudoaneurysm, dissection. 11% of patients may require reintervention for restenosis seen by CMR or CTA and supported by physical exam findings [4]. Patients who have undergone surgical patch repair are at a higher risk of developing aneurysms [4, 18].

Clinical Pearls

- Recurrent obstruction is defined as an upper extremity to lower extremity resting pressure gradient of >20 mmHg (i.e., right arm Systolic BP of 150 mmHg and left leg systolic BP of 110 mmHg—in this example the peak to peak gradient is 40 mmHg), and/or mean Doppler systolic gradient >20 mmHg [4].
- Recurrent obstruction may be amenable to balloon aortoplasty.
- If LV systolic function is decreased or aortic regurgitation is present, recurrent obstruction is defined as an upper extremity to lower extremity gradient of >10 mmHg or mean Doppler gradient >10 mmHg with collateral flow. (CMR or CT is used to help assess for anatomic evidence of recurrent Coarctation of the aorta) [4].
- Cerebral aneurysm can be present in up to 10% of patients with coarctation of the aorta [4, 19].

L-TGA

Anatomy and Physiology

Congenitally corrected transposition of the great arteries (CCTGA) or L-TGA describes the condition in which the right sided (subpulmonary) ventricle has the shape of the anatomic left ventricle (morphologic LV), and the left sided (sub aortic) ventricle has the shape of the anatomic right ventricle (morphologic RV). This physiology results in the patient having a systemic right ventricle. This defect can occur in isolation or can be associated with other defects such as atrial or ventricular septal defects or pulmonary stenosis. There is also a high incidence of Ebstein-like malformation of the left sided AV-valve, which is the anatomic tricuspid valve. This incidence is felt to be as high as 90%. This malformation can lead to progressive tricuspid (systemic) valve regurgitation [4, 20]. There is a 1% per year or 10% per decade risk of complete heart block [4, 21] with this condition.

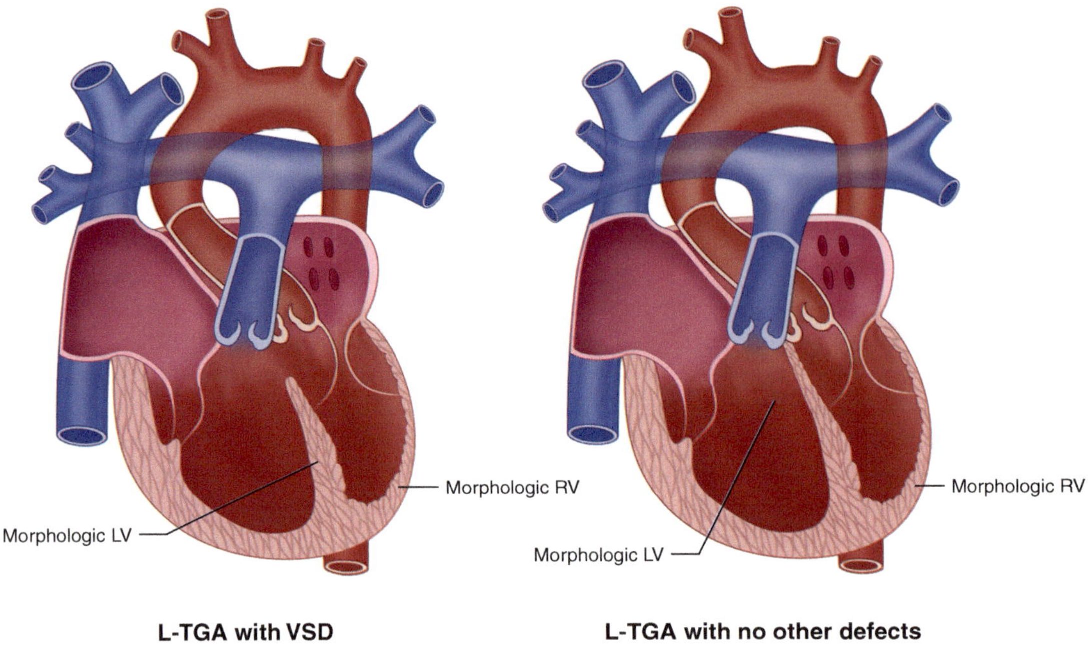

Physical Exam Correlations

Physical exam findings depend on other lesions present or prior surgery/palliation. If no other lesions, physical exam may be normal. Abnormalities in physical exam may show the presence of a systolic murmur in patients with PS and/or VSD.

Pathology/Description

Isolated L-TGA without other defects may present in the third or fourth decade with a new diagnosis of heart failure. More than 1/3 of patients with L-TGA and no other significant defects presents by the fifth decade with significant heart failure (systemic RV) or may present in complete heart block with a 10% per decade risk (i.e., 40% risk by age 40 years) [22, 23]. Patients with L-TGA with other significant associated defects and history of prior heart surgery have a significant risk of systemic ventricular failure, with 2/3 of these patients presenting by age 45 with heart failure [23].

Imaging

Cardiac MRI or Cardiac CT, and echocardiography are all used to evaluate the ventricular function, AV-valve regurgitation, as well as any other intracardiac lesions or anatomic repairs/palliations [4]. Given the likelihood for conduction abnormalities, patients will also need routine EKG monitoring as well as Holter monitoring [4].

Management

Surgical management of patients with L-TGA varies based on the additional defects involved. One operation that can be done for patients with L-TGA with or without VSD is called a "double switch." This operation consists of an atrial switch (Senning or Mustard procedure) to re-route the venous return to the appropriate ventricle, and then arterial switch to switch the great vessels so that they are then aligned with the re-routed systemic venous return to the appropriately shaped ventricle [4, 23]. Progressive systemic atrioventricular valve regurgitation (tricuspid valve) is common and tricuspid valve replacement should be considered early when there is severe tricuspid valve regurgitation to prevent further decline in systemic ventricular dysfunction (right ventricle).

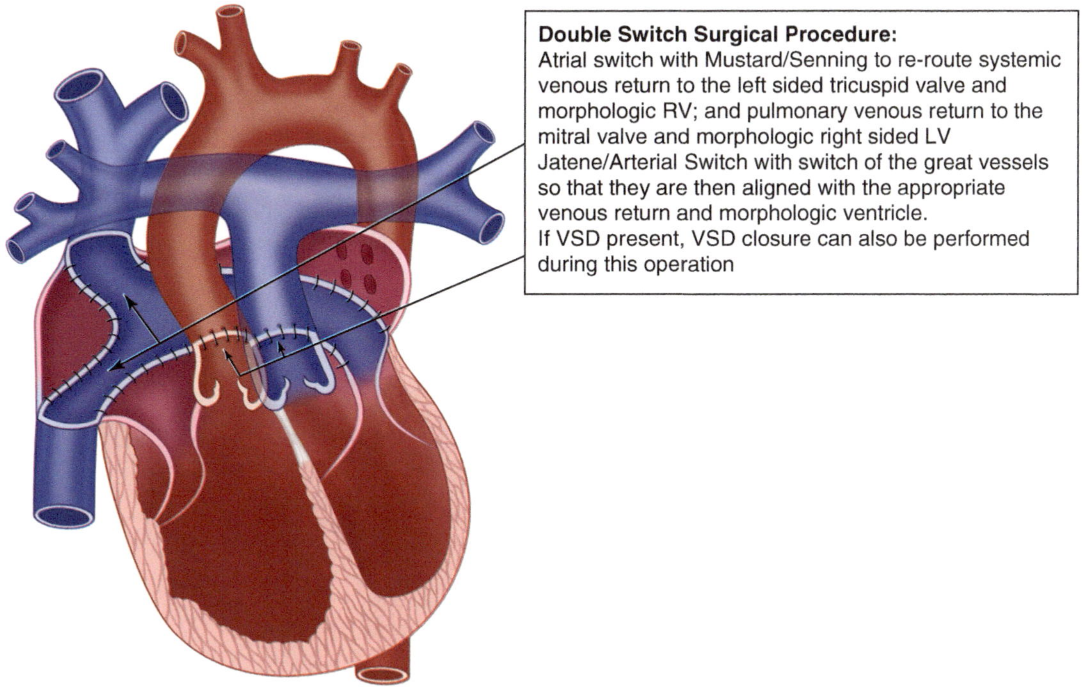

Clinical Pearls

- Disease progression and clinical course is primarily related to the presence and type of other defects and their severity. The presence of other defects also determines the type and complexity of the surgical repair/palliations needed.
- Tricuspid valve replacement in L-TGA should be considered at the earliest sign of RV dysfunction.
- These patients have a high risk of heart block as well as atrial arrhythmias.
- Failure of the systemic ventricle is higher with concomitant tricuspid regurgitation [23].
- May present later in life after asymptomatic period after birth.

D-TGA

Anatomy and Physiology

In d-TGA (dextro-transposition of the great arteries) the pulmonary artery and aorta are "switched," with the pulmonary artery arising from the left ventricle and the aorta arising from the right ventricle. This defect is often accompanied by an atrial septal defect and/or PFO. It may also have associated ventricular septal defect and coronary artery abnormalities [23, 24].

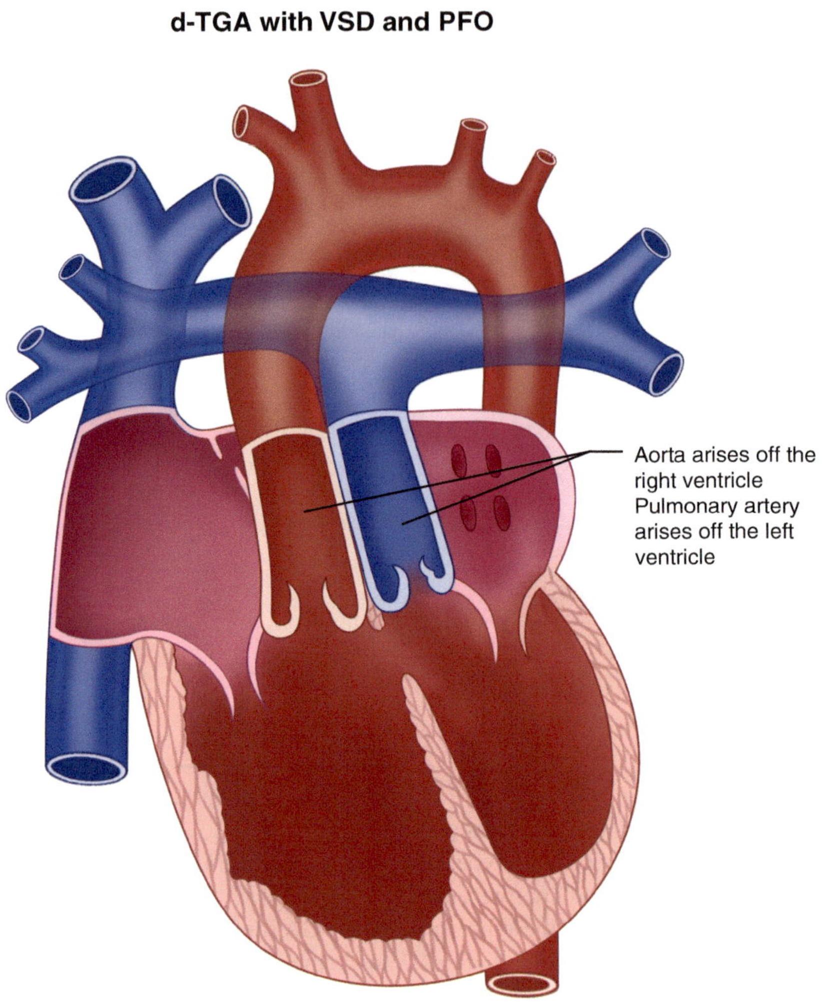

Physical Exam Correlations

A patient with repaired transposition, either with an arterial switch or an atrial switch, may have a normal physical exam. However, exam findings may include a single S2 (A2) (given anterior location of the aorta), and a systolic murmur if there is associated main or branch pulmonary artery stenosis [24]. Other physical exam findings are based on residual defects. In patients with atrial switch, assess ambulatory saturations to assess for baffle leaks and possible right to left shunting and desaturation [23].

Pathology/Description

In unrepaired d-TGA, there are two parallel circuits in which the deoxygenated systemic venous return is recirculated in the systemic circuit and oxygenated pulmonary venous return is recirculated in the pulmonary circuit. These parallel circuits are not compatible with life unless there is mixing, which can occur across an atrial defect, a VSD or PDA [23, 24]. The patent ductus arteriosus (PDA) needs to remain open in the neonatal period, which can be accomplished by an infusion of prostaglandin. Additionally, creation of an atrial defect with a balloon atrial septostomy procedure may need to be done if there is inadequate mixing prior to surgical repair [24].

Imaging

Echo, EKG, Cardiac MRI, Cardiac CT, and exercise testing are all used at routine intervals to evaluate patients with both arterial and atrial switch for d-TGA. The timing and type of additional testing such as Holter monitors, pulse oximetry vary between the two repair types [4].

Management

There are two common surgical repairs seen in adults who underwent repair as a child—the Arterial switch (Jatene switch with LeCompte Maneuver) and Atrial switch (also known as a Mustard or Senning operation) [4, 23].

Arterial (Jatene) switch and VSD closure

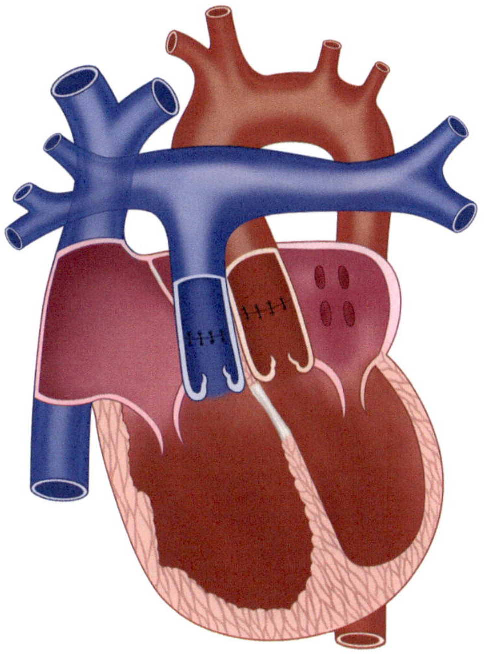

Present day Surgical Repair – arterial switch (Jatene switch) done around 3-5 days of age.
Jatene switch was developed and 1st done successfully in 1975, gained popularity and widespread use for d-TGA repair in the 1980's VSD/ASD/PFO closed (if present) Aorta and pulmonary artery transected above the sinus. Coronary buttons taken off and re-implanted on the neo-aorta. Pulmonary arteries are brought anterior to the aorta, and draped over the ascending (LeCompte Maneuver)

Long Term Consequences of the Arterial Switch
Stenosis at the arterial anastomotic sites, most commonly supravalvular PS Branch pulmonary artery stenosis Neoaortic root dilation Neoaortic valve regurgitation (native pulmonary valve) Coronary ostial stenosis/occlusion

Clinical Pearls

- Some patients with d-TGA s/p arterial switch who have early problems with pulmonary stenosis undergo RV to PA conduit placement (Rastelli), and can need further surgical revision of this conduit either in an open or transcatheter procedure [4, 24].
- Patients post Le-Compte maneuver as a part of the arterial switch may need branch PA plasty, which is often done in the cardiac cath lab using stent angioplasty technique [4].
- Patients post-arterial switch can develop coronary artery stenosis or occlusion given that the coronary arteries are moved as buttons in the arterial switch procedure [4].
- Patients undergoing arterial switch are at higher risk for neurodevelopmental problems and ADHD [24, 25].

Atrial Switch (Mustard/Senning)

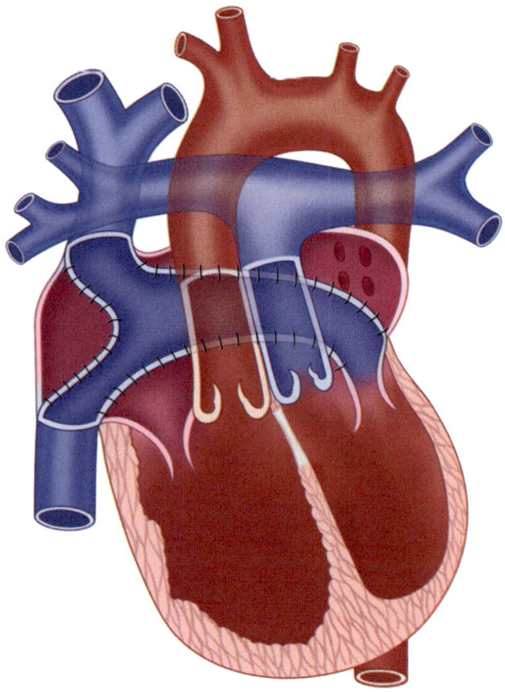

Senning: Developed by Dr. Ake Senning in 1957. Uses a complex reconstruction utilizing flaps from the atrial septum and atrial tissue to create the baffles

Mustard: Developed in 1963 by Dr. William Mustard. Resects the atrial septum and uses pericardial patch to create the baffles

Long Term Consequences of the Atrial Switch (Mustard/Senning)

Baffle leaks
Obstruction of the venous pathways
Arrhythmias
Need for pacemakers/defibrillators
Systolic dysfunction of the systemic right ventricle.

Clinical Pearls

- Patients post-atrial switch can develop leak or obstruction of their systemic venous or pulmonary venous baffles. If systemic SVC venous baffle obstruction occurs, they may present with SVC type syndrome—JVD, prominent veins on upper limbs and chest. Systemic IVC baffle obstruction may present with abdominal distension/ascites, prominent veins on abdomen, lower extremity edema, and no significant upper extremity symptoms. Baffle leak may present with systemic desaturation. Assessment for baffle leak can be done with agitated saline injection but must be done from upper and lower extremities to rule out upper (SVC) and lower (IVC) baffle leaks [4, 26].
- These patients can have a significant burden of atrial arrhythmias given multiple atrial suture lines [4, 26].
- Patients with d-TGA post Atrial switch may present in heart failure given failure of the systemic RV and require transplant evaluation [4].

Ebstein's Anomaly

Anatomy and Physiology

Ebstein's anomaly of the tricuspid valve is an uncommon congenital heart defect occurring in about 0.005% of live births [4]. It is a malformation of the tricuspid valve and right ventricle with varying severity. This defect is classically described as apical displacement of the septal and posterior tricuspid valve leaflets, leading to "atrialization" of the right ventricle [27]. It is associated with an ASD in more than 80% of patients [28]. Ebstein malformation of the tricuspid valve is often found in patients who also have L-TGA (congenitally corrected TGA).

Ebstein Anomaly

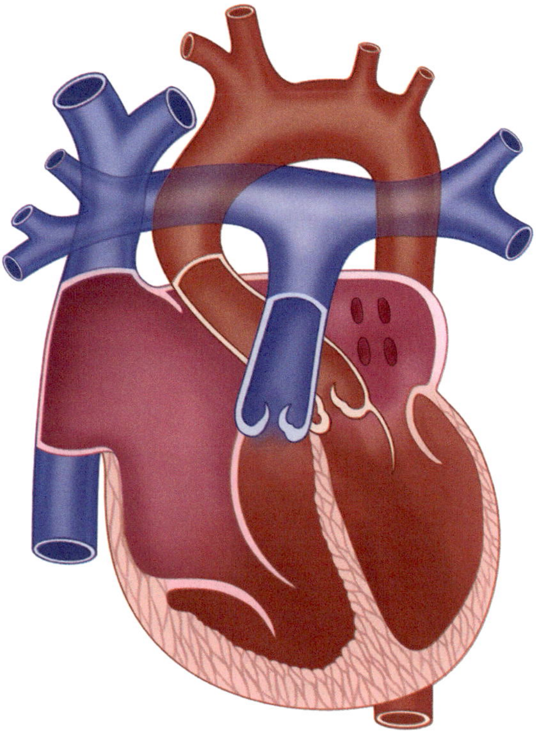

Apical displacement of the tricuspid valve leaflets with atrialization of the right ventricle

Physical Exam Correlations

The exam in these patients varies based on severity of the anatomy. Exam may include systolic AV-valve murmur secondary to the tricuspid regurgitation. The patient may have cyanosis secondary to right to left shunting across the atrial septum, if ASD/PFO present.

Pathology/Description

Ebstein's anomaly has apical displacement of the septal and posterior tricuspid valve leaflets. The valve may be tethered/have restricted motion or have a sail like appearance with abnormal chordal attachments, which can contribute to inappropriate coaptation leading to significant regurgitation [27]. The functional right ventricle can be very small and consist only of the RVOT in cases of severe apical displacement [27]. Conduction system abnormalities are common, and as many as 1/3 of patients with Ebstein anomaly have more than one accessory pathway. 5–25% of patients with Ebstein anomaly have Wolff Parkinson White syndrome [28, 29].

Imaging

EKG, Holter, Cardiac MRI, 2D, and 3D echocardiogram including TEE may all be helpful.

Management

Management for Ebstein Anomaly depends on the severity of the lesion. Intervention may include ablation of accessory pathways, or surgical management of these pathways at the time of surgery. Surgical repair can include tricuspid valve repair or replacement, plication of the atrialized right ventricle (Cone procedure), reduction atrioplasty, closure of atrial defect, and arrhythmia management [4]. Poorer outcomes are associated with delay of surgery until presentation of HF symptoms or RV systolic dysfunction [4].

Pearls

- Over half of the adult patients' initial presenting symptom is palpitations or arrhythmia [29].
- Patients can present with cyanosis, fatigue, dyspnea, arrhythmia, and/or symptoms of right heart failure [27].
- There is an association with accessory pathway tachycardia (WPW).

Single Ventricle/Fontan Physiology

Anatomy and Physiology

The term single ventricle physiology or Fontan physiology refers to complex intracardiac anatomy that is not amenable to 2-ventricule circulation, thus leaving the patient with a "single ventricle" for systemic circulation. This may be either a systemic right ventricle or systemic left ventricle.

1. Defects include, but are not limited to:
   (a) Hypoplastic left heart syndrome (HLHS)
   (b) Double inlet left ventricle (DILV)
   (c) Tricuspid atresia
   (d) Double outlet right ventricle (DORV)
   (e) Pulmonary atresia with intact ventricular septum (PA/IVS)
   (f) Ebstein anomaly
   (g) AV canal (unbalanced)
2. Fontan palliation is typically a three-stage operation over the first few years of life.
   (a) Stage I is typically creation of a shunt—either Blalock-Taussig (BT) or Sano to the pulmonary arteries.
   (b) Stage II is a bidirectional Glenn operation in which the SVC is disarticulated from the RA and sewn directly into the pulmonary arteries. The shunt, which was placed in stage I is taken down.
   (c) Stage III—or Fontan Completion—is the baffling of the IVC return to the pulmonary arteries via a conduit. There are many variations of this with the most common including: Classic Fontan, Lateral Tunnel, and extra-cardiac.

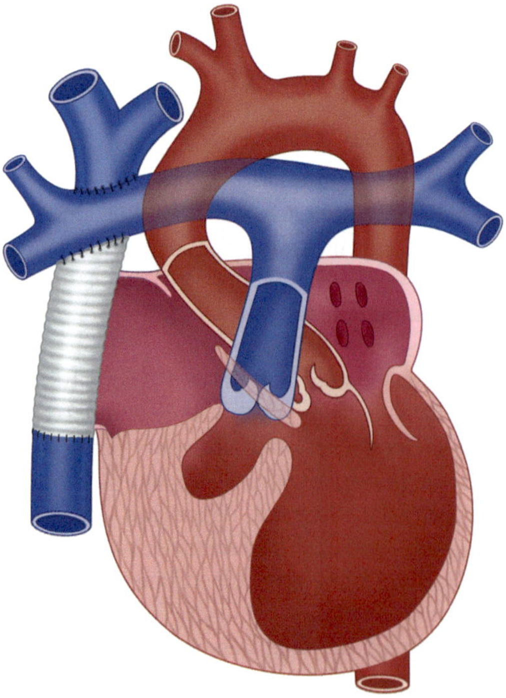

Hypoplastic Right ventricle with Tricuspid atresia, severe pulmonary stenosis, and VSD – s/p Bidirectional Glenn and Extra-cardiac Fontan completion

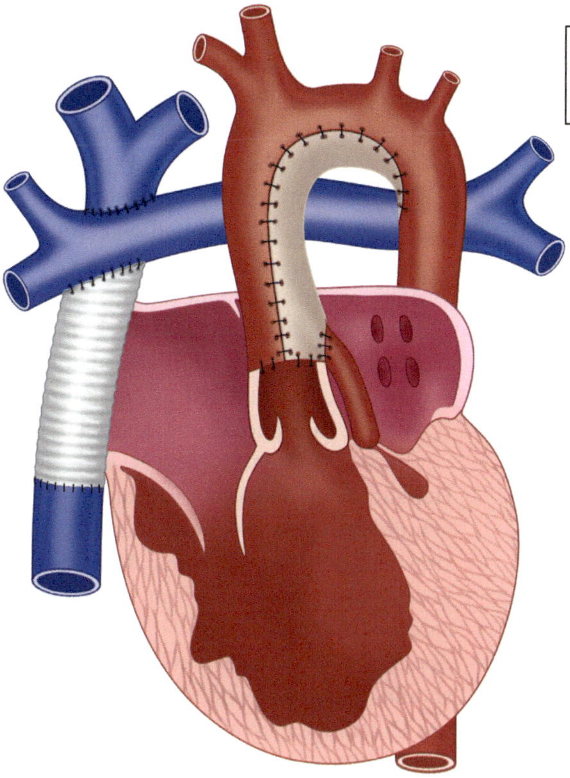

Hypoplastic Left ventricle with Aortic and mitral atresia – s/p Norwood, Bidirectional Glenn and Extra-cardiac Fontan completion

Physical Exam Correlations

In a well-functioning Fontan, the patient may have normal physical exam findings with normal oxygen saturation. Alternatively, there may be a murmur if there is significant valve disease, recurrent coarctation of the aorta, or a significant burden of aorto-pulmonary collaterals. Oxygen saturation may not be normal and may range between 88% and 92%, in the absence of significant venous abnormalities, depending on the physiology. Prominent abdominal vessels, distended abdomen, or lower extremity edema may be present if the Fontan pressures are elevated or if there is obstruction in the Fontan circuit. If a fenestration is present, the oxygen saturations may drop with ambulation.

Pathology/Description

In the unoperated patient, stage I or II single ventricle physiology, there is mixed blood circulation (mixed systemic venous and systemic arterial blood) through the body. This mixing occurs depending on structural abnormality but is typically across an atrial septal defect (ASD), ventricular septal defect (VSD) or patent ductus arteriosus (PDA). This mixing of the blood is necessary to maintain cardiac output [30]. Over the three palliative surgeries, the circulation is separated such that the venous blood is routed to the lungs by passive/gravitational flow and arterial blood is pumped to the body without mixing, allowing for the patient to have a relatively normal oxygen saturation. Adults with Fontan physiology have chronically low cardiac output given the passive cavo-pulmonary flow of the Fontan circuit. The Fontan circuit is not able to deliver normal amount of volume across the pulmonary vascular bed, which results in reduced ventricular filling and low stroke volume. This physiologic state is not able to augment stroke volume normally with exercise or other states of increased demand [31, 32]. Atrial tachycardias occur in 60% of adults with Fontan palliation. They are poorly tolerated and can be difficult to manage, thus they should be addressed promptly [4]. Sinus node dysfunction occurs in up to 45% of adults with Fontan palliation [4].

Imaging

EKG, transthoracic, Cardiac MRI, Cardiac CT, and stress testing are all used to evaluate the patient with a Fontan. Holter monitoring for arrhythmias is also used for evaluation.

Clinical Pearls

- Cardiac output for patients with Fontan physiology is not normal. They are limited by the passive flow to the lungs and the abnormal blood throughput in the pulmonary circuit. Over time the chronic volume depletion causes progressive decline in ventricular function, resulting in a cycle of increased end-diastolic pressure, systemic venous congestion, and low cardiac output [31, 32].
- Failing Fontan physiology:
  - Cyanosis: Patients with Fontan physiology are often mildly hypoxemic. This is caused by the presence of a surgically created fenestration or leaks in the fontan baffle itself, coronary sinus venous return to the atrium, pulmonary AV-malformations, and veno-venous collaterals which can drain into the pulmonary veins or directly into the left atrium [31].
  - Protein losing enteropathy (PLE) occurs in 5–15% of patients with Fontan physiology. This refers to the loss of serum proteins into the lumen of the gut leading to chronic diarrhea, abdominal discomfort, and peripheral edema. Lab values indicative of PLE are decreased serum albumin <3.5 g/dL and Total protein <6.0–6.3 g/dL, as well as augmented enteric protein loss with Fecal alpha-1-antitrypsin clearance >56 ml/24H (with diarrhea) and >27 ml/24 h (without diarrhea) [31].

    Management: decrease resistance in the Fontan circuit by alleviating any obstruction, reducing PVR, unfractionated heparin or budesonide to reduce enteric inflammation. Other medications that can help improve endothelial cell function and reduce inflammation such as Spironolactone and Octreotide (limited evidence) [31, 33].
  - Hepatic dysfunction: Elevated central venous pressure and systemic hypoperfusion lead to congestive hepatopathy, liver fibrosis to cirrhosis and even hepatocellular carcinoma [31].
  - Screening for hepatocellular carcinoma should be done with Alpha fetoprotein (AFP) and liver imaging (Ultrasound, liver MRI with Evoist or CT).
  - Thromboembolic complications: Risk of thromboembolism as high as 20% in patients with Fontan physiology. This is felt to be caused by lack of pulsatile flow in the pulmonary circuit and ensuing venous stasis leading to a hypercoagulable state which is made worse by deficiency of protein C, S, antithrombin III and increased platelet reactivity [31, 34].

Infective Endocarditis Prophylaxis

It should be discussed in detail with the patient the importance of infective endocarditis prevention. Infective endocarditis can be a potentially life-threatening condition with 10–20% mortality and prevention along antibiotic prophylaxis when indicated and early diagnosis is of paramount relevance. Recommendations of proper dental hygiene including teeth brushing three times a day, flossing once a day, visiting the dentist twice a year and following infective endocarditis prophylaxis guidelines with antibiotics when indicated. Also, for other procedures, infective endocarditis prophylaxis may need to be considered. Patients need to receive education regarding early symptoms of infective endocarditis that may include fever, myalgias, headache, arthralgias, or other symptoms. The condition could be confused with flu or COVID. Also, a low threshold for blood cultures in the absence of a clear diagnosis with fever and contacting the ACHD Care Center in collaboration with primary care providers to facilitate diagnostic and care pathways as needed. AHA infective endocarditis prophylaxis card must be given.

(Please see Chap. 19 for more details.)

References

1. Le Gloan L, Legendre A, Iserin L, Ladouceur M. Pathophysiology and natural history of atrial septal defect. J Thorac Dis. 2018;10(Suppl 24):S2854–63. https://doi.org/10.21037/jtd.2018.02.80. PMID: 30305945; PMCID: PMC6174151.
2. Redfield MM, Jacobsen SJ, Borlaug BA, et al. Age- and gender-related ventricular-vascular stiffening: a community-based study. Circulation. 2005;112:2254–62. https://doi.org/10.1161/CIRCULATIONAHA.105.541078.
3. Webb G, Gatzoulis MA. Atrial septal defects in the adult: recent progress and overview. Circulation. 2006;114(15):1645–53. https://doi.org/10.1161/CIRCULATIONAHA.105.592055. PMID: 17030704.
4. Stout KK, Daniels CJ, Aboulhosn JA, Bozkurt B, Broberg CS, Colman JM, Crumb SR, Dearani JA, Fuller S, Gurvitz M, Khairy P, Landzberg MJ, Saidi A, Valente AM, Van Hare GF. 2018 AHA/ACC guideline for the management of adults with congenital heart disease: a report of the American College of Cardiology/American Heart Association Task Force on Clinical Practice Guidelines. J Am Coll Cardiol. 2019;73(12):e81–e192. https://doi.org/10.1016/j.jacc.2018.08.1029. Epub 2018 Aug 16. Erratum in: J Am Coll Cardiol. 2019 May 14;73(18):2361–2362. PMID: 30121239.
5. Minette MS, Sahn DJ. Ventricular septal defects. Circulation. 2006;114(20):2190–7. https://doi.org/10.1161/CIRCULATIONAHA.106.618124. Erratum in: Circulation 2007 Feb 20;115(7):e205. PMID: 17101870.
6. Tretter JL, Benson L, Crucean A, Spicer DE, Anderson R. Ventricular septal defect. In: Wernovsky G, Anderson RH, Kumar K, Mussatto KA, Redington AN, Tweddell JS, editors. Anderson's pediatric cardiology. 4th ed. Phillidelphia, PA: Elsivier; 2020. p. 557–84.
7. Dakkak W, Oliver TI. Ventricular septal defect. [Updated 2022 May 10]. In: StatPearls [Internet]. Treasure Island, FL: StatPearls Publishing; 2022. Available from: https://www.ncbi.nlm.nih.gov/books/NBK470330/.
8. Corone P, Doyon F, Gaudeau S, et al. Natural history of ventricular septal defect. A study involving 790 cases. Circulation. 1977;55:908–15.
9. Mattila S, Kostiainen S, Kyllönen KE, et al. Repair of ventricular septal defect in adults. Scand J Thorac Cardiovasc Surg. 1985;19:29–31.
10. Mathieu P, Bossé Y, Huggins GS, Della Corte A, Pibarot P, Michelena HI, Limongelli G, Boulanger MC, Evangelista A, Bédard E, Citro R, Body SC, Nemer M, Schoen FJ. The pathology and pathobiology of bicuspid aortic valve: state of the art and novel research perspectives. J Pathol Clin Res. 2015;1(4):195–206. https://doi.org/10.1002/cjp2.21. PMID: 27499904; PMCID: PMC4939890.
11. Fernandes SM, Sanders SP, Khairy P, Jenkins KJ, et al. Morphology of bicuspid aortic valve in children and adolescents. J Am Coll Cardiol. 2004;44(8):1648–51. https://doi.org/10.1016/j.jacc.2004.05.063.
12. Siu SC, Silversides CK. Bicuspid aortic valve disease. J Am Coll Cardiol. 2010;55(25):2789–800. https://doi.org/10.1016/j.jacc.2009.12.068. PMID: 20579534.
13. Vincent F, Ternacle J, Denimal T, Shen M, Redfors B, Delhaye C, Simonato M, Debry N, Verdier B, Shahim B, Pamart T, Spillemaeker H, Schurtz G, Pontana F, Thourani VH, Pibarot P, Van Belle E. Transcatheter aortic valve replacement in bicuspid aortic valve stenosis. Circulation. 2021;143(10):1043–61. https://doi.org/10.1161/CIRCULATIONAHA.120.048048. Epub 2021 Mar 8. PMID: 33683945.
14. Ruckdeschel E, Kim YY. Pulmonary valve stenosis in the adult patient: pathophysiology, diagnosis and management. Heart. 2019;105:414–22.
15. Diaz-Frias J, Guillaume M. Tetralogy of Fallot. [Updated 2022 Jan 18]. In: StatPearls [Internet]. Treasure Island, FL: StatPearls Publishing; 2022. Available from: https://www.ncbi.nlm.nih.gov/books/NBK513288/.
16. Law MA, Tivakaran VS. Coarctation of the aorta. [Updated 2022 May 15]. In: StatPearls [Internet]. Treasure Island, FL: StatPearls Publishing; 2022. Available from: https://www.ncbi.nlm.nih.gov/books/NBK430913/.
17. Qureshi AM, McElhinney DB, Lock JE, et al. Acute and intermediate outcomes, and evaluation of injury to the aortic wall, as based on 15 years experience of implanting stents to treat aortic coarctation. Cardiol Young. 2007;17:307–18.
18. Hager A, Kanz S, Kaemmerer H, et al. Coarctation long-term assessment (COALA): significance of arterial hypertension in a cohort of 404 patients up to 27 years after surgical repair of isolated coarctation of the aorta, even in the absence of restenosis and prosthetic material. J Thorac Cardiovasc Surg. 2007;134:738–45.

19. Wiebers DO, Whisnant JP, Huston J, et al. Unruptured intracranial aneurysms: natural history, clinical outcome, and risks of surgical and endovascular treatment. Lancet. 2003;362:103–10.
20. Prieto LR, Hordof AJ, Secic M, et al. Progressive tricuspid valve disease in patients with congenitally corrected transposition of the great arteries. Circulation. 1998;98:997–1005.
21. Huhta JC, Maloney JD, Ritter DG, et al. Complete atrioventricular block in patients with atrioventricular discordance. Circulation. 1983;67:1374–7.
22. Graham TP Jr, Bernard YD, Mellen BG, Celermajer D, Baumgartner H, Cetta F, Connolly HM, Davidson WR, Dellborg M, Foster E, Gersony WM, Gessner IH, Hurwitz RA, Kaemmerer H, Kugler JD, Murphy DJ, Noonan JA, Morris C, Perloff JK, Sanders SP, Sutherland JL. Long-term outcome in congenitally corrected transposition of the great arteries: a multi-institutional study. J Am Coll Cardiol. 2000;36:255–61.
23. Warnes CA. Transposition of the great arteries. Circulation. 2006;114(24):2699–709. https://doi.org/10.1161/CIRCULATIONAHA.105.592352. PMID: 17159076.
24. Szymanski MW, Moore SM, Kritzmire SM, et al. Transposition of the great arteries. [Updated 2022 May 11]. In: StatPearls [Internet]. Treasure Island, FL: StatPearls Publishing; 2022. Available from: https://www.ncbi.nlm.nih.gov/books/NBK538434/.
25. Marino BS, Lipkin PH, Newburger JW, Peacock G, Gerdes M, Gaynor JW, Mussatto KA, Uzark K, Goldberg CS, Johnson WH, Li J, Smith SE, Bellinger DC, Mahle WT, American Heart Association Congenital Heart Defects Committee, Council on Cardiovascular Disease in the Young, Council on Cardiovascular Nursing, and Stroke Council. Neurodevelopmental outcomes in children with congenital heart disease: evaluation and management: a scientific statement from the American Heart Association. Circulation. 2012;126(9):1143–72.
26. Broberg CS. Cardiac magnetic imaging of the patient with an atrial switch palliation for transposition of the great arteries. Prog Pediatr Cardiol. 2014;38:49–55.
27. Brown ML, Dearani JA, Danielson GK, Cetta F, Connolly HM, Warnes CA, Li Z, Hodge DO, Driscoll DJ, Mayo Clinic Congenital Heart Center. The outcomes of operations for 539 patients with Ebstein anomaly. J Thorac Cardiovasc Surg. 2008;135(5):1120–36, 1136.e1–7.
28. Khositseth A, Danielson GK, Dearani JA, Munger TM, Porter CJ. Supraventricular tachyarrhythmias in Ebstein anomaly: management and outcome. J Thorac Cardiovasc Surg. 2004;128(6):826–33.
29. Fuchs MM, Connolly HM. Ebstein anomaly in the adult patient. Cardiol Clin. 2020;38(3):353–63.
30. Heaton J, Heller D. Single ventricle. [Updated 2022 May 1]. In: StatPearls [Internet]. Treasure Island, FL: StatPearls Publishing; 2022. Available from: https://www.ncbi.nlm.nih.gov/books/NBK557789/.
31. Mazza GA, Gribaudo E, Agnoletti G. The pathophysiology and complications of Fontan circulation. Acta Biomed. 2021;92(5):e2021260. https://doi.org/10.23750/abm.v92i5.10893. PMID: 34738582; PMCID: PMC8689331.
32. Gewillig M, Brown SC, Eyskens B, Heying R, et al. The Fontan circulation: who controls cardiac output? Interact Cardiovasc Thorac Surg. 2010;10:428–33.
33. John AS, Johnson JA, Khan M, Driscoll DJ, Warnes CA, Cetta F. Clinical outcomes and improved survival in patients with protein-losing enteropathy after the Fontan operation. J Am Coll Cardiol. 2014;64:54–62.
34. Monagle P, Karl TR. Thromboembolic problems after the Fontan operation. Semin Thorac Cardiovasc Surg Pediatr Card Surg Annu. 2002;5:36–47.

Part IX

Ambulatory/Preventative Cardiology

Prevention of Cardiometabolic Disease

30

Allison W. Dimsdale and Christopher Kelly

Introduction

Atherosclerotic cardiovascular disease (ASCVD) is a progressive, systemic disorder that affects vascular systems throughout the body and can lead to devastating complications such as myocardial infarction, stroke, and limb amputation. In the United States, ASCVD is the leading cause of death and generates >$200 billion per year in annual healthcare costs and lost productivity. A large share of the disease burden occurs because of failure to implement appropriate prevention strategies and control known risk factors in the general adult population [1]. This chapter will discuss the assessment and management of ASCVD risk, with a particular focus on coronary artery disease (CAD).

Assessment of Risk

All adults should be regularly assessed for their risk of developing ASCVD and, among those at increased risk, questioned regarding symptoms that would indicate such disease is already established. Most patients have an optimistic bias—i.e., they tend to judge their own risk as lower than predicted [2].

Although it is impossible to precisely quantify risk at the individual level, given the large number of pro-atherogenic genetic and other factors that remain poorly understood, it is possible to estimate risk by comparing an individual to a matched population from which longitudinal data have already been collected. Multiple screening tools exist to fuel and inform this critical conversation, so the clinician should be facile with the research and evidence as it changes.

It is important to recall that even though clinicians think frequently about risk and view most risk-reducing intervention favorably, patients have a wide range of attitudes toward risk and often have negative views of medications, especially when they do not treat a symptom or offer some other immediate benefit. Therefore, any discussion of risk should include an overview of how the risk has been determined, what the risk actually means, and the lifestyle changes or therapies available to reduce that risk (Fig. 30.1). Afterward, the clinician should learn about the patient's overall impression of that risk and assess their willingness to make changes, as well as the real and perceived costs of any medical interventions (e.g., statin therapy).

When discussing the concept of risk, one effective strategy to present this information is to state, "Eight out of 100 people like you will have a heart attack or stroke in the next ten years." Or,

A. W. Dimsdale (✉)
Duke University Health System, Durham, NC, USA
e-mail: Allison.dimsdale@duke.edu

C. Kelly
UNC Rex Hospital, UNC Health, Raleigh, NC, USA
e-mail: Christopher.Kelly@unchealth.unc.edu

R. Musialowski, K. Allshouse (eds.), *Cardiovascular Manual for the Advanced Practice Provider*,
https://doi.org/10.1007/978-3-031-35819-7_30

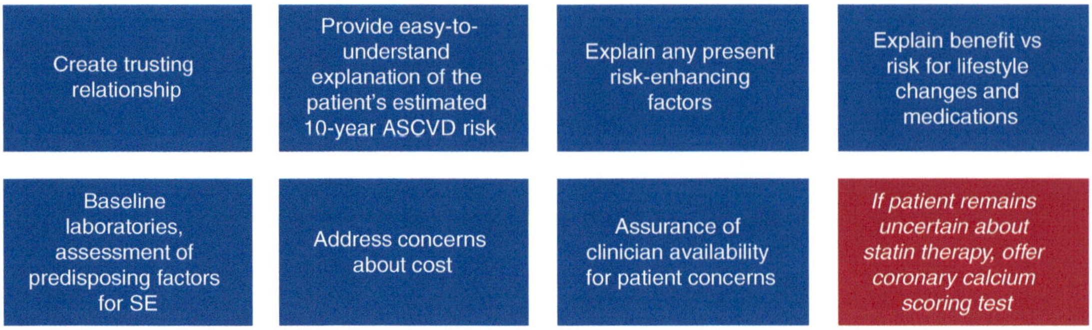

Fig. 30.1 Clinician-patient risk discussion

conversely, "92 out of 100 people like you will not have a heart attack or stroke in the next ten years." When the 10-year estimates are not compelling enough to motivate change, the lifetime estimates of risk can be more motivational. Of note, creative display of risk information such as pictograms does not necessarily improve patient understanding and, in one study, was actually shown to decrease the perception of risk [2].

It is important to clarify that a seemingly low risk of ASCVD—such as 8% over 10 years—is actually characterized as intermediate. Likewise, it can be useful to discuss relative rather than absolute risk reduction while discussing the implications of proposed therapies. A reduction in 10-year risk from 20% to 16% may not sound impressive to a patient, whereas a 20% reduction in their overall risk could be more compelling.

The risk score most often used in clinical practice is the pooled cohort equation (PCE) [3]. This calculator is used to estimate the 10-year risk of myocardial infarction and stroke, and it can be applied to adults age 40–75 years. Variables in this model include age, gender, race, systolic and diastolic blood pressure, total cholesterol, HDL and LDL cholesterol, diabetes status, smoking status, and the presence or absence of hypertension treatment, lipid-lowering treatment, and aspirin therapy. Notably, the equation does not consider a family history of ASCVD, novel risk markers such as lipoprotein(a), or the severity of diabetes. In addition, it performs best among non-Hispanic whites and blacks, and less accurately for other race groups. Nonetheless, the tool can serve as a useful starting point for discussions about risk and can help forecast the potential impact of interventions such as statin therapy or smoking cessation. In addition, risk can be reassessed at follow-up visits. This information can increase patient engagement in guideline-directed changes in lifestyle and medication strategies by allowing them to witness the impact of their choices on their risk estimate.

Several alternatives to the PCE are also available, including the Framingham [4] and Reynolds [5] scores. In general, however, most patients in contemporary practice are evaluated using the PCE and then further assessed to determine if other risk-enhancing factors are present.

Risk-Enhancing Factors

When a patient's 10-year risk is borderline (5% to <7.5%) or intermediate (>7.5% to <20%), the presence or absence of risk-enhancing factors can help further refine the estimation [1]. Such factors include family history of early-onset ASCVD, familial hypercholesterolemia, metabolic syndrome, chronic kidney disease, inflammatory conditions (such as rheumatoid arthritis), premature menopause, history of pregnancy-associated conditions such as preeclampsia, high-risk race/ethnicity such as South Asian ancestry, abnormal ankle-brachial index (<0.9), and lipid biomarkers associated with increased ASCVD risk including lipoprotein(a) and apolipoprotein B (Fig. 30.2a, b).

a Risk Enhancing factors for Clinician-Patient Risk Discussion

Risk-Enhancing Factors
Family history of premeture ASCVD (males, age <55; females age <65)
Primary hypercholesterolemia (LDL-C, 160-189 mg/dl (4.1-4.8 mmol/L), non HDL-C 190-219 mg/dl (4.9-5.6 mmol/L))
Metabolic syndrome (incrased waist circumference,elevated triglycerides (>150 mg/dL, nonfasting), elevated blood pressure, elevated glucose, and low HDL-C(<40 mg/dL in men; <50 md/dL in women) are factors; a tally of 3 makes the diagnosis
Chronic kidney disease (eGFR 15-59 mL/min/1.73 m2 with or without albumineuria; not treated with dialysis or kidney transplantation
History of premature menopause (before age 40) and history of pregnancy-associated conditions that increase later ASCVD risk, such as preeclampsia
High-risk race/ethnicity (eg, South Asian ancestry)
Lipids/biomakers: associated with increased ASCVD risk
Persistently elevated primary hypertriglyceridemia (>175 mg/dL, nonfasting)
If measured:
Elevated high-sensitivity C-reactive protein (>2.0 mg/L)
Elevated Lp(a): A relative indication for its measurement is family history of premature ASCVD. An Lp(a) >50 mg/dL or >125 nmol/L cinstitutes a risk-enhancing factor, especially at higher levels of Lp(a)
Elevated apoB (>130 mg;dL): A relative indication for its measurement would be triglyceride>200 mg/dL A level >130 mg/dL corresponds to an LDL-C<160 mg/dL and constitutes a risk-enhancing factor
ABI (<0.9)

Fig. 30.2 (**a**) Risk-enhancing factors for clinician-patient risk discussion. (**b**) Risk enhancing factors

Fig. 30.2 (continued)

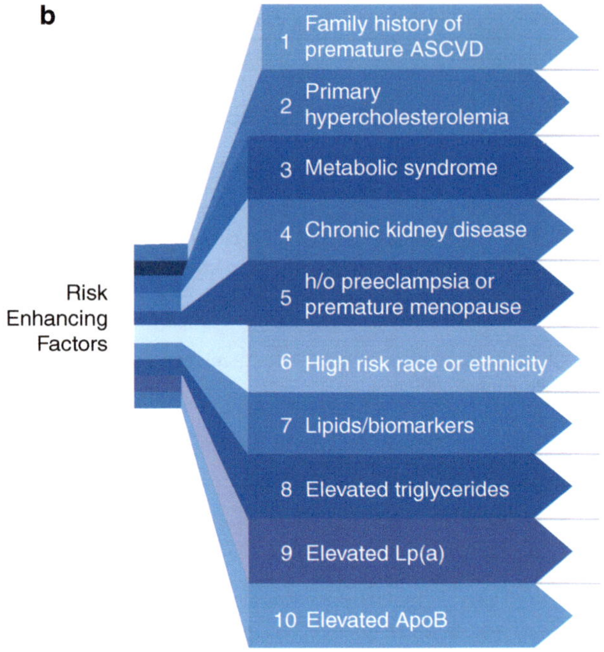

Risk-Enhancing Factors

When a patient's 10-year risk is borderline (5% to <7.5%) or intermediate (>7.5% to <20%), the presence or absence of risk-enhancing factors can help further refine the estimation [1]. Such factors include family history of early-onset ASCVD, familial hypercholesterolemia, metabolic syndrome, chronic kidney disease, inflammatory conditions (such as rheumatoid arthritis), premature menopause, history of pregnancy-associated conditions such as preeclampsia, high-risk race/ethnicity such as South Asian ancestry, abnormal ankle-brachial index (<0.9), and lipid biomarkers associated with increased ASCVD risk, including lipoprotein(a) and apolipoprotein B (Figs. 30.2a, b).

Calcium Scoring

When an asymptomatic patient's risk estimate remains uncertain or is in the intermediate range, a coronary artery calcium (CAC) score often helps inform the discussion by providing a snapshot of the patient's existing burden of coronary atherosclerosis. This score is calculated from a non-contrast CT scan of the chest gated to the ECG. Because calcium hyperattenuates and is easily seen on a CT scan, the degree of coronary calcification correlates fairly well with the total amount of atherosclerosis. The calcium score is quantified using the Agatston method and reported both as a total number and as subtotals for each coronary artery.

CAC is particularly helpful when deciding whether to initiate preventive medical therapies such as a statin or aspirin. Moreover, this test converts the abstract concept of risk into the more concrete concept of coronary plaque burden and the risk of a clinical event. If the CAC is zero, the patient is unlikely to derive any benefit from statin therapy, and the risk can be reassessed after 10 years. In contrast, if the score is greater than 400, stress testing may be warranted for an inactive patient to ensure there is no obstructive disease. A calcium score of any value can be entered alongside other patient characteristics in the MESA risk estimator to assess its impact on the 10-year risk [6–8].

The CAC is easily available, often without a prescription. As such, people may obtain this score out of interest and then present to their provider with the score to discuss how to manage further preventive efforts [6, 9]. The average cost of a CAC is $43.00–$246.00 [10].

Additional patient groups that may benefit from learning their calcium score include those who are reluctant to initiate statin therapy as well as those who have discontinued statins because of side effects and are concerned about reattempting lipid-lowering therapy.

Modification of Risk

Social Determinants of Health

In 2008, the World Health Organization's Commission on the Social Determinants of Health defined such determinants as the "conditions in which people are born, grow, live, work and age." The Healthy People 2030 initiative [11] further classified these determinants into five groups: economic stability, education access/quality, healthcare access/quality, neighborhood and built environment, and social and community context.

A discussion of the patient's social determinants of health is a useful starting point for the conversation about how to modify risk [1]. The CDC has developed a framework to be used as a screening tool to assess housing instability, food insecurity, transportation difficulties, utility assistance needs, and interpersonal safety [12]. Of course, if a patient lacks transportation to appointments or the grocery store, cannot afford (or identify) healthy fresh food, or cannot afford medications, discussions regarding lifestyle changes and medications are likely futile.

Even among patients not facing such fundamental barriers, additional determinants may compromise efforts to modify risk. Barriers to heart-healthy diets include access to fresh food, living in an inner-city or rural environment, socioeconomically disadvantaged status, cultural practices and traditions, and advanced age. Exercise may be limited if individuals do not have access to appropriate venues such as sidewalks, malls, or gyms. Issues such as sleep hygiene, work hours, psychosocial stressors and support, financial well-being, and exposure to second-hand smoke are also essential to consider in all patients.

Nutrition and Diet

There are innumerable diets and dietary fads in popular culture, most of which have never been shown to improve cardiovascular health. The shift over time from high-carbohydrate/low-fat diets to low-carbohydrate/high-fat diets—and now, even zero carb, ketogenic diets—has left many patients confused and frustrated [13].

In contrast, the current recommendations from the American College of Cardiology and American Heart Association and (ACC-AHA) incorporate simple and clear guidelines based on data whenever possible. Although there are not many randomized clinical trials of diets that have included clinically meaningful endpoints, multiple observational studies have associated increased CVD risk with the consumption of refined grains, trans- and saturated fats, sodium, red meats, processed meats, and sugar [14, 15]. Meanwhile, the Adventist Health Study [16] demonstrated that replacing meat with seeds and nuts was associated with a significant reduction in cardiovascular risk, while the PREDIMED Mediterranean diet study [17] demonstrated reduced mortality among patients assigned to a Mediterranean-style diet rich with olive oil and nuts. There is an ever-growing body of evidence showing that plant-based and whole food diets are associated with decreased mortality [18].

The current ACC-AHA recommendations include the following five diet strategies:

1. Eating a diet which emphasizes eating vegetables, fruits, legumes, nuts, whole grains, and fish.
2. Replacing saturated fat—which is solid at room temperature and found in meat, coconut oil, and cheese—with dietary monounsaturated and polyunsaturated fat.
3. Reducing intake of dietary cholesterol and sodium (<2000 mg daily).
4. Minimizing the intake of processed meats (e.g., deli meats, hot dogs), refined carbohy-

drates (e.g., high fructose corn syrup), and sweetened beverages.

5. Reducing trans fats, which are found in prepared foods and occur naturally, albeit to a small degree, in meat and dairy.

Physical Activity and Obesity

Physical activity and exercise are essential for maintaining or improving cardiovascular health. Multiple clinical trials have shown that regular physical activity can increase life expectancy by 0.4 to 6.9 years [19]. Aerobic and resistance exercise can also improve glycemic control, decrease weight, and lower blood pressure [15]. When discussing an exercise prescription, it is essential to understand the patient's current baseline. A sedentary or obese individual should begin with low-intensity exercise such as slow walking and then gradually increase to recommended levels. It is also essential that any functional impairment (musculoskeletal pain, low vision, lack of safe places to exercise) be addressed before starting an exercise program.

The current ACC/AHA guidelines recommend that the average adult engage in 150 minutes weekly of moderate-intensity exercise, or 75 min weekly of vigorous-intensity physical activity. If an adult cannot meet these goals, engaging in even some moderate- or lower-intensity activity can still reduce the risk of ASCVD. Defining high and low intensity for patients can help them assess their own lifestyle. It can be helpful to share the definition of METs and their associated values (Fig. 30.3). The take-home message for these patients is that any improvement upon a sedentary lifestyle is likely to reduce ASCVD risk [15]. Annual assessment of BMI and waist circumference may help patients see the results of their intentions and actions, creating a positive feedback cycle that encourages further progress.

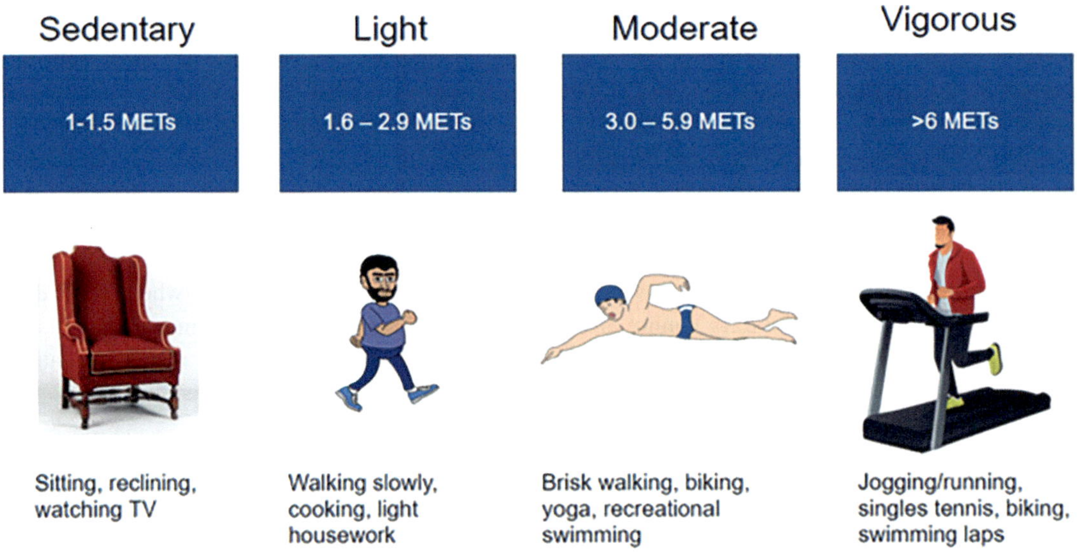

Fig. 30.3 Definitions of varying intensity of physical activity. (Adapted from: "Leather Recliner #723" by DesignFolly.com is licensed under CC BY-SA 2.0 "Person Walking Through Fall Leaves Foreground in focus, person soft focus" by ShebleyCL is licensed under CC BY 2.0 "2017-08-08-Matt_Duboff-Men's Swimming-47" by 2017 Canada Games //Jeux du Canada 2017 is licensed under CC BY 2.0 "Carrera Regency" by @jluisro is licensed under CC BY-NC-SA 2.0)

Type 2 Diabetes Mellitus

Type 2 diabetes mellitus (T2DM) is a metabolic disorder defined by insulin resistance leading to hyperglycemia. This condition is highly prevalent in the United States, affecting nearly one in eight adults. More than one third of American adults have prediabetes and are at high risk of developing T2DM. Moreover, adults with diabetes are two to four times more likely to die of heart disease than adults without diabetes [20].

Important interventions in treating and managing T2DM include diet, exercise, weight loss, and pharmacotherapies such as metformin. Mediterranean, low sodium, and vegetarian diets have all been shown to improve glycemic control [15]. Clinicians can take a multidisciplinary approach with diabetic patients to provide education, exercise prescriptions including aerobic and resistance strategies, diet oversight, medication management, and assessment of social determinants in order to decrease the risk of developing clinical ASCVD.

Management of Blood Cholesterol

Several cholesterol markers—including LDL, lipoprotein B, and lipoprotein(a)—strongly predict ASCVD risk. Therefore, defining and targeting cholesterol goals for all patients is essential. The concept of a single "normal" cholesterol threshold remains popular among patients but is no longer used in contemporary practice. Instead, an individual's target cholesterol values are determined based on their global risk of either developing clinical ASCVD or experiencing a recurrence. The current guidelines for setting and then achieving such goals were established in the "2018 Cholesterol Clinical Practice Guidelines." [1]

For the purposes of primary prevention, the clinician will typically determine the need for lipid lowering with the 10-year ASCVD risk as calculated using the PCE. If the risk is intermediate or higher, and the LDL is ≥70 mg/dl, lipid-lowering therapy is recommend to reduce the LDL by at least 30–50%. Of note, however, lipid-lowering therapy is also recommended in all adults with an LDL > 190 mg/dl regardless of the overall ASCVD risk score, as well as adults with T2DM. Among those with diabetes, an LDL goal of <70 mg/dl is appropriate (Fig. 30.4).

Among lipid-lowering drugs, statins have the strongest evidence for reducing the incidence of a first clinical ASCVD event. The various agents and available doses are generally divided into "moderate-" and "high-" intensity regimens, with the latter recommended for those with the highest LDL levels or highest risk (e.g., those with

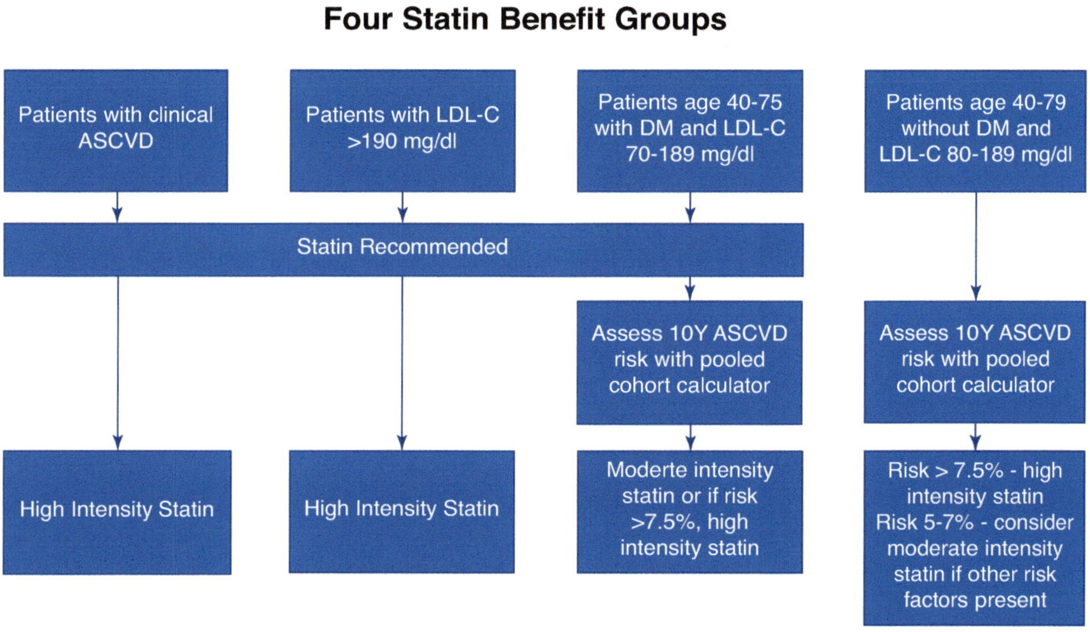

Fig. 30.4 Management of blood cholesterol

High Intensity Statin Therapy	Moderate Intensity Statin Therapy	Low Intensity Statin Therapy
Daily dose lowers LDL-C on average by approximately >50%	Daily dose lowers LDL-C on average by approximately 30<50%	Daily dose lowers LDL-C on average by <30%
Atorvastatin 40-80 mg	Atorvastatin 10-20 mg	Simvastatin 10 mg
Rosuvastatin 20-40 mg	Rosuvastatin 5-10 mg	Pravastatin 10-20 mg
	Simvastatin 20-40 mg	Lovastatin 20 mg
	Pravastatin 40-80 mg	Fluvastatin 20-40 mg BID
	Lovastatin 40 mg	Pitavastatin 1 mg
	Fluvastatin XL 80 mg	
	Fluvastatin 40 mg BID	
	Pitavastatin 20 mg	

Fig. 30.5 Intensity of statin medications. (Adapted from Grundy et al. [1])

T2DM) (Fig. 30.5). Other agents—such as ezetimibe, bempedoic acid, and PCSK9 inhibitors—are currently used only when patients are unable to achieve adequate lipid lowering with statins, either because of inefficacy or intolerable side effects.

When initiating lipid-lowering therapy, it is important to discuss the potential risk reduction, possible adverse effects, drug-drug interactions, and cost. Adherence to the prescribed regimen should be assessed at each visit. Myalgia is the most common side effect of statin therapy and can affect adherence. Prior to initiating statin therapy, baseline CK and myalgia assessment should be completed. Review of systems will include muscle aching, pain, stiffness, tenderness, weakness, fatigue, or cramps (Fig. 30.6). The clinician may also evaluate other reasons for myalgias in order to establish a causal relationship. These may include hypothyroidism, low vitamin D, recent exercise, or alcohol/drug abuse [21]. Note that there is no evidence that statins adversely affect cognition. If a patient develops confusion or memory impairment while on statin, consider all causes.

Randomized clinical trials have repeatedly demonstrated that the benefits of moderate- or high-intensity statin outweigh the risks in nearly all patients, excepting those with significant adverse effects such as myositis. Regardless, patients tend to focus on potential side effects—the most common of which include myalgias, dysglycemia, and cognitive impairment. A patient experiencing side effects with one statin should

Fig. 30.6 How to evaluate for myalgias in patients on statins

Assessing for myalgia

- Prior to initiating and during statin therapy
- Baseline CK for increased risk (elderly, meds that increase myopathy risk
- No routine assessment
- ROS:
  - Muscle aching
  - Pain
  - Stiffness
  - Tenderness
  - Weakness
  - Fatigue
  - Cramps
- Evaluate other reasons for myalgias-establish causal relationship
  - Hypothyroidism
  - Low vitamin D
  - Recent exercise
  - Alcohol/drug abuse

generally be transitioned to a different statin, often at a lower intensity, and then retitrated. Patients should generally not be labeled as statin intolerant until they have failed at least three different agents. For the clinician, it can be difficult to convince a patient to accept a medication that causes adverse effects, even if only perceived, in order to prevent a theoretical future risk.

Blood Pressure

Hypertension accounts for more ASCVD fatalities than any other modifiable risk factor, largely because of its high and rising prevalence [22]. In a meta-analysis of 61 studies, a log-linear association was observed between SBP levels <115 to >180 mmHg and DBP levels <75 to 105 mmHg and the risk of ASCVD across an age spectrum of 30–80 years. Thus, all clinicians must diligently help patients achieve target blood pressure levels to decrease their cardiac risk.

The definition of hypertension has evolved over the past several decades, and many professional organizations continue to offer slightly differing thresholds and goals. Unlike cholesterol, where lower values are almost always better, the relationship between mortality and blood pressure is clearly U-shaped, and overtreatment is a common challenge.

The current guidelines categorize blood pressure as normal, elevated, or hypertension, which is then further divided into stages 1 and 2 (Fig. 30.7). Previously, a blood pressure of <130/80 was considered normal, and clinicians may find patients are confused by the newer, lower goals.

For most patients, the diagnosis of hypertension requires abnormal readings on two separate occasions [15]. An exception may be made for patients with especially high blood pressure (e.g., SBP greater than 160 mm Hg or DBP > 100 mm Hg) on a single occasion, provided the measurement has been repeated under appropriate conditions and after an adequate period of rest.

BP Category	SBP		DBP
Normal	<120 mm Hg	and	<80 mm Hg
Elevated	120-129 mm Hg	and	<80 mm Hg
Hypertension			
Stage 1	130-139 mm Hg	or	80-89 mm Hg
Stage 2	>140 mm Hg	or	<90 mm Hg

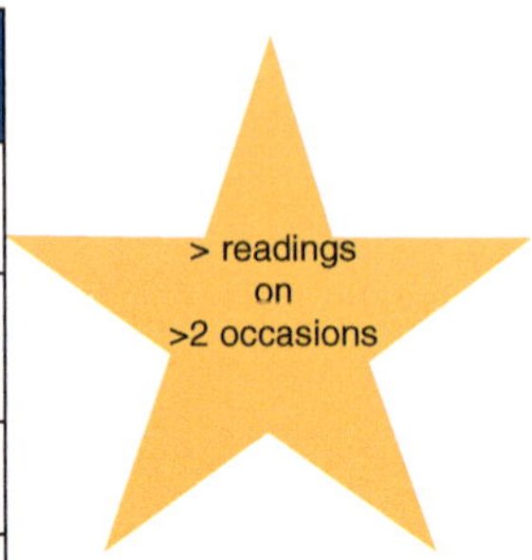

Guideline now defines hypertension to be above 130 mmHg systolic, or 80 mmHg diastolic

More patients (46% vs 32% based on JNC7) will be diagnosed with hypertension

Fig. 30.7 Blood pressure definitions

Patients with normal BP (<120/80 mmHg) should continue to pursue healthy lifestyle habits. Patients with elevated BP (120–129/<80 mmHg) or stage I hypertension (BP 130–139/80–89 mmHg) with an estimated 10-year ASCVD risk <10% should consider lifestyle changes and nonpharmacological therapies. Patients with stage 2 hypertension (>140/90 mmHg), as well as those with stage 1 hypertension and a 10-year risk >10%, should pursue both nonpharmacological and pharmacological therapies [23].

Nonpharmacologic approaches to blood pressure management can be very effective, though long-term adherence is challenging [15]. The most effective interventions include weight loss, a plant-based diet, reduced dietary sodium intake, increased dietary potassium intake, physical activity, and reduction of alcohol consumption. In addition, patients may need to reduce or avoid the use of certain medications and supplements that can raise blood pressure, including decongestants, antidepressants, caffeine, oral contraceptives, nonsteroidal anti-inflammatory drugs (NSAIDs), corticosteroids, licorice, anise, black cohosh, ginger, ma huang, ginseng, and St. John's wort.

The antihypertensive medications currently available for use include ACE inhibitors or angiotensin receptor blockers, diuretics (loop, potassium sparing, aldosterone antagonists), calcium channel blockers, beta blockers (cardioselective, vasodilatory, combined), direct renin inhibitors, and alpha blockers. The clinician should choose therapies based on the amount of blood pressure lowering that is required, the patient's other comorbidities, dosing frequency, side effects, and cost (Fig. 30.8).

Every hypertensive patient should have a clear and detailed plan of care that outlines their treatments and their personalized, achievable goals. They should know how to measure their blood pressure at home, how to record it, and whom to contact when questions arise. An interprofessional collaborative care team including a clinician (physician, nurse practitioner, or physician assistant), nurse, medical assistant, pharmacist, and perhaps trainer or exercise physiologist should assume shared responsibility for this effort. The reassessment frequency should depend on the level and stability of control, and the patient should always leave the office with a follow-up appointment scheduled.

Thiazide diuretics	Chlorthalidone, hydrochlorothiazide, metolazone, indapamide	• Monitor for hyponatremia and hypokalemia, uric Acid and calcium, careful with gout • chlorthalidone is preferred diuretic due to long half life and proven risk reduction
Ace Inhibitors	Benazepril, enalapril, lisinopril, ramipril etc.	• May cause ARF in patients with bilateral renal artery stenosis, watch for angioedema at any time • Do not combine with ARB or direct renin inhibitor, increased risk of hyperkalemia in CKD • Do not use in pregnancy
Angiotensin Receptor Blocker	Candesartan, irbesartan, olmesartan, valsartan, etc.	• Do not combine with ACEi
CCB – dihydropyridine	Amlodipine, febdipine, nifedipine, nisoldipine	• Avoid in HFrEF • More common in women • Associated with dose-related pedal edema
CCB – nondihydropyridine	Diltiazem, verapamil	• Avoid routine use with BB drug interactions with diltiazem and verapamil • Associated with bradycardia and heart block • Avoid in HFrEF
Diuretics – loop	Bumetanide, furosemide, torsemide	• Preferred diuretic in patient with symptomatic HF • Preferred over thiazides in patients with moderate to severe CKD (GFR <30ml/min)
Diuretics – aldosterone antagonists	Eplerenone, spironolactone	• Spironolactone associated with increased gynecomastia and impotence • Common add-on in resistant htn • Avoid use with K+ supplements
		• Eplerenone often requires BID dosing • Preferred in primary aldosteronism and resistant hypertension
Beta blockers – cardioselective	Atenolol, bisoprolol, metoprolol	• Not recommended as first line agents unless patient has CAD or HFrEF • Bisoprolol preferred to treat HTN + bronchospastic airway disease • Bisoprolol and metoprolol succinate preferred in HTN with HFrEF • Avoid abrupt cessation
Beta blockers – cardioselective and vasodilatory	Nebivolol	• Induces nitric oxide-induced vasodilation • Avoid abrupt cessation
Beta blockers – non cardioselective	Nadolol, propranolol	• Avoid with reactive airway disease • Avoid abrupt cessation
Beta blockers – combined alpha and beta receptor	Carvedilol, labetalol	• Preferred in patients with HFrEF
Direct renin inhibitor	Aliskaren	• Long acting • Increased risk of hyperkalemia • Watch for acute renal failure with renal artery stenosis • Avoid in pregnancy • Targets renin angiotensis sytem • Do not combine with ACEi/ARB
Alpha-1 blockers	Doxazosin, prazosin, terazosin	• May consider as second line agent with concomitant BPH • Associated with orthostatic hypotension
Central alpha2-agonist and other centrally acting drugs	Clonidine, methyldopa, guanfacine	• Reserved as last line due to CNS adverse effects especially in older adults • Avoid abrupt discontinuation of clonidine which may induce hypertensive crisis, must be tapered
Direct vasodilators	Hydralazine, minoxidil	• Associated with sodium and water retention, and reflex tachydardia • Minoxidil associated with hirsutism – use with loop diuretic, can induce pericardial effusion • Must be used with diuretic and beta blocker

Fig. 30.8 Classes of oral antihypertensives

Tobacco Use

Tobacco use is the leading preventable cause of death, disease and disability in the United States, and even secondhand smoke contributes to the risk of ASCVD and stroke. Although the risks of cigarettes are now well-known, newer, electronic nicotine delivery systems (e-cigarettes) also emit aerosols containing particulates, nicotine, and noxious gases that can increase the risk of cardiovascular and pulmonary diseases [24].

Many clinicians are daunted by the challenge of delivering effective tobacco cessation therapy, given the chronic and relapsing nature of tobacco addiction. The assessment should cover frequency of use, lifelong exposure, and readiness to quit, often at each ambulatory encounter. Appropriate questions to ask the patient include: "Have you smoked any tobacco products in the past 30 days? Have you vaped or Juul'ed in the past 30 days? Have you used any tobacco products in the past 30 days, even a puff?" Such questions are far more effective than, "Do you smoke?".

The pharmacologic arsenal for helping patients defeat tobacco addiction includes FDA-approved pharmacotherapies—including varenicline, bupropion, nortriptyline—and several approved forms of nicotine replacement, such as patches, gums, lozenges, and inhalers [25]. These interventions should always be combined with cognitive behavioral skills training and appropriate encouragement and incentives. Formal tobacco cessation clinic referrals should be considered if available.

Aspirin Use

Aspirin has long been recommended for the prevention of ASCVD. Aspirin reduces the risk of atherosclerosis by inhibiting platelet function, but this also increases the risk of bleeding [26]. Its importance for secondary prevention remains unchallenged, but its role in primary prevention has become more controversial. Historically, low-dose aspirin was recommended for primary prevention among adults aged 40–70 years at increased risk of ASCVD and low risk of bleeding.

In current practice, however, most guidelines favor the use of low-dose aspirin only in a small cohort of patients [27]. Aspirin use for prevention in adults aged 40–59 years who have a 10% or greater 10-year CVD risk has a small net benefit. The use of aspirin for primary prevention of CVD events should be avoided in adults 60 years or older, adults with an increased risk of bleeding, and adults younger than 59 with a <10% 10-year ASCVD risk estimate [27].

Factors consistent with an increased risk of bleeding include a history of GI bleed, peptic ulcer disease, bleeding at other sites, thrombocytopenia, coagulopathy, chronic kidney disease, or concurrent use of other medications that may increase bleeding (NSAIDS, steroids, anticoagulants, warfarin, or fish oil) (Fig. 30.9). In the future, precision medicine may help clinicians understand a patient's platelet phenotype, and relative risk versus benefit, when making decisions about antiplatelet use [27].

Fig. 30.9 Contraindications to aspirin use in primary prevention

Contraindications to aspirin use in primary prevention
History of GI bleed
Peptic Ulcer Disease
Bleeding at Other sites
Age > 70 years
Thrombocytopenia
Coagulopathy
Chronic kidney disease
Concurrent medications that may increase bleeding (NSAIDS, steroids, anticoagulants, fish oil, warfarin)

Conclusion

Many ASCVD events are avoidable with effective primary prevention. The best way to prevent ASCVD is to promote a lifelong, healthy lifestyle. Tobacco avoidance is critical, and all adults should seek to engage in brisk physical activity as often as possible. A diet high in fruits, vegetables, and whole grains is preferred. Although a plant-based diet is preferred, fish and poultry are the preferred sources of protein among meat eaters. It is important to minimize trans fats, added sugars, red and processed meats, and excessive sodium.

Clinicians should work with patients to assess their readiness for change as well as their ability to assess and understand their personal risk factors. Practice models are more effective if they include an interprofessional team working together to encourage and guide the patient. Lastly, awareness of the social determinants of health must undergird every recommendation. Clinicians must consider their patient's health literacy, education level, and psychosocial support to maximize the change of their recommendations being implemented.

References

1. Grundy SM, Stone NJ, Bailey AL, et al. 2018 AHA/ACC/AACVPR/AAPA/ABC/ACPM/ADA/AGS/APhA/ASPC/NLA/PCNA guideline on the Management of Blood Cholesterol. J Am Coll Cardiol. 2019;73(24):e285–350. https://doi.org/10.1016/j.jacc.2018.11.003.
2. Navar AM, Wang TY, Mi X, et al. Influence of cardiovascular risk communication tools and presentation formats on patient perceptions and preferences. JAMA Cardiol. 2018;3(12):1192. https://doi.org/10.1001/jamacardio.2018.3680.
3. American College of Cardiology, American Heart Association ASCVD Risk Estimator. Available at: https://tools.acc.org/ascvd-risk-estimator-plus/#!/calculate/estimate/. Accessed 5 Apr 2022. https://tools.acc.org/ascvd-risk-estimator-plus/#!/calculate/estimate/
4. D'Agostino RB, Vasan RS, Pencina MJ, et al. General cardiovascular risk profile for use in primary care: the Framingham heart study. Circulation. 2008;117(6):743–53. https://doi.org/10.1161/CIRCULATIONAHA.107.699579.
5. Ridker PM, Buring JE, Rifai N, Cook NR. Development and validation of improved algorithms for the assessment of global cardiovascular risk in women: the Reynolds risk score. JAMA. 2007;297(6):611. https://doi.org/10.1001/jama.297.6.611.
6. Miedema MD, Duprez DA, Misialek JR, et al. Use of coronary artery calcium testing to guide aspirin utilization for primary prevention: estimates from the multi-ethnic study of atherosclerosis. Cardiovascul Qual Outcom. 2014;7(3):453–60. https://doi.org/10.1161/CIRCOUTCOMES.113.000690.
7. Mitchell JD, Fergestrom N, Gage BF, et al. Impact of statins on cardiovascular outcomes following coronary artery calcium scoring. J Am Coll Cardiol. 2018;72(25):3233–42. https://doi.org/10.1016/j.jacc.2018.09.051.
8. Explaining ASCVD risk scores for primary prevention. https://www.acc.org/-/media/Non-Clinical/Files-PDFs-Excel-MS-Word-etc/Tools-and-Practice-Support/Risk-Communications/3-Explaining-ASCVD-Risk-Scores-for-Primary-Prevention.pdf?la=en&hash=FBAA16BC5DC66F56CB2BA718825628C462FDCC23. Accessed 5 Apr 2022.
9. Parikh P, Shah N, Ahmed H, Schoenhagen P, Fares M. Coronary artery calcium scoring: its practicality and clinical utility in primary care. CCJM. 2018;85(9):707–16. https://doi.org/10.3949/ccjm.85a.17097.
10. Pletcher MJ, Pignone M, Earnshaw S, et al. Using the coronary artery calcium score to guide statin therapy: a cost-effectiveness analysis. Circ Cardiovasc Qual Outcomes. 2014;7(2):276–84. https://doi.org/10.1161/CIRCOUTCOMES.113.000799.
11. U.S. Department of Health and Human Services, Office of Disease Prevention and Health Promotion. Healthy people 2030. https://health.gov/healthypeople/objectives-and-data/social-determinants-health. Accessed 1 Aug 2021.
12. Centers for Medicare and Medicaid Services, Billioux A, Verlander K, et al. Standardized screening for health-related social needs in clinical settings: the accountable health communities screening tool. NAM Perspectives. 2017;7(5) https://doi.org/10.31478/201705b.
13. Lichtenstein AH, Appel LJ, Vadiveloo M, et al. 2021 dietary guidance to improve cardiovascular health: a scientific statement from the American Heart Association. Circulation. 2021;144(23):e472–87. https://doi.org/10.1161/CIR.0000000000001031.
14. Reedy J, Krebs-Smith SM, Miller PE, et al. Higher diet quality is associated with decreased risk of all-cause, cardiovascular disease, and cancer mortality among older adults. J Nutr. 2014;144(6):881–9. https://doi.org/10.3945/jn.113.189407.
15. Arnett DK, Blumenthal RS, Albert MA, et al. ACC/AHA guideline on the primary prevention of cardiovascular disease: a report of the American College of Cardiology/American Heart Association Task Force on Clinical Practice Guidelines. Circulation.

2019;2019:140(11). https://doi.org/10.1161/CIR.0000000000000678.
16. Tharrey M, Mariotti F, Mashchak A, Barbillon P, Delattre M, Fraser GE. Patterns of plant and animal protein intake are strongly associated with cardiovascular mortality: the Adventist Health Study-2 cohort. Int J Epidemiol. 2018;47(5):1603–12. https://doi.org/10.1093/ije/dyy030.
17. Martínez-González MA, Sánchez-Tainta A, Corella D, et al. A provegetarian food pattern and reduction in total mortality in the Prevención con Dieta Mediterránea (PREDIMED) study. Am J Clin Nutr. 2014;100(suppl_1):320S–8S. https://doi.org/10.3945/ajcn.113.071431.
18. Kim H, Caulfield LE, Rebholz CM. Healthy plant-based diets are associated with lower risk of all-cause mortality in US adults. J Nutr. 2018;148(4):624–31. https://doi.org/10.1093/jn/nxy019.
19. Reimers CD, Knapp G, Reimers AK. Does physical activity increase life expectancy? A review of the literature. J Aging Res. 2012;2012:1–9. https://doi.org/10.1155/2012/243958.
20. Benjamin EJ, Virani SS, Callaway CW, et al. Heart disease and stroke statistics—2018 update: a report from the American Heart Association. Circulation. 2018;137(12):e67. https://doi.org/10.1161/CIR.0000000000000558.
21. Birtcher K. When compliance is an issue-how to enhance statin adherence and address adverse effects. Curr Atheroscler Rep. 2015;17(1):471.
22. Danaei G, Ding EL, Mozaffarian D, et al. The preventable causes of death in the United States: comparative risk assessment of dietary, lifestyle, and metabolic risk factors. PLoS Med. 2009;6(4):e1000058. https://doi.org/10.1371/journal.pmed.1000058.
23. Whelton PK, Carey RM, Aronow WS, et al. 2017 ACC/AHA/AAPA/ABC/ACPM/AGS/APhA/ASH/ASPC/NMA/PCNA guideline for the prevention, detection, evaluation, and management of high blood pressure in adults. J Am Coll Cardiol. 2018;71(19):e127–248. https://doi.org/10.1016/j.jacc.2017.11.006.
24. Bhatnagar A. Cardiovascular perspective of the promises and perils of E-cigarettes. Circ Res. 2016;118(12):1872–5. https://doi.org/10.1161/CIRCRESAHA.116.308723.
25. Barua RS, Rigotti NA, Benowitz NL, et al. 2018 ACC expert consensus decision pathway on tobacco cessation treatment. J Am Coll Cardiol. 2018;72(25):3332–65. https://doi.org/10.1016/j.jacc.2018.10.027.
26. Guirguis-Blake JM, Evans CV, Senger CA, O'Connor EA, Whitlock EP. Aspirin for the primary prevention of cardiovascular events: a systematic evidence review for the U.S. Preventive Services Task Force. Ann Intern Med. 2016;164(12):804. https://doi.org/10.7326/M15-2113.
27. Lloyd-Jones DM. USPSTF report on aspirin for primary prevention. JAMA Cardiol. 2022; https://doi.org/10.1001/jamacardio.2022.0935.

Part X

Emergency Department Evaluation of Chest Pain

Musialowsk Musialowski

There are approximately 130 million emergency department (ED) visits annually, many of which are due to a cardiovascular cause [1]. Cardiovascular complaints frequently require hospital admission. Congestive heart failure is the second leading cause of emergency department (ED) visits requiring hospital admission, comprising 4.1% of all hospital admission [2]. Acute myocardial infarction (AMI) and cardiac dysrhythmias are also among the top ten admission diagnoses with 2.5% and 2.2% of all hospital admissions, respectively [2]. Cardiac disease remains the leading cause of death in the USA, accounting for 211.5 deaths per 100,000.

Patients presenting with chest pain may have a wide array of potential diagnoses with varying severity and urgency. This spectrum can range from a non-cardiovascular etiology of symptoms to a life-threatening emergency requiring immediate diagnosis and intervention. A provider in the ED must exclude life-threatening diagnoses via a rapid and thorough evaluation prior to the consideration of more benign etiologies. The high prevalence of cardiovascular disease in patients presenting to the ED has prompted many guideline-directed care pathways. These guidelines and pathways are essential to rapidly evaluate and triage the acuity of the patient.

Patients can present to healthcare locations other than an ED. Patients with STEMI may present to the office or any ambulatory setting. The same principles apply to the evaluation of patient complaints in any setting. The following chapter will evaluate the common presenting complaint of cardiovascular disease: chest pain. The common theme will be focusing on pertinent elements of patient history, physical examination, laboratory, and diagnostic testing which will guide rapid diagnosis and treatment. Always remember to exclude the most dangerous and life-threatening etiologies before considering a less severe or even noncardiovascular etiology.

M. Musialowski
Sanger Heart and Vascular Institute, Atrium Health, Charlotte, NC, USA
e-mail: Richard.musialowski@atriumhealth.org

References

1. https://www.cdc.gov/nchs/fastats/emergency-department.htm
2. https://www.hcup-us.ahrq.gov/reports/statbriefs/sb277-Top-Reasons-Hospital-Stays-2018.pdf#:~:text=%E2%96%A0%20The%20most%20frequent%20principal%20diagnoses%20for%20hospitalizations,stays%29%20and%20the%20costliest%20%28%2441.5%20billion%20in%20aggregate%29

Acute Evaluation of Chest Pain

31

Devin Stives and Richard Musialowski

Introduction

Chest pain accounts for approximately 5% of all ED visits. Noncardiac chest pain will be identified in over 50% of these patients [1]. ED clinicians should always consider cardiovascular pathologies when evaluating a patient complaining of chest pain. However, several pathologies involving the pulmonary, musculoskeletal, and gastrointestinal systems share similar symptoms with cardiovascular disease. Afferent pain fibers originating from intrathoracic organs course with afferent sympathetic nerves to paravertebral ganglion before entering the spinal cord. The destination for visceral pain sensation is the thalamus. No area within the cerebral cortex localizes visceral pain. The lack of brain stem localization results in patients unable to localize a specific origin of their visceral pain and symptoms can overlap between different organ systems [2]. The involvement of sympathetic nerves in cardiac pain sensation was known as early as 1921, when angina pectoris was successfully treated with sympathectomy [3]. This practice is no longer used today due to the numerous superior medical and invasive treatment options (see Part II).

D. Stives (✉)
Cardiovascular Disease Fellow, Aurora St. Lukes Medical Center, Milwaukee, WI, USA
e-mail: Devin.Stives@aah.org

R. Musialowski
Sanger Heart and Vascular Institute, Atrium Health, Charlotte, NC, USA
e-mail: Richard.musialowski@atriumhealth.org

Etiologies of Chest Pain

We recommend an anatomic approach to establishing a differential diagnosis for chest pain as outlined in Table 31.1. Besides cardiovascular causes, there are numerous noncardiac etiologies including pulmonary, gastrointestinal, and musculoskeletal diseases. ED providers will need to evaluate for any life-threatening causes in a timely manner prior to consideration of a more benign diagnosis. Patient history and examination is insufficient to establish a diagnosis and typically requires further testing.

Myocardial Ischemia

Cardiac causes of chest pain can be due to ischemia attributable to coronary disease such as acute coronary syndrome, coronary vasospasm, spontaneous coronary artery dissection, or increased myocardial demand in the setting of a flow limiting lesion. Noncoronary cardiovascular etiologies such as aortic dissection, heart failure, or myopericarditis should also be considered [4].

There are several mechanisms of myocardial injury and elevated troponin. Type I MI refers to coronary occlusion due to acute atherosclerotic

R. Musialowski, K. Allshouse (eds.), *Cardiovascular Manual for the Advanced Practice Provider*,
https://doi.org/10.1007/978-3-031-35819-7_31

Table 31.1 Differential diagnosis of chest pain

Cardiovascular	– Acute myocardial infarction (type I MI)
	– Acute coronary ischemia (type II MI)
	– Aortic dissection
	– Cardiac tamponade
	– Pericarditis
	– Coronary vasospasm/spontaneous coronary artery dissection (SCAD)
	– Valvular heart disease
	– Hypertrophic cardiomyopathy
	– Stress cardiomyopathy
Respiratory	– Pulmonary embolus
	– Tension pneumothorax
	– Pneumonia
	– Malignancy
Gastrointestinal	– Esophageal rupture
	– Esophageal spasm
	– Gastroesophageal reflux disease
	– Peptic ulcer
	– Hiatal hernia
	– Pancreatitis
	– Cholecystitis
Chest wall	– Costochondritis
	– Chest wall trauma
	– Herpes zoster
	– Musculoskeletal strain
Psychiatric	– Anxiety
	– Panic disorder

Disease processes that require urgent or immediate evaluation and intervention are underlined

plaque rupture, and type 2 MI refers to myocardial oxygen supply/demand mismatch [5]. Type I MI is due to an acute coronary syndrome that often necessitates invasive angiography and percutaneous coronary intervention (PCI) or coronary artery bypass grafting (CABG) if indicated. For full details, see Part II on CAD.

A detailed history including prior coronary evaluation, family history of early myocardial infarction as defined as age in men <45 or women <55, and risk factors for CAD should be obtained. "Typical" chest pain will be described as substernal chest pain provoked by exertion or emotional stress and relived by rest. Patients will describe chest pain as a heaviness, pressure, or squeezing sensation that originates retrosternal and may radiate to the left arm or jaw. Pain described as sharp or worsening with inspiration decreases your likelihood of myocardial ischemia as the origin for their pain. Improvement of a patient's chest pain in response to nitroglycerin was classically taught as diagnostic for angina. However, newer data suggests that response to nitroglycerin does not provide diagnostic accuracy and should not weigh heavily as a predictor of coronary-related chest pain [6]. Current guidelines for chest pain recommend distinguishing chest pain as "cardiac," "possible cardiac," and "noncardiac" to describe the suspected cause of a patient's chest pain and recommend against the use of "atypical" [7]. Attention should be given to the uniqueness of the ischemic presentation in women, diabetics, elderly patients. This cohort is more likely to experience associated symptoms such as shortness of breath, nausea or vomiting, lightheadedness, confusion, presyncope, syncope, or vague abdominal symptoms. Women with AMI are more likely to present with "typical symptoms" compared to men but also have a higher frequency of associated symptoms such as nausea, vomiting, and palpitations [8].

Pericardial Disease

Pericarditis is a common cause of chest pain in the emergency department and occurs due to inflammation of the pericardial layers due to systemic inflammatory or infectious processes. However, the most common cause is idiopathic as seen in about 90% of patients. Pericarditis is typically a benign etiology of chest pain. However, complications such as pericardial effusion with tamponade and/or pericardial constriction warrant further investigation [9]. See Chap. 23 for full discussion on pericarditis.

Vascular Causes

An acute aortic dissection is an uncommon but life-threatening cause of chest pain in the ED. Aortic dissections occur due to a tear within the tunica intima and formation of a false lumen due to shear stress on the intimal wall, most commonly due to underlying hypertension and atherosclerosis. Other risk factors including underlying connective tissue disorders (Marfan syndrome or Ehlers-Danlos syndromes), cocaine use, pregnancy, and known aortic aneurysm also increase risk of aortic dissection as an etiology [10]. Aortic dissections are classified by the Stanford classification, with type A involving the ascending aorta and type B without ascending aortic involvement. This distinction is crucial as it drives management.

Patients will classically describe pain as a severe "tearing," "ripping," or "stabbing" sensation. Pain is often sudden onset. According to the International Registry of Acute Aortic Dissection (IRAD), "tearing" or "ripping" was found to not be as reliable descriptor as previously thought [11]. Examination may reveal an uncomfortable appearing, hypertensive patient. A diastolic murmur may be heard in up to 40% of patients with a type A aortic dissection. Asymmetric pulses were only present in 30% of type A aortic dissections and 20% of type B aortic dissections [11]. See Chap. 28 for full discussion on aortic dissection.

Pulmonary Causes

Several pulmonary pathologies can result in chest pain. Pain will commonly be described as pleuritic and worsens with inspiration. Associated dyspnea or cough may be seen. Tension pneumothorax is an uncommon but life-threatening cause of chest pain to the ED due to air within the intrapleural space. Patients with tension pneumothorax are typically hypoxic and may progress to respiratory and hemodynamic failure. Signs on physical exam of a tension pneumothorax may include tracheal deviation away from the pneumothorax, absent or diminished lung sounds ipsilaterally, and subcutaneous emphysema [12]. This is a surgical emergency requiring urgent decompression of the trapped air.

Pulmonary embolism (PE) is a common consideration for patients presenting with chest pain in the emergency department and significant contributor to global disease burden [13]. Commonly, pulmonary emboli originate from a deep vein thrombosis in the lower extremities with embolization to the pulmonary arteries [14]. Patients with a pulmonary embolism are at risk for acute respiratory and right ventricular failure resulting in hemodynamic collapse. Patients with an acute PE may report chest pain, dyspnea, hemoptysis, or presyncope. These are nonspecific findings, and their absence does not exclude PE. Risk factor assessment is a crucial element in patients with suspected PE. Recent fracture of a lower limb, hip, or knee replacement; major trauma or surgery; and prior spinal cord injury has an odds ratio of >10 for venous thromboembolism [15]. Prior VTE, malignancy, and oral contraceptives are also significant risk factors for VTE (see Chap. 22).

Gastrointestinal

Gastrointestinal causes of chest pain can mimic cardiovascular chest pain but are often due to benign etiologies. Esophageal perforation or perforated peptic ulcer can be life-threatening. Nitroglycerin is often used for patients with suspected chest pain due to cardiac ischemia, and the medication may be helpful for patients with esophageal spasm. Attention to precipitating factors such as relation to meals or associated dysphagia may be an indicator that a patient's pain is due to a gastrointestinal etiology. Eructation and flatus improving the symptoms suggest a GI etiology as well. Symptoms such as odynophagia, GI bleeding, unintentional weight loss, or vomiting may warrant further esophageal evaluation.

History

Detailed history is commonly insufficient to establish a clear diagnosis. Attention should also be given to a patient's past medical history and underlying risk factors (Table 31.2). Features of chest pain carry significant overlap, although history and physical examination will likely drive additional testing and evaluation. History should be obtained in a standardized format with a focus on high yield questioning based on most likely etiology.

1. **Onset**: The events leading up to the onset of pain can provide helpful indicators for an etiology. Pain that started during physical or emotional stress and builds gradually is typi-

Table 31.2 Risk factors for common causes of chest pain

Acute coronary syndrome	Aortic dissection	Pulmonary embolism	Pericarditis	Pneumothorax
Coronary artery disease Diabetes mellitus Tobacco use Hypertension Advanced age	Hypertension Atherosclerosis Pregnancy Bicuspid aortic valve Connective tissue disease (Marfan syndrome, Ehlers-Danlos syndrome) Aortic aneurysm Tobacco use Cocaine use	Hypercoagulable state Malignancy Lower limb fracture Hip replacement Knee replacement Spinal cord injury Major trauma or surgery Oral contraceptives Prolonged immobility	Prior pericarditis Autoimmune disease Recent type I MI Uremia Radiation therapy	Prior pneumothorax Chronic lung disease Tobacco use

cal for ischemic heart disease. Pain that began abruptly may indicate an acute aortic dissection, pneumothorax, or PE. Chest pain that began after eating or drinking is more commonly due to a gastrointestinal cause.

2. **Nature**: Angina symptoms can be described in many ways such as pain, discomfort, pressure, or squeezing like sensation. A sharp or stabbing pain may indicate pneumothorax or acute pericarditis. A “ripping” or “tearing” sensation is classic for aortic dissection, although these features lack sensitivity to be used reliably.
3. **Location and radiation**: Pain due to ischemic heart disease is most likely retrosternal. Patients may report radiation to the arm or jaw. Associated back pain may be seen in aortic dissection. Pain involving the trapezius muscle may be due to phrenic nerve irritation and pericarditis.
4. **Precipitating factors:** Chest pain that worsens with exertion or emotion is most likely due to myocardial ischemia. Pain that worsens with lying flat usually occurs with acute pericarditis. Pain that worsens with positional changes or worsening of pain with chest wall palpation may be seen in musculoskeletal etiologies. Symptoms after eating are often not cardiovascular and suggest a GI etiology.
5. **Palliating factors:** Resolution of the symptoms with cessation of an activity is very suggestive of coronary ischemia. Newer data suggests that relief from nitroglycerin is not as reliable as previously thought and should not be used as diagnostic criteria. Improvement with change of position may be musculoskeletal in origin.
6. **Associated symptoms:** Symptoms that may be associated with ACS include dyspnea, palpitations, diaphoresis, presyncope, or abdominal pain. Hemoptysis may be a sign of PE, although this is not a common complaint.

Physical Examination

Physical exam rarely leads to a solidified type I MI diagnosis without additional testing. Patients may be diaphoretic and either tachycardic or bradycardic. A new murmur may represent a mechanical complication of MI. Signs of volume overload such as jugular venous distention, S3 gallop, rales, or peripheral edema suggest depressed LV function as a cause of their symptoms.

Patients with an aortic dissection typically appear distressed and are often tachycardic and hypertensive. Assessment of upper extremity peripheral pulses bilaterally should be performed and assessed for differences. This pulse difference was only present in 30% of patients with aortic dissection and should not be used to exclude aortic dissection. A new diastolic murmur may be heard indicating aortic insufficiency.

In acute pulmonary embolism, patients are commonly tachycardic and short of breath. A low-grade fever may be present. Despite the patient’s shortness of breath, lung auscultation typically reveals clear lungs. A pleural rub may be heard. JVD may be a sign of more severe disease.

In acute pericarditis, a pericardial friction rub is one of four diagnostic criteria. Tachycardia and low-grade fever are common. If a pericardial effusion is large enough, it may produce pericardial tamponade which will present as tachycardia, hypotension, and JVD.

Pneumothorax can be identified with absent lung sounds unilaterally, tracheal deviation, and respiratory distress. Tension pneumothorax may produce obstructive shock and JVD on exam. With gastrointestinal causes of chest pain, there may also be epigastric tenderness. Clinicians should not neglect direct visualization of the patient's skin to look for vesicles, erythema as signs of herpes zoster infection.

Diagnostic Testing During the Acute Presentation

Electrocardiogram

An electrocardiogram (ECG) should be performed within 10 min of patient presentation for all patients complaining of chest pain (Fig. 31.1). The ECG is crucial for the identification of STEMI to facilitate timely coronary reperfusion in type I MI. If an initial EKG is nondiagnostic but clinical suspicion remains high for ACS, serial ECGs may increase the sensitivity in detecting potential candidates for coronary reperfusion [16]. The universal definition of myocardial infarction defines STEMI as new ST elevation at the J point in at least two contiguous leads of ≥2 mm (0.2 mV) in men or ≥1.5 mm (0.15 mV) in women in leads V2-V3 and/or of ≥1 mm (0.1 mV) in other contiguous chest leads or the limb leads in the absence of left ventricular hypertrophy or left bundle-branch block (LBBB) [17]. Paced rhythm and underlying LBBB make the ECG difficult to evaluate for STEMI. ST depressions in V1-V4 may prompt a clinician to perform a repeat ECG including leads V7-V9 to evaluate for posterior STEMI (see Part II CAD).

The ECG will provide additional information in the setting of acute PE. The most common ECG finding in PE is sinus tachycardia. Patients with "S1Q3T3" are threefold more likely to have

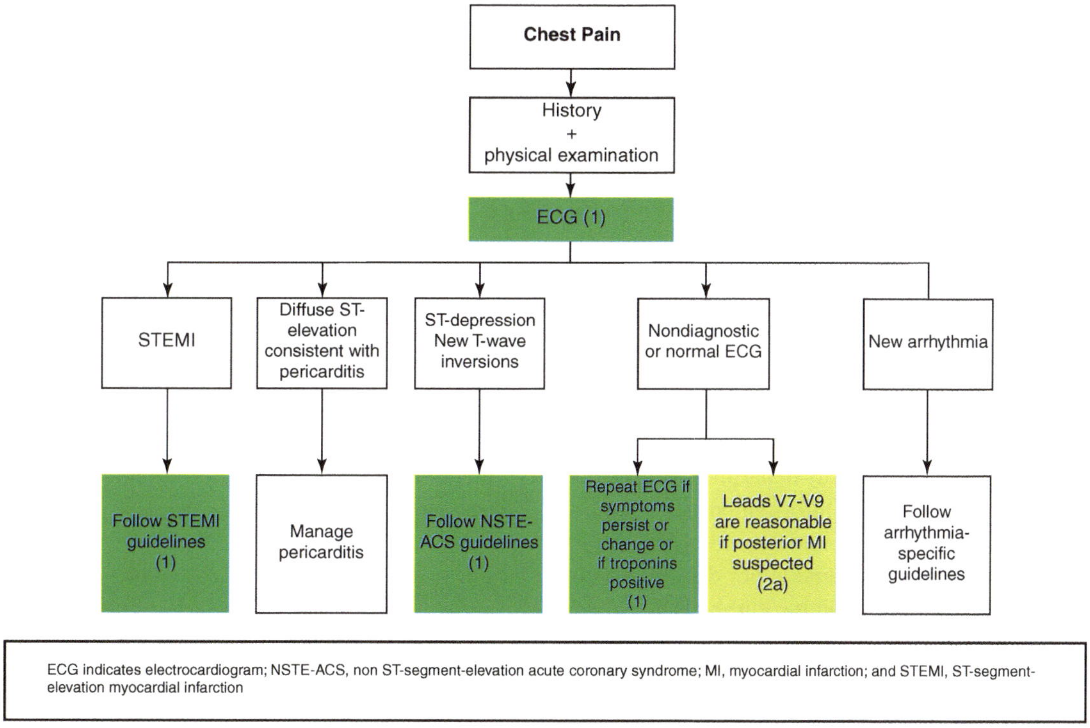

Fig. 31.1 Ekg and chest pain decision tool. (Adapted from 2021 AHA/ACC/ASE/CHEST/SAEM/SCCT/SCMR Guideline for the Evaluation and Diagnosis of Chest Pain: A Report of the American College of Cardiology/American Heart Association Joint Committee on Clinical Practice Guidelines)

a PE than patients who do not. Right bundle branch block, inverted T waves in V1-V4, and ST elevation in aVR are concerning features for patients with PE [18]. The ECG may clue a clinician toward a diagnosis of acute pericarditis if diffuse ST elevations and PR depression are seen. Nonspecific ST and T wave changes may be seen in as many as 42% of patients with acute aortic dissection, and up to 5% of patients with an acute aortic dissection may also have an acute inferior MI due to extension into the RCA.

Chest Radiography

Chest radiograph is a quick, noninvasive test that should be performed with patient's complaining of chest pain. Chest radiographs often do not change management in acute coronary syndrome but are beneficial for evaluating other potential etiologies of chest pain. A pneumothorax can be readily identified on chest X-ray by a visible visceral pleura edge seen as a thin, sharp white line without lung markings peripheral to this line. Mediastinal deviation from midline suggests tension physiology and warrants urgent intervention. Subcutaneous emphysema may also be seen. A widened mediastinum may be seen in acute aortic dissection, although this lacks sensitivity and does not exclude the possibility of aortic dissection. Bacterial pneumonia may be seen as a focal opacity which may produce symptoms of chest pain. Other parenchymal lung diseases like malignancy may be identified.

Ultrasonography

Point-of-care ultrasound (POCUS) has grown in popularity in the emergency department setting due to the rapid high-yield information that may be obtained. Cardiac ultrasound has developed into a vital instrument used by emergency department clinicians with proper training in bedside image acquisition and interpretation to guide rapid diagnosis and clinical decision-making in symptomatic patients with cardiovascular disease. According to the American College of Emergency Physicians and American Society of Echocardiography, the use of focused cardiac ultrasound (FOCUS) provides great utility for the assessment of global cardiac systolic function, marked ventricular chamber enlargement, or the assessment for the presence of a pericardial effusion. In cases of uncertain volume status, FOCUS may be used to aid in the assessment of intravascular volume assessment. FOCUS should also be used for guidance during pericardiocentesis and confirmation of a transvenous pacing wire placement [19].

In the case of an AMI, segmental wall motion abnormalities should only be evaluated under comprehensive echocardiography and interpreted by experienced readers. FOCUS may be used to establish the presence of a pericardial effusion in acute pericarditis but does not replace comprehensive echocardiography for monitoring of effusion size. In the case of an acute aortic dissection, comprehensive echocardiography should be used to evaluate aortic valve function and measure aortic root dilation. Pericardial effusion may also be seen in as many as 18% of patients with a type A aortic dissection.

Echocardiography should be obtained in patients with suspected or confirmed pulmonary embolus. This can be useful to assess for RV size, function, or the presence of a right-sided thrombus. A classic finding is "McConnel's sign" which refers to preserved apical RV function with hypokinesis to akinesis of RV free wall. This finding is highly specific for pulmonary embolism. The echocardiographic findings for pulmonary embolism lack sensitivity and should not be used to exclude the diagnosis.

Cardiac Biomarkers

Troponin

Troponin is a protein highly specific for myocardium. Under normal physiologic states, troponin should be undetectable in the serum. Elevated troponin levels often indicate myocardial injury or inflammation. While acute myocardial infarction is one of the most considered conditions for troponin elevation, several other conditions include chronic kidney disease, congestive heart failure, pulmonary hypertension, skeletal myopathies, chemotherapeutic agents, hypertrophic cardiomyopathy, and infiltrative processes such as cardiac amyloid, hemochromatosis, or cardiac sarcoidosis which have been linked to elevated troponin levels [20]. Troponin assay is recommended in all patients who present to the emergency department for chest pain unless an obvious noncardiac etiology is present [7]. Newer high-sensitivity assays have replaced traditional troponin assays which have markedly improved the early diagnosis of acute myocardial infarction [21]. Troponins have tremendous negative predictive value to rule out AMI. The negative predictive value for myocardial infarction within 30 days in patients with undetectable high-sensitivity troponin and no ischemic ECG changes with 99.8% and the negative predictive value for death was 100% [22]. Two consecutive high-sensitivity troponins below detection on high-sensitivity assays effectively exclude acute coronary syndrome. Patients who presented with chest pain with an initial high-sensitivity troponin that was undetectable had a less than 1% risk of MI at 30-day follow-up. High-sensitivity troponin has utility in noncoronary pathologies as well. Troponin can be elevated and acute pericarditis in up to 40% of cases. Elevated troponin may also be seen in the cases of acute aortic dissection and pulmonary embolism. In the case of a pulmonary embolism, troponin elevation is a sign of RV strain, myocardial injury, and increased disease severity. Significantly elevated troponin with a nondiagnostic EKG also warrants consideration for myocarditis.

D-Dimer

D-dimer is produced by the body by natural breakdown of clot. Therefore, this biomarker will be elevated during the acute phase of thrombus. D-dimer is recommended for use in low and intermediate risk of PE. A patient with low or intermediate risk of PE and a low serum D-dimer effectively excludes PE as a diagnosis.

BNP

Cardiac brain natriuretic peptide (BNP) is a peptide originally isolated from porcine brain tissue, giving it its name. BNP is also found in human blood with the primary source being cardiac myocytes. Myocyte injury and/or stretch causes the biomarker to be released and detectable in the blood. Cardiac BNP is not used in the diagnosis of acute myocardial infarction in the emergency department. The most common cause of elevated cardiac BNP is due to decompensated heart failure and volume overload. Cardiac BNP should be obtained in the setting of a diagnosed PE for risk stratification and to guide urgency for anticoagulation/thrombolytics.

Clinical Decision Pathways

Once STEMI has been ruled out, patients with acute chest pain and suspected ACS require further risk stratification [25]. The ACC/AHA guidelines recommend the use of clinical decision-making pathways summarized in Table 31.3. Each of these pathways stratifies patients into low, intermediate, and high risk to guide further workup in management. No decision-making pathway is known to be superior. Patients identified as low risk have a 30-day risk of death or major adverse cardiac events of <1% and are often safe to discharge from the emergency department. Patients identified as intermediate risk may be managed in an observation unit for cardiac monitoring, serial troponins, and additional diagnostic evaluation such as echocardiography or stress testing (see Chap. 5). Invasive coronary angiography is recommended for patients who are recommended as high risk for short-term major adverse cardiac events. This may be identified by an elevated risk score in clinical decision-making pathway but also includes new ischemic ECG changes, acute myocardial injury identified by elevated troponin levels, new-onset left ventricular dysfunction <40%, newly diag-

Table 31.3 Summary of current clinical decision pathways

	HEART pathway	EDACS	ADAPT	NOTR	2020 ESC/ hs-cTn	2015 ESC/GRACE
Variables used	History ECG Age Risk factors Troponins	Age Sex Risk factors History Troponin	TIMI score 0–1 No ischemic ECG changes Troponins	Age Risk factors Previous AMI or CAD Troponin	History ECG hs-cTn	Age HR, SBP Serum Cr Cardiac arrest ECG Cardiac biomarker Killip class
Low risk	HEART score <3 Negative troponin at 0 and 2–3 h	EDACS score <16 Negative troponin at 0 and 2 h No ischemic ECG changes	TIMI score 0 Troponin negative at 0 and 2 h No ischemic ECG changes	Age <50 <3 risk factors Negative troponin at 0 and 2 h	Initial troponin is "very low" and symptom onset >3 h prior OR Initial troponin is "low" and 2 h troponin change is "low"	Chest pain free and GRACE <140 Sx <6 h and troponin <ULN at 0 and 3 h Sx >6 h and troponin <ULN on arrival
Intermediate risk	HEART score 4–5	NA	TIMI score 2–4	NA	Initial troponin is between "low" and "high"	0 h high sensitivity troponin = 12–52 ng/L or 1 h change = 3–5 ng/L
High risk	HEART score 7–10	NA	TIMI 5–7	NA	Initial high sensitivity troponin is "high" Or 1 or 2 h high sensitivity troponin change is "high"	Initial high-sensitivity troponin >52 ng/L or 1 h change >5 ng/L
Performance	AMI sensitivity 100% Increased ED discharged by 21% Decreased length of stay by 12 h Decreased 30-day objective testing by 12%	AMI sensitivity 100% More patients identified as low risk vs ADAPT (42% vs 31%)	AMI sensitivity 100% More patients discharged <6 h (19% vs 11%)	AMI sensitivity 100% 28% eligible for ED discharge	AMI sensitivity >99%	AMI sensitivity >99%

Adapted from 2021 AHA/ACC/ASE/CHEST/SAEM/SCCT/SCMR Guideline for the Evaluation and Diagnosis of Chest Pain: A Report of the American College of Cardiology/American Heart Association Joint Committee on Clinical Practice Guidelines nosed moderate-severe ischemia on stress testing, or hemodynamic instability.

Management

Even benign etiologies of chest pain may have potentially life-threatening complications, i.e., pericardial tamponade in pericarditis. As such, assessment and stabilization of hemodynamics, mentation, and airway should precede additional testing or evaluation. Due to the broad etiologies of chest pain with varying degrees of acuity, patients with acute chest pain should be transported to the nearest ED by emergency medical services. All patients should be evaluated promptly, and an EKG should be obtained within minutes of patient presentation. After assessment of vital signs, it is reasonable to administer sublingual nitroglycerin (0.4 mg every 3–5 min) and 325 mg aspirin if there is initial concern for myocardial infarction.

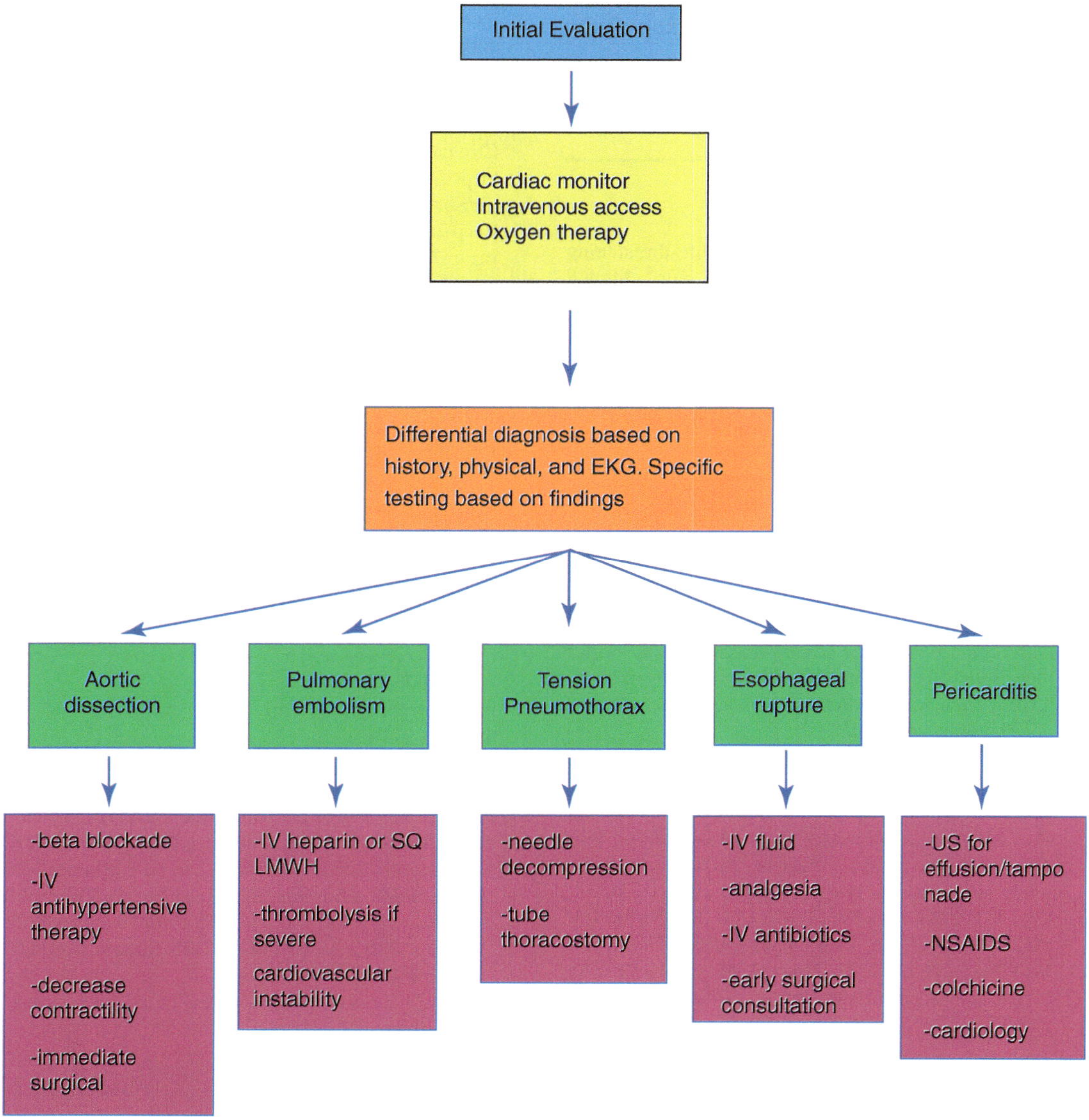

Clinical Pearls

- Start with a thorough history, physical examination, and 12-lead ECG.
- Clinical suspicion drives further workup and testing to include biomarkers and radiographic imaging.
- Consider and exclude the diagnosis with highest morbidity and mortality.
- A troponin measurement of zero does not exclude ACS.
- A markedly abnormal troponin does not confirm type I MI and ACS.
- Cardiovascular chest pain is not exclusively ACS and Type I MI.

References

1. A national study of the prevalence of life-threatening diagnoses in patients with chest pain. https://jamanetwork.com/journals/jamainternalmedicine/fullarticle/2527387
2. Chest pain: anatomic pathways and physiologic mechanisms. https://www.ahajournals.org/doi/abs/10.1161/01.cir.16.4.644
3. Jonnesco T. Traitment chirurgical de I'angine de poitrine par la resection du sympathetique cervicothoracique. Presse Méd. 1921;29:193–5.
4. Chest pain: differentiating cardiac from noncardiac causes. https://www.researchgate.net/profile/Mark-Holden-3/publication/237244124_Chest_Pain_Differentiating_Cardiac_from_Noncardiac_Causes/links/549306530cf22d7925d62a09/Chest-Pain-Differentiating-Cardiac-from-Noncardiac-Causes.pdf
5. https://www.jacc.org/doi/10.1016/j.jacc.2019.02.018
6. https://www.sciencedirect.com/science/article/abs/pii/S0196064404018062
7. 2021 AHA/ACC/ASE/CHEST/SAEM/SCCT/SCMR guideline for the evaluation and diagnosis of chest pain: a report of the American College of Cardiology/American Heart Association joint committee on clinical practice guidelines. https://www.jacc.org/doi/10.1016/j.jacc.2021.07.053?_gl=1*11f07hk*_ga*MTk3OTk1NDA3Ny4xNjMyODcwMzkx*_ga_2V8VW4Y237*MTY2MzQ1MjY2MS41LjEuMTY2MzQ1MjcyMy42MC4wLjA.&_ga=2.12283956.1217772748.1663452661-1979954077.1632870391
8. https://www.sciencedirect.com/science/article/pii/S1936878X16000462
9. https://www.jacc.org/doi/10.1016/j.jacc.2019.11.021
10. https://www.ncbi.nlm.nih.gov/pmc/articles/PMC2676130/
11. https://www.ahajournals.org/doi/10.1161/CIRCULATIONAHA.117.031264?url_ver=Z39.88-2003&rfr_id=ori:rid:crossref.org&rfr_dat=cr_pub%20%200pubmed
12. https://journals.lww.com/annalsofsurgery/FullText/2015/06000/Clinical_Presentation_of_Patients_With_Tension.9.aspx
13. Management of pulmonary embolism: an update—ScienceDirect.
14. 2019 ESC Guidelines for the diagnosis and management of acute pulmonary embolism developed in collaboration with the European Respiratory Society (ERS) | European Heart Journal | Oxford Academic (oup.com).
15. Risk Factors for Venous Thromboembolism | Circulation (ahajournals.org)
16. https://www.sciencedirect.com/science/article/abs/pii/S0735675708004816?via%3Dihub
17. https://www.jacc.org/doi/pdf/10.1016/j.jacc.2012.11.019?_gl=1*fpev5s*_ga*MTk3OTk1NDA3Ny4xNjMyODcwMzkx*_ga_2V8VW4Y237*MTY2MzgwOTQwOC43LjEuMTY2MzgwOTQzMy4zNS4wLjA.&_ga=2.147404785.799435267.1663809408-1979954077.1632870391
18. https://www.ncbi.nlm.nih.gov/pmc/articles/PMC5306533/
19. A consensus statement of the American Society of Echocardiography and American College of Emergency Physicians. J Am Soc Echocardiogr. 2010;23(12):1225–30. https://www.sciencedirect.com/science/article/pii/S0894731710008710
20. Insight on the Etiologies of Chronically Elevated Troponin - ScienceDirect
21. https://www.nejm.org/doi/full/10.1056/nejmoa0900428
22. https://www.sciencedirect.com/science/article/pii/S0735109714017264
23. https://www.cdc.gov/nchs/fastats/emergency-department.htm
24. https://www.hcup-us.ahrq.gov/reports/statbriefs/sb277-Top-Reasons-Hospital-Stays-2018.pdf#:~:text=%E2%96%A0%20The%20most%20frequent%20principal%20diagnoses%20for%20hospitalizations,stays%29%20and%20the%20costliest%20%28%2441.5%20billion%20in%20aggregate%29
25. https://jamanetwork.com/journals/jama/article-abstract/2468896

Part XI

Cardiovascular Disease in Pregnancy

Cardiovascular Disease in Pregnancy

32

Cindy Sing and Malissa J. Wood

Introduction

In the USA, the leading cause of mortality in pregnancy is cardiovascular disease, and the numbers continue to rise despite global improvements in healthcare. This is due to the increase in women surviving congenital heart disease to childbearing age, the upsurge of pregnancies at an advanced maternal age, chronic medical conditions (obesity, hypertension, and diabetes mellitus), as well as disparities related to race and ethnicity. To improve cardiovascular outcomes and reduce maternal mortality, an early and specialized multidisciplinary cardio-obstetrics team is vital to render a comprehensive patient review and counsel regarding maternal cardiovascular risks [1]. Counseling should ideally start prior to pregnancy, and preferably in specialized centers managed by the cardio-obstetrics interdisciplinary team [2]. This team is usually comprised of obstetricians, anesthetists, maternal-fetal medicine experts, cardiologists, and nursing. The cardio-obstetrics team's primary goal is to focus on the progress of the pregnancy and create a safe delivery plan. Prompt referrals of pregnant women with any type of cardiovascular disease can improve outcomes [3].

C. Sing
Atrium Health Pulmonary and Critical Care Consultants, Charlotte, NC, USA
e-mail: cindy.sing@atriumhealth.org

M. J. Wood (✉)
Corrigan Minehan Heart Center, Massachusetts General Hospital, Boston, MA, USA
e-mail: MJWOOD@mgh.harvard.edu

Physiological Changes During Pregnancy

Expected hemodynamic and structural changes during pregnancy include vascular adaptations, hormonal changes, increases in heart rate (HR), volume, and cardiac output (CO), increased hypercoagulability and decreased systemic vascular resistance (SVR) [3]. In pregnancy, the renin-angiotensin-aldosterone system is activated, along with hormonal fluctuations, leading to an increase in plasma volume, rise in CO, and decrease in SVR [1]. An increase in blood volume compared to red cell mass results in normal physiologic anemia. In early pregnancy, ejection fraction (EF) increases, CO increases by 30–50% due to increased stroke volume, and SVR decreases via prostacyclin and nitric oxide (NO). In the second trimester, CO is 50% above baseline, increasing HR, minute ventilation, and pulse pressure. Blood pressure also starts to rise in the second trimester. Lastly, by the third trimester, HR peaks about 15 bpm above baseline, EF

R. Musialowski, K. Allshouse (eds.), *Cardiovascular Manual for the Advanced Practice Provider*,
https://doi.org/10.1007/978-3-031-35819-7_32

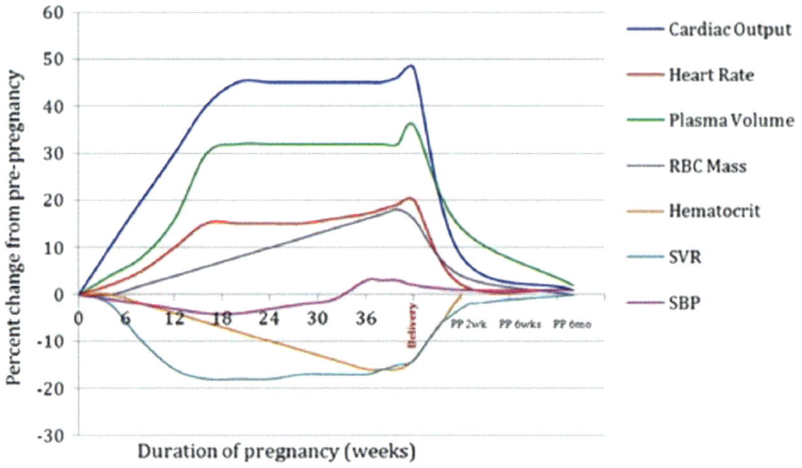

Fig. 32.1 Hemodynamic changes in Pregnancy. (Yucel, E., DeFaria Yeh, D. Pregnancy in Women with Congenital Heart Disease. Curr Treat Options Cardio Med 19, 73 (2017). https://doi.org/10.1007/s11936-017-0572-0)

decreases, CO and SVR both increase thereby increasing BP above pre-pregnancy levels [4]. See Fig. 32.1.

Chest Pain in Pregnancy

The anatomic and physiologic changes described above are often the main cause of chest pain and shortness of breath (SOB) in pregnancy. However, these complaints require further investigation to rule out pathologic conditions that can affect maternal and/or fetal health. Differential diagnosis for chest pain during pregnancy include ischemic heart disease such as spontaneous coronary artery dissection (SCAD), pulmonary embolism, musculoskeletal issues, gastrointestinal reflux disease (GERD), and acute coronary syndrome (ACS) [5]. An often-missed diagnosis in pregnant patients with chest pain is aortic dissection and therefore should also be considered in the differential [1].

Spontaneous Coronary Artery Dissection (SCAD)

Less than 1% of total hospitalizations for ACS are due to SCAD. However, pregnancy related SCAD (P-SCAD) accounts for 2–8% of all SCAD cases and a little over 40% of ACS cases in this population. The main difference between SCAD and most cases of ACS is that SCAD is due to rupture of the vasa vasorum and intramural hematoma formation with coronary dissection. This is different from rupture of atherosclerotic plaque and thrombosis. Hormonal changes are suspected to increase the risk for SCAD, as progesterone reduces collagen and elastin strength of the coronary arteries. Therefore, pregnancy, multiparity, breastfeeding, and fertility treatments are also considered risk factors. While P-SCAD only comprises a small amount of the total number of SCAD cases, its worse prognosis is due to having more proximal involvement along with involvement of multiple vessels, resulting in larger myocardial injury. Most cases of P-SCAD have been reported in the third trimester or post-partum [6]. In P-SCAD, percutaneous coronary intervention has been linked to iatrogenic dissections, propagation of existing dissections, and low success rate. Therefore, conservative management needs to be considered in P-SCAD when patients are stable [7].

The most common symptoms of P-SCAD include chest pain and SOB. One study revealed that 75% of these patients presented with ST-segment elevation MI (STEMI) and about 25% with non-STEMI. The most common location of the STEMI was anterior and anterolateral. Some of the patients with STEMI also developed ventricular fibrillation. The average left ventricular ejection fraction (LV EF) was 40% to 49%, and cardiogenic shock was seen in approximately

25% of patients. These led to higher rates of fetal and maternal mortality [7].

Catheter-based reperfusion therapy in SCAD is controversial, as one study shows over 50% of patients with low success rate with percutaneous coronary intervention (PCI) requiring emergency coronary artery bypass graft (CABG) surgery. The reason behind this was higher incidence of complex coronary anatomy and hemodynamic instability. Approximately a third of the patients were managed conservatively and developed recurrent symptoms, eventually requiring revascularization procedures. Half of the patients in this study were treated with aspirin, a third with a second antiplatelet agent (prasugrel or clopidogrel), and some with anticoagulation. Concerns for fetal and maternal safety must be weighed against the potential benefits of these medications. Thrombolytic therapy is also controversial due to the risk of dissection extension with approximately 60% of patients with SCAD-associated MI developing clinical deterioration after thrombolytic therapy. These findings suggest that a diagnosis without invasive procedures and conservative management in stable low risk pregnant women should be considered. Moreover, close, and long-term follow-up is recommended in women with P-SCAD, as many show persistence of SCAD or involvement of new vessels even at their 1-year follow-up visit. Lastly, future pregnancies are not recommended in women with P-SCAD due to the high incidence of recurrence and coronary artery vulnerability [7].

Pulmonary Embolism in Pregnancy

Venous thromboembolism (VTE) has a higher incidence both during pregnancy and in the postpartum period. The highest risk of VTE occurs specifically after a cesarean section [2]. VTE can manifest as a lower extremity deep venous thrombosis (DVT) or a pulmonary embolism (PE). VTE represents a significant cause of pregnancy related morbidity and mortality. In the USA, the sixth leading cause of maternal mortality is PE [8].

Having risk factors such as previous VTE, family history of VTE, obesity, smoker, preeclampsia, known thrombophilia, cesarean section, or immobility can heighten the risk of VTE during and after pregnancy [2].

Clinical Presentation

PE has a non-specific presentation during pregnancy as clinical signs and symptoms are similar to normal physiologic changes (i.e., dyspnea, chest pain, tachycardia, and sweating). These similarities make it challenging to identify PE and requires a high index of suspicion for a timely diagnosis [8].

Diagnosis

Echocardiograms, arterial blood gases, and D-dimer levels are usually performed, however, they are neither sensitive nor specific diagnostically during pregnancy. For example, respiratory alkalosis is common in both PE and pregnancy. Additionally, d-dimer levels slowly rise with each trimester. An echocardiogram is sometimes used in this population to evaluate the size of the right ventricle after a PE is confirmed but this has not been officially evaluated in pregnancy. Echocardiograms are also used to rule out cardiomyopathy related to pregnancy [8]. Therefore, when the diagnosis cannot be confirmed or ruled out, a computed tomographic pulmonary angiography (CTPA) or a lung scintigraphy (ventilation/perfusion scan [V/Q]) should be performed. Both modalities provide radiation exposure to the fetus (V/Q scan>CTPA) but below the limit considered dangerous [2]. Thyroid function is the major concern of administering iodinated contrast, but studies have shown an exceptionally low risk of neonatal hypothyroidism secondary to fetal exposure to iodine [8].

Due to insufficient data on diagnostic modalities, the following approach is suggested:

- All patients with respiratory symptoms concerning for PE should undergo chest radiograph.
- In the context of a normal chest radiograph, V/Q scan is both sensitive and specific for PE diagnosis.
- If chest radiograph is abnormal or V/Q scan is indeterminate, CTPA is suggested.

In certain circumstances, more than one modality will be required, and it is often case specific, depending on availability of tests, renal insufficiency, allergies to contrast, and weight limitations [8].

Treatment

Treatment for PE in pregnancy is unique. Thrombolytics have a high risk of maternal hemorrhage and should only be used when acute PE is life-threatening. Initial considerations include the following:

- If there is low or moderate clinical suspicion for PE, potential empiric anticoagulation should be considered.
- -If there is a high clinical suspicion for PE, anticoagulation is indicated even before diagnostic evaluation.
- If anticoagulation is contraindicated but PE is suspected, prompt diagnostic evaluation is of utmost importance and if VTE is confirmed, inferior vena cava filter is indicated.
- If only DVT is suspected, and diagnostics can be done in a timely manner, hold anticoagulation therapy, particularly if diagnostic tests confirm VTE.

If anticoagulation (AC) is clinically indicated, heparin should be started. The options available include unfractionated heparin (UFH) either subcutaneous or intravenous, as well as low molecular weight heparin (LMWH). Avoid direct oral anticoagulants (DOACs) as there is not enough information on their safety profile in pregnancy and in some cases, miscarriage has been reported [9]. See Table 32.1.

If a patient has decreased cardiopulmonary reserve because of an acute PE, and stopping anticoagulation is not possible, an IVC filter can be used. IVC filter can also be used if significant bleeding has occurred, and anticoagulation needs to be stopped. Otherwise, if labor is unforeseen, proceed with delivery [9].

Heparin is recommended for a minimum of 6 weeks after delivery and a total duration of 3–6 months. Long-term therapy can consist of subcutaneous UFH, subcutaneous LMWH or coumadin. If the latter is selected, both warfarin and heparin should be administered for a minimum of 5 days until a therapeutic INR is reached. Warfarin is safe during breastfeeding but DOACs should be avoided. Side effects of heparin should be closely monitored. These include osteoporosis, heparin-induced thrombocytopenia, skin necrosis and bleeding. These can manifest with long-term use but also with prophylactic doses [9].

Musculoskeletal Chest Pain

A myriad of physiologic and anatomic changes occur during pregnancy. Some examples include increase in chest wall diameters (anterior–posterior and transverse), subcostal angle, as well as overall increase of the circumference of the chest wall. These changes can impact the musculoskeletal system and can cause chest wall pain due to hormonal changes, the new body habitus, and the pressure from the uterus in the lower rib area. One of the rare causes of pregnancy-specific musculoskeletal chest pain is rib fractures, often in those pregnant women with pregnancy-associated osteoporosis. If chest wall discomfort occurs with other cardiac associated symptoms, prompt evaluation is paramount [10].

GERD

GERD is common in pregnancy, reported in 40–85% of pregnant women in all three trimesters. It is unclear if the secretion of gastric acid is shifted during pregnancy, but mechanical and intrinsic factors affect the tone of the lower esophageal sphincter causing GERD. During all

Table 32.1 Anticoagulants for PE

	Subcutaneous LMWH	IV UFH	Subcutaneous UFH
When to use	• Preferred for initial AC in pregnancy • Higher efficacy • Better safety profile	• Preferred in severe renal failure • Preferred in patients with increased risk of bleeding or persistent hypotension 2/2 PE because short half-life	Preferred in severe renal failure
Weight adjusted dosing	• Enoxaparin 1 mg/kg q12h • Dalteparin 200 μ/kg daily • Tinzaparin 175 units/kg daily	• Bolus of 80 units /kg • Then continuous infusion 18 units/kg/hr. • Titrate every 6 h until therapeutic aPTT level is reached	• Initiate at 17,500 units q12h • Then titrate to reach therapeutic aPTT level
AC monitoring	• Anti Xa level monitoring controversial • If given BID check levels 4 h after third and fourth • If given daily check levels after second or third dose • Recheck every 1–3 months after reaching adequate anti-Xa levels	• Monitor AC activity • Once therapeutic level is reached monitor once or twice daily	• Monitor AC activity • aPTT first measured 6 h after second dose • Once a stable dose is reached, measure after 3–4 days of treatment • Then measure every few weeks • Closer monitoring in last 10 weeks of pregnancy
Discontinue	• Discontinue 24 h before delivery, particularly if epidural anesthesia will be used	• Discontinue 4–6 h before delivery	
Restart after delivery	If no significant bleeding restart: • 6 h after vaginal birth • 12 h after cesarean delivery	If no significant bleeding restart: • 6 h after vaginal birth • 12 h after cesarean delivery	If no significant bleeding restart: • 6 h after vaginal birth • 12 h after cesarean delivery

trimesters, the pressure of the lower esophageal sphincter is lower than normal, and may be explained by hormonal changes, particularly in progesterone [11]. This relaxation allows the food to "reflux" back up the esophagus from the stomach (with stomach acid) causing the burning sensation. Indigestion can occur concurrently with GERD and cause chest pain, that initially starts in the epigastric region and moves upward [12].

Initial management includes dietary and lifestyle modifications including avoiding dietary triggers (mint, chocolate, tomatoes, oranges), as well as elevating the head of the bed. If symptoms persist, treatment should begin with antacids, alginates, or sucralfate. These are safe both in pregnancy and while breastfeeding. If symptoms are still not well controlled, histamine 2 receptor antagonist (H2RA) and proton pump inhibitors (PPI) can be used. PPIs are safe during pregnancy, but not enough data exist on their secretion in breastmilk. Preferred PPIs are pantoprazole, omeprazole, lansoprazole if symptoms persist with H2RAs. Upper endoscopy should be reserved for severe cases such as severe gastrointestinal bleeding and postponed until the second trimester if possible [13].

Aortic Diseases

Aortic disease can present prior to or during pregnancy and the hemodynamic and hormonal changes of pregnancy can result in further aortic enlargement. Most of the pregnancy-related aortic dissections involve the ascending aorta and occur in the third trimester (50%) or the postpartum period (33%). Heritable thoracic aortic disorders that predispose patients to aortic dissection or aneurysm formation include Marfan syndrome, Ehlers-Danlos syndrome, bicuspid aortic valve, and other familial forms of aortic

Table 32.2 Heritable disorders that affect the thoracic aorta

Disorder	Risks/Risks factors	Considerations/management
Bicuspid aortic valve	50% of patients have dilatation of ascending aorta. Dissection less often than Marfan's	• Distal part of ascending aorta, not visualized by echo, MRI or CT before pregnancy. If diameter >50 mm, consider pre-pregnancy surgery
Ehlers-Danlos syndrome	Exclusive to autosomal dominant trait type IV-so pregnancy is contraindicated. Rupture of large vessels or uterus may occur	• Increased bruising • Prophylactic surgery not well established because it can lead to poor wound healing, tissue fragility and increase hemorrhage • Early cesarian delivery advised
Turner syndrome	Prevalence of cv malformations 25–50% Dissection risk is higher if other risk factors such aortic dilatation, HTN etc.	• If the diameter is >27 mm, consider pre-pregnancy surgery

dissection. Advanced maternal age and hypertension are common risk factors for aortic pathology. Pregnant patients at elevated risk for aortic complications include those with previous aortic dissection. Patients with known familiar aortic pathology or diagnosed with Marfan syndrome, should have counseling, a thorough evaluation, and imaging of the aorta prior to pregnancy as they are at higher risk for dissection [1].

Marfan Syndrome

The diameter of the aortic root of those patients with Marfan syndrome determines risk and management. For example, those with a normal diameter have a 1% risk of severe complications or dissection. However, when the diameter is >40 mm, the risk for dissection increases. Moreover, pregnancy is not recommended when the diameter is >45 mm, particularly for those with a family history of dissection, as life-threatening aortic dissection may occur. Other potential complications include worsening of mitral regurgitation that can further lead to heart failure or supraventricular arrythmias [1].

Management

Typically, pregnant patients with aortic disease undergo echocardiogram at 4–12-week intervals depending on the diameter of the aorta as well as at 6 months after delivery. These patients require specialized supervision by a team aware of the potential complications. Beta blockers have been used in Marfan's disease to reduce the rate of aortic dilatation and prevent dissection, although recent studies do not confirm this benefit. Beta blockers should also be taken in the peripartum period. When the mother is on beta blockers, the growth of the fetus should be closely monitored. If dilatation progresses during pregnancy before a viable fetus, an aortic repair with fetus in utero should be considered. Once the fetus is viable, the recommendation is cesarean section followed by aortic surgery in a hospital with a specialized cardio-obstetrics team available. Ascending aortic dissection is considered a surgical emergency. For patients with ascending aorta enlargement, with an aorta diameter > 40–45 mm, it is recommended that they undergo vaginal delivery with regional anesthesia to prevent increases in blood pressure. If necessary, cesarean section is also advised, particularly in those with a diameter >45 mm [1]. See Table 32.2.

Hypertension in Pregnancy

In the USA, hypertensive disorders of pregnancy are common, and the number of cases has increased over the last five decades. Factors contributing to this increased rate include older maternal ages (>35 years), diabetes, and obesity [14]. Maternal risks of pregnant women with chronic hypertension include pulmonary edema, renal failure, cerebrovascular accidents (CVA), gestational diabetes, and disseminated intravascular coagulation. These risks were 5–6 times more likely to occur in this population than in those pregnant women without hypertension. Chronic hypertension in pregnancy also has been correlated with worse perinatal outcomes [15].

The fetus is at risk of growth restriction, congenital abnormalities, preterm labor, placental abruption, and fetal demise. These risks were 2–4 times higher than in non-hypertensive women [14].

Two confirmed elevated blood pressure readings (SBP ≥140 or DBP ≥90) on two separate occasions are necessary for the diagnosis of hypertension in pregnancy. It is recommended to monitor these women with basic laboratory studies including liver enzymes, urinalysis, blood count, hematocrit, serum uric acid, and serum creatinine. If there is suspicion of pheochromocytoma, ultrasound of the adrenals as well as urine catecholamine assays (urine metanephrines) should be considered, as this can be fatal if not diagnosed before labor. Also, a doppler ultrasound of the uterine arteries after 16 weeks gestation can be used to detect uteroplacental hypoperfusion associated with a higher risk of pre-eclampsia [2].

Classifications by the American College of Obstetricians and Gynecologists (ACOG) of hypertensive disorders include chronic hypertension, pre-eclampsia/eclampsia, gestational hypertension, and chronic hypertension with superimposed pre-eclampsia [1]. Please see Table 32.3.

Table 32.3 Definitions of hypertensive disorders

Type of HTN	Diagnostic criteria
Chronic HTN	BP ≥ 140/90 mmHg Present before 20 weeks of gestation
Gestational HTN	BP ≥ 140/90 mmHg Onset after 20 weeks gestation
Preeclampsia	BP ≥ 140/90 mmHg Onset after 20 weeks with proteinuria
Severe preeclampsia	BP > 160/110 mmHg Excessive proteinuria
Chronic HTN with superimposed preeclampsia	BP ≥ 140/90 mmHg Present before 20 weeks of gestation New onset proteinuria

Adapted from the American College of Obstetricians and Gynecologists (ACOG)

Pre-eclampsia

This occurs when the systolic blood pressure is ≥140 mmHg or diastolic blood pressure is ≥90 mmHg in previously normotensive women, after 20 weeks of gestation, with evidence of proteinuria (≥30 mg/mmol urinary creatinine in a random urine sample or ≥0.3 g/day in a 24 h urine collection) as well as poor organ perfusion. This typically resolves within 42 days postpartum [2]. Compared to normal cohorts, women with pre-eclampsia have a >70% increased risk of mortality due to CVD, fourfold increased risk of heart failure, and a little over twofold increased risk of coronary disease. Pre-eclampsia also occurs more frequently during the first pregnancy, in women with diabetes or in pregnancies with multiple fetuses. It is the most common cause of prematurity [2].

Signs and symptoms of severe pre-eclampsia include right upper quadrant pain secondary to liver fullness, occipital lobe blindness, visual disturbances accompanied by headaches (cerebral edema), clonus/hyperreflexia, pulmonary edema, elevated creatinine without other etiology, and HELLP syndrome (hemolysis, elevated liver enzymes, and low platelet count). Management focuses on recognizing the condition and delivery of the placenta [2].

Eclampsia

Defined as new onset of a clonic-tonic seizure in women with pre-eclampsia, typically lasting 60–90 s. Seizures can happen antepartum, 20 weeks after gestation, during delivery and up to 6-weeks post-partum. This is a serious complication of pre-eclampsia related to increased morbidity and mortality of both mother and fetus when it is not recognized or diagnosed promptly [16].

Pre-existing Hypertension

Defined as BP 140/90 mmHg present before pregnancy or develops before 20 weeks of gestation and persist >42 days after delivery. This may go unrecognized in women not previously diagnosed with hypertension because the physiological decrease in BP in the first trimester.

Pre-existing Hypertension with Overlapping Gestational Hypertension

This occurs when pre-existing hypertension is concomitant with BP worsening and protein excretion ≥3 g/day in 24-hour period after 20 weeks' gestation. About a quarter of these cases proceed to pre-eclampsia and it is vital to recognize for long-term prognosis.

Treatment

A strategy with a multidisciplinary team to include lifestyle changes such as diet, exercise, smoking cessation, and algorithms targeting cardiovascular risk factors was recently highlighted by both ACOG and AHA. Many studies have suggested regular exercise can improve vascular function and prevent pre-eclampsia, but more studies are needed to analyze the possible reversal of endothelial dysfunction [1].

Other non-pharmacologic strategies include low impact exercise, a normal diet without sodium restriction, especially when close to delivery as it may reduce intravascular volume. In pre-eclampsia, delivery of the fetus at 37 weeks should be considered with the hope of preventing peripartum pre-eclampsia. Lastly, for obese women, aggressive weight loss is not recommended [4].

For those with pre-existing hypertension, consider continuing their current therapy except for direct renin inhibitors, angiotensin receptor blockers (ARBs) or angiotensin-converting-enzyme inhibitors (ACE-Is) due to severe toxicity to the fetus, particularly in the second and third trimesters [2]. Monitor for pre-eclampsia if medications are discontinued. Avoid diuretics as it reduces the blood flow to the placenta and are not recommended in pre-eclampsia. In the multicenter Chronic Hypertension and Pregnancy (CHAP) trial, 2408 pregnant women enrolled at <23 weeks of gestation with non-severe chronic hypertension were randomly assigned to receive antihypertensive therapy at a threshold of 140/90 mmHg (active treatment) or no treatment until development of severe hypertension (systolic BP ≥ 160 or diastolic BP≥ 105 mmHg). The rate of the primary composite outcome (pre-eclampsia with severe features, medically indicated preterm birth at <35 weeks of gestation, abruption, or fetal or neonatal death) was reduced in the active treatment group and was not associated with a significant difference in rates of fetal growth restriction or serious neonatal or maternal morbidity [17].

When severe hypertension is confirmed (blood pressure ≥160/110 mmHg that persists for 15 min) prompt treatment should be started to decrease the risk of maternal heart failure, renal disease, MI, or stroke. A rapid IV infusion is recommended with reduction of BP within 60 min, avoiding DBP below 80 mmHg, to prevent interruption of placental blood flow. In these cases, treatment with intravenous hydralazine or labetalol is recommended. Hydralazine is slower in onset and longer in duration. Immediate-release dose nifedipine is the drug of choice if no immediate IV access is available. When there is pulmonary edema associated with pre-eclampsia, the drug of choice is IV nitroglycerin. Intravenous magnesium sulfate is recommended to prevent eclampsia as well as treating seizures. First-line antihypertensive medications include methyldopa, labetalol and nifedipine for less severe hypertension. Second line antihypertensive agent include hydrochlorothiazide [1].

Assume all antihypertensive agents are present in breast milk [4]. It is also important to monitor BP in the first 1–2 weeks post-partum and continue antihypertensive therapy for those with persistent hypertension (≥150/110 mmHg). Lastly, adjust to maintain a BP not higher than 150/110 mmHg [1].

Arrhythmias

Studies have shown that there has been an increase in the number of pregnancy related hospitalizations due to arrhythmias because of the increase advanced maternal age, particularly in women between 41 and 50 years old [1]. Sustained tachyarrhythmias and premature extra beats become more frequent and sometimes manifest for the first time during pregnancy. While most palpitations are benign, new onset ventricular tachycardia (VT) is worrisome and should be further investigated for possible structural heart disease [2]. Palpitations secondary to atrial and ventricular ectopy as well as sinus tachycardia (ST) are usually benign, self-terminating and resolve without pharmacological treatment. However, a cardio-obstetrics team should be used to manage more complex arrythmias as this may require not only antiarrhythmic therapy but also radiofrequency ablation or other electrophysiological studies [2].

Arrhythmias during pregnancy are often attributed to hormonal, hemodynamic, and autonomic changes. For example, the rise in intravascular volume increases preload on the ventricles and in turn increases the size of the atria and ventricles. Moreover, increase in myocardial stretch can initiate arrythmias [18].

Antiarrhythmic drugs should be assumed to be potentially toxic to the fetus, which is a major concern. The greatest teratogenic risk is during the first trimester, however, other adverse effects on fetal growth and development later in pregnancy can also occur including the increased risk of pro-arrhythmia. Patients with congenital heart disease during pregnancy are more likely to develop supraventricular and ventricular arrhythmias requiring treatment. For example, atrial flutter is not well tolerated and can lead to hypoperfusion of the fetus [1].

Supraventricular tachycardia (SVT) is the most prevalent arrhythmia during pregnancy. For those women with no pre-existing structural heart disease the most common cause behind paroxysmal SVT is atrioventricular nodal reentrant tachycardia (AVNRT). AVNRT during pregnancy should be initially treated with the use of vagal maneuvers [19]. Stable supraventricular tachycardias should be treated the same way as that in the nonpregnant patient (see Chap. 9). If vagal maneuvers do not work, proceed to use intravenous adenosine (first choice). If adenosine fails, then IV metoprolol is recommended to terminate the tachycardia. For intolerable symptoms or if tachycardia leads to hemodynamic compromise, use prophylactic antiarrhythmic drugs [1]. Wolf-Parkinson-White (WPW) syndrome can also further deteriorate during pregnancy and IV procainamide is typically used for wide-complex tachyarrhythmias. If medical therapy fails, consider catheter ablation for atrial arrythmias, ideally with minimal exposure to radiation and only if medical therapy does not work, during pregnancy [2].

When hyperthyroidism or structural heart disease are present during pregnancy, atrial flutter and atrial fibrillation may also be present. During pregnancy, life-threatening ventricular arrythmias are uncommon [1].

Fetal Arrhythmias

While fetal arrhythmias have been reported to occur in up to 1% of pregnancies, sustained arrhythmias are much less common and occur in approximately 0.1% of pregnancies. The most encountered fetal arrhythmias include supraventricular tachycardia (SVT), atrial flutter, and atrial tachycardia. Propranolol is the usual first-line agent for fetal tachycardia. Flecainide may also be used in fetal SVT, particularly in refractory or complicated cases. Other drugs that have been successfully used in the management of fetal arrhythmias include digoxin and sotalol. Procainamide is also safe to use in pregnancy but is less commonly used to treat fetal arrhythmias [20, 21].

Syncope

Also known as transient loss of consciousness, syncope may be due to many clinical conditions ranging from benign vasovagal episodes to more serious and potentially deadly conditions such as arrythmias. The incidence of syncope during pregnancy is approximately 1%. Prognostic information tends to correlate with timing of the syncopal episodes during pregnancy. For example, higher preterm births were found when the first syncopal episode occurred during the first trimester. Moreover, syncope during pregnancy seemed to correlate with higher rates of syncope and cardiac arrythmias 1-year post-partum, when compared to those women without syncope during pregnancy [22].

During pregnancy, the expectant mother undergoes many hemodynamic changes that predisposing her to the development of syncope. These changes include decreased systemic vascular resistance secondary to a vasodilatory state, eccentric hypertrophy of the left ventricle, as well as increased heart rate and blood volume. These changes can lead to an exaggerated vasovagal response. Other potential causes include inferior vena cava compression by the enlarged uterus causing reduced venous return to the heart or stimulation of the nerve plexus (behind the uterus) [22].

Some arrythmias that may result in syncope during pregnancy include Mobitz type II block below the AV node and congenital complete heart block. There is no clear association between pregnancy and complete heart block. Moreover, syncope in pregnancy is rarely caused by severe arrythmia. For those women with a high degree AV block and symptoms (such as syncope), inpatient monitoring and implantation of a pacemaker is recommended. The most frequent concern in these cases is the exposure to radiation due to the use of fluoroscopy during implantation. However, the average radiation dose to the fetus is <1 mGy which has not shown to increase the risk [23].

Edema

More than half of pregnant women are affected by edema, starting around weeks 22 and 27 of gestation. This is due to the increase in body fluids because of increase in total blood flow, and venous congestion from superior vena cava compression. Infrequently, leg edema can be due to a DVT, which can be life-threatening if it dislodges causing a PE [24].

When DVT occurs, it typically affects the left leg because the growing uterus compresses the left iliac vein at the point where it crosses the right iliac artery [2]. DVT is manifested by leg pain, erythema, or heaviness, particularly felt when standing up [24]. When DVT is suspected, the diagnostic imaging of choice is compression ultrasound. This test has a high specificity and sensitivity for proximal DVT but less for distal DVT. If a proximal DVT is detected, treatment should be initiated (see Chap. 27) [2].

Moreover, excessive swelling can be a sign of pre-eclampsia when it occurs along with facial edema, elevated blood pressure, protein in the urine and rapid weight gain [25].

To help prevent edema during pregnancy, women can elevate their legs, stay active by walking or swimming, avoid prolonged periods of sitting or standing, avoid stockings that are too restrictive, sleep on the left side preferably and wear comfortable shoes [24].

Peripartum Cardiomyopathy

Pregnancy-associated cardiomyopathy, also known as peripartum cardiomyopathy (PPCM), is a rare cause of heart failure typically toward the end of pregnancy or 5 months post-partum, without another identifiable cause of heart failure and with a left ventricular ejection fraction (EF) of <45% [26]. Predisposing factors include family history, smoking, ethnicity, pre-eclampsia, diabetes, hypertension, multiparty, advanced maternal age, malnutrition, multiple childbirths as well as prolonged use of beta agonists. Heart failure in PCCM can develop briskly and though it is rare, it can result in severe complications [2].

Signs and symptoms of PPCM can be vary and may be like other forms of heart failure. These may include dyspnea, orthopnea, cough, paroxysmal nocturnal dyspnea, pedal edema, hemoptysis, displaced apical impulse, elevated jugular venous pressure, a third heart sound as well as a mitral regurgitation murmur [26].

Treatment

Women with PCCM during pregnancy require a specialized team of obstetric and cardiac care, considering possible adverse effects on the fetus. For those women with advanced heart failure with hemodynamic instability, and urgent delivery should be considered. Once the baby is delivered, and hemodynamic stability is reached, standard therapy for heart failure can be applied. For example, anticoagulation should be started immediately following delivery of the baby (and after bleeding has stopped) as those with a low EF tend to have peripheral embolism including ventricular thrombi and cerebral embolism. This is secondary to the increase in procoagulant activity in the peripartum stage [2]. Echocardiogram and EKG should be completed [26]. See Table 32.4 for medical treatment.

Consider transferring to a facility with a specialized cardio-obstetrics team for those that are inotrope dependent as interventions such as ventricular assist device (VAD), balloon pump counter pulsation or transplant consults may be needed [2].

The prognosis of PCCM is different from other cardiomyopathies such as dilated cardiomyopathy (DCM) as most patients with PCCM have a normalization of their EF within 6 months after diagnosis. For women with persistent symptoms and severe LV dysfunction 6 months after initial presentation, despite optimal medical treatment, consider implantable cardioverter defibrillator (ICD) or cardiac resynchronization therapy. Also, for women who do not recover after 6–12 months of mechanical circulatory support, heart transplant should be considered [2].

Table 32.4 Treatment for PCCM in pregnancy

Medical Treatment	• To reduce afterload, use hydralazine and nitrates instead of ACE-I • If inotropes needed use dopamine and levosimendan • Beta-1 selective drugs (metoprolol) are preferred • Diuretics only if pulmonary congestion (furosemide and HCTZ)
Avoid	• ACE-I, ARBS and renin inhibitors during pregnancy because of fetotoxicity • Atenolol • Aldosterone antagonist
During breastfeeding	• If ACE-I needed, enalapril, captopril, and benazepril are preferred
Anticoagulation	• For those with low EF LMWH or oral anticoagulation • For those with intracardiac thrombus and/or atrial fibrillation

Delivery

If the patient is hemodynamically stable, vaginal delivery is preferred over cesarean delivery with close hemodynamic monitoring. The preferred method of analgesia is an epidural. With advanced heart failure and hemodynamic instability despite medical treatment, consider urgent delivery regardless of gestation duration. In this case, cesarean section with both spinal and epidural anesthesia is recommended [2].

Counseling for Future Pregnancy

Contraception choices and risk for future pregnancies should be part of the education for those with PCCM as successive pregnancies have a 30–50% risk of recurrence of PCCM. Subsequent pregnancies should be discouraged when the EF has normalized [2].

Pulmonary Edema Post-Delivery with Normal LV Function

Approximately 0.5% of women experience acute pulmonary edema during pregnancy as well as post-partum and can be due to pre-eclampsia or iatrogenic volume overload. In the post-partum period, pulmonary edema involves a complex chain of events including increased vascular permeability, increased intravascular hydrostatic pressures, decreased intravascular colloid osmotic pressures that can lead to fluid extravasation into the pulmonary interstitium [27].

In one study, half of the cases of pulmonary edema were due to cardiac disease or tocolytic medications (terbutaline) used to inhibit preterm labor [27]. Beta 2 adrenergic receptors are stimulated with the use of tocolytics. This increases cardiac output and pulse rate leading to hemodilution. Uterine contractions during delivery cause autotransfusion, increasing venous tone and blood pressure resulting in pulmonary edema post-partum [27]. The use of tocolytics is more frequent in multiparity or maternal infections. Tocolytic pulmonary edema is usually caused by fluid overload from large IV fluid amounts administered when peripheral vasodilatation causes hypotension. However, increased permeability of the capillaries and cardiac dysfunction can also contribute to the overall pulmonary edema [28].

Signs and symptoms of tocolytic-related pulmonary edema include basilar crackles, tachycardia, hypoxemia, dyspnea, tachypnea and occasionally chest pain, fever, and cough. Chest X-ray shows airspace disease bilaterally [28].

Women receiving tocolytic medications who develop the signs above, without an alternative explanation, are diagnosed with tocolytic-related pulmonary edema. Most women respond well to supplemental oxygen, discontinuation of tocolytic therapy, diuresis, and fluid restriction. Most cases resolve within 24 hours, but mechanical ventilation may be needed. Tocolytic use of calcium channel blockers like nifedipine and nicardipine can also result in pulmonary edema [28].

Amniotic Fluid Embolism (AFE)

An unusual and potentially fatal condition in the peripartum period is amniotic fluid embolism. This occurs after the woman's exposure to an unknown stimulating antigen with symptoms of sudden hypoxia, seizures, and cardiovascular collapse, in the absence of other explanations [29].

The pathogenesis of this rare condition is not clear, but AFE occurs after the amniotic fluid enters the maternal systemic circulation when the breach of maternal/fetal interface results in a systemic inflammatory response. This in turn, causes an acute increase in pulmonary pressure, increasing RV pressure and RV failure from cellular components and debris from the amniotic fluid [29].

Potential risk factors include pre-eclampsia/eclampsia, abnormalities of the placenta, cesarean delivery, or instrumented vaginal delivery. Signs and symptoms develop abruptly and progress rapidly including sudden hypotension, hypoxia, and cardiorespiratory compromise. Many times, this may be followed by non-cardiogenic pulmonary edema and bleeding related to disseminated intravascular coagulopathy [29].

For unstable patients, a specialized multidisciplinary approach should be used, focusing on controlling hemorrhage, performing high-quality CPR, excluding other etiologies and delivery of the fetus. Initial testing to exclude other etiologies include EKG, bedside ultrasounds, portable chest-X-ray, CBC with platelets, CMP, BNP, ABG, blood type and screen, troponin. After delivery and once patients are stable, it is recommended to monitor closely in the intensive care unit as many patients may require intubation, fluid resuscitation, vasopressors, as well as venous or arterial access [29].

AFE is a leading cause of maternal mortality and those who survive have a poor prognosis. Hypoxemia causes about half of the deaths, and others die from cardiac arrest or cardiogenic shock [29].

Clinical Pearls

- Coronary artery dissection in pregnancy is often treated conservatively but some women need CABG. PCI is high risk.
- Future pregnancies are not recommended with P-SCAD due to high recurrence risk.
- Risk of VTE is highest after c-section.
- In PE, heparin is used, rather than DOACs.
- In HTN in pregnancy, ACE-I and ARBs should be avoided as they cause severe toxicity to the fetus.
- Arrhythmias, most frequently SVT, are common in pregnancy.
- Pregnancy-related cardiomyopathy can cause heart failure from the end of pregnancy up to 5-months post-partum.

References

1. Mehta LS, et al.. Cardiovascular consideration in caring for pregnant patients. A Scientific statement from the American Heart Association. 2020.
2. Regitz-Zagrosek V. ESC guidelines on the management of cardiovascular diseases during pregnancy. Eur Heart J. 2011;32:3147–97. https://doi.org/10.1093/eurheartj/ehr218.
3. Davis MB, Walsh MN. Cardio-obstetrics. Circ Cardiovasc Qual Outcomes. 2019;12:e005417. https://doi.org/10.1161/CIRCOUTCOMES.118.005417.
4. Vidaeff A, Espinoza J, Simhan H, Pettker CM. Chronic hypertension in pregnancy. Clinical management guidelines for obstetrician-gynecologists. ACOG Pract Bull. 2019;133:1.
5. Wagner SM, Waldman IN, Karikari KA, Kunsellmen AR, Smith ER, Deimling TA. The Impact of pregnancy in the evaluation of chest pain and shortness of breath in the emergency department. J Acute Med. 2018. https://www.ncbi.nlm.nih.gov/pmc/articles/PMC7517890/.
6. Chen S, Merchant M, Mahrer KN, Ambrosy AP, Lundstrom RJ, Naderi S. Pregnancy-associated spontaneous coronary artery dissection: clinical characteristics, outcomes, and risks during subsequent pregnancy. J Invasive Cardiol. 2021;33:E457. https://www.hmpgloballearningnetwork.com/site/jic/articles/pregnancy-associated-spontaneous-coronary-artery-dissection-clinical-characteristics-outcomes-and-risk-during-subsequent-pregnancy.
7. Havakuk O, Goland S, Mehra A, Elkayam U. Pregnancy and the risk of spontaneous coronary artery dissection an analysis of 120 contemporary cases. Circ Cardiovasc Interv. 2017;10(3):e004941. https://www.ahajournals.org/doi/pdf/10.1161/CIRCINTERVENTIONS.117.004941.
8. Malhotra A, Weinberger SE. Diagnosis of pulmonary embolism in pregnancy. UpToDate. 2022. https://www.uptodate.com/contents/diagnosis-of-pulmonary-embolism-in-pregnancy?search=diagnosis%20of%20pulmonary%20embolism%20in%20pregnancy&source=search_result&selectedTitle=1~150&usage_type=default&display_rank=1.
9. Malhotra A, Weinberger SE. Diagnosis of pulmonary embolism in pregnancy: treatment. UpToDate. 2022. https://www.uptodate.com/contents/diagnosis-of-pulmonary-embolism-in-pregnancy?search=diagnosis%20of%20pulmonary%20embolism%20in%20pregnancy&source=search_result&selectedTitle=1~150&usage_type=default&display_rank=1.
10. Bermas BL. Maternal adaptations to pregnancy: musculoskeletal changes and pain. UpToDate. 2022. https://www.uptodate.com/contents/maternal-adaptations-to-pregnancy-musculoskeletal-changes-and-pain?search=maternal%20adaptations%20to%20pregnancy&source=search_result&selectedTitle=6~107&usage_type=default&display_rank=6.
11. Bianco A. Maternal adaptations to pregnancy: gastrointestinal tract. UpToDate. 2022. https://www.uptodate.com/contents/maternal-adaptations-to-pregnancy-gastrointestinal-tract?search=maternal%20adaptations%20to%20pregnancy&source=search_result&selectedTitle=1~107&usage_type=default&display_rank=1.
12. 2016 Heart and vascular health. Chest pain during pregnancy: when to worry. 2022. https://share.upmc.com/2016/12/chest-pain-during-pregnancy/.
13. Kahrilas PJ. Medical management of gastroesophageal reflux disease in adults. UpToDate. 2022. https://www.uptodate.com/contents/medical-management-of-gastroesophageal-reflux-disease-in-adults?search=medical%20management%20of%20GERD%20in%20adults&source=search_result&selectedTitle=1~150&usage_type=default&display_rank=1.
14. Musialowski R. Hypertension in pregnancy (PowerPoint slides).
15. ACOG Practice Bulletin clinical management guidelines for obstetrician–gynecologists number 203. Obstet Gynecol. 2019;133(1).
16. Magley M, Hinson MR. Eclampsia. National Library of Medicine; 2022. https://www.ncbi.nlm.nih.gov/books/NBK554392/.
17. Tita AT, Szychowski JM, Boggess K, Dugoff L, Sibai B, Lawrence K, Hughes BL, Bell J, Aagaard K, Edwards RK, Gibson K, Haas DM, Plante L, Metz T, Casey B, Esplin S, Longo S, Hoffman M, Saade GR, Hoppe KK, Foroutan J, Tuuli M, Owens MY, Simhan HN, Frey H, Rosen T, Palatnik A, Baker S, August P, Reddy UM, Kinzler W, Su E, Krishna I, Nguyen N, Norton ME, Skupski D, El-Sayed YY, Ogunyemi D, Galis ZS, Harper L, Ambalavanan N, Geller NL, Oparil S, Cutter GR, Andrews WW, Chronic Hypertension and Pregnancy (CHAP) Trial Consortium. Treatment for mild chronic hypertension during pregnancy. N Engl J Med. 2022;386(19):1781–92. https://doi.org/10.1056/NEJMoa2201295. PMID: 35363951.
18. Silversides C, Harris L, Yap S. Supraventricular arrythmias during pregnancy. UpToDate. 2022. https://www.uptodate.com/contents/medical-management-of-gastroesophageal-reflux-disease-in-adults?search=medical%20management%20of%20GERD%20in%20adults&source=search_result&selectedTitle=1~150&usage_type=default&display_rank=1.
19. Enriquez AD, Economy KE, Tedrow UB. Contemporary management of arrhythmias during pregnancy. Circ Arrhythm Electrophysiol. 2014;7:961–7.
20. Gozar L, Gabor-Miklosi D, Toganel R, Fagarasan A, Gozar H, Toma D, Cerghit-Paler A. Fetal tachyarrhythmia management from digoxin to amiodarone-a review. J Clin Med. 2022;11(3):804. https://doi.org/10.3390/jcm11030804. PMID: 35160256; PMCID: PMC8836967.

21. Joglar JA, Page RL. Management of arrhythmia syndromes in pregnancy. Curr Opin Cardiol. 2014;29:36–44.
22. Chatur S, Islam S, Moore LE, Sandhu RK, Sheldon RS, Kaul P. Incidence of syncope during pregnancy: temporal trends and outcomes. J Am Heart Assoc. 2019;8:e011608. https://doi.org/10.1161/JAHA.118.011608.
23. Harris L, Yap SC, Silversides C. Maternal conduction disorders and bradycardia during pregnancy. UpToDate. 2022. https://www.uptodate.com/contents/maternal-conduction-disorders-and-bradycardia-during-pregnancy?search=Maternal%20conduction%20disorders%20and%20bradycardia%20during%20pregnancy&source=search_result&selectedTitle=1~150&usage_type=default&display_rank=1.
24. O'Connor A. Edema (swelling of the ankles and feet) during pregnancy. 2020. https://www.whattoexpect.com/pregnancy/symptoms-and-solutions/edema.aspx#:~:text=During%20pregnancy%2C%20edema%20occurs%20when,blood%20from%20your%20lower%20limbs.
25. August P, Sibai BM. Preeclampsia: clinic features and diagnosis. UpToDate. 2022. https://www.uptodate.com/contents/preeclampsia-clinical-features-and-diagnosis?search=Preeclampsia:%20clinic%20features%20and%20diagnosis&source=search_result&selectedTitle=1~150&usage_type=default&display_rank=1.
26. Tsang W, Lang RM. Peripartum cardiomyopathy: etiology, clinical manifestations, and diagnosis. UpToDate. 2022. https://www.uptodate.com/contents/peripartum-cardiomyopathy-etiology-clinical-manifestations-and-diagnosis?search=Peripartum%20cardiomyopathy:%20etiology,%20clinical%20manifestations,%20and%20diagnosis&source=search_result&selectedTitle=1~64&usage_type=default&display_rank=1.
27. Randhawa JS, Ashraf H, Colombo JP, Kudla P. Postpartum respiratory distress due to hypertension related pulmonary edema. Cureus. 2021;13(9):e18179. https://doi.org/10.7759/cureus.18179. https://www.cureus.com/articles/70641-postpartum-respiratory-distress-due-to-hypertension-related-pulmonary-edema#:~:text=Acute%20pulmonary%20edema%20occurs%20in,to%20be%20multifactorial%20%5B14%5D.
28. Clardy PF, Reardon CC. Acute respiratory failure during pregnancy and the peripartum period. UpToDate. 2022. https://www.uptodate.com/contents/acute-respiratory-failure-during-pregnancy-and-the-peripartum-period?search=Acute%20respiratory%20failure%20during%20pregnancy%20and%20the%20peripartum%20period&source=search_result&selectedTitle=1~150&usage_type=default&display_rank=1.
29. Baldisseri MR, Clark SL. Amniotic fluid embolism. UpToDate. 2022. https://www.uptodate.com/contents/amniotic-fluid-embolism?search=Amniotic%20fluid%20embolism&source=search_result&selectedTitle=1~50&usage_type=default&display_rank=1.

Index

R. Musialowski, K. Allshouse (eds.), *Cardiovascular Manual for the Advanced Practice Provider*,
https://doi.org/10.1007/978-3-031-35819-7

D

Q

R

S

T

U

GPSR Compliance

The European Union's (EU) General Product Safety Regulation (GPSR) is a set of rules that requires consumer products to be safe and our obligations to ensure this.

If you have any concerns about our products, you can contact us on ProductSafety@springernature.com

In case Publisher is established outside the EU, the EU authorized representative is:

Springer Nature Customer Service Center GmbH
Europaplatz 3
69115 Heidelberg, Germany

Batch number: 10731403

Printed by Printforce, the Netherlands